PRAISE FOR THE BOOK THAT PARENTS AND DOCTORS TRUST

◆ ◆ ◆ ◆ ◆

"Excellent. I recommend it to all my new patients.
I have a seventeen-month-old.
This book was a bible even for me—a pediatrician."
—CLAUDIA SOMES, M.D.

◆ ◆ ◆

"*What to Expect When You're Expecting* has been
my pregnancy bible."
—CYNTHIA CRAVENS ALLEN,
KENTUCKY

◆ ◆ ◆

"Wonderful. Well organized, readable."
—CATHERINE C. WILEY, M.D.

◆ ◆ ◆

"Your book . . . has been a godsend.
I've faithfully read each chapter prior to beginning that month and have
been reassured by your calm and compassionate writing."
—CAROL ROZNER, CALIFORNIA

◆ ◆ ◆

"Contains useful information not available
in other books."
—JIM WILEY, M.D.

◆ ◆ ◆

"Your calm and confident style fills me with courage
for our transition to parenthood."

—DIANE WHEELER, CALIFORNIA

◆ ◆ ◆

"Very reassuring to the new mother."

—RALPH MINEAR, M.D.

◆ ◆ ◆

"Your books have not left my night table for 18 months
(except when they went to the hospital with me)!
Your information is always *right on schedule,* clear, concise
and unbiased."

—LORI SLAYTON, NEW JERSEY

◆ ◆ ◆

"Excellent—we used it as our bible during pregnancy."

—BRUCE ORAN, M.D.

◆ ◆ ◆

"[It] has seen me through my first pregnancy . . . providing a
concise, user-friendly source of information . . . Thanks to your book,
I feel our daughter had a head start on life."

—VICTORIA SCHEI, ONTARIO

◆ ◆ ◆

"Extremely helpful. I've used this book as a
valuable resource with my patients."

—SAUNDRA SCHOICHET, PH.D.
CLINICAL PSYCHOLOGIST

◆ ◆ ◆

WHAT TO EXPECT® WHEN YOU'RE EXPECTING

♦ ♦ ♦ ♦

Heidi Murkoff, Arlene Eisenberg & Sandee Hathaway, B.S.N.

*Medical Consultant: Dr. Richard Aubry, M.D., M.P.H.,
Professor and Director of Academic and Community Obstetrics
for the State University of New York
Upstate Medical University at Syracuse*

Research Consultant: Sharon Mazel

WORKMAN PUBLISHING • NEW YORK

To EMMA, WHO INSPIRED THIS BOOK WHILE STILL IN THE WOMB,
WHO DID HER BEST TO KEEP US FROM WRITING IT ONCE SHE WAS OUT, AND
WHO, WE TRUST, WILL PUT IT TO GOOD USE ONE DAY.

To HOWARD, ERIK, AND TIM, WITHOUT WHOM THIS BOOK WOULD NOT
HAVE BEEN POSSIBLE—IN MORE WAYS THAN ONE.

To RACHEL, WYATT, AND ETHAN,
WHO SHOWED UP A LITTLE LATE FOR OUR FIRST EDITION,
BUT WHOSE GESTATIONS CONTRIBUTED PLENTY TO THE SECOND ONE,
AND TO ELIZABETH,
WHOSE GESTATION OFFERED US EVEN MORE FOR THE THIRD.

AND TO ARLENE, WITH SO MUCH LOVE, FOR EVERYTHING.

◆ ◆ ◆ ◆

Library of Congress Cataloging-in-Publication Data
Murkoff, Heidi.
What to expect when you're expecting / Heidi Murkoff, Arlene Eisenberg,
and Sandee Hathaway; with a foreword by Richard Aubry.
—3rd ed., completely rev. & updated.
p.   cm.
Includes index.
ISBN-13: 978-0-7611-2132-9; ISBN-10: 0-7611-2132-3 (pbk.: alk. paper)
ISBN-13: 978-0-7611-2549-5; ISBN-10: 0-7611-2549-3 (hd.: alk. paper)
1. Pregnancy. 2. Childbirth. 3. Postnatal care.
I. Murkoff, Heidi Eisenberg. II. Hathaway, Sandee Eisenberg. III. Title.
    RG525.E36 2002 618.2'4—dc21   2001043523
                                                     CIP

Book Design: Lisa Hollander, Kathy Herlihy Paoli, Susan Aronson Stirling
Cover Illustration: Judith Cheng
Interior Illustrations: Judy Francis

Workman books are available at special discounts when purchased in bulk
for premiums and sales promotions as well as for fund-raising or educational use.
Special editions or book excerpts can be created to specification.
For details, contact the Special Sales Director at the address below.

Workman Publishing Company, Inc.
708 Broadway
New York, NY 10003-9555
www.workman.com

Printed in the U.S.A.

Third edition first printing: March 2002
45 44 43 42 41 40

SO MANY TO THANK
AND THE THANKS KEEP COMING . . .

In the eighteen years since we put fingers to keyboard to write the first edition of *What to Expect When You're Expecting*, we've learned a lot—not just about what goes into the making of a healthy baby, but what goes into the making of a healthy baby (or pregnancy) book. Lesson number one: we couldn't have done it alone. So many friends and colleagues have helped us, supported us, and guided us through the creation and re-creation of this book—more than we can possibly mention, at least without devoting an entire chapter in this third edition. We gratefully thank you all, including:

Suzanne Rafer, the best friend and editor an author ever had—for her enthusiasm, dedication to detail (long may those pink flags wave), her good humor, her great insights, her love and her caring, and most of all, for always being there when we need her.

Peter Workman, an extraordinary publisher, for his commitment to excellence in publishing, and his commitment to a little series that could—and did. We truly couldn't have done it without you, or without . . .

Lisa Hollander for the refreshed design; Judith Cheng for creating the "Mona Lisa" of pregnancy, and then bringing her beautifully into the 21st century; Judy Francis for the terrific new illustrations. Jenny Mandel, Carolan Workman, Bruce Harris, Kate Tyler, Jim Eber, Pat Upton, Saundra Pearson, Beth Doty, and all the members of the Workman family who make it the special place it is—hugs and kisses to all of you. Thanks, too, to all those who helped out with the first and second editions but who've since moved on.

Sharon Mazel, for saving the day. Your tireless (even when you're exhausted) efforts, your research, and your insights not only made this edition possible, they helped make it far better. Thanks, too, to Kira, for being in the right uterus at the right time, and to Daniella and Arianne for sharing their mom.

Lisa Bernstein, Executive Director of the What to Expect Foundation, for absolutely everything she does, which means just about absolutely everything. Nobody does as much, and nobody does it better—and we love you for that and for a million other reasons. Also, to Zoe and Oh-That-Teddy Bernstein, and Dan Dubno, for your patience and understanding—and for letting mommy talk on the phone so much.

Richard Aubry, M.D., Professor of Obstetrics and Gynecology, and our esteemed medical advisor. Dick's breadth of knowledge and depth of caring make him not only a remarkable physician, an extraordinary teacher, and an outstanding advocate for pregnant women and their babies, but an invaluable resource for us.

Marc Chamlin, for being the greatest lawyer, and even a greater friend; to Ellen Goldsmith-Vein (with XO's) for managing it all and then some, for always believing, and for always being so much fun to be with; to Alan Nevins for being the best; and to all my other friends at Artists Management Group.

All the wonderful, dedicated people at The American College of Obstetricians and Gynecologists and the American Academy of Pediatrics, for always giving us the answers we need to keep the What to Expect books up-to-date, and to the countless physicians who've clarified points, answered questions, filled out questionnaires—and helped make this book the best it could be.

Three men without whom this book (and those that followed) would literally not have been possible: Howard Eisenberg, Erik Murkoff, and Tim Hathaway. You're the best fathers and husbands around, and we'll always love you. And to Mildred and Harry Scharaga, Victor Shargai, and John Aniello, for your love and support.

All those who were so instrumental in the success of our first and second editions, including Henry Eisenberg, M.D., Elise and Arnold Goodman, Susan Stirling, and Carol Donner.

All the doctors, midwives, and nurses who care for pregnant women. And most of all, to our readers—who are and will always be our greatest resource and inspiration.

◆ ◆ ◆

About the
What to Expect® Foundation

◆ ◆ ◆

We're proud to announce the birth of the
What to Expect® Foundation, a nonprofit organization dedicated
to providing information, support, and resources to pregnant women in need—
so that what every mother can expect
is a healthy pregnancy and a healthy baby.

◆

To find out more, visit our Web site at
www.whattoexpect.org

CONTENTS

Part 1
IN THE BEGINNING

Chapter 1: Are You Pregnant? 2
What You May Be Concerned About 2

> *Vitamin Reminder* ◆ Diagnosing Pregnancy ◆ *Testing Smart*
> ◆ *Possible Signs of Pregnancy* ◆ *Probable Signs of Pregnancy* ◆
> *Positive Signs of Pregnancy* ◆ Making the First Appointment
> ◆ *If You're Not Pregnant . . .* ◆ *Pregnancy Timetable* ◆ Due Date

What It's Important to Know:
CHOOSING (AND WORKING WITH) YOUR PRACTITIONER 9

> A Look Back ◆ What Kind of Patient Are You? ◆ Obstetrician?
> Family Practitioner? Nurse-Midwife? ◆ Types of Practice ◆ Find-
> ing a Candidate ◆ Birthing Alternatives ◆ Making Your Selection
> ◆ Making the Most of the Patient-Practitioner Partnership ◆
> *So You Won't Forget*

Chapter 2: Now That You're Pregnant 20
What You May Be Concerned About 20

> Your Gynecological History ◆ *This Book's for You* ◆ Previous
> Abortions ◆ Your Obstetrical History Repeating Itself ◆
> Pregnancies Too Close Together ◆ The Second Time Around
> ◆ Having a Big Family ◆ Repeat Cesareans ◆ Vaginal Birth
> After Cesarean (VBAC) ◆ Obesity ◆ Rh Incompatibility ◆ Being a
> Single Mother ◆ Having a Baby After Thirty-Five ◆ Age and
> Testing for Down Syndrome ◆ The Father's Age ◆ Fibroids ◆
> Endometriosis ◆ Incompetent Cervix ◆ In Vitro Fertilization (IVF)

—————————— *Part 2* ——————————

NINE MONTHS AND COUNTING
From Conception to Delivery

Chapter 5: The First Month

Part 3
LAST BUT NOT LEAST

—— *Part 4* ——

OF SPECIAL CONCERN

—————————— *Part 5* ——————————
THE NEXT BABY

Another Word from the Doctor

I wouldn't have thought it possible. The best just got better.

In my position as professor, as well as a daily provider of maternity care for more than forty years, I have come to realize the fundamental importance of healthy childbearing to the health and vitality of society. These precious new lives, when nurtured by loving parents, become healthy, contributing members of a new generation. There is no book that better prepares parents for that important job of nurturing those young lives—a job that begins even before sperm meets egg—than *What to Expect When You're Expecting.*

For seventeen years, I've watched the development of the previous editions of *What to Expect,* while observing the impact the book has had on a generation of expectant parents, including those in my care. As medical advisor, I've consulted with the authors, vetted the manuscripts, crossed every biologic "t" and dotted every anatomic "i." When the first revised edition arrived on my desk some ten years ago, I marveled at the improvements that had been made in a book I thought was groundbreaking when I originally read it—and with this brand-new third edition, I've marveled once again.

It's hard to stay on the cutting edge of the rapidly evolving field of obstetrics, and it's even harder to convey this sometimes complex information in a manner that women (and their partners) who don't happen to be medical professionals can understand and relate to and be reassured by, but as I have come to expect, the authors have succeeded. And it's harder still, perhaps, to provide this detailed and medically sound advice in a way that augments rather than conflicts with advice parents-to-be get from their maternity care providers—but, once again, they have managed to. As before, *What to Expect When You're Expecting* will appeal to those on both sides of the exam table, embraced by parents and health care providers alike. It's not only recommended (or given) to new patients by many ob-gyns and midwives, but used by those practitioners and their spouses at home. My young residents—and many others in programs across the country—read it to learn what patients are wondering and worrying about, so they'll be better prepared when they begin their own practice.

Finally, this edition of *What to Expect When You're Expecting* continues the tradition of cheering expectant parents on as they venture off to face this life-changing experience, providing them with the inspiration that they "can do it."

Miracles happen—best wishes on yours.

—*Richard Aubry, M.D., M.P.H.*

A Word from the Doctor

These are the best years in history to be expecting a baby. In recent decades, there has been a remarkable improvement in the outcome of human pregnancy—for mothers as well as for infants. Women enter pregnancy healthier; they get better, more complete prenatal care; and the hospital maternity wing has replaced the kitchen table and the four-poster as the place to have a baby.

Yet more can be done. To those of us in academic medicine it is becoming increasingly clear that superior doctors and superior equipment aren't enough. Further reductions in pregnancy and childbirth risks will require actively participating expectant couples as well. In order to participate more fully, couples will have to be more completely and accurately informed, not just about the climactic birth experience, but about the all-important nine months that precede it; not just about the risks that pregnancy presents, but about the steps parents can take to minimize and eliminate risks; not just about the medical aspects of pregnancy, but about psycho-social and lifestyle factors as well.

How can parents become so informed? High schools and colleges have no time or place in their curricula for Babymaking 101. Professionals who provide obstetrical care have a time problem, too. And they are sometimes overly scientific in their explanations and insufficiently sensitive to the psychological and emotional needs of expectant parents.

Consumer advocates have vaulted into the void with books, magazine articles, and classroom instruction. They are often tremendously helpful, but almost as often they're medically inaccurate, unnecessarily alarming, and/or disproportionately focused on the inadequacies of the health care profession, driving a wedge of suspicion and doubt between parents and their obstetrical caregivers.

The need for a book that provides accurate, up-to-date, and medically sound information with proper emphasis on nutrition, lifestyle, and the emotional aspects of pregnancy has long been apparent. Now, I believe, that need has been met in a highly readable and eminently practical month-by-month format.

The three authors—each an experienced "consumer" of maternity care—have given us that essential consumer perspective. They have wisely concentrated on giving expectant parents the information that will allow them to intelligently play their central role in the entire process, without threatening the doctors and nurse-midwives with whom they must work closely and congenially.

What to Expect When You're Expecting is lively in style, accurate, current, and well-balanced overall. But four aspects of its structure and content deserve special comment:

♦ The book's thoughtful family-centered approach to childbearing—with involvement of the husband throughout the pregnancy process and with a chapter responding to his special needs and problems—is excellent and important.

♦ Its practical chronological arrangement—sensibly answering all the big and little, trying and troubling questions that come up month after month—makes for timely reassurance and easy bedside-table reference.

♦ The book's emphasis on pre-pregnancy and pregnancy nutrition and lifestyle, and its commonsense approaches to lactation and the psychosocial dimensions of motherhood, make it particularly valuable and unique.

♦ Its accurate and up-to-the-minute medical detail—particularly the clarity of its sections on genetics, teratology, preterm labor, delivery, cesarean section, and again, lactation—is outstanding.

All in all, I believe that this excellent book, should be *required reading* not only for expectant parents, but for doctors and nurses who are training to provide obstetrical care and for professionals already providing it. That is, I know, a long way out on a limb for a generally cautious medical school professor to go. But I say it out of strong conviction: the belief that only with properly informed and responsible consumers and providers working together can we draw near our common goal—healthy babies, mothers, and families. And, ultimately, a healthy society.

—*Richard Aubry, M.D., M.P.H.*

Why This Book Was Born Again...and Again

Eighteen years ago I gave birth to a daughter and a book within a few short hours of each other. Nurturing both those babies, Emma and *What to Expect When You're Expecting* (as well as my son Wyatt, and—along with my co-authors—the other "offspring" that followed, the *What to Expect* sequels, the What to Expect Foundation, and the *What to Expect Kids* series), as they've grown and evolved over the years has been at once exhilarating and exhausting, fulfilling and confounding, heartwarming and nerve-wracking. It's been an incredible (and always challenging) journey, and like any parent, I wouldn't trade a day of it. (Though there was that week when Emma was thirteen . . .)

And now, we've delivered again: a brand-new, third edition of *What to Expect When You're Expecting*. Although frequent printings allow us to update our books with important new information, the birth of this third edition has provided us with the welcome opportunity to write a complete start-to-finish revi-sion, adding and subtracting and incorporating the latest in obstetrical innovations, from the high-tech to the complementary and alternative, so that *What to Expect* can continue to be as comprehensive and up-to-date as expectant parents need it to be.

There are so many changes that we're excited about. We've made the book even more practical, incorporating sections for the expectant working woman, insights for the family on managed care, more tips for staying beautiful inside and out while you're expecting, more advice for second- (and third-) time moms, and an expanded section that outlines a preconception strategy for both moms and dads who are getting ready to make a baby. Rounding out our new edition are more questions about more symptoms, a monthly visual peek at both you and your baby, and a bigger and (we think) better father's chapter. We've also cooked up a kinder, gentler, and more realistic Pregnancy Diet that you may find easier to follow and easier to apply to your chronically time-challenged life. Even our cover woman has been refreshed; after seventeen years of enduring a 1980s perm and a potato sack of a dress, she has enjoyed a sleek hair-to–cute shoe makeover. *And* she gets to wear pants.

But just as important as what's different in this third edition is what has stayed precisely the same. When I first co-wrote *What to Expect When You're Expecting,* I saw my work as a personal crusade with a single goal: I never wanted any expectant parent to ever worry as much during their pregnancy as I (and my husband Erik) had during mine. That sentiment still holds true today, and *What to Expect When You're Expecting*'s third edition was written, as the first one was, to inform, reassure, and help parents get that better night's sleep (or at least as good a night's sleep as urinary frequency, leg cramps, and backache will allow).

Of course, no sooner than the ink dries on this third edition we'll probably be tackling a fourth. In doing that we will, as always, welcome any and all suggestions you would like to make.

What to Expect is, after all, an ever-evolving book and other parents continue to be our most valuable resource in that work in progress.

Wishing you the healthiest of pregnancies, and a lifetime of happy parenting.

—*Heidi Murkoff*

ANY QUESTIONS?

We've tried to answer them all, and hopefully we've managed to answer most. But since every pregnancy (like every expectant parent) is different, it's likely we may have missed a few. If, in reading this book, you find that we've overlooked any of your questions or concerns, we'd like to know. That way we'll be able to include them in our next edition in plenty of time, we hope, for *your* next addition. Write to us at Workman Publishing, 708 Broadway, New York 10003.

How This Book Was Born

I was pregnant, which about one day out of three made me the happiest woman in the world. And for the remaining two, the most worried.

Worried about the wine I'd sipped nightly with dinner, and the gin and tonics I'd downed more than a few times before dinner in my first six weeks of pregnancy—after two gynecologists and a blood test convinced me that I wasn't pregnant.

Worried about the seven doses of Provera one of the doctors had prescribed to bring on what she was certain was just a tardy period, but which proved two weeks later to be a nearly two-month gestation.

Worried about the coffee I'd drunk, and the milk I hadn't; the sugar I'd eaten, and the protein I hadn't.

Worried about the cramps in my third month, and the four days in my fifth month when I felt not even a flicker of fetal movement.

Worried about the time I fainted while touring the hospital I was to deliver in (I never did get to see the nursery), my middle-of-the-street belly-flop in the eighth month, and a bloody vaginal discharge in the ninth.

Worried, even, about feeling *good* ("But I'm not constipated. . . . I don't have morning sickness. . . . I'm not urinating more frequently—something must be wrong!").

Worried that I wouldn't be able to tolerate the pain during labor, or stand the sight of blood at delivery. And worried that because I couldn't squeeze out a drop of the colostrum all my books told me should fill my breasts by the ninth month, I wouldn't be able to breastfeed.

Where could I turn to find reassurance that all would be well? Not to the ever-growing stack of pregnancy books piled high on my bedside table. As common and normal as a few days of no fetal activity is in the fifth month, I couldn't find a single reference to it. As often as pregnant women take a tumble—almost always without harming their babies—I could find no mention of accidental falls.

When my symptoms, problems, or fears *were* discussed, it was usually in an alarming way which only compounded my concern. *Never* take Provera unless you would "absolutely abort," warned one volume—without adding that a woman who has taken the drug has so slight an increased risk of birth defects in her baby that an unwanted abortion need never be considered. "There is evidence that a single drinking 'binge' during pregnancy may affect some babies, depending on the stage of development they have reached," cautioned another book ominously—disregarding studies showing that a few drinking sprees in early pregnancy, when many women indulge unknowingly, appear to have no effect on a developing embryo.

I certainly couldn't find relief for my worries by opening a newspaper, flipping on the radio or television, or browsing through magazines. According to the media, threats to the pregnant lurked everywhere: in the air we breathed, in the food we ate, in the water we drank, at the dentist's office, in the drugstore, even at home.

My doctor offered some solace, of course, but only when I was able to summon up the courage to phone. (I was either afraid my worries would sound silly or afraid of what I would hear. Besides, how could I spend two days out of three on the phone badgering her?)

Was I (and my husband, Erik—who worried about everything I worried about, and then some) alone in my fears? Far from it. Worry, according to one study, is one of the most common complaints of pregnancy, affecting more expectant women than morning sickness and food cravings combined. Ninety-four out of every hundred women worry about whether their babies will be normal, and 93% worry about whether they and their babies will come through delivery safely. More women worry about their figures (91%) than their health (81%) during pregnancy. And most worry that they worry too much.

But though a little worry is normal for pregnant women and their mates, a lot of worry is an unnecessary waste of what should be a blissfully happy time. Despite all that we hear, read, and worry about, never before in the history of reproduction has it been safer to have a baby—as Erik and I discovered some seven and a half months of worrying later, when I gave birth to a healthier and more beautiful baby girl than I'd dared to dream possible.

Thus, out of our concerns, *What to Expect When You're Expecting* was born. It is dedicated to expectant couples everywhere, and written with the hope that it will help fathers- and mothers-to-be worry less and enjoy their pregnancies more.

—*Heidi Murkoff*

Part 1

IN THE BEGINNING

CHAPTER 1

Are You Pregnant?

Maybe your period's just a day overdue. Or maybe it's going on three weeks late. Maybe your only symptom so far is that missed period. Or maybe you've already developed every possible first trimester symptom, and then some. Maybe you've been giving baby making everything you've got for six months or longer. Or maybe that night two weeks ago was the first contraceptive-free encounter. Or maybe you weren't trying at all. No matter what the circumstances are that have brought you to this book, you're bound to be wondering: Am I pregnant?

VITAMIN REMINDER

If you're trying to conceive or believe you might be pregnant, be sure to take a *prenatal* vitamin pill containing folic acid, iron, and calcium (see page 93).

What You May Be Concerned About

DIAGNOSING PREGNANCY

"My doctor said the exam and pregnancy test showed I wasn't pregnant, but I really feel I am."

As remarkable as modern medical science is, when it comes to pregnancy diagnosis, it still sometimes takes a backseat to a woman's intuition. The accuracy of the different pregnancy tests varies, and many do not indicate pregnancy as early as some women begin to "feel" that they are pregnant—which is sometimes within a few days after conception.

The home pregnancy test. Like the urine test done in a lab or the doctor's office, the home pregnancy test diagnoses pregnancy by detecting the presence of the hormone hCG (human chorionic gonadotropin) in the urine. These tests can tell you if you're pregnant in just minutes, with an any-time-of-the-day urine sample—fewer than fourteen days after conception (and as early as the first day you've missed your period). Results, however, are more accurate if you wait until your period is at least a few days late—one or two weeks late may even be better. An at-home test performed correctly is as accurate as a urine test done in a doctor's office or laboratory, with a positive result more likely to be correct than a negative one.

Home tests offer the advantage of privacy and virtually immediate results. And because they provide a very accurate diagnosis early in pregnancy—earlier than you would probably consider consulting a physician or midwife—they can give you the opportunity to start taking optimum care of yourself within days of conception. But they can be relatively expensive, and because you're less likely to feel confident in the results, you're more apt to want a retest, increasing the cost to you. (Some brands include a second test in the package.)

The major drawback with home pregnancy tests is that if a test produces a false negative result and you actually are pregnant, you may postpone seeing a practitioner and taking appropriate care of yourself. And even with a positive result, you may postpone the office visit because you assume that getting a diagnosis is the only reason to see your practitioner at this point. So if you use such a test, keep in mind that it is not designed to take the place of a consultation with, and examination by, a medical professional. Medical follow-up to the test is essential. If the result is positive, you should have it confirmed by a physical exam and then get a complete prenatal checkup. If it is negative and your period still hasn't started within a week, do a retest. If the second test is negative, you and your doctor need to find out why. And while the issue is explored, you should "act pregnant" (avoiding alcohol, cigarettes, and so on) until you know for sure that you're not.

The in-office urine test. Like the at-home variety, this test can detect hCG in the urine with an accuracy of close to 100 percent—and as early as seven to fourteen days after conception. Unlike the home test, it is performed by a professional, who is, at least theoretically, more likely to do it correctly. The in-office test does not require a first-morning urine sample. Urine tests are less expensive than blood tests, but they do not provide as much information.

The blood test. The more sophisticated blood pregnancy test can detect pregnancy with virtually 100 percent accuracy as early as one week after conception (barring lab error), using just a few drops of blood. It can also help to date the pregnancy by measuring the exact amount of hCG in the blood, since hCG values change as pregnancy progresses. Most practitioners order both a urine and a blood test to be doubly certain of the diagnosis.

The medical exam. No matter which test you use, the chances of the diagnosis being correct are enhanced when the test is followed by a medical examination. Some of the physical signs of pregnancy—including softening of the uterus and a change in the texture of the cervix—may be apparent to your doctor or midwife as early as four to six weeks into your pregnancy. As with tests, a practitioner's diagnosis of "pregnant" is more likely to be correct than one of "not pregnant"—though false negative results are fairly uncommon with a full medical exam.

If you are experiencing the symptoms of early pregnancy (a missed period or two, breast fullness and tenderness, morning sickness, frequent urination, fatigue) and feel, test or no test, exam or no exam, that you are pregnant, act as though you are, taking all prenatal precautions, until you find out definitely otherwise. Neither tests nor medical practitioners are infallible. You know your own body—at least externally—better than your practitioner does. Ask for a retest (preferably a blood test) and another exam in a week or so; in your case, it may just be too early for an accurate diagnosis. More than one full-term baby has arrived seven and a half or eight months after a pregnancy test and/or a doctor concluded that the mother wasn't pregnant.

If the tests continue to be negative but you still haven't begun to menstruate, be sure to check with your doctor to rule out an ectopic pregnancy, one that takes place outside of the uterus. (See page 124 for warning signs of this kind of pregnancy.)

It is possible, of course, to experience all the signs and symptoms of early pregnancy and not be pregnant at all. After all, none of them alone—or even in combination—is absolute proof positive of pregnancy. After a second pregnancy test and a physical exam determine that you are not pregnant, you and your doctor should investigate other biological causes of your symptoms. If those are ruled out as well, you should consider that the "pregnancy" may have psychological roots—possibly that you very strongly do, or don't, want to have a baby.

TESTING SMART

Home pregnancy tests are easier to use and more reliable than ever. The following tips may seem obvious, but in the excitement of the moment (will I be? won't I be?), don't forget to:

◆ Read the directions for the test thoroughly before you use it (even if you've used it, or another test, in the past). Then reread them, just to be sure.

◆ Have an easy-to-read clock, watch, or timer ready so that you can time the test precisely.

◆ Be sure containers, dipsticks, or any other equipment to be used with the test are clean when you begin the test.

Don't reuse these if you want to try again.

◆ If a waiting period is required, place the sample on a flat surface away from the heat and in a place where it won't be disturbed.

◆ Read the test after the recommended waiting period; not waiting long enough—or waiting too long—can affect the result.

◆ If the kit you've purchased contains a second test, or if you buy a second kit, wait at least a few days before trying a retest.

POSSIBLE SIGNS OF PREGNANCY

You can have all of the signs and symptoms of early pregnancy and not be pregnant. Or you can have only a few of them and be very definitely pregnant. The various signs and symptoms of pregnancy are only clues—it's important to pay attention to them, but you can't rely on them for absolute confirmation.

SIGN	WHEN IT APPEARS	OTHER POSSIBLE CAUSES
Amenorrhea (absence of menstruation)*	Following conception	Travel, fatigue, stress, fear of pregnancy, hormonal problems, illness, extreme weight gain or loss, going off the Pill, breastfeeding
Morning sickness (nausea, with or without vomiting, any time of day) †	2–8 weeks after conception	Food poisoning, emotional stress, infection, a variety of illnesses
Frequent urination	As early as 2–3 weeks after conception	Urinary tract infection, diuretics, stress, diabetes
Tingling, tender, swollen breasts	As early as a few days after conception	Birth control pills, impending menstruation
Darkening of areola (area around nipple) and elevation of tiny glands around nipple	First trimester	Hormonal imbalance or effect of prior pregnancy
Blue and pink lines under skin on breasts and later on abdomen	First trimester	Hormonal imbalance or effect of prior pregnancy
Food cravings	First trimester	Poor diet, stress, impending menstruation
Darkening of line from navel to pubis (*linea nigra*)	4th or 5th month	Hormonal imbalance or effect of prior pregnancy

*Some women have periodic staining or bleeding during the first months of pregnancy; others may have some bleeding during implantation of the embryo in the uterus.
†More than half of all women experience morning sickness.

PROBABLE SIGNS OF PREGNANCY

SIGN	WHEN IT APPEARS	OTHER POSSIBLE CAUSES
Changes in color of vaginal and cervical tissue to bluish violet*	First trimester	Impending menstruation
Softening of cervix and uterus*	About 6 weeks	A delayed menstrual period
Enlarging uterus* and abdomen	8–12 weeks after conception	Fibroids, tumor
Palpable uterine artery pulsation*	Early in pregnancy	Fibroids, tumor
Fluttering sensation in lower abdomen (fetal movement)	First noted at 16–22 weeks of pregnancy	Gas, bowel contractions

*Signs of pregnancy looked for in medical examination.

POSITIVE SIGNS OF PREGNANCY

SIGN	WHEN IT APPEARS	OTHER POSSIBLE CAUSES
Visualization of embryo or gestational sac through ultrasound*	As early as 4–6 weeks after conception	None
Fetal heartbeat*	10–20 weeks of pregnancy†	None

*Signs of pregnancy looked for in medical examination.
†Depending on device used; Doppler detects as early as 10 to 12 weeks.

MAKING THE FIRST APPOINTMENT

"The home pregnancy test I just took came back positive. When should I schedule the first visit with my practitioner?"

Good prenatal care is one of the most important ingredients in making a healthy baby. So don't delay. As soon as you suspect you might be pregnant, or have a positive home pregnancy test result, call your practitioner to schedule an appointment. Just how soon you'll be able to come in for that appointment may depend on office traffic and policy. Some practitioners will be able to fit you in right away, while some very busy offices may not be able to accommodate you for several weeks or even longer. At other practitioners' offices, it's actually routine procedure to wait until a woman is six weeks pregnant for that first prenatal visit. But even if your official prenatal care has to be postponed, that doesn't mean you should put off taking care of yourself and your baby.

IF YOU'RE NOT PREGNANT . . .

If your pregnancy test is negative this time, but you'd very much like to become pregnant soon, start making the most of the preconception period by taking the steps outlined in Chapter 21. Good preconception preparation will help ensure the best possible pregnancy outcome when you do conceive.

Regardless of when you get in to see your practitioner, as soon as you see that pink line or plus sign on the home pregnancy test, start taking your prenatal vitamins (if you aren't doing so already) and start acting pregnant (no alcohol or smoking, start eating right, and so on). If you feel you may be a high-risk case (because of a history of miscarriage or ectopic pregnancies) or if you would just feel more comfortable seeing your practitioner earlier than he or she usually sees pregnant patients, check with the office to see if

PREGNANCY TIMETABLE

While most women count their pregnancies in months, your doctor or midwife will do his or her calculations in weeks. And that's where things can get a little tricky. The average pregnancy lasts 40 weeks, but because counting begins from the first day of your last period—and ovulation and conception don't take place until two weeks after that (if your periods are regular)—you actually become pregnant in week 3 of your pregnancy. In other words, you've already clocked two weeks by the time sperm meets egg. This may sound very confusing, but as your pregnancy progresses and

you experience pregnancy milestones traditionally marked by weeks (baby's heartbeat heard with Doppler around 10 weeks; the top of the uterus reaches your belly button at 20 weeks), you'll start to make sense of the weekly calendar.

Though this book is organized in chapters by month, corresponding weeks are also provided. Keep in mind: Weeks 1 to 13 (approximately) make up the first trimester and include months 1 to 3; weeks 14 to 27 (approximately) comprise the second trimester and include months 4 to 6; and weeks 28 to 40 (approximately) the third trimester, and include months 7 to 9.

the rules can be bent and if you can come in earlier. (For more on what to expect from your first prenatal visit, see page 106.)

DUE DATE

"I am trying to plan my pregnancy leave. How do I know if my due date is really correct?"

Life would be a lot simpler if you could be certain that your due date is actually the day you will deliver, but life isn't that simple very often. According to most studies, only one in twenty babies are actually born on their due date. Because a normal full-term pregnancy can last anywhere from 38 to 42 weeks, most are born within two weeks either way of that date.

Because so few women actually deliver on the day they're "due"—causing much needless anxiety—some in the obstetrics field propose that women be given an "assigned week of delivery" instead. For the first timer, the assigned week would be between 40 and 41 weeks. But until such an assigned week of delivery is put into practice, most practitioners rely on a "due date" or EDD, *estimated* date of delivery. The date your practitioner gives you is only an educated estimate. It is usually calculated this way: Subtract three months from the first day of your last menstrual period (LMP), then add seven days— that's your due date. For example, say your last period began on April 11. Count backward three months, which gets you to January, and then add 7 days. Your due date would be January 18.

This dating system works well for women who have a fairly regular menstrual cycle. But if your cycle is irregular, this dating system may not work for you at all. Say you typically get your period every six to seven weeks and you haven't had one in three months. On testing,

you find out you're pregnant. When did you conceive? Because a reliable EDD is important, you and your practitioner will have to try to come up with one. Even if you can't pinpoint conception or aren't sure when you last ovulated, there are clues that can help.

The very first clue is the size of your uterus, which will be noted when your initial internal pregnancy examination is performed. It should conform to your suspected stage of pregnancy. Later on, there are other milestones that together can more accurately gauge just how pregnant you are: the first time the fetal heartbeat is heard (at about 10 to 12 weeks with a Doppler device, or at about 18 to 20 weeks with a stethoscope); when the first flutter of life is felt (at about 20 to 22 weeks with a first baby, or 16 to 18 with subsequent ones); the height of the fundus (the top of the uterus) at each visit (for example, it will reach the navel at about week 20). If all of these indications seem to correspond to the due date you and your practitioner have calculated, you can be pretty sure that it is close to accurate—that is, that you are quite likely to deliver within two weeks of that date. Your practitioner may also decide to do an ultrasound before week 12 to pinpoint more closely the gestational age of your fetus (see page 49). Some doctors will do an ultrasound routinely, to obtain the most accurate date possible.

As delivery nears, there will be other clues to the date of the big event: painless contractions may become more frequent (and possibly become uncomfortable), the fetus will drop into the pelvis (engagement), your cervix may begin to thin and shorten (effacement), and last of all, your cervix will begin to dilate. These clues will be helpful, but still not definitive—only your baby knows for sure what his or her birthday will be. And baby's not telling.

What It's Important to Know: CHOOSING (AND WORKING WITH) YOUR PRACTITIONER

We all know it takes two to conceive a baby, but it takes a minimum of three—mother, father, and at least one health care professional—to make that transition from fertilized egg to delivered infant a safe and successful one. Assuming you and your spouse have already taken care of conception, the next challenge you face is selecting that third member of your pregnancy team and making sure that it's a selection you can live with—and labor with. (Of course you can, and ideally should, make this selection even before you conceive.)

A LOOK BACK

The selection of a pregnancy caregiver wasn't a major consideration for mothers-to-be a half century ago. Those were the days of no-questions-asked obstetrical care, when the few choices there were in childbirth were left up to the doctor. As far as selecting an obstetrician was concerned, one seemed pretty much like the next. And besides, since you were likely to be unconscious during delivery, it didn't ultimately matter much whether you had rapport with your doctor. Instead of being a participating team member, the mother-to-be was more or less a spectator, sitting obediently on the bench while the obstetrical captain called the plays.

Today there are almost as many choices in childbirth—yours for the choosing—as there are doctors in the yellow pages. The trick is in matching yourself up with a compatible practitioner.

WHAT KIND OF PATIENT ARE YOU?

Your first step in figuring out the kind of practitioner that is right for you is to give some thought to the kind of patient you are.

Do you believe that "doctor knows best" (after all, he or she's the one who went to medical school)? Would you prefer that your physician make most decisions about your treatment without consulting you (after all, that's why you chose someone with more expertise and experience than you)? Do you feel most secure and most comfortable when all the latest medical technology is being used in your care—whether it's really necessary or not? In your medical fantasies, does the person in the white lab coat taking your pulse fit an image of the fatherly physician you've seen on old television show reruns? If so, you may be most comfortable with an obstetrician who has a traditional practice, a paternal persona (even if she's a woman), and an unswerving dedication to his or her own obstetrical philosophy.

Or do you believe that your body and your health are by and large your business? Do you have definite ideas about pregnancy and childbirth and feel you'd like to call the shots based on those ideas—with minimal interference from your health professional? Then skip over the traditional types, and look for a physician or midwife who's willing to let you run the show as much as possible. Someone who will let you make as many of the childbirth decisions as is medically practical, who is dogmatic only when it comes to giving the patient a controlling vote.

Or perhaps your style as a patient is somewhere in the middle. Maybe you'd like your relationship with your practitioner to be a partnership—one in which each partner contributes what they know and do best. You'd prefer a practitioner who will make decisions based on his or her experience and knowledge, as well as your medical best interest, but will always include you and your wishes in the process. If so, the practitioner for you is probably one who is neither a slave to medical gospel nor putty in your hands; one who doesn't automatically either give or withhold medication; one whose first choice would be to proceed naturally through labor and delivery but who won't hesitate to bring on the medical interventions should they prove necessary for your safety or your baby's.

OBSTETRICIAN? FAMILY PRACTITIONER? NURSE-MIDWIFE?

Narrowing your ideal practitioner down to one of three general personality types makes your search easier, but exam-table-side manner and philosophy aren't everything. You'll also have to give some thought to what kind of medical credentials would best meet your needs or requirements.

The obstetrician. Are you looking for a practitioner who is trained to handle every conceivable aspect of pregnancy, labor, delivery, and the postpartum period—from the most obvious question to the most obscure complication? Then you'll want to look to an obstetrician-gynecologist. Ob-gyns not only provide complete obstetrical care; they can also take care of all your nonpregnancy female health needs (Pap smears, breast exams, and so on). Some also offer general medical care, and thus can act as your primary physician as well.

If yours is a high-risk pregnancy,[1] you will very likely need and want to seek out an ob-gyn. You may even want to find a specialist's specialist, an obstetrician who specializes in high-risk pregnancies and is certified in maternal-fetal medicine. But if your pregnancy looks pretty routine, you may still want to select an obstetrician for your care—more than 80 percent of women do. If you've been seeing an ob-gyn you like, respect, and feel comfortable with for your gynecological care, there may be no reason to switch now that you're pregnant. If you haven't been seeing an ob-gyn, or you're not sure the one you've been seeing is the practitioner you want to spend your pregnancy with, it's time to start shopping around.

The family practitioner. Like the general practitioner of years ago, a family practitioner (FP) of today provides one-stop medical service for the whole family. Unlike the obstetrician, who has had postmedical school training in women's reproductive and general health only, the FP has had training in primary care, obstetrics, and pediatrics after receiving an MD. If you decide on an FP (about 10 to 12 percent of pregnant women use one), he or she can serve as your internist, obstetrician/gynecologist, and, when the time comes, pediatrician. Ideally, an FP will become familiar with the dynamics of your family, will be interested in all

---

1. Traditionally, a high-risk pregnancy is one in which the expectant mother has had a problem pregnancy before; has a preexisting medical problem such as diabetes, hypertension, autoimmune disease, or heart disease; or has an Rh or genetic problem.

aspects of your health, not just your pregnancy, and will view pregnancy as a normal part of the life cycle. If complications occur, an FP may send you to an obstetrician but remain involved in your care.

The certified nurse-midwife. If you are looking for a practitioner whose emphasis is on you the person rather than you the patient, who will take extra time to talk with you about your feelings and problems, and who will be oriented toward the "natural" in childbirth, then a certified nurse-midwife (CNM) may be right for you (though, of course, many physicians meet those requirements, too). Although a CNM is a medical professional, she is more likely to treat your pregnancy as a human condition rather than as a medical one.

A certified nurse-midwife is a registered nurse who has completed graduate-level programs in midwifery, and is certified by the American College of Nurse-Midwives. A CNM is thoroughly trained to care for women with low-risk pregnancies and to attend uncomplicated births. In some cases, a CNM may provide continuing routine gynecological care and, sometimes, newborn care. She may work in a hospital, at a birthing center, and/or do home births. Though CNMs have the right in most states to prescribe pain medication, a birth attended by a CNM is less likely to include medication and routine medical interventions. Studies show that for low-risk pregnancies, deliveries by CNMs are as safe as those by physicians.

If you choose a certified nurse-midwife (about 9 percent of expectant mothers do), be sure to select one who is certified and licensed (all fifty states now license nurse-midwives). Most CNMs use a physician as a backup in case of complications; many practice with one or with a group that includes several.

Direct-entry midwives. These midwives are trained without first becoming nurses, though they may hold degrees in other health care areas. Direct-entry midwives are more likely than CNMs to do home births, though some also deliver babies in birthing centers. Those who are evaluated and certified through the North American Registry of Midwives (NARM) are called Certified Professional Midwives (CPM); other direct-entry midwives are not certified. Licensing for direct-entry midwives is also currently offered in certain states; in some of those states, the services of a CPM are reimbursable through Medicaid and private health plans. In other states, direct-entry midwives cannot practice legally. For more information, call the Midwives Alliance of North America at (888) 923-6262 or check their Web site at www.mana.org.

TYPES OF PRACTICE

You've decided on an obstetrician, a family practitioner, or a nurse-midwife. Next you've got to decide which kind of medical practice you would be most comfortable with. The most common kinds of practices, and their possible advantages and disadvantages, are:

Solo medical practice. In such a practice, a doctor works alone, using another doctor to cover when he or she is away or otherwise unavailable. An obstetrician or a family practitioner might be in solo practice; a nurse-midwife, in almost all states, must work in a collaborative practice with a physician. The major advantage of a solo practice is that you see the same practitioner at each visit. This way, you get to know and, hopefully, feel more comfortable with this person before delivery. The major disadvantage is that if your doctor is not available, a physician you don't know may deliver your baby (although arranging to meet the covering physician in advance remedies this potential drawback). A solo practice may also be a problem if, midway in the pregnancy, you find you're not really crazy about the doctor. If that happens and you decide to switch doctors, you'll have to start from scratch again searching for a practitioner who suits your needs.

Partnership or group medical practice. In this type of practice, two or more doctors in the same specialty care jointly for patients, seeing them on a rotating basis. Again, you can find both obstetricians and family doctors in this type of practice. The advantage of this arrangement is that by seeing a different doctor each time, you will get to know them all, and when those labor pains are coming strong and fast, there will be a familiar face in the room with you. The disadvantage is that you may not like all of the doctors in the practice equally, and you usually won't be able to choose the one who attends your child's birth. Also, depending on whether you find it reassuring or unsettling, hearing different points of view from the various partners may be an advantage or a disadvantage.

Combination practice. A group practice that includes one or more obstetricians and one or more nurse-midwives is considered a combination practice. The advantages and disadvantages are similar to those of any group practice. There is the added advantage of having at some of your visits the extra time and attention a midwife may offer and at others the security of a physician's extensive training and expertise. You may have the option of a midwife-coached delivery, plus assurance that if a problem develops, a physician you know is in the wings.

Maternity center– or birth center–based practice. In these practices, certified nurse-midwives provide the bulk of the care, and physicians are on call as needed. Some maternity centers are based in hospitals with special birthing rooms, and others are separate facilities. All maternity centers provide care for low-risk patients only.

The advantage of this type of practice is obviously great for those women who prefer certified midwives as their primary practitioners. The potential disadvantage is that if a complication arises during pregnancy, you may have to switch to a physician and start developing a relationship all over again. If a complication arises during labor or delivery, you may need to be delivered by the doctor on call, who may be a complete stranger. And finally, if you are delivering at a freestanding maternity center and complications arise, you may have to be transported to the nearest hospital for emergency care.

Independent certified nurse-midwife practice. In the states in which they are permitted to practice independently, CNMs offer women with low-risk pregnancies the advantage of personalized pregnancy care and a low-tech natural delivery (sometimes at home, but more often in birthing centers or hospitals). An independent CNM should have a physician available for consultation as needed and on call in case of emergency—during pregnancy, childbirth, and postpartum. Care by an independent CNM is covered by most health plans, though only some insurers will cover midwife-attended home births or births in a facility other than a hospital.

FINDING A CANDIDATE

When you have a good idea of the kind of practitioner you want and the type of practice you prefer, where can you find some likely candidates? The following are all good sources:

- Your gynecologist or family practitioner (if he or she doesn't do deliveries) or your internist, assuming you're happy with his or her style of practice. (Doctors tend to recommend others with philosophies similar to their own.)

- Friends who have had babies recently and whose childbearing philosophies are similar to yours.

- An obstetrical nurse who practices locally, if you're lucky enough to know one.

- The county medical society, which can give you a list of names of physicians who deliver babies, along with information on their medical training, specialties, special interests, type of practice, and board certification. The society may also be able to tell you whether or not a specialist will be helpful in your situation and, if so, what kind of specialist.

- The *Directory of the American Medical Association* or the *Directory of Medical Specialties,* often available at your public library or doctor's office.

- The *American College of Obstetricians and Gynecologists Physician's Directory* for the name of an obstetrician-gynecologist or a maternal-fetal specialist; 409 12th Street SW, PO Box 96920, Washington, DC 20090-6920. Web site: www. ACOG.org.

- The American College of Nurse-Midwives, 818 Connecticut Avenue NW, Suite 900, Washington, DC 20006, if you are looking for a CNM. Web site: www. ACNM.org, or call (202) 728-9860.

- The local La Leche League, especially if you're strongly interested in breast-feeding.

- A nearby hospital with facilities that are important to you—for example, birthing rooms with Jacuzzis, rooming-in for both baby and Dad, or a neonatal intensive care unit—or a local maternity or birth center. Ask them for the names of attending physicians.

- The International Childbirth Education Association, PO Box 20048, Minneapolis, MN 55420. Web site: www. ICEA.org, or call (612) 854-8660; or the American Society for Prophylaxis in Obstetrics (ASPO)/Lamaze, 1840 Wilson Boulevard, Suite 204, Arlington, VA, 22201. Web site: www. Lamaze-childbirth.com, or call (800) 368-4404 if you are interested in a practitioner who emphasizes prepared childbirth.

- If all else fails, the yellow pages, under Physicians, looking for the headings Obstetrics and Gynecology, Maternal-Fetal Medicine, or Family Practice.

If your HMO or health insurance hands you a list of practitioners, try to check them out with friends, acquaintances, or another physician to find the one in the bunch that seems right for you. If that's not possible, visit and meet with several of the candidates personally. In most cases, you should be able to find someone who is compatible. If not, you may, finances permitting, want to see if you can switch plans.

BIRTHING ALTERNATIVES

Never before have women had so much control over having babies. For millennia it was largely nature's whims that decided a woman's obstetrical fate. Then, early in the twentieth century, it became the physician who decided how she was to deliver. Today, though nature still holds a few cards and physicians still have a say, more and more of the decisions are falling to women and their spouses. It is becoming increasingly possible for a woman to choose the best time to conceive (thanks to better birth control methods and kits that let you pinpoint ovulation) and, often, how she will give birth. The array of birthing options is dizzying, even in a hospital setting. Leave the hospital, and there's yet more to select from.

Though your delivery preferences shouldn't be your only criteria in choosing a practitioner, they should certainly come into play. (Keep in mind, however, that no firm birthing decisions can be made until further into your pregnancy, and many can't be finalized until the delivery itself.) The following options are among those that expectant parents today can consider and might want to ask about before picking a practitioner and hospital:

Family-centered care. What many feel is the ideal in hospital maternity care—complete family-centered care—is not yet a reality in every hospital, though there's definitely a trend in that direction. ASPO/Lamaze has set criteria for this ideal, which include: an official hospital policy of family-centered maternity care; childbirth education programs that reflect such a policy; management of labor without unnecessary technological interference and with attention to psychosocial needs; an atmosphere in which questions, self-help, and self-knowledge are encouraged, in which adaptations are made for cultural differences, and in which breastfeeding is encouraged within one hour of birth unless medically contraindicated; and a program that assesses a mother's basic infant care skills (including satisfactory initiation of breastfeeding, if applicable) prior to discharge. According to ASPO/Lamaze criteria,

patient rooms should have a door (for privacy), comfortable furnishings, private toilet and bath/shower facilities, as well as sufficient space to accommodate family (including siblings) and other support persons, professional personnel and medical equipment, personal possessions, a newborn crib and supplies, and a sofa bed for family members staying overnight. There should be an area nearby for support persons to take relaxation breaks away from the scene of the labor. Many hospitals and most birthing centers (facilities independent from or close to a hospital where women labor, deliver, and recover) provide this type of family-centered care.

Birthing rooms. For much of the twentieth century, every woman about to have a baby labored in a labor room, delivered in a delivery room, and recovered in a postpartum room. Her newborn was immediately whisked from her after birth and tucked away in a nursery to be cared for behind glass windows. Today, the availability of birthing rooms in most hospitals makes it possible for you to stay in the same bed from labor through recovery, sometimes even for your entire hospital stay, and for your baby to remain at your side from birth on.

Some birthing rooms are used just for labor, delivery, and recovery (LDRs). If an LDR is used, the newly delivered mother (and her baby, if she's rooming in) is moved from the birthing room to a postpartum room after an hour or so of largely uninterrupted family togetherness. But in more and more hospitals, LDRP (labor, delivery, recovery, postpartum) rooms make it possible for mothers and babies—and often Dad and even siblings—to stay put from check-in to checkout.

Most birthing rooms boast an "at-home-in-the-hospital" look, with soft lighting, rocking chairs, pretty wallpaper, soothing pictures on the wall, curtains on the windows, and beds that look more as if they came out of an Ethan Allen showroom than a hospital supply catalog. Though the rooms are thoroughly equipped for low-risk births and even unexpected emergencies, medical equipment is usually stowed out of sight behind the doors of armoires and other bedroomlike cabinetry. The back of the birthing bed can be raised to support the mom in a squatting or semi-squatting position and the foot of the bed snaps off to make way for the birthing attendants. After delivery, a change of linens, a few flipped switches, and presto, you're back in bed. Many hospitals and birthing centers also offer showers and/or Jacuzzi tubs in or adjacent to the birthing rooms, both of which can offer hydrotherapy relief during labor. Tubs for water birth are also available in some birthing centers and hospitals. (See below for more on water birth.)

Birthing rooms at some hospitals are available only for women who are at low risk for childbirth complications; if you don't meet this criterion, you may have no choice but to go to a traditional labor and delivery room, where more technology is at hand. Fortunately, with the increasing availability of birthing rooms for most women, odds are great that you'll be able to experience unrushed, family-friendly, noninterventionist labor and delivery within a traditional hospital setting.

Birthing chairs. A birthing chair is designed to support a woman in a sitting or squatting position during delivery, allowing for an assist from gravity, theoretically speeding labor. Many women find that squatting aids during the pushing stage. Another plus: mothers get to see more of the birth in this position.

Leboyer births. When the French obstetrician Frederick Leboyer first propounded his theory of childbirth without violence, the medical community scoffed. Today many of the procedures he proposed, aimed at making a newborn's arrival in the world more tranquil, are common practice. Many babies are delivered in birthing rooms, without the bright lights once deemed necessary, on the theory that gentle lighting can make the transition from the dark uterus to the bright outside world more gradual and less jolting. Upending and slapping the newborn is no longer routine anywhere; less violent procedures are preferred for establishing breathing when it doesn't start on its own. In some hospitals, the umbilical cord isn't cut immediately; instead, this last physical bond between mother and baby remains intact while they get to know each other for the first time. And though the warm bath Leboyer recommended for soothing the new arrival and smoothing the transition from a watery home to a dry one isn't common, being put immediately into Mother's arms is.

In spite of the growing acceptance of many Leboyer theories, a full-blown Leboyer birth—with soft music, soft lights, and a warm bath for baby—isn't widely available. If you're interested in one, though, ask about it when you're interviewing practitioners.

Water birth. The concept of delivering underwater to simulate the environment of the womb is not widely used in the medical community, but it is more accepted among midwives. Advocates of water birth say the water eases the baby from the warm, wet womb into another warm, wet environment, offering familiar comfort after the stresses of delivery. The baby is pulled out of the water and placed in the mother's arms immediately after birth. And since breathing doesn't begin until the baby is exposed to the air, there is little risk of drowning. Water births can be done at home, in birthing centers, and in some hospitals. Many spouses join the mother in the tub, often holding her from behind to provide support.

Most women with low-risk pregnancies can choose a water birth. If you're in a high-risk category, however, it's not a wise option, and it's unlikely you'll find even a midwife who will allow you to try a water birth.

Even if you don't find the idea of a water birth inviting (or don't have the option of one open to you), you might welcome the opportunity to labor in a Jacuzzi or tub. Most women find that the water not only provides relaxation but even facilitates the progression of labor. Some hospitals and most birthing centers offer tubs in the birthing rooms.

Home birth. For some women, the idea of being hospitalized when they aren't sick isn't appealing. If you are one of them, you might want to consider a home birth. The newborn arrives amid family and friends in a warm and loving atmosphere. The downside is that if something unexpectedly goes wrong, the facilities for an emergency cesarean or resuscitation of the newborn will not be close at hand. For this reason, many women find a maternity center or a hospital birthing room an ideal compromise, combining the intimate atmosphere of a home birth with the high-tech backup of a hospital.

If you are considering a home birth, you should, according to the American College of Nurse-Midwives, meet these guidelines:

♦ Be in a low-risk category—no hypertension, diabetes, or other chronic medical problems, and no history of a previous difficult labor and/or delivery.

♦ Be attended by a physician or a CNM. If using a CNM, a consulting physician should be available, preferably one who has seen the mother during pregnancy and who has worked with the nurse-midwife.[2]

♦ Have transportation available and live within thirty miles of a hospital, if the roads are good and traffic negligible, or ten miles if these standards aren't met.

For more information on home births, check www.home-birth.org.

MAKING YOUR SELECTION

Once you've secured a prospective practitioner's name, call to make an appointment for an interview. Go prepared with questions that will enable you to sense if your philosophies are in sync and if your personalities mesh comfortably. Don't expect that you will agree on everything—that doesn't happen even in the happiest of marriages. If it's important that your doctor be a good listener or a careful explainer, does this one seem to fulfill those requirements? If you're concerned about the emotional aspects of pregnancy, will this practitioner take your concerns seriously? Ask about his or her positions on issues that you feel strongly about. These might include unmedicated childbirth versus pain relief as needed in childbirth; breastfeeding; induction of labor; use of fetal monitoring, enemas, forceps, or routine IVs; cesarean sections; or anything else that concerns you. (See A Birthing Plan on page 274 for other subjects to discuss.) That way there won't be any unpleasant last-minute surprises.

Perhaps the most important thing you can do at this first meeting is to let the practitioner know what kind of patient you are. You can judge from the

---

2. Direct-entry midwives typically practice without physician backup.

response whether he or she will be comfortable with—and responsive to —you.

You will also want to know something about the hospital the practitioner is affiliated with. Does it provide features that are important to you—for example, plenty of LDR or LDRP rooms, breastfeeding support, the latest fetal monitoring equipment, a neonatal intensive care unit? Is there flexibility about procedures that concern you (say, routine IVs)? Are siblings allowed in the birthing rooms? Are fathers allowed during a surgical delivery?

Before you make a final decision, think about whether the practitioner inspires a feeling of trust. Pregnancy is one of the most important voyages you'll ever make; you'll want a skipper (or first mate) in whom you have complete faith.

MAKING THE MOST OF THE PATIENT-PRACTITIONER PARTNERSHIP

Choosing the right practitioner is only the first step. For the vast majority of women—those who are neither ready to cede all responsibility to the practitioner nor to take over entirely themselves—the next step is nurturing a good working partnership with that professional. Here's how:

♦ When a question or concern comes up between visits, write it down on a notepad, in the back of this book, or in the *What to Expect When You're Expecting Pregnancy Organizer,* and take it to your next appointment. (It may help to keep pads in convenient places—the refrigerator door, your purse, your desk at work, your bedside table—so that you'll always be within jotting distance of one; consolidate the lists before each doctor's visit.) That way you can be sure that you won't forget to ask all your questions and report all your symptoms —and that you won't be wasting your time, or your practitioner's, while you try to remember what it was you wanted to ask. Along with your list of questions, bring a pen and pad (or the *Pregnancy Organizer*) to each office visit so you can record your practitioner's recommendations. If your practitioner doesn't volunteer adequate information, make inquiries before you leave, so there's no confusion once you get home. Ask about such things as side effects of treatments, when to stop taking a medication if one is prescribed, when to check back about a problem situation. If possible, quickly review your notes with the doctor to be sure they are accurate.

♦ Though you don't want to call your practitioner at every pelvic twinge, you shouldn't hesitate to call about worries that you can't resolve by checking in a book such as this one, and that you feel can't wait until the next visit. Don't be afraid that your concerns will sound silly. Doctors and midwives have seen and heard it all before. Be prepared to be very specific about your symptoms. If you are experiencing pain, be precise about its location, duration, quality (is it sharp, dull, crampy?), and severity. If possible, explain what makes it worse or better—changing positions, for example. If you have a vaginal discharge, describe its color (bright red, dark red, brownish, pinkish, yellowish), when it started, and how heavy it is. Also report accompanying symptoms, such as fever, nausea, vomiting, chills, or diarrhea. (See When to Call the Practitioner, page 130.)

◆ Keep up-to-date. But also realize that you can't believe everything you read. When you read about something new in obstetrics, don't brandish the clipping in front of your practitioner saying, "I must have this." Instead, ask if he or she feels there is any value to this new procedure or validity to that new theory. Often the media reports medical advances prematurely, before they are proven safe and effective through controlled studies. If indeed it is a legitimate advance, your practitioner may already be aware of it or may want to find out more about it. You may both learn something through the exchange.

◆ When you hear something that doesn't correspond to what your practitioner has told you, ask for an opinion on what you've heard—not in a challenging way, just in order to get more information.

◆ If you suspect that your practitioner may be mistaken about something (for example, okaying intercourse when you have a history of incompetent cervix), speak up. You can't assume that he or she, even with your chart in hand, will always remember every aspect of your medical and personal history. As partner in your health care, you share the responsibility of making sure errors are not made.

◆ Ask for explanations. Find out what the potential side effects of a prescribed medication are. Be sure you know why a test is ordered, what it will involve, what its risks are, and how and when you'll learn the results.

◆ If you find your practitioner doesn't seem to have time to respond to all your questions or concerns, try providing a written list. If it isn't possible

SO YOU WON'T FORGET

Because there'll be times when you'll want to do a little writing with your reading, jot down a symptom so you can share it with your doctor, make a note of this week's weight so you can compare it to next week's, record what needs recording so you'll remember what needs remembering—you'll find note pages starting on page 555.

for you to get a complete response at the visit, ask if you can get the answers you need through a follow-up phone call or e-mail or a longer visit next time.

◆ Tell the whole truth, and nothing but the truth. Don't give your practitioner a false or incomplete general, gynecological, or obstetrical medical history. Make sure he or she knows about any drugs—prescription or non- (including herbal), legal or illegal, medicinal or recreational, including alcohol and tobacco—that you are currently taking or have taken recently, as well as about any past or present illnesses or operations. Remember, what you tell your doctor is confidential; no one else will know.

◆ Don't reject recommended ultrasounds, tests, or medications unless you have a solid medical or personal reason that backs up your decision. Discuss your reason with your practitioner.

◆ Follow instructions carefully when undergoing a medical procedure.

◆ Follow your practitioner's recommendations as to appointment schedule, weight gain, bed rest, exercise, medication, vitamins, and so on.

- Always alert a practitioner to an obvious adverse effect of a medication or treatment, as well as to any other worrisome symptoms that you experience in your pregnancy.

- Take good care of yourself, following the Pregnancy Diet (see Chapter 4), getting adequate rest and exercise, and absolutely avoiding alcohol, tobacco, and other nonprescribed drugs and medications, once you find out you're pregnant, or better still, once you start trying to conceive.

- If you have a gripe about anything (from being kept waiting to not getting answers to your questions), air it, in as nice a way as possible. Letting it fester will jeopardize the practitioner-patient relationship.

- Insurance companies will often serve as mediators between patient and practitioner when there is a conflict or complaint. If you have a problem with your practitioner that good communication isn't solving, contact your health organization for help.

If you feel you can't follow your practitioner's instructions or go along with the recommended course of treatment, you clearly have little faith in the person you've chosen to care for you and your baby during your pregnancy, labor, and delivery. In such a case—or if, for some other reason, your relationship with your practitioner breaks down irreparably—all sides will be better served if you find a replacement (assuming that's financially feasible and your medical plan permits it).

◆ ◆ ◆

CHAPTER 2

Now That You're Pregnant

The test results are back; the news has (sort of) sunk in. Excitement is growing, and so is your list of concerns: Will my age or the baby's father's age have an effect on my pregnancy and on our baby? How about chronic medical problems or family genetic problems? Will our past lifestyles make a difference? Will my previous obstetrical history (if any) repeat? What can I do to lower any risks my history may present?

Now that you're pregnant, you'll want answers to these questions and more. So read on.

What You May Be Concerned About

YOUR GYNECOLOGICAL HISTORY

"I haven't mentioned a previous pregnancy to my practitioner because it happened before I was married. Is there any reason I should?"

This is one time when you definitely shouldn't try to put your past behind you. Previous pregnancies, miscarriages, abortions, surgery, or infections may or may not have an impact on what happens in this pregnancy, but any information you have about them—or any aspect of your obstetrical and gynecological history— should be passed on to your practitioner. The more he or she knows about you, the better care you'll get. Your history, of course, will be handled with confidentiality. And don't worry about what your practitioner might think. It's the job of the physician or midwife to help, not to judge.

THIS BOOK'S FOR YOU

As you read *What to Expect When You're Expecting*, you'll notice many references to traditional family relationships—to "wives," "husbands," "spouses." These references are not meant to exclude expectant mothers (and their families) who may be somewhat "untraditional"—for example, those who are single, who have same-sex partners, or who have chosen not to marry their live-in partners. These terms are, rather, a way of avoiding phrases (for instance, "your husband or significant other") that are more inclusive but also more cumbersome to read. Our thought is that you will mentally edit out any phrase that doesn't fit and replace it with one that's right for you and your situation.

PREVIOUS ABORTIONS

"I've had two abortions. Will they affect this pregnancy?"

It's all about timing. Multiple first-trimester abortions aren't likely to have an effect on future pregnancies. So if your abortions were performed before the 14th week, chances are there's no cause for concern. Multiple second-trimester abortions (performed between 14 and 27 weeks), however, do appear to increase the risk of premature delivery. If you had your abortions after the third month, see page 270 for tips on reducing the risks of premature birth.

In either case, be sure your practitioner knows about the abortions. The more familiar he or she is with your complete obstetrical and gynecological history, the better care you will receive.

YOUR OBSTETRICAL HISTORY REPEATING ITSELF

"My first pregnancy was very uncomfortable—I must have had every symptom in the book. Will I be that unlucky again?"

In general, your first pregnancy is a pretty good predictor of future pregnancies, all things being equal. So you are a little less likely to breeze comfortably through pregnancy than someone who already has. Still, there's always the hope that your luck will change for the better. All pregnancies, like all babies, are different. If, for example, morning sickness or food cravings plagued you in your first pregnancy, they may be barely noticeable in the second (or vice versa). While luck, genetic predisposition, and the fact that you've experienced certain symptoms before have a lot to do with how comfortable or uncomfortable this pregnancy will be, other factors— including some that are within your control—can alter the prognosis to some extent. The factors include:

General health. Being in good all-around physical condition gives you a better shot at having a comfortable pregnancy. Ideally, attend to chronic conditions (allergies, asthma, back problems) and clear up lingering infections (such as urinary tract infections or vaginitis) before conception. Once you become pregnant, continue to take good care of yourself as well as your pregnancy.

Diet. While it can't offer any guarantees, following the Pregnancy Diet (see Chapter 4) improves every pregnant woman's chances of having a comfortable pregnancy. Not only can it better your chances of avoiding or minimizing the miseries of morning sickness and indigestion, it can help you fight excessive fatigue, combat constipation and hemorrhoids, and prevent urinary tract infections and iron-deficiency anemia. (And even if your pregnancy turns out to be uncomfortable anyway, by eating well you'll have bestowed on your baby the best chances of developing well and being born healthy.)

Weight gain. Gaining weight at a steady rate and keeping the gain within the recommended boundaries (between 25 and 35 pounds) can improve your chances of escaping or minimizing such pregnancy miseries as hemorrhoids, varicose veins, stretch marks, backache, fatigue, indigestion, and shortness of breath.

Fitness. Getting enough and the right kind of exercise (see page 190 for guidelines) can help improve your general well-being. Exercise is especially important in second and subsequent pregnancies because abdominal muscles tend to be more lax, making you more susceptible to a variety of aches and pains, most notably backache.

Lifestyle pace. Leading a harried and frenetic life, as so many women do today, can aggravate or sometimes even trigger one of the most uncomfortable of pregnancy symptoms—morning sickness—and exacerbate others, such as fatigue, headache, backache, and indigestion. Getting some help around the house, taking more breaks away from whatever frazzles your nerves, cutting back on job responsibilities, letting low-priority tasks go undone for the time being, or learning relaxation techniques can bring some relief (see page 125 for more tips).

Other children. Some pregnant women with other children at home find that keeping up with their offspring keeps them so busy that they barely have time to notice pregnancy discomforts, major or minor. But for many others, having one or more older children tends to aggravate pregnancy symptoms. For example, morning sickness can increase during times of stress (the getting-to-school or the getting-dinner-on-the-table rush, for instance); fatigue can be heightened because there doesn't seem to be any time to rest; backaches can be aggravated if you're doing a lot of child toting; even constipation becomes more likely if you never have a chance to use the bathroom when the urge strikes. You are also more likely to come down with colds and other illnesses, caught from your older child. (See Chapter 18 for preventing and dealing with such illnesses.)

What's the key to lessening the toll that caring for your other child can take on your pregnant body? Finding more time to take care of yourself—an elusive goal, but one worth pursuing. Take advantage of any potential helper you can find (paid or volunteer) to lighten your load and to help free up personal time.

"My first pregnancy was rough, with several serious complications. Will this one be just as rough?"

While it's possible that this pregnancy will be similar to your previous one, one complicated pregnancy doesn't necessarily predict another. Often a woman who weathered high seas the first time around is rewarded with smooth sailing the next. If it was a onetime event, such as an infection or an accident, that caused the complications, then they aren't likely to recur. Nor will they recur if they were caused by lifestyle habits that you've now changed (like smoking, drinking, or using drugs), an exposure to an environmental hazard (such as lead) to which you are no longer exposed, or by failure to seek medical care early in pregnancy (assuming you've sought care early on this time).

If the cause was a chronic health problem, such as diabetes or high blood pressure, correcting or controlling the condition prior to conception or very early in pregnancy can greatly reduce the risk of repeat complications.

Discuss with your practitioner the complications you had last time and what can be done to prevent them from being repeated. No matter what the problems or their causes (even if no cause was ever pinpointed), the tips in the response to the previous question can help make your pregnancy more comfortable and safer for both you and your baby.

"With my first child, I had a very uneventful pregnancy. That's why the forty-two-hour labor with five hours of pushing came as such a shock. Is that what I'm in for again?"

Relax, enjoy your pregnancy, and put thoughts of another difficult labor out of your mind. Thanks to a more experienced uterus and a more lax birth canal, second and subsequent deliveries are almost always easier than first ones, barring a less than ideal fetal position or some other unforeseen complication. All phases of labor tend to be shorter, and the amount of pushing necessary to deliver generally decreases dramatically.

PREGNANCIES TOO CLOSE TOGETHER

"I became pregnant again just ten weeks after I delivered my first child. What effect will this have on my health and on the baby I'm now carrying?"

Conceiving again before you've fully recovered from a recent pregnancy and delivery puts enough strain on your body without your adding the debilitating effects of worry. So, first of all, *relax*. Though conception in the first three

postpartum months is rare (especially if the new baby is exclusively breast-fed), it's taken other women by surprise, too. And most have delivered normal, healthy infants, little the worse for wear themselves.

Still, studies indicate that two to two and a half years is the medically ideal space between pregnancies. So it's essential to be aware of the toll two closely spaced pregnancies can take, and to do everything possible to compensate, including:

♦ Getting the best prenatal care, starting as soon as you think you're pregnant. And you should be scrupulous about following the practitioner's orders and not missing office visits.

♦ Following the Pregnancy Diet (see Chapter 4). It's possible your body has not had a chance to rebuild its stores and you may still be at a nutritional disadvantage, particularly if you are still nursing. You may need to overcompensate nutritionally to be sure both you and the baby you are carrying will not be deprived. Pay particular attention to protein (have at least 75 grams or three servings daily) and iron (you should take a supplement).

♦ Adequate weight gain. Your new fetus doesn't care whether or not you've had time to shed the extra pounds his or her sibling put on you. The two of you need the same 25- to 35-pound gain this pregnancy. So don't even think about losing weight, not even early on. A carefully monitored gradual weight gain will be relatively easy to take off afterward, particularly if it was gained on the highest-quality diet, and especially once you have a toddler and an infant to keep up with. Be certain, too, that you don't let lack of time or energy keep you from eating enough. Feeding and caring for the child you already have shouldn't keep you from feeding and caring for your child-to-be. Watch your weight gain carefully, and if you're not progressing as you should, monitor your calorie intake more closely and follow the tips for increasing weight gain on page 159.

◆ Fair-share feeding. If you are breastfeeding your older baby, you can continue as long as you feel up to it. If you are utterly exhausted, you may want to supplement with formula or consider weaning completely. Discuss the options with your practitioner. If you decide to continue breastfeeding, be sure to get enough extra calories to feed both your baby and your fetus (about 500 to 800 extra calories daily), as well as adequate amounts of protein (5 servings), calcium (6 servings), and fluids (1 cup an hour during waking hours). You will also need plenty of rest. For more tips, see *What to Expect the First Year.*

◆ Rest. You need more than may be humanly (and new-motherly) possible. Getting it will require not only your own determination but help from your spouse and others as well—who should take over as much of the cooking, housework, and baby care (particularly tasks that involve a lot of heavy lifting or carrying) as possible. Set priorities: let less important chores or work go undone, and force yourself to lie down when your baby is napping. If you're not breastfeeding, let Daddy take over nighttime feedings.

◆ Exercise. But just enough to keep you in shape and relax you, not enough to overtax you. If you can't seem to find the time for a regular pregnancy exercise routine, build physical activity into your day with your baby. Take him or her for a brisk walk in the stroller. Or enroll in a pregnancy exercise class (see page 198 for tips on choosing one) or swim at a club or community center that offers baby-sitting services. But avoid strenuous exercise.

◆ Eliminating or minimizing all other pregnancy risk factors, such as smoking and drinking. Your body and the baby in your womb shouldn't be subjected to any additional stress.

THE SECOND TIME AROUND

"This is my second pregnancy. How will it be different from the first?"

Since no two pregnancies are exactly alike, there's no predicting how different (or how similar) these nine months will be from the last. There are some generalities, however, about second and subsequent pregnancies that hold true at least some of the time (like all generalities, none will hold true all of the time):

◆ You'll probably "feel" pregnant sooner. Most second-timers are more attuned to the early symptoms of pregnancy, and more apt to recognize them. The symptoms themselves may vary from last time—you may have more or less morning sickness, indigestion, and other tummy troubles; you may be more tired (especially likely if you were able to nap in your first pregnancy but now barely have the chance to sit down) or less tired (perhaps because you're too busy to notice how tired you really are or because you're so used to being tired); you may have more urinary frequency or less (though it's likely to appear sooner).

Some symptoms that are typically less pronounced in second and subsequent pregnancies include food cravings and aversions, breast enlargement and sensitivity, and worry (since you've already been there, done that, and lived to tell about it, pregnancy is less likely to induce panic).

◆ You'll "look" pregnant sooner. Thanks to abdominal and uterine muscles that are more lax, you're likely to "pop" much sooner than you did the first time. You may notice, too, that you'll carry differently than you did with baby number one. Baby number two (or three or four) is liable to be larger than your firstborn, so you may have more to carry around. Another potential result of those "loosened-up" abdominals: backache and other pregnancy pains may be exacerbated.

◆ You'll feel movement sooner. Something else to thank those looser muscles for—chances are you'll be able to feel baby kicking much sooner this time around, as early as 16 to 18 weeks. You're also more likely to know it when you feel it, having felt it before.

◆ You may not feel as excited. Of course you're thrilled to be expecting again. But you may notice that the excitement level (and that compulsion to tell everyone you pass in the street the good news) isn't quite as high. This is a completely normal reaction (again, you've been here before) and in no way reflects on your love for this baby.

◆ You may be in for an easier labor and a faster delivery. Here's the really good part about those laxer muscles. All that loosening up (particularly in the areas involved in childbirth), combined with the prior experience

of your body, may help ensure a speedier exit for baby number two. Every phase of labor and delivery is likely to be shorter, with pushing time significantly reduced. (That is, of course, barring any complicating circumstances, such as a harder-to-deliver baby position.)

◆ You may wonder how to tell baby number one about the new baby who's on the way. Realistic, empathetic, and age-appropriate preparation for your firstborn to make the life-changing transition from only child to older child should begin during pregnancy. For tips, see *What to Expect the First Year* and *What to Expect the Toddler Years*. Reading *What to Expect When Mommy's Having a Baby* and *What to Expect When the New Baby Comes Home* to your child will also help prepare him or her.

"I had a perfect first baby. Now that I'm pregnant again, I can't shake the fear that I won't be so lucky this time."

Your chances of hitting the jackpot again are excellent. A mother who has had a "perfect" baby isn't only likely to win again, her odds are better than they were before she had a successful pregnancy under her belt. In addition, with each subsequent pregnancy, she has the chance to improve her odds a little—by eliminating any existing negatives (smoking, drinking, drug use) and accentuating all positives (proper diet, exercise, and medical care).

HAVING A BIG FAMILY

"I'm pregnant for the sixth time. Does this pose any additional risk for my baby or for me?"

It had long been believed in medical circles that women who had six or more children were putting both themselves and their babies at increased risk with each additional pregnancy. But with today's obstetrical advances, women receiving good prenatal care have an excellent chance of having healthy, normal babies in sixth or later pregnancies. Recent studies show that the only factors that increase in such pregnancies is a small jump in the incidence of multiple births (twins, triplets, and so on) and a *very slightly increased* risk of having a baby born with trisomy 21, a chromosomal disorder (though it's unclear if this has to do with the mother's advancing age or her number of pregnancies).

So enjoy your pregnancy *and* your large family. But do take a few precautions:

♦ Consider prenatal testing if you are thirty years old or older (rather than waiting until you're thirty-five), since the incidence of offspring with chromosomal problems appears to increase earlier in women with many pregnancies.

♦ Be sure to get all the help you can, and drop nonessential chores for the duration. Teach your older children to be more self-sufficient (preschoolers can certainly dress and undress themselves, put away toys, and so on). Exhaustion isn't good for any pregnant woman, particularly not one with a large brood to look after.

♦ Watch your weight. It's not uncommon for women who've had several pregnancies to put on a few extra pounds with each baby. If that's been the case with you, be particularly careful to eat efficiently and not gain too much. Being overweight does increase some risks, particularly that of having a difficult labor, and it can complicate cesarean delivery and recovery. On the other hand, make sure you're not so busy you don't eat enough to gain adequate weight.

REPEAT CESAREANS

"When I had my first baby by cesarean I was told I could never deliver vaginally because of my abnormal pelvis. I want to have six kids just like my mother did. Is there a limit on the number of cesareans a woman can have?"

The shape of your pelvis doesn't necessarily have to affect the size of your family. Limits are no longer arbitrarily placed on the number of cesareans a woman can undergo, and having numerous cesareans is generally considered a much safer option than it once was. Just how safe depends on the type of incision made, as well as on the scars that are formed following the procedure. Discuss your concern with your obstetrician, because only someone fully familiar with your clinical history can predict whether there are any factors that might stand in the way of your having a large family.

If you do have multiple cesareans, however, you may, because of numerous scars or the type of uterine incision, be at increased risk for uterine rupture caused by labor contractions. For this reason, you should be particularly alert for the signs of oncoming labor (contractions, bloody show, ruptured membranes; see page 334) in the final months of pregnancy. Should they occur, notify your doctor and go to the hospital immediately. You should also notify him or her at *any* time in your pregnancy if you have bleeding or unexplained, persistent abdominal pain.

VAGINAL BIRTH AFTER CESAREAN (VBAC)

"I had my last baby by cesarean. I'm pregnant again and I'm wondering what my chances are of having a vaginal delivery."

Until fairly recently, "once a cesarean, always a cesarean" was an obstetrical edict, engraved in stone—or rather, in the uteruses of women who'd had one or more surgical deliveries. It is now recognized that repeat cesareans need not be considered routine and that Vaginal Birth After Cesarean (VBAC) is generally worth a try, at least under the right circumstances (i.e. with a practitioner who is willing to give it a try and in a hospital that allows it). Studies show that 75 percent of women who have had cesareans are able to go through a normal labor and a vaginal delivery in subsequent deliveries. Even women who have had more than one cesarean or are carrying twins have a good chance of being able to deliver vaginally, as long as the proper precautions are taken.

Whether or not you will be able to try VBAC will depend on the type of uterine incision made in your previous c-section and on the reason your baby was delivered surgically. If you had a low-transverse uterine incision (across the lower part of the uterus), as 95 percent of women do today, your chances of succeeding at VBAC are good; if you had a classic vertical incision (down the middle of your uterus), as was popular in the past and is still occasionally needed, you will probably not be allowed to attempt a vaginal delivery because of the risk of uterine rupture. If the reason for your c-section was one that isn't likely to repeat (fetal distress, premature separation of the placenta, faulty placement of the placenta, infection, breech, preeclampsia), it's very possible that you can try for a vaginal delivery this time. If it was a chronic disease (diabetes, high blood pressure, heart disease) or an uncorrectable problem (a badly contracted pelvis, for example), you will probably require a repeat cesarean. Don't rely on your recollection of the type of uterine incision you had or the reason you needed a cesarean last time—check, or have your practitioner check, the medical records of your prior cesarean delivery.

If you feel strongly about wanting a vaginal delivery this time—and your obstetrical or medical history doesn't automatically disqualify you—discuss the possibility with your practitioner now. You may also want to discuss—and get your practitioner's feedback on—a recent study that has reopened the argument for routine repeat cesareans; it has some doctors who encouraged VBAC in the past now rethinking their position. The study found a higher risk of uterine rupture and other complications among women who had VBAC—three times higher when labor was spontaneous, five times higher when induced without prostaglandins (a substance used to ripen the cervix), and fifteen times higher when it was induced with prostaglandins. Still, the relative risk of such complications during VBAC—though statistically significant—was shown to be low: approximately 5 per 1,000 among women who had spontaneous labor, and approximately 24 per 1,000 among women with prostaglandin-induced labor. Some women will conclude, in discussion with their practitioner, that the added risk of a VBAC labor definitely isn't worth the benefits of avoiding a cesarean; others will conclude that it definitely is—especially if the potential for problems is lowered substantially by avoiding induction.

To give your VBAC the best odds of success, you'll need to find a doctor who backs you up on your decision. But your role in ensuring a safe vaginal delivery will be important, too. You should:

◆ Make sure your doctor has detailed records of your previous cesarean.

◆ Be informed. Learn everything you can about VBAC, including what your options are. You can get information from childbirth organizations and/or your practitioner.

◆ Take childbirth education classes and take them seriously, so that you will be able to labor as efficiently as possible to minimize the stress on your body.

◆ Plan on delivering in a hospital fully equipped and staffed for emergency cesarean sections, should one become necessary.

◆ Ask your doctor to avoid using prostaglandins or other hormonal stimulants to induce labor, if possible. Keep in mind that if your labor does end up having to be induced, your practitioner may veto VBAC, for safety's sake.

◆ Discuss with your doctor whether pain medication will be an option for you. Some practitioners limit medication during VBAC to avoid masking signs of an impending rupture, though most studies have found that epidurals are safe to use during VBAC if labor is closely monitored.

◆ Be sure that your doctor will be with you from the beginning of labor through delivery. Careful monitoring lowers the potential risks substantially.

Though your chances of having a normal, safe vaginal delivery are good—especially if the right precautions are taken—even the woman who has never had a cesarean has approximately a 20 percent chance of needing one. So don't

be disappointed if, despite your best efforts (and your practitioner's), you end up with a repeat. After all, the safest possible birth of that wonderful baby of yours is what this is all about.

Don't feel guilty, either, if you decide ahead of delivery (in consultation with your practitioner) that you'd rather schedule an elective second cesarean than attempt VBAC. One-third of all cesareans are repeats, and many are actually performed at the request of the mother. Again, what's best for your baby—and best for you—is what matters.

OBESITY

"I'm about 60 pounds overweight. Does this put me and my baby at higher risk during pregnancy?"

Most overweight mothers[1] and their babies come through pregnancy and delivery safe and sound. Still, it's important to be aware of the possible complications that extra weight could lead to and what you can do about them. For one thing, there is an increased risk of gestational diabetes and of high blood pressure. Accurately dating a pregnancy may be tricky because ovulation is often erratic in obese women and because some of the yardsticks doctors traditionally use to estimate the date (the height of the fundus, the size of the uterus, hearing the heartbeat) may be difficult to read because of layers of fat. That padding can also make it impossible for the doctor to determine a fetus's size and position manually, so that technological assistance might be necessary to avoid surprises during delivery. And delivery difficulties can

---

1. Definitions vary, but usually a woman is considered obese if her weight is 20 percent over her ideal weight, very obese if it measures 50 percent over. Thus a woman who should weigh 120 pounds is obese at 144 and very obese at 180 pounds.

result if the fetus is much larger than average, which is often the case with obese
mothers (even among those who don't
overeat during pregnancy, and particularly with those who are diabetic). Finally,
if a cesarean delivery is necessary, the over-
ample abdomen can complicate both the
surgery and recovery from it.

The good news is that, as with other
high-risk pregnancies, top-notch medical and self-care can greatly minimize
the risks for both you and your baby.
Medically, you will probably undergo
more tests than the typical low-risk pregnant woman: ultrasound early on to
more accurately date your pregnancy,
and later to determine the baby's size and
position; at least one glucose tolerance
test or screening for gestational diabetes
to determine if you are showing any signs
of developing diabetes; and, toward the
end of your pregnancy, nonstress and
other diagnostic tests to monitor your
baby's condition.

There's also plenty you can do for
yourself and your baby. Eliminating all
pregnancy risks that are within your control—such as drinking and smoking—
will be particularly important for you.
Avoiding excessive pregnancy weight
gain will be, too. It's likely that under
your doctor's supervision you will be able
to gain less than the generally recommended 25 to 35 pounds without compromising your baby's birthweight or
health. But your daily diet will have to
contain at least 1,800 calories, and be
packed with foods that are concentrated
sources of vitamins, minerals, and protein
(see the Pregnancy Diet in Chapter 4).
Making every bite count and being efficient in your food choices will help you
and your baby get the most nutrition for
the calories you consume. (And you
should be particularly scrupulous about
taking a prenatal vitamin containing folic
acid.) Getting regular exercise, within
the guidelines recommended by your

doctor, will also help keep your weight
gain in check without your having to reduce food intake drastically.

For your next pregnancy, if you are
planning on one, try to get as close as
possible to your ideal weight *prior* to
conception. It will make the course of
your pregnancy a lot easier.

RH INCOMPATIBILITY

*"My doctor said my blood tests show I
am Rh negative. What does that mean
for my baby?"*

It means there's the potential for problems—but, fortunately, they're problems that can be easily prevented. A little
biology background may help you understand why.

Each cell in the body has numerous
antigens, or antenna-like structures, on
its surface. One such antigen is the Rh
factor. Everyone inherits blood cells that
either have the Rh factor (which makes
the person Rh positive) or lack the factor
(which makes them Rh negative). In a
pregnancy, if the mother's blood cells do
not have the Rh factor (she's Rh negative) while the fetus's blood cells do have
it (making the fetus Rh positive), the
mother's immune system will view the
fetus (and its Rh-positive blood cells) as
a "foreigner." In a normal immune response, her system will mobilize armies
of antibodies to attack this foreigner.
This is known as Rh incompatibility.

All pregnant women are tested for
the Rh factor early in pregnancy, usually
at the first prenatal visit. If a woman turns
out to be Rh positive, as 85 percent are,
the issue of compatibility is moot because
whether the fetus is Rh positive or Rh
negative, there are no foreign antigens on
the fetus's blood cells to cause the
mother's immune system to mobilize.

When the mother is Rh negative, as
you are, the baby's father is tested to

determine whether he is Rh positive or negative. If your spouse turns out to be Rh negative, your fetus will be Rh negative, too (since two "negative" parents can't make a "positive" baby), which means that your body will not consider it "foreign." But if your spouse is Rh positive, there's the possibility that your fetus will inherit the Rh factor from him, creating an incompatibility between you and baby.

This incompatibility is usually not even a potential problem in a first pregnancy. Trouble starts to brew if some of the baby's blood enters the mother's circulation during her first delivery (or abortion or miscarriage). The mother's body, in that natural protective immune response, produces antibodies against the Rh factor. The antibodies themselves are harmless—until she becomes pregnant again with another Rh positive baby. During the subsequent pregnancy, these new antibodies could potentially cross the placenta into the baby's circulation and attack the fetal red blood cells, causing very mild (if maternal antibody levels are low) to very serious (if they are high) anemia in the fetus. Only very rarely do these antibodies form in first pregnancies, in reaction to fetal blood leaking back through the placenta into the mother's circulatory system.

Prevention of the development of Rh antibodies is the key to protecting the fetus when there is Rh incompatibility. Most practitioners use a two-pronged attack. At 28 weeks, an expectant Rh negative woman is given a vaccine-like injection of Rh-immune globulin, known as Rhogam, to prevent the development of antibodies. Another dose is administered within 72 hours after delivery if blood tests show the baby is Rh positive. If the baby is Rh negative, no treatment is required. Rhogam is also administered after a miscarriage, an ectopic pregnancy, an abortion, CVS, amniocentesis, uterine

bleeding, or trauma during pregnancy. Giving Rhogam as needed at these times can head off serious problems in future pregnancies.

If an Rh negative woman was not given Rhogam during her previous pregnancy and tests reveal that she has developed Rh antibodies capable of attacking an Rh positive fetus, amniocentesis can be used to check the blood type of the fetus. If it is Rh negative, mother and baby have compatible blood types and there's no cause for concern or treatment. If it is Rh positive, and thus incompatible with the mother's blood type, the maternal antibody levels are monitored regularly. If the levels become dangerously high, tests will be done to assess the condition of the fetus. If at any point the safety of the fetus is threatened because hemolytic or Rh disease has developed, a transfusion of Rh-negative blood to the fetus may be necessary. When the incompatibility is severe, which is rare, the fetal transfusion can take place while the fetus is still in the uterus. More often it can wait until immediately after delivery. In mild cases, when antibody levels are low, a transfusion may not be needed. But doctors will be ready to do one at delivery if necessary.

The use of Rhogam has greatly reduced the need for transfusions in Rh-incompatible pregnancies to less than 1 percent, and in the future may make this lifesaving procedure a medical miracle of the past.

A similar incompatibility can arise with another factor in the blood, the Kell antigen (another "antenna" found on blood cells), though it is much more rare than Rh incompatibility. If the father has the antigen and the mother does not, there is again potential for problems. A standard screening, part of the first routine blood test, looks for the presence of circulating anti-Kell antibodies in the mother's blood. If anti-Kell antibodies are found, the father of the baby is tested to see if he is Kell-positive, in which case the management is the same as with Rh incompatibility.

BEING A SINGLE MOTHER

"I'm single, I'm pregnant, and I'm happy about it—but I'm also a little nervous about going through this alone."

Just because you don't have a husband doesn't mean you have to go through pregnancy alone. The kind of support you'll need can come from sources other than a spouse. A good friend or a relative you feel close to and comfortable with can step in to hold your hand, emotionally and physically, throughout pregnancy. That person can, in many ways, play the role of the "father" during the nine months and beyond—accompanying you to prenatal visits and childbirth education classes, lending an ear when you need to talk about your concerns and fears as well as your joyous anticipation, helping you get both your home and life ready for the new arrival, and acting as coach, supporter, and advocate during labor and delivery. You might also consider joining a support group for single mothers both during and after your pregnancy.

HAVING A BABY AFTER THIRTY-FIVE

"I'm thirty-eight and pregnant with my first—and probably last—baby. It's so important that it be healthy, but I've read so much about the risks of pregnancy after thirty-five."

Becoming pregnant after thirty-five puts you in good—and growing—company. While the pregnancy rate has dropped slightly in recent decades among women in their twenties, it has nearly doubled among women over thirty-five. And though the number of babies born to women in their forties remains relatively small, their ranks have also doubled in recent years.

If you've lived for more than thirty-five years, you're probably aware that nothing in life is completely risk free. Pregnancy, at any age, certainly isn't. And though these days the risks are very small to begin with, they do increase slightly and gradually as age advances—from your teens on. Most older mothers, however, feel that the benefits of starting a family at the time that's right for them far outweigh any risks. And they are buoyed by the fact that new medical discoveries are rapidly reducing these risks.

The major reproductive risk faced by a woman in your age group is that she might not become pregnant at all because of decreased fertility. Once she's overcome that and become pregnant, she also faces a somewhat greater chance of having a baby with Down syndrome. The incidence increases with the mother's age: 1 in 10,000 for twenty-year-old mothers, about 3 in 1,000 for thirty-five-year-old mothers, and 1 in 100 for forty-year-old mothers. It's speculated that this and other chromosomal abnormalities, though still relatively rare, are more common in older women because their ova are older, too (every woman is born with a lifetime supply of eggs), and have had more exposure to x-rays, drugs, infections, and so on. (It is now known, however, that the egg is not always responsible for such chromosomal abnormalities. An estimated minimum 25 percent of Down syndrome cases can be linked to a defect in the father's sperm.)

While Down syndrome isn't preventable at this time, it can be identified in utero, through prenatal diagnosis (see page 47). Such diagnostic testing is now routine for mothers over thirty-five and others in high-risk categories, including those who have abnormal readings on one or more prenatal screening tests.

There are a handful of other risks that increase slightly with age. Being older, particularly over forty, means that a woman is more likely to develop high blood pressure (particularly if she's overweight), diabetes, or cardiovascular disease during pregnancy—but all of these conditions are more common in older groups in general, and all are usually controllable. Older mothers are also somewhat more subject to miscarriage (because of their older ova), preeclampsia, and preterm labor (which can often be prevented). Labor and delivery, *on average,* are longer and slightly more likely to be complicated, with cesarean section and other forms of assisted delivery (such as forceps or vacuum extraction) more common. In some older women, a decrease in muscle tone and joint flexibility may contribute to labor difficulties—but for many others, especially those who are in excellent physical shape thanks to regular exercise routines and healthy eating, this doesn't seem to be the case.

But in spite of these slightly increased risks, there's lots of good news for expectant moms over thirty-five, too. Today's older mothers have more going for them than ever before. Evaluations for birth defects can be done in utero through a variety of screening and diagnostic tests, which means that the risk that a mother-to-be over thirty-five will bear an infant with a severe birth defect can be reduced to a level comparable to that for a younger woman. Chronic conditions that are more common in older moms can be well controlled. Drugs and close medical supervision can sometimes forestall preterm labor. And medical breakthroughs continue to decrease risks in the delivery room.

But as successful as these advances have been in helping older mothers have safer pregnancies and healthier babies, they pale next to the strides women themselves have taken to improve their odds through exercise, diet, and quality prenatal care. Advanced reproductive age alone does not necessarily put a mother in a high-risk category, but an accumulation of many individual risks can. When the older mother makes a concerted effort to eliminate or minimize as many risk factors as possible, she can take years off her pregnancy profile—making her chances of delivering a healthy baby virtually as good as those of a younger mother.

And there may be some additional pluses. It's been theorized that this new breed of women—better educated (more than half of older mothers have gone to college), career-oriented, and more settled—make better parents, thanks to their maturity and stability. Because they are older and have probably had their share of the fast lane, they are now less likely to resent being tied down by a baby. One study showed that these mothers were generally more accepting of the demands of parenting and displayed more patience and other qualities that are beneficial to the development of their children. And though they may have less physical stamina than when they were younger, the joys of parenting more than make up for any energy deficits.

So relax, enjoy your pregnancy, and be reassured. There's never been a better time to be over thirty-five and expecting a baby.

AGE AND TESTING FOR DOWN SYNDROME

"I'm thirty-four now, but I'm due to deliver just two months before my thirty-fifth birthday. Should I consider testing for Down syndrome?"

The chances of having a baby with Down syndrome don't escalate suddenly on a woman's thirty-fifth birthday. The risk increases gradually from the early twenties on, with the greatest jump coming when you pass forty. So there is no clear scientific answer to whether or not it makes sense to undergo prenatal diagnosis when you are just shy of thirty-five. Thirty-five is simply an arbitrary date selected by doctors trying to detect as many fetuses with Down syndrome as possible without exposing more mothers and babies than necessary to the slight risk some of these prenatal diagnostic procedures pose. Some practitioners advise women who will turn thirty-five during pregnancy to consider prenatal diagnosis, such as amniocentesis; others don't.

In many cases, the practitioner will suggest that one or more of the screening tests (see page 48) be performed and evaluated first, before a woman under thirty-five undergoes amniocentesis. An abnormal reading on a screening test can indicate the possibility—but not the probability—of Down syndrome and sometimes other abnormalities in the fetus, and the doctor probably will suggest that a follow-up amniocentesis is a good idea. If the screening reading is normal, on the other hand, amniocentesis may no longer be necessary, assuming there are no indications for it other than the age of the mother (see page 52). Discuss the options, and your concerns, with your practitioner or genetic counselor.

THE FATHER'S AGE

"I'm only thirty-one, but my husband is over fifty. Does advanced paternal age pose risks to a baby?"

Throughout most of history, it was believed that a father's responsibility in the reproductive process was limited to fertilization. Only during the 20th century (too late to help those queens who lost their heads for failing to produce a male heir) was it discovered that a father's sperm held the deciding genetic vote in determining his child's gender. And only in the last few years have researchers postulated that an older father's sperm might contribute to an increased risk of miscarriage or birth defects such as Down syndrome. Like the older mother's ova, the older father's primary oocytes (undeveloped sperm) have had longer exposure to environmental hazards and might conceivably contain altered or damaged genes or chromosomes. And from the studies that have been done, there is some evidence that in about 25 or 30 percent of Down syndrome cases, the faulty chromosome can be traced to the father. It also appears that there is an increase in the incidence of Down syndrome when the father is over fifty or fifty-five, though the association is weaker than in the case of maternal age.

But the evidence remains inconclusive—mostly because of the inadequacy of the existing research. Setting up the kind of large-scale studies required to obtain conclusive results has been difficult so far, for two reasons. First of all, Down syndrome is relatively rare (about 1 in 700 births). Second, in the majority of cases, older fathers are married to older mothers, making it tricky to clarify the independent role of paternal age.

So the question of whether or not Down syndrome and other birth defects can be linked to advanced paternal age remains largely unanswered. Experts believe that there probably is some connection (although it's not clear at what age it begins), but the risk is almost certainly very small. At this time, genetic counselors do not recommend amniocentesis on the basis of paternal age alone, though if you're going to spend the rest of your pregnancy worrying about the possible—though unlikely

—effects of your husband's age on your baby, it makes sense to ask your practitioner for a screening test (see page 48), if one isn't already scheduled. If that turns out normal, you can relax without having to go through amniocentesis.

FIBROIDS

"I've had fibroids for several years, and they've never caused me any problems. Will they, now that I'm pregnant?"

Chances are your fibroids won't stand between you and an uncomplicated pregnancy. In fact, most often these small nonmalignant growths on the inner walls of the uterus (which are more common in women over thirty-five) don't affect a pregnancy at all.

Occasionally, however, fibroids do cause problems, increasing slightly the risk of miscarriage, preterm birth, breech birth, and other complications. To minimize these risks, you should:

◆ Be under the care of a physician

◆ Discuss the fibroids with your physician so that you become better informed on the condition in general and the risks in your particular case

◆ Reduce other pregnancy risks

◆ Be particularly attentive to symptoms that could signal impending trouble (see page 130)

Sometimes a woman with fibroids notices pressure or pain in the abdomen. It should be reported to the doctor, but it usually isn't anything to worry about. Bed rest for four or five days along with the use of safe pain relievers (ask your practitioner to recommend one) usually brings relief.

Sometimes the fibroids degenerate or twist, causing abdominal pain, often accompanied by fever. Rarely, surgery may be needed to remove such a degenerating fibroid or one that is otherwise causing problems. If doctors suspect that the fibroids could interfere with a safe vaginal delivery, they may opt to deliver by cesarean section. In most cases, however, even a large fibroid will move out of the fetus's way as the uterus expands during pregnancy.

"I had a couple of fibroids removed a few years ago. Will that affect my pregnancy?"

In most cases, surgery for the removal of small uterine fibroid tumors doesn't affect a subsequent pregnancy. Extensive surgery for large fibroids could, however, weaken the uterus enough so that it would be unable to tolerate labor. If, on reviewing your surgical records, your physician decides this might be true of your uterus, a cesarean delivery will be planned. You should become familiar with the signs of early labor in case contractions begin before the planned surgery (see page 334). And you should have an emergency plan for getting to the hospital immediately if you do go into labor.

ENDOMETRIOSIS

"After years of suffering with endometriosis, I'm finally pregnant. Will I have problems with this pregnancy?"

Endometriosis is typically associated with two challenges: difficulty in conceiving, and pain. Congratulations! Becoming pregnant means that you've overcome the first of those challenges. And the good news gets even better. Being pregnant may actually help with the second challenge.

The symptoms of endometriosis, including pain, do improve during pregnancy. This seems to be due to hormonal changes. When ovulation ceases, the endometrial implants generally become smaller and less tender. There are psychological benefits, too. Since pregnancy is something a normal woman's body does naturally, someone who has struggled with endometriosis may feel "normal" perhaps for the first time since puberty.

Improvement is greater in some women than in others. Many women are symptom free during the entire pregnancy; others may feel increasing discomfort as the fetus grows and begins packing a stronger punch—particularly if those punches and kicks reach tender areas. Fortunately, however, having endometriosis doesn't seem to raise any risks during pregnancy or childbirth (unless uterine surgery has been performed, in which case the risk of uterine rupture is slightly increased).

The less happy news is that pregnancy only provides a respite from the symptoms of endometriosis, not a cure. After pregnancy and nursing (and sometimes earlier), the symptoms usually return.

INCOMPETENT CERVIX

"I had a miscarriage in the fifth month of my first pregnancy. The doctor said it was caused by an incompetent cervix.[2] I just had a positive home pregnancy test and I'm worried that I will have the same problem again."

Now that your incompetent cervix has been diagnosed, your physician should be able to take steps to prevent it from causing another miscarriage. An incompetent cervix, one that opens prematurely under the pressure of the growing uterus and fetus, is estimated to

occur in 1 or 2 of every 100 pregnancies; it is believed responsible for 20 to 25 percent of all second-trimester miscarriages. An incompetent cervix can be the result of genetic weakness of the cervix; exposure of the mother to DES (diethylstilbestrol; see page 43) when she was in her mother's womb; extreme stretching of or severe lacerations to the cervix during one or more previous deliveries; a cone biopsy for cervical cancer; or cervical surgery or laser therapy. Carrying more than one fetus can also lead to incompetent cervix, but if it does, the problem will not usually recur in subsequent single-fetus pregnancies.

Incompetent cervix is usually diagnosed when a woman miscarries in the second trimester after experiencing progressive painless effacement (shortening and thinning) and dilation of the cervix without apparent uterine contractions or vaginal bleeding. It may also be diagnosed when ultrasound or a vaginal examination shows that the cervix is shortening or opening prematurely.

Be sure your practitioner for this pregnancy knows about your condition. It is likely that cerclage (suturing, or stitching closed, the opening of the cervix) will be performed between the 12th and 16th weeks to prevent a repeat of this tragedy. Although recent studies are questioning the effectiveness of cerclage, it's likely your doctor will still perform it until more is known. The simple procedure is performed through the vagina under local anesthesia. Twelve hours after surgery, the patient can resume normal activities, though sexual intercourse may be prohibited for the duration of the pregnancy, and frequent exams by the doctor may be necessary. (Treatment may also be initiated when ultrasound or a vaginal examination shows that the cervix is opening, even if there was no previous late miscarriage.) When the sutures will be removed

---

2. The cervix is the outlet of the uterus, through which a baby is delivered.

will depend partly on the doctor's preference and partly on the situation. Usually they are removed a few weeks before the estimated due date; in some cases they may not be removed until labor begins unless there is infection, bleeding, or premature rupture of the membranes.

With cerclage, you will have to be alert for signs of an impending problem in the second or early third trimester: pressure in the lower abdomen, vaginal discharge with or without blood, unusual urinary frequency, or the sensation of a lump in the vagina. If you experience any of these, go immediately to the doctor's office or the emergency room. (For more on second-trimester miscarriage, see page 496.)

IN VITRO FERTILIZATION (IVF)

"I conceived my baby through in vitro fertilization. Are my chances of having a healthy baby as good as anyone else's?"

The fact that you conceived in a laboratory rather than in bed doesn't affect your chances of having a healthy baby. Recent studies have shown that all other factors being equal (age, DES exposure, the condition of the uterus, the number of fetuses, for example), there is no significant increase in pregnancy and labor complications in IVF mothers. Nor does there appear to be more risk of a baby being born with abnormalities—even if the embryo was frozen at one point.

The statistics show there is a slightly higher miscarriage rate among IVF mothers, but this is probably due to the fact that women who have IVF are so closely monitored that every pregnancy is diagnosed very early and therefore every miscarriage noted. This is not the case in the general population, where many miscarriages occur before pregnancy is suspected and go unobserved or unreported.

There will, however, be some differences between your pregnancy and others, at least in the beginning. Because a positive test doesn't necessarily mean a pregnancy, because trying again can be so emotionally and financially draining, and because it's not known right off how many of the test-tube embryos are going to develop into fetuses, the first six weeks of an IVF pregnancy are usually more nerve-wracking than most. In addition, if an IVF mother has miscarried in previous tries, intercourse and other physical activities may be restricted, or complete bed rest may even be ordered. And the hormone progesterone may be prescribed to help support the developing pregnancy during the first two months. But once this period is past, you can expect that your pregnancy will be pretty much like everyone else's—unless you're carrying more than one fetus, as 5 to 25 percent of IVF mothers do. If you are, see page 164.

And, as with everyone else, your chances of having a healthy baby can be improved significantly by good medical care, excellent diet, moderate weight gain, a healthy balance of rest and exercise, and avoidance of alcohol, tobacco, and unprescribed drugs.

HERPES

"I'm really happy to be pregnant, but I'm also worried because I have genital herpes. Can my baby catch it from me?"

Having genital herpes during pregnancy is cause for concern, but definitely not for fear. While it's true that babies can contract this sexually transmitted disease through an infected birth canal—and that the condition can be serious in newborns, whose immune systems are immature—the chances are excellent that your baby will arrive safe, sound, and completely unaffected by herpes, particularly if you and your practitioner take protective steps during pregnancy and delivery.

First of all, infection in a newborn is quite rare. A baby has only a 2 to 3 percent chance of contracting the condition if the mother has a recurrent infection during pregnancy (that is, she's had herpes before). Second, though a primary infection (one that appears for the first time) early in pregnancy increases the risk of miscarriage and premature delivery, such infection is uncommon. Even for babies at greatest risk—those whose mothers have their first herpes outbreak as delivery nears—there is an up to 75 percent chance that they will escape infection. Finally, the disease, though still serious, seems to be somewhat milder in newborns nowadays than it was in the past.

So, if you picked up your herpes infection before pregnancy, which is most likely, the risk to your baby is very low. And with good medical care it can be lowered still further.

To protect their babies, women who have a history of herpes and have active lesions at the onset of labor are usually delivered by cesarean. Some doctors test weekly for active infection when a woman develops lesions close to her due date, and continue doing cultures into labor; others simply check for active lesions (or signs that an active infection is about to erupt) as labor begins. Both approaches can reduce the possibility that an unnecessary cesarean will be performed. Because of the slight risk of fetal infection when the protection of the amniotic sac is gone, cesarean delivery is usually carried out within four to six hours after the membranes rupture if there are active lesions.

At birth, newborns at risk for herpes infection are usually isolated from other newborns to prevent the possible spread of infection. In the unlikely event that infection does occur, treatment with an antiviral drug will reduce the risk of permanent damage. If the mother has an active infection, she can still care for her baby and even breastfeed if she takes special precautions to avoid transmitting the virus.

SIGNS AND SYMPTOMS OF GENITAL HERPES

It is during a primary, or first, episode that genital herpes is most likely to be passed on to the fetus, so your doctor should be informed if you experience the following symptoms of the disease: fever, headache, malaise, achiness for two or more days, accompanied by genital pain, itching, pain on urination, vaginal and urethral discharge, and tenderness in the groin, as well as lesions that blister and then crust over. Healing generally takes place within two to three weeks, during which time the disease can still be transmitted.

If you have genital herpes, be careful not to pass it on to your partner (and he should likewise be careful if he's infected). Avoid intercourse when either of you has lesions; wash your hands thoroughly with mild soap and water after using the toilet or having sexual relations; shower or bathe daily; keep lesions clean, dry, and dusted with cornstarch; wear cotton underpants and avoid wearing clothes that are tight in the crotch area.

If you test negative for herpes, taking steps to prevent a first-time infection (such as practicing safe sex if you're not in a monogamous relationship) is important.

OTHER STDS (SEXUALLY TRANSMITTED DISEASES)

"I've heard that herpes can harm the fetus. Is this also true of other sexually transmitted diseases?"

The bad news: yes, there are other STDs that present a hazard to the fetus (and to the mother as well). The good news: most are easily diagnosed and treated safely, even during pregnancy. But because women are often unaware of being infected, the Centers for Disease Control (CDC) recommends that *all* pregnant women be tested early in pregnancy for *at least* the following STDs: chlamydia, gonorrhea, hepatitis B, HIV, and syphilis.

Keep in mind that STDs don't happen just to one group of people or only at a certain economic level. They can occur in women (and men) in every age group, of every race and ethnic background, at every income level, and among those living in small towns as well as in big cities. The major STDs include:

Gonorrhea. Gonorrhea has long been known to cause conjunctivitis, blindness, and serious generalized infection in a fetus delivered through an infected birth canal. For this reason, pregnant women are routinely tested for the disease, usually at their first prenatal visit (see page 106). Sometimes, particularly in women at high risk for STDs, the test is repeated late in pregnancy. If infection with gonorrhea is found, it is treated immediately with antibiotics. Treatment is followed by another culture, to be sure the woman is infection free. As an added precaution, an antibiotic ointment is squeezed into the eyes of every newborn at birth. (This treatment can be delayed for as long as an hour—but no longer—if you want to have some unblurry eye-to-eye contact with your baby first.)

Syphilis. Testing for this disease (which can cause a variety of birth defects as well as stillbirth) is also routine at the first prenatal visit. Antibiotic treatment of infected pregnant women before the fourth month, when the infection usually begins to cross the placental barrier, almost always prevents damage to the fetus. The very good news is that mother-to-baby transmission of syphilis is down dramatically. In fact, the CDC is optimistic that this trend is a sign that syphilis will soon be wiped out in the United States.

Chlamydia. Though recognized more recently as a potential danger to the fetus and a possible risk to mothers, chlamydia is now reported to the CDC more often than gonorrhea. Sexually active women under twenty-five are particularly susceptible. Chlamydia is the most common infection passed from mother to fetus, which is why chlamydia screening in pregnancy is a good idea, particularly if you have had multiple sexual partners in the past, increasing your chance of infection. Since about half the women with chlamydial infection experience no symptoms, it often goes undiagnosed if not tested for.

Prompt treatment of chlamydia prior to or during pregnancy can prevent chlamydial infections (pneumonia, which fortunately is most often mild, and eye infection, which is occasionally severe) from being transmitted by the mother to the baby during delivery. Though the best time for treatment is prior to conception, administering antibiotics to the pregnant infected mother can also be effective in preventing infant infection. Antibiotic ointment used at birth protects the newborn from chlamydial, as well as gonorrheal, eye infection.

Bacterial vaginosis (BV). Although not technically an STD, BV can be spread by sexual contact (though it can also be trasmitted in other ways). BV can cause pregnancy complications such as premature rupture of the membranes and intraamniotic infection, which may lead to premature labor. It may also be associated with low birthweight. Possible symptoms of the condition include a foul, musty, or "fishy" vaginal odor, and/or a thin milky white or gray discharge. Itching and irritation are rare and many women don't notice any symptoms at all. While some doctors test for BV only in women who are at high risk for preterm delivery, other doctors believe that all pregnant women should be screened for bacterial vaginosis, so it may be among the infections you are tested for at your first visit. Treatment of symptomatic BV with antibiotics is effective.

Venereal, or genital, warts. These sexually transmitted warts may appear anywhere in the genital area and are caused by the human papilloma virus (HPV). In appearance, they can vary from a barely visible lesion to a soft, velvety, flat bump or a cauliflower-like growth; colors range from pale to dark pink. Highly contagious, venereal warts are particularly important to treat. While they are rarely transmitted to the baby, 5 to 15 percent of cases go on to produce inflammation of the cervix, which can progress to cervical cancer. Treatment may include a prescribed topical medication safe for use in pregnancy. *Do not use* over-the-counter wart remedies. If necessary, large warts may be removed late in pregnancy by freezing, electrical heat, or laser therapy; in some cases, this treatment may be delayed until after delivery.

Trichomoniasis. The symptoms of this parasite-caused STD (also referred to as trichomonas infection or "trich") are a greenish, frothy vaginal discharge with an unpleasant fishy smell and, often, itching. About half of those affected have no symptoms at all. Though the disease does not usually cause serious illness, it can predispose the pregnant woman to preterm delivery, so treatment is important. The oral medication generally prescribed is considered safe, even early in pregnancy.

HIV infection. Infection in pregnancy by the HIV virus, which causes Acquired Immune Deficiency Syndrome (AIDS), is a threat not just to the expectant mother but to her baby as well. A large proportion (estimates range from 20 to 65 percent) of babies born to mothers who are HIV positive develop the infection in the first six months of life, and it is suspected that pregnancy itself could speed up the progress of the disease in the mother. For these reasons, some infected women choose to terminate their pregnancies. Before taking any action, anyone who tests HIV positive should consider retesting (tests are not always accurate and can sometimes be positive in someone who does not have the virus, particularly if she has borne several children). If a second test is positive, then formal counseling about AIDS and the treatment options is absolutely imperative. Treating the HIV-positive mother with AZT (also known as Zidovudine—ZDV—or Retrovir) or other antiretroviral drugs and, possibly, vitamin A can dramatically reduce the risk of her passing the infection on to her child—apparently without any damaging side effects. Delivering by elective cesarean section (before contractions begin and before membranes rupture) can reduce the risk of transmission to close to zero.

If you suspect that you may have been infected with any sexually transmitted disease, check with your practitioner to see if you've been tested; if you haven't, ask to be. If a test turns out to be positive, be sure that you—and your partner, if necessary—are treated. Treatment will protect not only your health but that of your baby.

FEAR OF AIDS

"Both my husband and I had a number of partners before we met. Since AIDS sometimes doesn't show up for years, how can I be sure I don't have it—and that I won't give it to my baby?"

Even if you've had multiple partners, the chance that you or your husband contracted the human immunodeficiency virus (HIV) that causes AIDS before you met is slight if neither one of you is in a high-risk group (hemophiliacs, IV drug users, those who've had sex with bisexual or homosexual males or with IV drug users). A test for HIV will probably relieve your worry. In the very unlikely event that the test turns out positive, you can be treated immediately, which could help not just you but your baby as well (see HIV Infection, page 39).

"I was surprised when my doctor asked if I wanted to be tested for HIV—I don't think I'm in a high-risk category."

It is becoming increasingly routine for pregnant women to be tested for HIV, whether or not they have a prior history of high-risk behavior. Many states actually require doctors to offer HIV counseling and an HIV test to pregnant women, and the American College of Obstetricians and Gynecologists recommends that all pregnant women, regardless of risk, be tested for HIV. So don't be offended; be glad your practitioner cares enough to recommend the test.

RUBELLA ANTIBODY LEVELS (TITER)

"I was vaccinated against rubella as a child, but my prenatal blood test shows my rubella antibody levels are low. Should I be concerned?"

No, but you should be cautious. Especially in the first trimester, when the risk that a baby will suffer serious harm from a rubella infection is greatest (see page 466), take extra care to avoid being exposed to the illness. (Which is not all that difficult, since most children and adults have been immunized.)

IMMUNIZATIONS IN PREGNANCY

Since infections of various sorts can cause pregnancy problems, it's a good idea to take care of all necessary immunizations *before* conceiving. Most immunizations using live viruses are not recommended during pregnancy, including the MMR (measles, mumps, rubella) and varicella (chicken pox) vaccines. Other vaccines, according to the Centers for Disease Control (CDC), shouldn't be given routinely, but can be given if they are needed. These include hepatitis A and pneumococcal vaccine. You also can be immunized safely after the first trimester against tetanus, diphtheria (Td), and hepatitis B with vaccines containing dead, or nonactive, viruses. The CDC also recommends that every woman who will be pregnant during flu season (generally October through March) receive a flu shot. Check with your doctor about which vaccines are safe during pregnancy and which, if any, you may need.

Though you won't be immunized during pregnancy, you will be given a new rubella vaccine right after you deliver, before you even leave the hospital. It's safe then, even if you're breastfeeding.

HEPATITIS B

"I'm a carrier of hepatitis B and just found out that I'm pregnant. Will my being a carrier hurt my baby?"

Knowing that you're a carrier for hepatitis B (as are an estimated 40,000 other pregnant women) is the first step in making sure that your condition won't hurt your baby. Depending on the results of testing for hepatitis B surface antigen, you may be treated with both hepatitis B immune globulin (HBIG) and hepatitis B vaccine. Your baby will be treated within twelve hours of birth with both the immune globulin and the vaccine; this treatment can almost always prevent infection from developing. So be sure your practitioner knows that you're a carrier and that your baby is treated as needed. For more information on hepatitis infections, see page 467.

AN IUD STILL IN PLACE

"I've been wearing an IUD for six months and just discovered that I'm pregnant. We want to be able to keep the baby; is it possible?"

Getting pregnant while using birth control is always a little unsettling, but it does happen. The odds of its happening with an IUD are less than 1 in 100, depending on the type of device used and whether or not it has been properly inserted. A woman who conceives with an IUD in place and doesn't want to terminate her pregnancy has two choices, which she should discuss as soon as possible with her practitioner: leaving the IUD in place or having the IUD withdrawn. Which of these is preferable usually depends on whether or not, on examination, the removal cord is found to be visibly protruding from the cervix. If it isn't visible, the pregnancy has a very good chance of proceeding uneventfully with the IUD in place. The IUD will simply be pushed up against the wall of the uterus by the expanding amniotic sac surrounding the baby and, during childbirth, will usually deliver with the placenta. If, however, the IUD string is visible early in pregnancy, the risk of infection is increased. In that case, chances of a safe and successful pregnancy are greater if the IUD is removed as soon as feasible, once conception is confirmed. If it isn't removed, there is a significant chance that the fetus will spontaneously miscarry; when it is removed, the risk is only 20 percent. If that doesn't sound reassuring, keep in mind that the rate of miscarriage in all known pregnancies is estimated to be about 15 to 20 percent.

If you do continue your pregnancy with the IUD left in, you should, during the first trimester, be especially alert for bleeding, cramps, or fever, because the IUD puts you at higher risk for early pregnancy complications (see Ectopic Pregnancy, page 124, and Miscarriage, page 121.) Notify your practitioner of such symptoms promptly.

BIRTH CONTROL PILLS IN PREGNANCY

"I got pregnant while using birth control pills. I kept taking them for over a month because I had no idea I was pregnant. Will this affect my baby?"

Ideally you should stop using oral contraceptives three months, or for at least two normally occurring menstrual cycles, before you try to become pregnant. But conception doesn't always wait for ideal conditions, and occasionally a woman becomes pregnant while taking the Pill. In spite of warnings you might have read on the package insert, there's no reason for alarm. Statistically, there is no good evidence of an increased risk to a baby when the mother has conceived while on oral contraceptives. A discussion of the subject with your practitioner should further relieve your concern.

SPERMICIDES

"I conceived while using a spermicide with my diaphragm, and used it several times again before I knew I was pregnant. Could the chemicals have damaged the sperm before conception, or the embryo after it?"

It is estimated that between 300,000 and 600,000 women who become pregnant each year used spermicides around the time of conception and/or in the early weeks of pregnancy, before finding out that they'd conceived. So the question of what effects spermicides may have during conception and pregnancy is of great significance to a great many expectant couples—and to those choosing a method of birth control.

Fortunately, the answers have been reassuring. No more than a tentative link has ever been suggested between the use of spermicides and the incidence of birth defects. And the most recent and most convincing studies have found no increase in the incidence of defects even with the repeated use of spermicides in early pregnancy. So according to the best information available, you and the other 299,999 to

599,999 mothers-to-be (and fathers-to-be) can relax.

You may, however, be more comfortable with a different, and perhaps more reliable, method of birth control in the future. And because exposing an embryo or fetus to uneccessary chemicals is never a good idea, if you do continue to use a spermicide, you should plan on discontinuing its use before you decide to become pregnant again—assuming your next pregnancy is planned.

PROVERA

"Last month my doctor gave me Provera to bring on a late period. It turns out that I was pregnant. The package insert warns that pregnant women should never take this drug. Could my baby be malformed?"

Taking a progesterone drug, such as Provera, during pregnancy isn't recommended. But it's no reason to worry. The drug company's warnings are not only for your protection but also for theirs, in case of a lawsuit. It's true that some studies show a 1 in 1,000 risk of certain birth defects when an embryo or fetus has been exposed to such a drug, but that risk is only minimally higher than the risk of the same defects occurring in any pregnancy.

Whether a progesterone drug can actually cause birth defects or not isn't even certain. Some physicians believe that it only *appears* to cause defects, by occasionally enabling a woman to sustain a blighted pregnancy that would have otherwise miscarried. It will probably take years of more study on hundreds of thousands of pregnant women to definitely determine the effects—if any—of progesterone drugs on the fetus. But from what is presently known, it is believed that if progesterone is actually a teratogen (a substance that can harm an embryo or fetus), it is a very weak one (see Putting Risk in Perspective, page 79). Cross this one off your worry list.

DES

"My mother took DES when she was pregnant with me. Can this affect my pregnancy or my baby in any way?"

Before the dangers of using the synthetic estrogen drug diethylstilbestrol (DES) to prevent miscarriage were known, more than a million pregnant women took it. The result: many of their daughters were born with structural abnormalities of the reproductive tract (the majority of abnormalities so minor that they are of no gynecological or obstetrical significance). While some of these DES babies are now past the age of childbearing, others, like you, are not— and are concerned about the effects these DES-induced abnormalities may have on their own pregnancies. Happily, these effects appear to be minimal for most women; it is estimated that at least 80 percent of DES-exposed women have been able to have children.

The women with the most severe abnormalities, however, do appear to have an increased risk of certain pregnancy problems: ectopic pregnancy (probably because of malformed fallopian tubes) and second-trimester miscarriage or preterm birth (usually because of a weakened, or incompetent, cervix, which can open prematurely under the weight of a growing fetus). Because of the risks involved with all of these complications, it's important that you advise your physician of your DES exposure.[3]

---

3. Because of the slightly increased risk of pregnancy complications, DES-exposed women are probably better off having an obstetrician oversee their pregnancy care.

It is also important for you to be aware of the symptoms of these pregnancy mishaps and, should they appear, to report them to your doctor at once. If an incompetent cervix is suspected, one of two courses will probably be taken. Either a preventive stitch will be placed around the cervix between the twelfth and sixteenth weeks of your pregnancy, or your cervix will be examined regularly for signs of premature opening, and then, if such signs are noted, steps will be taken to prevent further progression toward premature delivery (see page 35).

LIVING AT A HIGH ALTITUDE

"I'm concerned because we live at a high altitude, and I've heard that this can cause problems in pregnancy."

Since you're accustomed to breathing the thinner air where you live, you're far less likely to encounter an altitude-induced problem in your pregnancy than if you'd just moved there after thirty years at sea level. Though women who live at high altitudes run a *very slightly* increased chance of developing pregnancy complications such as hypertension and water retention, and of giving birth to a somewhat smaller than average baby, good prenatal care coupled with sensible self-care (eating a top-notch diet, gaining adequate weight, abstaining from alcohol and other drugs) can greatly minimize these risks. So can avoiding tobacco smoke—yours and/or anybody else's. Smoking, which deprives babies of oxygen and optimum development at any altitude, appears to do still further damage at higher elevations, more than doubling the decrease in average birthweight. Strenuous exercise can also rob your baby of oxygen in high altitudes, so choose brisk walking over jogging, for example, and—this goes for *all* pregnant women—quit before you reach exhaustion.

Though you should be able to handle the high altitude without any trouble, women accustomed to living at low altitudes may have difficulty handling pregnancy high above sea level. Some doctors suggest postponing a contemplated move or visit from low altitude to high until after delivery (see page 223). And scaling Mt. Rainier is definitely out for now.

LACK OF INSURANCE

"I'm pregnant and very excited about having the baby. But I don't have health insurance and I'm not sure if I'll be able to afford to see a doctor or pay for delivery."

Having a baby these days can definitely be an expensive proposition. Still, no expectant mother needs to go through pregnancy and childbirth without the proper care, even if she's uninsured. If you can't afford to pick up health insurance now, here are some other ways to find that care at a price you can afford:

◆ Check your yellow pages. Look under "Clinics" or "Health Care Centers." Most communities provide health services through organizations such as Planned Parenthood and at women's health centers. Many of these can provide some free care, and most will offer care on a sliding pay-what-you-can basis.

◆ Look to the government. If your income is low enough, you may qualify for Medicaid. Through this program, you'll be entitled to prenatal care. If you don't qualify for Medicaid, there are low-cost health insurance programs

(that will cover your pregnancy as well as your child's health care after delivery) offered through the government. Ask at any clinic or call (877) KIDS-NOW—(877) 543-7669. If affording nutritious food is an issue—or will be once you're feeding another mouth—contact WIC (Women, Infants, and Children), a government program that provides pregnant and nursing mothers with food and nutrition counseling. For information contact WIC, 3101 Park Center Drive, Alexandria, VA 22302; (703) 305-2746.

◆ Call your local hospital. Some hospitals provide a certain amount of free or low-cost obstetrical care to women who need it. Childbirth classes may also be available at little or no cost to women who can't afford to pay full price for them.

◆ As a last resort, try the ER. If you do go into labor before you've been able to secure a practitioner, go to the ER of the nearest hospital immediately. By law, they have to treat you.

RELIGIOUS OBJECTIONS TO MEDICAL CARE

"Because of my religious beliefs, I am opposed to seeking medical care. That holds especially for pregnancy, which after all is a natural process. My in-laws insist that this is dangerous."

They're right—it can be dangerous. Though pregnancy is a natural process, it's one that, without appropriate medical care, can be risky to mother and baby—and you have to decide if the risks are worth taking. And beyond the personal risk, are you willing to subject yourself to the legal risk if any harm befalls your baby that you might have prevented by seeking prenatal care? Some courts will hold a mother responsible for behavior potentially damaging to the fetus she is carrying.

It's not likely that your in-laws are saying that your religious principles aren't important; rather, that human life—not only yours, but that of your precious baby—is at stake here. Finally, it may help you to know that almost all religious convictions are fully compatible with good and safe obstetrical care. Discuss your convictions with two or three prospective practitioners. It's very possible that you can find a physician or nurse-midwife who will be able to find ways to safely adapt your pregnancy care to your religious rules, perhaps with help from your clergyperson.

YOUR FAMILY HISTORY

"I recently discovered that my mother and one of her sisters both lost babies shortly after delivery. No one knows why. Could that happen to me?"

It used to be that family histories of infant illness or death were often concealed, as though losing a baby or a child were something to be ashamed of. But now we realize that exposing the history of past generations can help protect today's generation. Though the deaths of the two babies under similar circumstances may just be coincidental, it would certainly make sense to see a genetic counselor or maternal-fetal specialist to get some advice. Your practitioner can recommend one.

Any couple that does not have information on possible hereditary defects in their families might be wise to make an effort to learn more, possibly by questioning older family members. Because prenatal diagnosis is possible for many hereditary disorders, being armed with such information beforehand may make it possible to prevent problems before

they occur or make it easier to treat them when they do.

"There are several stories in our family about babies who seemed fine at birth but then started to get sicker and sicker. Eventually they died in early infancy. Should I be concerned?"

Among the major causes of infant illness and death in the first few days and weeks of life are what are known as inborn errors of metabolism. Babies born with this type of genetic defect are missing an enzyme or other chemical substance, making it impossible for them to metabolize a particular dietary element; which element depends on which enzyme is missing. Ironically, the baby's life is in jeopardy as soon as feeding begins.

Fortunately, most such disorders can be diagnosed prenatally or tested for at birth, and many can be treated. There are currently tests available for thirty neonatal diseases that can be done at birth (though these tests are not routine and must be specifically requested by parents; see page 289). And there's proof that early diagnosis and intervention can make a huge difference in the prognosis of such diseases. So consider yourself lucky to be aware of this family history in advance, and be sure to discuss it with your practitioner and, if recommended, with a genetic counselor.

GENETIC COUNSELING

"I keep worrying that I might have a genetic problem and not know it. Should I get genetic counseling?"

Probably all of us carry at least one gene for a genetic disorder. But fortunately, because most disorders require a matched pair of genes, one from Mom and one from Dad, they often don't show up in our children. One or both parents can be tested for some of these disorders before or during pregnancy. But testing usually makes sense only if there is a better-than-average possibility that both parents are carriers of a particular disorder. The clue is often ethnic or geographic. For example, it has recently been recommended that all Caucasians be tested for cystic fibrosis (since a CF mutation is carried by about 1 in 25 Caucasians of European descent). Jewish couples whose forebears came from Eastern Europe should be tested for Tay-Sachs and possibly Canavan's disease. (Tay-Sachs has also been noted in other ethnic groups, including Irish Americans, Louisiana Cajuns, and French Canadians.) Similarly, black couples should be tested for the sickle-cell anemia trait and those of Mediterranean descent for thalassemia (a hereditary form of anemia). In most cases, testing will be recommended for one parent; testing the second parent becomes necessary only if the first tests positive.

Diseases that can be passed on via a single gene from one carrier parent (hemophilia, for example) or by one affected parent (Huntington's chorea) have usually turned up in the family before, but it may not be common knowledge among your family. That's why it's important to keep family health history records.

Most expectant parents, happily, are at low risk for transmitting genetic problems and need never see a genetic counselor. In many cases an obstetrician will talk to a couple about the most common genetic issues, referring to a genetic counselor or a maternal-fetal medicine specialist those with a need for more expertise:

◆ Couples whose blood tests show they are carriers of a genetic disorder that they might pass on to their children

◆ Parents who have already borne one or more children with genetic birth defects

◆ Couples who have experienced three or more consecutive miscarriages

◆ Couples who know of a hereditary disorder on any branch of either of their family trees. In some cases (as with cystic fibrosis or certain thalassemias), doing DNA testing of the parents before pregnancy makes interpreting later testing of the fetus much easier

◆ Couples in which one partner has a congenital defect (such as congenital heart disease)

◆ Pregnant women who have had positive screening tests (see page 48) for the presence of a fetal defect

◆ Closely related couples; the risk of inherited disease in offspring is greatest when parents are related (for example, 1 in 9 for first cousins)

◆ Women over thirty-five

A genetic counselor is trained to give such couples the odds of their having a healthy child, based on their genetic profiles. The counselor can guide them in deciding whether or not to have children, or if they are already pregnant, suggest appropriate prenatal testing.

Genetic counseling has saved hundreds of thousands of high-risk couples from the heartbreak of bearing children with serious problems. The best time to see a genetic counselor is before getting pregnant, or, in the case of close relatives, before getting married. But it's not too late even after pregnancy is confirmed.

If testing uncovers a serious defect in a fetus, expectant parents are faced with the decision of whether or not to continue with the pregnancy. Though the decision is theirs, a genetic counselor can provide important input. (See page 54 for more information.)

YOUR OPPOSITION TO ABORTION

"My spouse and I don't believe in abortion. Why should I have to go through prenatal diagnosis just because I'm thirty-seven?"

The best reason for prenatal diagnosis is the reassurance it almost always brings. The vast majority of babies whose possibly-at-risk moms undergo such testing will receive a clean bill of health.

And although some couples do opt for terminating the pregnancy in the rare instances when the news is very bad, testing can also be valuable when abortion is not an option. When the defect discovered is a fatal one, it gives the parents time to grieve before the birth and minimizes the sense of shock later. When other kinds of defects are present, it provides parents a head start on preparing for life with a special-needs child. Testing

may also be useful in deciding where, when, or how the baby should be delivered.

Parents can also begin working through the inevitable reactions (denial, resentment, guilt) that come with discovering their baby has a problem, rather than waiting until after delivery, when such feelings can compromise parent-child bonding, as well as affect a couple's relationship. They can learn about the particular problem in advance and prepare to ensure the best possible life for their child. They may even discover that the defect is treatable in the uterus or that special precautions at or after birth will increase the odds that the baby will be okay. For parents who feel unable to cope, knowing in advance will allow them to consider a special-needs adoption.

So, if prenatal diagnosis is indicated, don't reject it out of hand. Talk to your practitioner, a genetic counselor, or a maternal-fetal medicine specialist to help you clarify your options before you make your decision. And don't necessarily let your opposition to abortion deprive you and your doctors of potentially valuable information.

What It's Important to Know: ABOUT PRENATAL DIAGNOSIS

Is it a boy or a girl? Will it have blond hair like Grandma, green eyes like Grandpa? Daddy's voice and Mommy's flair for figures or—uh-oh!— the other way around? The questions of pregnancy far outnumber the answers, providing lively material for nine months of dinner table debate, neighborhood speculation, and office betting pools.

But there's one question that isn't a topic for casual wagering. It's the one

most parents hesitate to talk about at all: "Is my baby okay?"

Until recently, that question could be answered only at birth. Today it can, to some extent, be answered as early as the first trimester, through prenatal diagnosis.

Because of inherent risks, small as they are, prenatal diagnosis isn't for everyone. Most parents will continue to play the waiting game, with the happy assurance that the odds are overwhelming that their babies are indeed "okay." But for those whose concerns represent more than normal expectant-parent jitters, the benefits of prenatal diagnosis can far outweigh the risks. Women who are good candidates for such testing include those who:

- Are over thirty-five

- Have a family history of genetic disease and/or have been shown to be carriers of such a disease

- Have a genetic disorder themselves (such as cystic fibrosis or congenital heart disease)

- Have been exposed to infection (such as rubella or toxoplasmosis) that could cause a birth defect

- Have been exposed since conception to a substance or substances that they fear might have been harmful to their developing baby. (Consultation with a physician can help determine whether prenatal diagnosis is warranted in a particular case.)

- Have had unsuccessful pregnancies previously, or have had babies with birth defects

- Have tested positive on a prenatal screening test

Screening Tests

Because there are potential risks attached to some forms of prenatal diagnosis, most women go through screening tests before deciding to undergo prenatal diagnosis. While some practitioners offer screening tests to women over thirty-five or those in high-risk categories, other practitioners recommend that these women skip the screening tests and go straight to CVS (chorionic villus sampling) or amniocentesis. The more common screening tests are the triple screen (Alpha-Fetoprotein, hCG, and estriol) or quad screen (Alpha-fetoprotein, hCG, estriol, inhibin-A) and ultrasound (which is most often performed in the second trimester but can also be used earlier or later). Screening during the first trimester is a promising new approach that is not widely available yet, though researchers and doctors hope that such early screening will soon be the standard of care.

FIRST-TRIMESTER SCREENING

First-trimester screening for Down syndrome involves an ultrasound test to check for an increased space in the back of the fetal neck; an increased diameter is associated with chromosomal abnormalities) and a blood test for high levels of PAAP-A and hCG, two hormones produced by the fetus and passed into the mother's bloodstream. (Researchers are looking, too, at whether the absence of a nasal bone in the fetus, as shown on ultrasound, may also indicate a higher risk of Down syndrome.) Women whose results are abnormal would be offered amniocentesis.

When is it done? Blood test between weeks 9 and 11; ultrasound between weeks 11 and 13; follow-up blood test and results reported between weeks 16 to 18.

How is it done? Both ultrasound and the blood test are simple procedures.

SECOND-TRIMESTER SCREENING

Second trimester screening involves a simple blood test (triple screen) that measures three hormones produced by the fetus and passed into the mother's bloodstream: alpha-fetoprotein (AFP), hCG, and estriol. Some doctors also measure another hormone, inhibin-A, making it the quad screen. (This blood test can also be used in conjunction with first trimester screening—called "integrated screen"—for the highest detection rate of chromosomal abnormalities; not all practitioners are equipped to test this way yet.) Elevated levels of the hormones in the mother's blood can indicate a neural tube defect in the baby such as spina bifida (a deformity of the spinal column).[5] Abnormally low levels suggest an increased risk of Down syndrome or other chromosomal defect. The triple screen cannot *diagnose* a birth defect; it can only indicate an increased risk. And because this is only a screening test, any abnormal result simply means that further testing is needed. In fact, the false positive rate for the triple screen is extremely high. Only 1 or 2 out of 50 women with abnormally high readings will eventually prove to have an affected fetus. In the other 48, further testing will reveal that the reason the hormone levels are abnormal is that there is more than one fetus, that the fetus is either a few weeks older or younger than originally thought, or that the results of the test were just wrong. If the woman is carrying only one fetus and the ultrasound shows the dates are correct, an amniocentesis is offered as follow-up.

---

5. Studies show that the risk of having a baby with a neural tube defect is greatly reduced if the mother takes prenatal vitamins containing folic acid before and during the early weeks of pregnancy.

When is it done? Between the 15th and 18th weeks. The results are usually available within one week.

How safe is it? Since the triple screen requires only a blood sample, it is completely safe. The major risk of the test is that a false positive result may lead to follow-up procedures that present greater risk—and, in rare cases, to therapeutic or accidental abortion of normal fetuses. Before you consider taking any action on the basis of prenatal testing, be sure an experienced physician or genetic counselor has evaluated the results. Get a second opinion if you have any doubts.

ULTRASOUND

The advent of sonography has made obstetrics a much more precise science and pregnancy a much less worrisome experience for many expectant parents. Using sound waves so high they can't be heard by the human ear, sonography allows visualization and "examination" of the fetus without X rays. Though sonography tends to be fairly accurate for most uses, in diagnosing birth defects the test can yield some false negatives (it seems as though everything is fine, but it's not) and some false positives (it looks as though there is a problem, but there isn't).

A level 1 ultrasound is usually done to date a pregnancy and is performed before 12 weeks. A more detailed, or level 2, ultrasound is used for sophisticated diagnostic purposes and is usually performed between 18 and 22 weeks. Besides dating a pregnancy and looking for abnormalities, ultrasound may be used to:

♦ Determine the cause of bleeding in early or mid-late pregnancy

♦ Locate an IUD that was in place at the time of conception

♦ Locate the fetus prior to CVS or amniocentesis

◆ Determine the condition of the fetus if no heartbeat has been detected by the 14th week with a Doppler device, or if there has been no fetal movement by the 22nd week

◆ Determine if the mother is carrying more than one fetus

◆ Measure the amount of amniotic fluid

◆ Check for fibroids if uterine growth is abnormal

◆ Measure the size of the fetus when preterm delivery is being contemplated or when the baby is believed to be late

◆ Detect cervical changes that might predict preterm labor

◆ Identify the location, size, maturity, or possible abnormalities of the placenta

◆ Evaluate the condition of the fetus through observation of fetal activity, breathing movements, amniotic fluid volume (see Biophysical Profile, page 325)

◆ Verify breech presentation or other uncommon fetal or cord position prior to delivery

When is it done? Anytime during the pregnancy, depending on the reason for performing one.

How is it done? Ultrasound examination may be performed through the abdomen or through the vagina; sometimes, when there's a special need, the doctor may have a look both ways. The procedures are quick (lasting from five to thirty minutes) and painless, except for the discomfort of the full bladder necessary for the first-trimester transabdominal exam.

During either exam, the expectant mother lies on her back. For the transabdominal, the woman's bare abdomen is spread with a film of gel that will improve the conduction of sound. A transducer is then moved slowly over the abdomen. For the transvaginal, the transducer is inserted into the vagina. In both procedures, the instruments record echoes of sound waves as they bounce off parts of the baby and translate them into pictures on a viewing screen. With the help of the technician or doctor, you may be able to differentiate the beating heart; the curve of the spine; the head, arms, and legs. You may even catch sight of your baby sucking its thumb. In many cases, you may get a "photo" or videotape, see a 3-D image of your baby, or even "touch" a computer-generated model of your unborn baby thanks to new technology. Nowadays, as images become clearer, even nonexperts (like parents) are able to distinguish head from buttocks, and more. Often, even the genital organs are distinguishable and the sex can be surmised, although with less than 100 percent reliability. (If you don't want to know your baby's sex yet, inform the doctor or technician in advance.)

How safe is it? After many years of clinical use and study, no known risks and a great many benefits have been associated with the use of ultrasound. And many practitioners order ultrasound exams routinely, at least once in a woman's pregnancy. Still, it's generally recommended by most experts that ultrasound be used in pregnancy only when a valid indication exists.

Recent research has shown that fetuses might actually be able to hear the high-pitched sound generated by sonography. It seems sound waves from the ultrasound "tap" the fetal ear with frequencies comparable to the high notes on a piano. Hearing the sound doesn't harm the fetuses, but it may stimulate their senses enough to make them shift around during the exam. And since the sound is very localized, the fetus can avoid it just by moving its head.

Diagnostic Tests

Along with ultrasound (which can be used as a screening or diagnostic tool), there are a number of prenatal diagnostic tests that you may be offered during your pregnancy. The two most common diagnostic tests are CVS and amniocentesis.

CHORIONIC VILLUS SAMPLING (CVS)

Because CVS is performed in the first trimester, it can give results (and most often, reassurance) earlier in pregnancy than amniocentesis, which is usually performed after the 16th week. The earlier diagnosis is particularly helpful for those who might consider a therapeutic pregnancy termination if something is seriously wrong, since an earlier abortion is less complicated and traumatic.

It is believed that chorionic villus sampling will eventually be able to detect virtually all of the 3,800 or so disorders for which defective genes or chromosomes are responsible. And in the future it may make possible the treatment or correction in utero of many of these conditions. At present, CVS is useful only to detect disorders for which the technology exists, such as Tay-Sachs, sickle-cell anemia, most types of cystic fibrosis, and Down syndrome. CVS cannot test for neural tube and other anatomical defects. Testing for specific diseases (other than Down syndrome) is usually done only when there is a family history of the disease or the parents are known to be carriers. The indications for doing the test are the same as those for amniocentesis. Occasionally, both CVS and amniocentesis may be needed. (See Amniocentesis, page 52.)

When is it done? Between the 10th and 13th weeks of pregnancy.

How is it done? CVS is most often performed in a hospital. Depending on the location of the placenta, the sample of cells is taken via the vagina and cervix (transcervical CVS) or via a needle inserted in the abdominal wall (transabdominal CVS). Neither method is entirely pain free; the discomfort can range from very mild to severe.

In the transcervical procedure, the expectant mother lies on an examining table and a long thin tube is inserted through the vagina into the uterus. Guided by ultrasound imaging, the doctor positions the tube between the uterine lining and the chorion, the fetal membrane that will eventually form the fetal side of the placenta. A sample of the chorionic villi (fingerlike projections of the chorion) is then snipped or suctioned off for diagnostic study.

In the transabdominal procedure, the patient also lies on an examining table, tummy up. Ultrasound is used to determine the location of the placenta and to view the uterine walls, and then to help the physician find a safe spot in which to insert the needle. Under ultrasound guidance, a guide needle is inserted through the abdomen and the uterine wall to the edge of the placenta. Then a narrower needle, which will draw up the cells, is inserted through the guide needle. The narrow needle is rotated and pushed in and out 15 or 20 times per sampling, then withdrawn with the sample of cells to be studied.

Since the chorionic villi are of fetal origin, examining them can give a complete picture of the genetic makeup of the developing fetus. Test results are available in three to five days.

How safe is it? Though most studies so far conclude CVS is safe and reliable, the procedure is slightly riskier than amniocentesis, can somewhat increase the risk of miscarriage, and has been linked to isolated cases of limb deformities. According to most studies, however, inexperience of the technician performing the procedure appears to be the cause of these rare complications. These risks have to be weighed against the benefit of earlier diagnosis with CVS. Choosing a testing center with a good safety record and waiting until after your 10th week can reduce the risks associated with CVS.

Some vaginal bleeding can occur after CVS and should not be a cause for concern, though it should be reported to your doctor. Your doctor should also be informed if the bleeding lasts for three days or longer. Since there is also a very slight risk of infection, be sure to report any fever in the first few days following the procedure.

Many women feel physically and emotionally drained following CVS (it's not unusual to fall into bed and sleep around the clock), so it's generally recommended that those undergoing the procedure arrange to have someone drive them home afterward and that they make no other plans for the rest of the day.

AMNIOCENTESIS

The fetal cells, chemicals, and microorganisms in the amniotic fluid surrounding the fetus provide a wide range of information about the new human being, such as genetic makeup, present condition, and level of maturity. Being able to extract and examine some of the fluid through amniocentesis has been one of the most important advances in prenatal diagnosis. Amniocentesis is more than 99 percent accurate in diagnosing—or ruling out, which is far more likely—Down syndrome. It is recommended when:

- The mother is over age thirty-five. Between 80 and 90 percent of all amnioceteses are performed solely on the basis of advanced maternal age, primarily to determine if the fetus has Down syndrome, which is most prevalent among children of older mothers. (More advanced screening tests, now being perfected by researchers, may, in the near future, eliminate the need for amniocentesis performed on the basis of age alone.)

- The couple has already had a child with a chromosomal abnormality, such as Down syndrome, or with a metabolic disorder, such as Hunter's syndrome.

- The couple has another child or a close relative with a neural tube defect.

- The mother is a carrier of an X-linked genetic disorder, such as hemophilia (which she has a 50-percent chance of passing on to any son she bears). In the case of hemophilia, amniocentesis can identify the sex of the fetus, as well as whether the baby has inherited the gene.

- Both parents are carriers of an autosomal recessive inherited disorder, such as Tay-Sachs disease or sickle-cell anemia, and thus have a 1 in 4 chance of bearing an affected child.

- A parent is known to have a condition such as Huntington's chorea, which is passed on by autosomal dominant inheritance, giving the baby a 1 in 2 chance of inheriting the disease.

- Toxoplasmosis, fifth disease, or other fetal infection is suspected.

- Results of a screening test (usually the triple screen or ultrasound) turn out

AN AMNIO COMPLICATION

Although complications with amniocentesis are rare, it is estimated that following about 1 in 100 procedures there is some leakage of amniotic fluid. If you should notice such leakage from your vagina, report it to your practitioner at once. The chances are very good that the leakage will stop after a few days, but bed rest and careful observation are usually recommended until it does.

to be abnormal, and evaluation of the amniotic fluid is necessary to determine whether or not there actually is a fetal abnormality.

◆ It is necessary to assess the maturity of the fetal lungs late in pregnancy (among the last organs ready to function on their own).

When is it done? Diagnostic amniocentesis is usually performed between the 16th and 18th weeks of pregnancy, but occasionally as early as the 14th or as late as the 20th week. Studies on earlier amniocentesis (between the 11th and 14th weeks) have so far shown a significant increase in complications. Test results are usually back in one week. Amniocentesis can also be performed in the last trimester to assess the maturity of fetal lungs.

How is it done? After changing into an examination gown, the expectant mother is positioned on the examining table on her back, her body draped so that only her abdomen is exposed. The fetus and placenta are then located via ultrasound, so that the doctor will be able to steer clear of them during the procedure. The abdomen is swabbed with antiseptic solution, and sometimes the area is numbed with an injection of a local anesthetic similar to the novocaine used by dentists. (But, because this injection is as painful as the passage of the amniocentesis needle itself, most practitioners omit it.) Then a long, hollow needle is inserted through the abdominal wall into the uterus and a small amount of fluid is withdrawn from the sac that surrounds the fetus. (The fetus produces more amniotic fluid to replace the fluid that is withdrawn.) The slight risk of accidentally pricking the fetus during this part of the procedure is further reduced by the use of simultaneous ultrasound guidance. The mother's vital signs and the fetal heart tones are checked before and after the procedure, which, from start to finish, shouldn't take more than thirty minutes. Rh-negative women are usually given an injection of Rh-immune globulin (Rhogam) after an amniocentesis to be sure the procedure does not result in Rh problems (see page 29).

Unless it's a necessary part of the diagnosis, parents have the option of learning the baby's gender when they receive the test results, or waiting to find out the old-fashioned way, in the delivery room. (If you choose the first, keep in mind that mix-ups, though rare, do occur.)

How safe is it? Most women experience no more than a few minutes to a few hours of mild pain or cramping after the procedure. Some doctors recommend resting for the remainder of the day, while others don't. Rarely, there is slight vaginal bleeding or amniotic fluid leakage. In very few cases, women experience infection or other complications that may lead to miscarriage, so amniocentesis should be used only when benefits outweigh risks.

WHEN A PROBLEM IS FOUND

In more than 95 percent of cases, prenatal diagnosis turns up no apparent abnormalities. In the remainder, the expectant couple's discovery that something is wrong with their baby isn't comforting. But, teamed with expert genetic counseling, the information can be used to make vital decisions about this and future pregnancies. Possible options include:

Continuing the pregnancy. This option is often chosen when the defect uncovered is one the couple feels that both they and the baby they are awaiting can live with, or when the parents are opposed to abortion under any circumstance. Even if abortion is not an acceptable option, having some idea of what is to come allows parents to make preparations (both emotional and practical) for receiving a child with special needs into the family, for coping with the inevitable loss of a child, or for considering a special-needs adoption.

Terminating the pregnancy. If testing suggests a defect that will be fatal or extremely disabling, and retesting and/or interpretation by a genetic counselor confirms the diagnosis,* many parents opt to terminate the pregnancy. In such a case, fetal tissue will be carefully examined; this may be helpful in determining the chances that the abnormality will repeat in future pregnancies. Most couples, armed with this information and the guidance of a physician or genetic counselor, do try again, with the hope that the tests and the pregnancy will be completely normal next time around. And most often they are.

* It's *very important* to get a second opinion and additional testing as advised before going ahead with termination.

Prenatal treatment of the fetus. This option is available in only a few instances, though in the future it can be expected to become more and more common. Treatment may consist of blood transfusion (as in Rh disease), surgery (to drain an obstructed bladder, for instance), or administration of enzymes or medication (such as steroids to accelerate lung development in a fetus who must be delivered before term). As technology advances, more kinds of prenatal surgery, genetic manipulation, and other fetal treatments may also become commonplace.

Donating the organs. If diagnosis indicates that the fetal defects are not compatible with life, it may be possible to donate one or more healthy organs to an infant in need. Some parents find that this provides at least some small consolation for their own loss. A maternal-fetal specialist or neonatologist may be able to provide helpful information in such a situation.

As far as prenatal diagnosis has come, it's still important to remember that it's far from infallible. Mistakes and mix-ups happen, even in the best of laboratories and facilities, even with the most skilled professionals wielding the most high-tech equipment—with false positives much more common than false negatives. That's why further testing and/or consultation with additional professionals should always be used to confirm a result that indicates there is something wrong with the fetus.

It's also important to keep in mind that for the vast majority of couples, it will never come to that. Most expectant mothers who undergo prenatal testing will receive the diagnosis they're hoping for right from the start: that all is well with their baby and their pregnancy.

OTHER TYPES OF PRENATAL DIAGNOSES

The field of prenatal diagnosis is expanding so rapidly that new methods are constantly being evaluated. In addition to the standard methods listed above, there are other prenatal diagnostic tests that are being used experimentally or only occasionally. These include:

Percutaneous umbilical blood sampling (PUBS). This test of fetal umbilical cord blood, performed after the 18th week of pregnancy, is useful for diagnosing several blood and skin diseases that amniocentesis can't detect. It is also used to check abnormal amniocentesis results, diagnose causes of growth retardation late in pregnancy, or learn if the fetus has been infected by a potentially harmful disease, such as rubella, toxoplasmosis, or fifth disease. Since this test is new, there's no definitive research on its reliability, but it's thought to be highly accurate.

The PUBS test is done in a manner similar to amniocentesis, except that the ultrasound-guided needle is inserted into a blood vessel of the unborn infant's umbilical cord rather than the amniotic sac to obtain a tiny sample of fetal blood. It usually takes three days to get results. PUBS poses risks slightly greater than amniocentesis, and is associated with a slight, additional risk of premature delivery or early rupture of the membranes.

Maternal blood test to determine fetal gender. Though still experimental, this test could be valuable in screening for certain hereditary conditions that affect male offspring only.

Fetal skin sampling. A tiny sample of fetal skin is taken and studied in order to detect certain skin disorders.

Cervical swabs. Taking a sample of the cervical mucous of a pregnant woman during the first trimester, researchers are able to isolate a single cell from the fetus to test for abnormalities. Though still in its early stages of research, this method could minimize the need for more invasive procedures such as amniocentesis or CVS.

Magnetic resonance imaging (MRI). This method is still investigational but offers promise of being able to give a clearer picture of the fetal condition and any abnormalities than ultrasound can provide. Researchers are working on improving the equipment to get pictures quicker; right now (because fetuses don't hold still very long) getting a useful picture is tricky. Its use during pregnancy appears to be safe.

Echocardiography. This is a method by which defects in the fetal heart can be detected, using targeted ultrasound that also shows the flow of blood within and around the heart.

◆ ◆ ◆

CHAPTER 3

Throughout Your Pregnancy

Pregnant women have always worried. What they worry about, however, has changed considerably over the generations, as obstetrical medicine—and expectant parents—have learned more and more about what does and does not affect the health and well-being of the unborn. Our foremothers, vulnerable to a variety of old wives' tales, feared that seeing a monkey during pregnancy would result in monkeylike offspring, or that slapping their bellies in fright would leave their babies with hand-shaped birthmarks.

Now we are exposed to a daily deluge of modern media tales (usually as frightening, often as unfounded as the old wives' tales), and have other fears: Is the air I'm breathing polluted? Is my drinking water safe? Is my job, or my husband's smoking, or that cup of coffee I had this morning hazardous to my baby's health? What about that X ray I had at the dentist's? As a basis for worry, these concerns can make pregnancy unnecessarily nerve-wracking. As a basis for action, they can give you an enhanced sense of control, improving even more the already excellent chances that all will go well. It will also help to keep remembering (and repeating) this reassuring mantra: There's never been a safer time in the history of reproduction to become pregnant and have a baby.

What You May Be Concerned About

ALCOHOL

"I had a few drinks on several occasions before I knew I was pregnant. Could the alcohol have harmed my baby?"

Wouldn't it be nice to get an instant message from your body alerting you the moment sperm and egg met up ("Just wanted to let you know we have a baby on board—time to start ordering Evian.")? But since that biotechnology doesn't exist (not yet, at least), most moms-to-be are oblivious that baby-making has begun until several weeks into their pregnancies. And in the meantime, they're apt to have done a few things they wouldn't have done if they'd only known. Like having a few, a few times too many. Which is why your concern is one of the most common ones brought to the first prenatal visit.

Fortunately, it's a concern that you can put aside. There's no evidence that a couple of drinks on a couple of occasions very early in pregnancy can harm a developing embryo. So you—and the other moms who didn't get the memo right away—can breathe a little easier.

That said, it's definitely time to change that drink order now. Continuing to drink regularly throughout pregnancy is associated with a wide variety of problems in the offspring. That's not surprising when you consider that alcohol enters the fetal bloodstream in approximately the same concentrations present in the mother's blood; each drink a pregnant woman takes is shared with her baby. Since it takes the fetus twice as long as its mother to eliminate the alcohol from its system, the baby can be at the point of passing out when the mother is just pleasantly tipsy.

Heavy drinking (generally considered to be the consumption of five or six drinks of wine, beer, or distilled spirits a day) throughout pregnancy can result, in addition to many serious obstetrical complications, in what is known as fetal alcohol syndrome (FAS). Described as "the hangover that lasts a lifetime," this condition produces infants who are born undersized, usually mentally deficient, with multiple deformities (particularly of the head and face, limbs, heart, and central nervous system) and a high mortality rate. Later, those who survive display learning, behavioral, and social problems, and generally lack the ability to make sound judgments. The sooner a heavy drinker stops drinking during pregnancy, the less risk to her baby.

The risks of continued drinking are certainly dose related: the more you drink, the more potential danger to your baby. But even moderate consumption (one to two drinks daily or occasional heavy bingeing on five or more drinks), if it occurs throughout pregnancy, is related to a variety of serious problems, including increased risk of miscarriage, prematurity, labor and delivery complications, low birthweight, stillbirth, abnormal growth, and developmental problems in childhood. Such drinking has also been linked to the somewhat more subtle fetal alcohol effect (FAE), characterized by numerous developmental and behavioral problems.

Although some women drink lightly during pregnancy—one glass of wine nightly, for instance—and still manage to deliver a healthy baby, there's no evidence to support that this is a completely safe bet. All that is known about alcohol and pregnancy has prompted the Surgeon General to advise that no amount of alcohol is safe for pregnant women. The research also leads to this suggestion: Although you shouldn't worry about what you drank before you knew you were pregnant, it would be prudent to abstain for the rest of your pregnancy—except perhaps for a celebratory half glass of wine on a very special occasion (taken *with* a meal, since food reduces the absorption of alcohol).

That's as easily done as said for some women—especially those who develop a distaste for alcohol in early pregnancy, which may linger through delivery. For others, particularly those who are accustomed to "unwinding" with cocktails at the end of the day or to drinking wine with dinner, abstinence may require a concerted effort, and may include a lifestyle change. If you drink to relax, for example, try substituting other methods of relaxation: music, warm baths, massage, exercise, or reading. If drinking is part of a daily ritual that you don't want to give up, try a Virgin Mary (a Bloody Mary without the vodka) at brunch, sparkling cider or grape juice or nonalcoholic malt beer at dinner, a juice spritzer (half juice, half carbonated water, with a twist), or a Mock Strawberry Daiquiri or Virgin Sangria (see pages 103–104)—served at the accustomed time, in the accustomed glasses, with the accustomed ceremony.[1] If your spouse joins you on the wagon (at least while in your company), the ride will be considerably smoother.

CIGARETTE SMOKING

"I've been smoking for ten years. Will this hurt my baby?"

Happily, there's no clear evidence that any smoking you've done prior to pregnancy—even if it's been for ten or twenty years—will harm a developing fetus. But it's well documented (as well as plastered on cigarette packs) that smoking during pregnancy, particularly beyond the third month, *is* hazardous.

In effect, when you smoke, your fetus is confined in a smoke-filled womb. Its heartbeat speeds, it coughs and sputters, and, worst of all, due to insufficient oxygen, it can't grow and thrive as it should.

The results can be catastrophic. Smoking has been linked to some 115,000 miscarriages and 5,600 infant deaths a year. It can also increase the risk of a wide variety of pregnancy complications. Among the more serious of these are vaginal bleeding, ectopic pregnancy, abnormal placental implantation, premature placental detachment, premature rupture of the membranes, and early delivery. As many as 14 percent of preterm

births in the United States are related to maternal cigarette smoking.

There is also strong evidence that an expectant mother's smoking adversely and very directly affects her baby's development in utero. The most widespread risks are low birthweight, shorter length, and smaller head circumference, as well as cleft palate or cleft lip. In industrialized nations, such as the United States and Britain, smoking is blamed for as many as a third of all the babies who are born too small. And being born too small is the major cause of infant illness and perinatal death (those that occur just before, during, or after birth).

There are other potential risks as well. Babies of smokers are more likely to suffer from apnea (breathing lapses) and are five times more likely to die of SIDS (sudden infant death syndrome, or crib death) than babies of nonsmokers. In general, babies of smokers aren't as healthy at birth as babies of nonsmokers, with three-pack-a-day maternal smoking associated with a quadrupled risk of low Apgar scores (the standard scale used to evaluate an infant's condition at birth). And there's evidence that, on average, these children will suffer long-term physical and intellectual deficits, especially if parents continue to smoke around them. They are particularly prone to respiratory diseases, ear infections, colic, TB, food allergies, asthma, short stature, and problems in school, including Attention Deficit Hyperactivity Disorder (ADHD). Studies also show that pregnant women who smoke are more likely to have children who are abnormally aggressive as toddlers and who continue to have behavioral problems into adulthood. Children of mothers who smoked while pregnant are hospitalized more often in their first year of life than children of mothers who did not smoke while pregnant. These children are also at higher risk of cancer and

1. Though substituting nonalcoholic lookalikes for favorite alcoholic beverages during pregnancy can work for the occasional drinker, the heavy drinker may find that these beverages serve to trigger a desire for alcohol. If they do in you, avoid any drink, or even setting, that reminds you of alcohol.

are more inclined to smoke themselves.

It was once believed that the reason for the difficulties these children display was poor prenatal nutrition: their mothers smoked rather than ate during their pregnancies. But recent studies disprove this theory; smoking mothers who eat as much and gain as much weight as nonsmoking mothers still give birth to smaller babies.

Studies show that the effects of tobacco use, like those of alcohol use, are dose related: tobacco use reduces the birthweight of babies in direct proportion to the number of cigarettes smoked, with a pack-a-day smoker 30 percent more likely to give birth to a lowbirthweight child than a nonsmoker. So cutting down on the number of cigarettes you smoke may help some. But cutting down can be illusory, because the smoker often compensates by taking more frequent and deeper puffs and smoking more of each cigarette. This can also happen when she tries to reduce the risk by using low-tar or low-nicotine cigarettes.

The news, however, isn't all bad. Some studies show that women who quit smoking early in pregnancy—no later than the third month—can reduce the risk of damage to the fetus to the level of a nonsmoker. Sooner is better, but quitting even in the last month can help preserve oxygen flow to the baby during delivery. For some smoking women, quitting will never be easier than in early pregnancy, when they might develop a sudden distaste for cigarettes—probably the warning of an intuitive body. If you're not lucky enough to develop such a natural aversion, see the tips for quitting on page 61.

Since nicotine is an addictive drug, most people experience withdrawal symptoms when they quit smoking, though the symptoms and their intensity vary from person to person. Some of the most common include a craving for tobacco, irritability, anxiety, restlessness,

AN EARLY BABY PRESENT

Chances are quitting smoking won't be easy, as you probably already know if you've tried to do it in the past. But a smoke-free environment—in utero and out—is the very best gift you can give to your baby.

tingling or numbness in the hands and feet, lightheadedness, fatigue, and sleep and gastrointestinal disturbances. Some people also find that both physical and mental performance is impaired at first. Most find that for a while they are coughing more, rather than less, because their bodies are suddenly better able to bring up all the secretions that have accumulated in the lungs.

To try to slow the release of nicotine and the nervousness that may result, increase your intake of fruit, fruit juice, milk, and mixed greens, and temporarily cut back on meat, poultry, fish, and cheese. You should also avoid caffeine, which can add to the jitters. Get plenty of rest (to counter fatigue) and exercise (to replace the kick you used to get from nicotine). Avoid activities that require a lot of focus and concentration, at least as much as possible, but keep busy by doing mindless tasks. Going to the movies or other places where smoking is prohibited may also help. If you experience serious depression as part of withdrawal, talk to your practitioner immediately.

The worst effects of withdrawal will last a few days to a few weeks. The benefits, however, will last a lifetime—for you and your baby.

"My sister-in-law smoked two packs a day through three pregnancies, and had no complications and big healthy babies. Why should I quit?"

Everyone has heard inspiring stories of someone beating the odds—a cancer patient given a 10 percent chance of survival who lived to a ripe old age, or a quake victim found alive after being trapped under rubble without food or drink for days. But there's something much less inspiring about an expectant mother who consciously stacks the odds against her unborn babies by choosing to smoke, yet manages to produce healthy offspring anyway.

There are no sure things when it comes to making a baby, but there are many ways of bettering your chances of having an uncomplicated pregnancy and delivery and a healthy baby. And giving up smoking is one of the most tangible ways to do this. Though there's the chance that you, too, can have a vigorous full-term baby even if you smoke your way through pregnancy, there's also a significant risk that your baby would suffer some or all of the effects detailed on page 58. Your sister-in-law was lucky (and this luck could have gotten a boost from heredity or other factors that might not hold for you); but do you really want to take the gamble that you will be lucky too? And then again, that luck may not be all that it seems to be. Some of the deficits—physical and intellectual—that afflict babies of smokers aren't apparent immediately. The seemingly healthy infant can grow into a child who is often sick, who is hyperactive, or who has trouble learning.

In addition to the effect smoking could have on your baby while you're still pregnant, there is an effect after he or she has moved from your smoke-filled womb to your smoke-filled rooms. Babies of parents (mothers and/or fathers) who smoke are sick more often than the babies of nonsmokers and are more likely to be hospitalized in infancy and childhood. They're also more likely to die from SIDS (Sudden Infant Death Syndrome).

So as you can see, quitting is your best bet—and your baby's too.

WHEN OTHER PEOPLE SMOKE

"I quit smoking, but my spouse still goes through two packs a day, and a couple of my co-workers smoke like chimneys. Will this hurt our baby?"

Smoking, it is becoming more and more apparent, doesn't affect just the person who is puffing away—it affects everyone around him, including a developing fetus whose mother happens to be nearby. So if your spouse (or anyone else who lives in your home or works near you) smokes, your baby's body is going to pick up nearly as much contamination from tobacco smoke by-products as if *you* were lighting up.

If your spouse says he can't quit

WEIGHT GAIN AND SMOKING

Though many women smoke in order to keep their weight down, there is no evidence that smoking actually accomplishes this. Many smokers are overweight. But it is true that *some,* not all, smokers gain weight while in the process of quitting. The average woman gains about eight pounds in the first four months of quitting (men about six); some gain more, some none at all. Interestingly enough, those who gain some weight while trying to break the smoking habit are more likely to succeed—and they find it fairly easy to drop those few pounds later. Dieting while trying to quit usually leads to failure in both arenas.

BREAKING THE SMOKING HABIT

Identify your motivation for quitting. When you're pregnant, that's easy.

Choose your method of withdrawal. Do you want to go cold turkey or taper off? Either way, pick a "last day" that isn't far off. Plan a full day of activities for that date—those you don't associate with smoking.

Identify your motivation for smoking. For example, do you smoke for pleasure, stimulation, or relaxation? To reduce tension or frustration? To have something in your hand or mouth? To satisfy a craving? Perhaps you smoke out of habit, lighting up without thinking about it. Once you understand your motivations, you should be able to find substitutes:

◆ If you smoke mainly to keep your hands busy, try playing with a pencil, beads, or a straw. Knit, play solitaire on the computer, knead some bread dough, catch up on your e-mail, play the piano, paint, do a crossword puzzle—anything that might make you forget to reach for a cigarette.

◆ If you smoke for oral gratification, try a substitute: a toothpick, gum, raw vegetables, popcorn, or a breadstick. Try to avoid empty-calorie nibbles.

◆ If you smoke for stimulation, try to get your lift from a brisk walk, an absorbing book, good conversation.

◆ If you smoke to reduce tension and relax, try exercise instead. Or relaxation techniques. Or listening to soothing music. Or a long walk. Or a massage. Or making love.

◆ If you smoke for pleasure, seek pleasure in other pursuits, preferably in no-smoke situations. Go to a movie, visit baby boutiques, tour a favorite museum, attend a concert or a play, have dinner with a friend who's a nonsmoker. Or try something more active, like a prenatal fitness class.

◆ If you smoke out of habit, avoid the settings in which you habitually smoke and friends who smoke; frequent places with no-smoking rules instead.

◆ If you associate smoking with a particular beverage, food, or meal, avoid the food or beverage, or eat the meal in a different location. (Say you smoke with breakfast but you never smoke in bed. Have breakfast in bed for a few days.)

◆ When you feel the urge to smoke, take several deep breaths with a pause between each. Hold the last breath while you strike a match. Exhale slowly, blowing out the match. Pretend it was a cigarette and crush it out.

If you do slip up and have a cigarette, don't despair. Just get right back on your program, knowing that every cigarette you *don't* smoke is going to help your baby.

Look at smoking as a nonnegotiable issue. When you were a smoker, you couldn't smoke in theaters, subways, or department stores, in many restaurants, and probably at your workplace. That was that. Now you have to tell yourself that you can't smoke, period. And that is that.

If at first you don't succeed . . . Try, try again. Many people don't succeed the first time around but do if they keep trying. Ask your practitioner about local resources that may give your efforts a boost. Look into hypnosis, acupuncture, and relaxation techniques, which work for many people. If you're comfortable with a group approach to quitting, you should consider programs run by Nicotine Anonymous (misery often loves company—and support), the American Lung Association, the American Cancer Society, and Smokenders (a for-profit group), which have helped millions of smokers break the habit.

Note: Using nicotine patches or gums during pregnancy is risky, but the risks of continued heavy smoking may be greater. Discuss this option with your practitioner.

smoking, ask him to at least do all his smoking out of the house, away from you and the baby. Quitting, of course, would be better, not just for his own health but also for the baby's long-term well-being. Parental smoking—mother's *or* father's—increases the risk of SIDS (Sudden Infant Death Syndrome) in infancy, of respiratory problems at all ages, and of damage to the lungs even into adulthood. And it ups the chances that the children themselves will become smokers one day.

You probably won't be able to get your friends and co-workers to kick the habit, but you may be able to get them to curtail smoking around you. If there are laws protecting nonsmokers where you live or work, then it will be relatively easy to do this. If there are no such laws, try tactful persuasion—show them the material in this book on the dangers of tobacco smoke to a fetus. If that fails, try to get a regulation passed where you work that limits smoking to certain areas, such as a lounge, and prohibits smoking in the vicinity of nonsmokers. If all else fails, try to move your office for the duration of your pregnancy.

MARIJUANA USE

"I've been a social smoker of marijuana—basically only at parties—for about ten years. Could this have caused harm to the baby I'm now carrying? And is smoking pot during pregnancy dangerous?"

Unlike cigarette smoking, not all the evidence on the effects of marijuana use is in yet. Consequently, those who choose to smoke marijuana today are taking a chance, testing a substance whose dangers may not be fully documented for some time to come. And since marijuana crosses the placenta, mothers who smoke it during pregnancy are taking chances with their unborn children as well.

It is usually recommended that couples trying to conceive abstain from marijuana use, since it can interfere with conception. But if you are already pregnant, you needn't worry about your past smoking—there is no present evidence that it will harm your fetus.

Continuing to smoke marijuana now that you've found out you're pregnant, however, might well be a story with a less happy ending. Some, though not all, studies show that women who use marijuana even as infrequently as once a month throughout pregnancy are more likely to gain inadequate weight; to suffer from hyperemesis (severe and chronic vomiting), which can interfere seriously with prenatal nutrition if not treated; to have dangerously rapid labor, prolonged or arrested labor, or a cesarean section; to show meconium in the amniotic fluid (a sign of possible fetal distress); and/or to have a baby that needs resuscitation after delivery. Maternal marijuana use may also damage genes, possibly resulting in birth defects or cancer in offspring, and lead to attention problems and other fetal alcohol syndrome–like characteristics (see page 57) as well as tremors, vision abnormalities, and withdrawal-like crying during the newborn period. Marijuana has also been shown to adversely affect placental function and the fetal endocrine system, potentially interfering with the successful completion of pregnancy.

So treat marijuana as you would any other drug during pregnancy: don't take it unless it is medically required and prescribed. But if you have already smoked early in your pregnancy, don't worry. Since most of the negative effects of marijuana appear to occur as pregnancy progresses, it's very unlikely any harm was done. If you're tempted to continue using it, try some of the suggestions for quitting tobacco—kicking one addiction is similar to kicking another. If you can't seem to break your marijuana habit, speak to your practitioner or seek other professional help as soon as possible.

COCAINE AND OTHER DRUG USE

"I did some cocaine a week before I found out I was pregnant. Now I'm worried about what that could have done to my baby."

Don't worry about past cocaine use; just make sure it was your last. On the up side: a single use of cocaine before you found out you were pregnant isn't likely to have had any effect. On the downside: continuing to use it during pregnancy could be catastrophic. Cocaine not only crosses the placenta, it can damage it, reducing blood flow to the fetus and restricting fetal growth, particularly that of the head. It can also lead to miscarriage, premature labor, stillbirth, and stroke at birth, as well as numerous long-term problems for your child. Among these are chronic diarrhea, irritability, excessive crying, neurological and behavior problems (such as difficulty with impulse control, with paying attention, and with responding to others), motor development deficits, and lower IQ scores. Certainly, the more often the expectant mother uses cocaine, the greater the risk to her baby. But even very occasional use later on in pregnancy can be hazardous. For instance, a single use in the third trimester can trigger contractions or an abnormal fetal heartbeat.

Tell your practitioner about any cocaine use since you've conceived. As with every aspect of your medical history, the more your doctor or midwife knows, the better care you and your baby will receive. If you have any difficulty giving up cocaine entirely, seek professional help immediately.

Pregnant women who use drugs of any kind—other than those that have been prescribed by a physician who knows they are pregnant—are putting their babies in jeopardy. Every known illicit drug (including heroin, methadone, crack, ecstasy, "ice," LSD, and PCP) and every prescription drug of abuse (including narcotics, tranquilizers, sedatives, and diet pills) can, with continued use, cause serious harm to a developing fetus and/or to your pregnancy. Check with your practitioner or another knowledgeable doctor about *any* drugs you've used during pregnancy, or call one of the hotlines listed in the Appendix (see page 552) to see what effect they could have had. Then, if you are still using drugs, get professional support (from a certified addiction counselor, an addictionologist, or a treatment center) to help you quit now. Enrolling in a drug-free pregnancy program *now* can make a tremendous difference in the outcome of your pregnancy.

CAFFEINE

"I use coffee to keep me going all day. Do I have to give up caffeine while I'm pregnant?"

While there is evidence to suggest that getting your get-up-and-go from caffeine isn't the best idea when you're pregnant, *light* coffee drinking doesn't seem to be a problem. Caffeine (found in coffee, tea, and some soft drinks) does cross the placenta and enter the fetal circulation, but to what extent (and at what dose) it affects the fetus is not completely clear. The latest studies indicate that women who drink two or even three cups of coffee a day are probably not putting their babies at risk. However, the miscarriage rate does increase slightly in women who have five to six cups of coffee a day.

More and more studies are being done on the affects of caffeine on the fetus. Until the tally is in on those, it probably makes sense to play it safe—either avoiding caffeine while you're expecting, or limiting your intake to no more than two servings a day. In calculating your intake, keep in mind that caffeine isn't just found in coffee—it's also in caffeinated soft drinks, coffee yogurt, tea, and chocolate (though the amount varies from product to product). Be aware, too, that dark brews sold in coffee houses contain far more caffeine than homemade; likewise, instant coffee contains less than drip does.

There are some additional reasons to consider giving up or cutting back on caffeinated beverages and foods during pregnancy. First, caffeine has a diuretic effect, drawing fluid and calcium—both vital to your health and your fetus's—from the body. If you're having a problem with frequent urination anyway, a high caffeine intake will compound it. Second, coffee and tea, especially when taken with cream and sugar, are filling and satisfying without being nutritious and can spoil your appetite for the nutritious food you need. Colas and other caffeine-filled sodas are not only filling but may contain questionable chemicals in addition to large quantities of unneeded sugar or artificial sweeteners. Third, caffeine can exacerbate your normal pregnancy mood swings and also prevent you from getting adequate rest, especially if you drink it after noon. Finally, caffeine may interfere with the absorption of the iron both you and your baby need.

How do you break (or cut down on) the caffeine habit? The first step, finding your motivation, is easy in pregnancy: you want to give your baby the healthiest possible start in life. Next you need to determine why you indulge, and which beverages you can safely substitute to satisfy this need. If

it's the taste of coffee or tea, or the comfort of a warm drink, that appeals to you, then switch to a decaffeinated replacement (which contains only a negligible amount of caffeine)—but don't let it take the place of your milk, orange juice, or other nutritious beverages.

If you drink a caffeinated beverage as part of a daily ritual (the coffee break, reading the paper, watching TV), switching to a decaf variety of the beverage should do the trick.

If you drink cola for the taste, you can substitute caffeine-free soft drinks occasionally, but soft drinks have no regular place in a pregnancy diet. Instead, explore the many varieties of flavored sparkling waters and unsweetened fruit juices (in addition to the ever popular orange and apple juices, consider berry, cherry, cranberry, mango, papaya, passion fruit, and so on, in the countless combinations available).[2] If it's refreshment you're thirsting for, you'll find that juices and plain or carbonated water (or juice and sparkling water mixed) are better thirst quenchers than colas.

If it's the lift you crave from your morning coffee, you'll get a more natural, longer-lasting boost from exercise and good food, especially complex carbohydrates and protein, or from doing something that exhilarates you, such as dancing, swimming, or making love. Though you'll doubtless sag for a few days after giving up or cutting back on caffeine, you'll soon feel better than ever. (Of course, you'll still experience the normal fatigue of early pregnancy.)

Minimizing caffeine withdrawal symptoms. As any caffeine addict is well aware, it is one thing to want to give

2. Some fruit combinations are mostly apple juice, which offers minimal nutrition; look at nutrition labels for juices that naturally contain or are fortified with some vitamin C, A, calcium, potassium, and/or iron.

up caffeine and another thing to do it. Caffeine is addictive, and heavy imbibers who quit cold turkey can expect to experience withdrawal symptoms, including headache, irritability, fatigue, and lethargy. That's why it's a good idea to ease off caffeine gradually. Start by cutting down to two cups daily (taken with food to buffer the effect on your system) for a few days. Then, once you've adjusted to two cups, gradually reduce your daily intake (assuming you want to quit entirely) a quarter of a cup at a time, down to one cup, and finally, as the need for the drug lessens, to none. Or switch temporarily to a half-and-half caffeinated-decaffeinated brew during the withdrawal period, gradually decreasing the proportion of caffeinated and increasing the proportion of decaf until your mug is virtually caffeine free.

If your taste buds miss the flavor of "regular" coffee, continue to satisfy them by using a good-quality brewed decaffeinated coffee. Even espresso lovers can be appeased—decaffeinated espressos are nearly as rich and flavorful as caffeinated ones.

Withdrawal will be less uncomfortable and easier to handle if you heed these energizing suggestions:

◆ Keep your blood sugar, and thus your energy level, up. Eat frequent small meals that are rich in protein and complex-carbohydrate foods. And be sure to take your pregnancy vitamins.

◆ Get some pregnancy-appropriate exercise every day (see page 190), venturing out-of-doors when possible.

◆ Be sure to get enough sleep—which will probably be easier without caffeine.

HERBAL TEA

"I drink a lot of herbal tea. Is it safe to keep drinking it while I'm pregnant?"

Unfortunately, since the effect of herbs in pregnancy has not been well researched, there's no definitive answer to your question yet. Until more is known, the FDA has urged caution on the use of most herbal teas in pregnancy and during lactation. And though many women have drunk a wide variety throughout pregnancy without problem, it is probably safest to stay away from, or at least limit, herbal teas while you're expecting—unless they've been specifically recommended or cleared by your practitioner.

To make sure your cup of tea is free of any herbs your practitioner hasn't approved, read labels carefully; some brews that seem to be fruit based also contain a variety of herbs. Stick to regular (black) tea (preferably caffeine free) that comes already flavored, or mix up your own by adding any of the following to boiling water or decaffeinated tea: orange, apple, pineapple, or other fruit juice; slices of lemon, lime, orange, apple, pear, or other fruit; mint leaves, cinnamon, nutmeg, or cloves. Green tea should probably be limited during pregnancy since it *may* interfere with cell development and growth. And *never* brew a homemade tea from a plant growing in your backyard unless you are absolutely certain what it is and that it's safe for use during pregnancy.

SUGAR SUBSTITUTES

"I'm trying not to gain too much weight. Can I use sugar substitutes?"

It usually comes as an unpleasant surprise to hopeful dieters, but the use of sugar substitutes rarely helps control weight. Maybe it's because the person who uses a substitute in her tea figures she's saved enough calories to have a few cookies with it. Even if sugar substitutes could guarantee weight control, however, expectant mothers would still be wise to proceed with caution. First of all, because so many commercially prepared items sweetened with sugar substitutes are nutritionally unworthy (they're often overloaded with additives and underloaded with nutrients), you should be selective when choosing among them. Choose those that offer nutrition (nonfat yogurt or whole-grain muffins, for example) along with sweetness. Second, research on some of these sweeteners, particularly in pregnant women, is inadequate. Here's how sugar substitutes stack up at the moment:[3]

Aspartame (Equal, NutraSweet). Aspartame is used in beverages, yogurt, and frozen desserts but not in baked goods or cooked foods (it doesn't survive when heated for long periods). Industry-funded studies have shown no harmful effects from the use of aspartame (composed of two common amino acids—phenylalanine and aspartic acid—plus methanol) during pregnancy,[4] but some experts question the quality of these studies and suggest that, until more is known, pregnant women be cautious in their use of this sweetener. Many practitioners will give you an okay for light or moderate use in pregnancy. Adding a packet to a cup of tea or coffee or downing a dish of aspartame-sweetened yogurt is probably fine. Regularly filling up on diet soft drinks or aspartame-sweetened desserts isn't.

Saccharin. Not much research has been done on saccharin use in human pregnancy, but animal studies show an

---

3. If you have developed gestational diabetes or had diabetes before you were pregnant, speak to your physician about which sweeteners are best to use.

4. Women with PKU (phenylketonuria) must limit their intake of phenylalanine and are generally advised not to use aspartame.

FRUIT JUICE CONCENTRATES

Unquestionably safe and nutritious, fruit juice concentrates are the smartest sweeteners to rely on during pregnancy. They're surprisingly versatile in the kitchen (you can substitute them for the sugar in most recipes; see the recipes starting on page 99, and in *What to Eat When You're Expecting*) and they're readily available in the supermarket. Look for them in a host of commercial products, from jams and jellies to whole-grain cookies, muffins, cereals, and granola bars, to pop-up toaster pastries, yogurt, and sparkling sodas. Unlike most products sweetened with sugar or other sugar substitutes, the majority of fruit-juice-sweetened products are made with nutritious ingredients, such as whole-grain flour, with small amounts of healthy fats, and without chemical additives. But read ingredient lists carefully, since juice concentrates are occasionally used to sweeten products that otherwise don't measure up nutritionally.

---

increase in cancer in the offspring of pregnant animals who ingest the chemical. Whether a similar risk exists for human offspring is unclear. Still, combined with the fact that the sweetener crosses the placenta in humans and is eliminated very slowly from fetal tissues, these studies suggest that it is sensible to avoid saccharin while preparing for pregnancy, around the time of conception, and during pregnancy itself. Don't worry, however, about saccharin you had before finding out that you were pregnant, since the risks, if any, are certainly extremely slight.

Sucralose (Splenda). Made from sugar, this sweetener has been used in other countries for years with no apparent ill effects. Studies in this country have shown it to be safe, and it can be found in a variety of products, including beverages, baked goods, and ice cream. Because it has been converted to a form not absorbable by the body, it provides sweetness with few calories; it is also approved for use by diabetics.

Acesulfame-K (Sunnette). This sweetener, 200 times sweeter than sugar, is approved for use in baked goods, gelatin desserts, chewing gum, and soft drinks. Until reliable and accurate studies are done (and there is no clear research to prove it is safe), it seems particularly wise to avoid this sweetener while you're expecting.

Sorbitol. This is a relative of sugar found naturally in many fruits and berries. With half the sweetness of sugar, it is used in a wide range of foods and beverages and is safe for use in pregnancy in moderate amounts. But it does present a problem in large doses: too much can cause diarrhea.

Mannitol. Less sweet than sugar, mannitol is poorly absorbed by the body and thus provides fewer calories than sugar. Like sorbitol, it is safe in modest amounts, but large quantities can cause diarrhea.

Lactose. This milk sugar is one-sixth as sweet as table sugar and adds light sweetening to foods. In those who are lactose-intolerant, it can cause uncomfortable symptoms; otherwise it's safe.

THE FAMILY CAT

"I have two cats at home. I've heard that cats carry a disease that can harm a fetus. Do I have to get rid of my pets?"

Don't send your feline friends packing. Since you've lived with cats for a while, the chances are pretty good that you've already contracted the disease toxoplasmosis (see page 461) and have developed an immunity to it. It's estimated that up to 40 percent of the American population has been infected, and the rates of infection are much higher among people who have cats, as well as among those who frequently eat raw meat or drink unpasteurized milk, both of which can also harbor and transmit the infection. If you weren't tested prenatally to see if you were immune, it's not likely you will be tested now, unless you show symptoms of the disease (and some practitioners will run regular tests on pregnant women who live with a lot of cats). If you were tested prenatally and were not immune, or if you're not sure whether you are immune or not, you should take the following precautions to avoid infection:

◆ Have your cats tested by a veterinarian to see if they have an active infection. If one or more do, board them at a kennel or ask a friend to care for them for at least six weeks—the period during which the infection is transmissible. If they are free of infection, keep them that way by not allowing them to eat raw meat, roam outdoors, hunt mice or birds (which can transmit toxoplasmosis to cats), or fraternize with other cats. Have someone else handle the litter box. If you must do it yourself, use disposable gloves and wash your hands when you're finished, as well as when you touch a cat. The litter should be changed daily.

◆ Wear gloves when gardening. Don't garden in soil in which cats may have deposited feces. Don't allow your children to play in sand that may have been used by cats.

◆ Wash fruits and vegetables, especially those grown in home gardens, rinsing very thoroughly, and/or peel or cook them.

♦ Don't eat raw or undercooked meat or unpasteurized milk. In restaurants, order meat well done.

♦ Wash your hands thoroughly after handling raw meats.

Some practitioners are urging routine testing before conception or in very early pregnancy for all women, so that those who test positive can relax, knowing they are immune, and those who test negative can take the necessary precautions to prevent infection. Others believe the financial cost of such testing may outweigh the benefits it may provide.

SPORTS

"I like to play tennis and swim. Is it safe to continue?"

In most cases, pregnancy doesn't mean giving up the sporting life; just remember that while you're carrying a new life, moderation makes sense. Most practitioners not only permit but encourage patients whose pregnancies are progressing normally to continue participating in sports they are proficient at for as long as is practical—but with several caveats. Among the most important: "Always check with your practitioner before continuing or beginning an exercise program" and "Never exercise to the point of fatigue." (See Exercise During Pregnancy, page 190, for more information.)

HOT TUBS AND SAUNAS

"We have a hot tub. Is it safe for me to use it while I'm pregnant?"

You won't have to switch to cold showers, but it's probably a good idea to refrain from long stays in the hot tub. Anything that raises the body temperature over 102°F (38.9°C) and keeps it there for a while—whether it's a dip in a hot tub or an extremely hot bath, too long a session in the sauna or steam room, or an overzealous workout in hot weather—is potentially hazardous to the developing embryo or fetus, particularly in the early months. Some studies have shown that a hot tub doesn't raise a woman's temperature to dangerous levels immediately—it takes at least ten minutes (longer if the shoulders and arms are not submerged or if the water is 102°F or less). But because individual responses and circumstances vary, play it safe by keeping your belly out of the hot tub. Feel free, however, to soak your feet.

If you've already had some brief sojourns in the hot tub, there is probably no cause for alarm. Studies show that most women spontaneously get out of a hot tub before their body temperatures reach 102°F, because they've become uncomfortable. It's likely you did too. If you are concerned, however, speak to your practitioner about the possibility of having an ultrasound exam or other prenatal test to help put your mind at ease.

Lengthy stays in the sauna may also be unwise. A pregnant woman is at greater risk for dehydration, dizziness, and lower blood pressure in general, and these are all symptoms that may be exacerbated by going into a sauna. And as with a hot tub, pregnant women should avoid anything that might potentially raise their body temperatures.

For more information on the safety of other types of spa treatments (massage, aromatherapy, and so on) see page 213.

MICROWAVE EXPOSURE

"I've read that exposure to microwave ovens is dangerous to a developing fetus. Should I unplug ours until after the baby's born?"

THROUGHOUT YOUR PREGNANCY

A microwave oven can be a mother-to-be's best friend, helping to make nutritious eating-on-the-run possible. But as with so many of our modern miracles, there's talk that it may also be a modern menace. Most research indicates that microwaves are safe. It is believed, however, that two types of human tissue—the developing fetus and the eye—are particularly vulnerable to the effects of microwaves because they have a poor capacity to dissipate the heat the waves generate. But rather than unplug your microwave oven, you should simply take some precautions in using it.

First of all, be sure your oven doesn't leak. Don't operate it if seals or gaskets around the door are damaged, if the oven doesn't close properly, or if something is caught in the door. Since inexpensive home devices for measuring radiation are unreliable, don't attempt to test for leaks yourself. Consult an appliance service center, the city or state consumer protection office, or your local health department. They may be able to do the testing for you, or recommend someone who can. Second, don't stand directly in front of the oven when it is on (at twenty inches you get 100 percent less exposure than at two inches). Finally, carefully follow the manufacturer's operating and cleaning directions.

ELECTRIC BLANKETS AND HEATING PADS

"We use an electric blanket all winter long. Is this safe for the baby we're expecting?"

Cuddle up to your sweetie instead, or if his toes are as cold as yours, invest in a down comforter, push up the thermostat, or heat the bed with the electric blanket and then turn it off before you get in. Electric blankets can raise body temperature excessively, and although

their use hasn't been clearly associated with pregnancy problems, the theory is there. So it would be prudent to try alternative routes to warmth. Don't, however, worry about nights you've already spent beneath an electric blanket; the chance that your baby was harmed is extremely remote, even in theory.

Be cautious, too, when using a heating pad. If treatment with one has been recommended by the practitioner, wrap it in a towel to reduce the heat it passes along, limit applications to fifteen minutes, and don't sleep with it.

CELL PHONES

"I spend hours a day on my cell phone. Could this have any effect on my baby?"

Cell phones have become an almost indispensable accessory of life in the fast lane, keeping us connected no matter where we roam. They may be particularly indispensable to a pregnant road warrior—allowing you to be available for that call from the doctor or midwife you can't wait for at home, to make consultation appointments with pediatricians while you're waiting at the obstetrician's, to alert a spouse at the first signs of labor without having to search for a pay phone. A cell phone may also allow you to be more flexible in your workday and in the amount of time spent chained to a desk (which might result in more time for needed rest and relaxation or baby preparations).

Whether or not cell phones and the radiation they emit pose a danger to those who use them is controversial. However, even the theoretical risks seem to be limited to the user—no link to miscarriage or birth defects has been suggested.

Of course, cell phones do pose one risk that isn't hypothetical. Driving while talking on a handheld cell phone is unsafe—at any speed *and* under any circumstances (and illegal in some areas)—but particularly when the hormone-induced fog of pregnancy leaves you more easily distracted than usual. Even a hands-free phone conversation can be risky if it takes your attention off the road. Play it smart, and pull over to a safe area before placing your calls.

X RAYS

"I had an X-ray series at the dentist's before I found out I was pregnant. Could this have hurt my baby?"

Routine dental X rays are usually put off until after delivery if a woman is known to be pregnant—just to be on the extra safe side. But having had dental X rays before you found out you were pregnant is nothing to worry about. First of all, dental X rays are directed far away from your uterus. Second, a lead apron shields the uterus and baby effectively from any radiation. Three factors affect whether or not radiation from X rays might be harmful:

1. The amount of radiation. Severe damage to the embryo or fetus occurs only at very high doses (50 to 250 rads). No damage appears to occur at doses lower than 10 rads. Since modern X-ray equipment rarely delivers more than 5 rads during a typical diagnostic exam, such exams should not present a problem in pregnancy.

2. When the exposure occurs. Even at high doses, there appears to be no risk of damage to the embryo before implantation (the sixth to eighth day postconception). There is a somewhat greater risk during the period of early development of a baby's organs (the third and fourth weeks after conception), and some continued risk of damage to the central nervous system throughout pregnancy. But again, only at very high doses.

3. Whether there is actual exposure of the uterus. Today's X-ray equipment is able to pinpoint precisely the area that needs to be viewed, which protects the rest of the body from radiation exposure. Most X rays can be done with the mother's abdomen and pelvis—and thus the uterus—shielded by a lead apron. But even an abdominal X ray is unlikely to be hazardous, since it practically never delivers more than 10 rads.

Of course, it still isn't wise to take unnecessary risks, no matter how small, so it's usually recommended that elective X rays be postponed until after delivery. Necessary risks are another matter. Since the likelihood of damage to the fetus from any X-ray exposure is slight, the health of the expectant mother shouldn't be endangered by putting off an X-ray procedure that is genuinely needed. Observing the following guidelines can minimize the already minimal hazards of an X ray during pregnancy:

♦ Always inform the doctor ordering the X ray and the technician performing it that you are pregnant.

♦ Do not have an X ray if a safer diagnostic procedure can be used instead.

♦ If an X ray is necessary, be sure that it's done in a licensed facility with well-trained technicians.

♦ The X-ray equipment should, when possible, be directed so that only the minimum area necessary is exposed to radiation. A lead apron should be used to shield your uterus, and a thyroid collar should be used to protect the pituitary gland in your neck when an X ray will be aimed at your head (as during dental X rays). Studies have shown that radiation to the pituitary gland during pregnancy can result in low birth weight babies.

♦ Follow the technician's directions precisely, being especially careful not to move while he or she is taking the picture, so retakes won't be needed.

♦ Most important, if you had an X ray before you found out you were pregnant—and weren't able to take these special precautions—don't worry. The risks to your baby are very remote.

HOUSEHOLD HAZARDS

"How much do I really have to worry about household hazards like cleaning products and bug sprays? And what about tap water—is it safe to drink while I'm pregnant?"

A little perspective goes a long way when you're expecting. Yes, there are environmental hazards to consider, even in your own backyard, but they quickly pale when compared to those faced by women when modern obstetrical medicine was in its infancy. All of today's environmental risks combined (alcohol, tobacco, and other drugs excepted) are far less of a danger to you and your baby than one untrained birth attendant with unwashed hands was to your ancestresses. In fact, pregnancy and childbirth have never been so safe. But while you won't have to trade in your home for a sterile room, a little caution is certainly warranted, even around the house:

Household cleaning products. Since many cleaning products have been in common use for decades and no correlation has ever been noted between clean homes and pregnancy problems or birth defects, it's unlikely that disinfecting your toilet bowl or polishing your dining-room table will in any way compromise the well-being of your baby. Actually, almost the opposite is probably true: the elimination of bacteria and other germs

by cleaning agents can protect your baby by preventing infection. No studies have proven that the occasional incidental inhalation of ordinary household cleansers has any detrimental effect on the developing fetus. So there's no reason for concern. But for the rest of your pregnancy, clean with care. Let your nose, and the following tips, be your guide in screening out potentially hazardous chemicals:

♦ If the product has a strong odor or fumes, don't breathe it in directly. Use it in an area with plenty of ventilation, or don't use it at all.

♦ Use pump sprays instead of aerosols. They're better for the environment anyway.

♦ Never (even when you're not pregnant) mix ammonia with chlorine-based products; the combination produces deadly fumes.

♦ Try to avoid using products such as oven cleaners and dry-cleaning fluids whose labels are plastered with warnings about toxicity.

♦ Wear rubber gloves when you're cleaning. Not only will they spare your hands a lot of wear and tear, they'll prevent the absorption through the skin of potentially toxic chemicals.

Lead. In recent years it's been discovered that lead—long known to reduce the IQ of children who ingest it from crumbling paint—can also affect pregnant women and their fetuses. Heavy exposure to the mineral can put a woman at increased risk of developing pregnancy-induced hypertension, and even of pregnancy loss. It can put her baby at risk for a variety of problems, ranging from relatively minor birth defects to serious behavioral and neurological problems. The risks multiply when a baby is exposed to lead in the uterus and then continues to be exposed after birth.

Fortunately, it's fairly easy to avoid lead exposure, along with all the problems it can cause. Here's how:

- Since drinking water is a common source of lead, be sure that yours is lead free (see below).

- Old paint is a major source of lead. If your home dates back to 1955 or earlier and layers of paint are to be removed for any reason, stay away from the house while the work is being done. If you find paint is flaking in an older home, see about having the walls repainted to contain the flaking lead paints, or have the old paint removed—again, stay away while the job is being done.

- Still another common source of lead is food or drink contaminated by lead leached from earthenware, pottery, or china. If you have pitchers or dishes that are home-crafted, imported, antique, just plain old (the FDA did not set limits on lead in dishes until 1971), or of otherwise questionable safety, don't use them for serving food or beverages, particularly those that are acidic (citrus, vinegar, tomatoes, wine, soft drinks).

Tap water. Water ranks second only to oxygen on the list of substances essential to life. Humans can survive for at least a week without food, but for only a few days without water. In other words, you've got more to worry about if you *don't* drink water than if you do.

It's true that water once posed a serious threat to the lives it sustained, often carrying deadly typhoid and other diseases. But modern water treatment has eliminated most such threats, at least in developed areas of the world.

Though most tap water is safe and drinkable, there are occasional lapses,

even in the United States. Some water is contaminated with lead as it passes through old lead pipes or newer pipes that were soldered with lead. Some is contaminated through seepage or other contact with bacteria (such as *E. coli,* shigella, or salmonella), viruses, or parasites. And in some areas, seepage of sewer wastes and chemicals from factories, toxic-waste sites, dumping grounds, underground storage tanks, and farms has also led to potentially hazardous contamination. Water that comes from an underground well is at least as subject to such contamination as water from rivers, lakes, and streams. To be sure that when you fill a glass of water you will be drinking to your—and your baby's—good health, do the following:

- Check with your local Environmental Protection Agency (EPA) or health department about the purity and safety of community drinking water or a well, if that is the source of your tap water. Or check with the EPA Water Safety Hotline at (800) 426-4791, a local environmental group, or the Environmental Defense Fund (www.edf.org, www.scorecard.org, or [212] 505-2100). If there is a possibility that the quality of your water (because of pipe deterioration, because your home borders on a waste disposal area, or because of odd taste or color) might differ from the rest of the community's, arrange to have it tested—your local EPA or health department (check the blue pages of your phone book) can tell you how.

- If your tap water fails the test, invest in a filter (what kind depends on what turns up in your water). The filter will last longer if it is used only for cooking and drinking and not for the dishwasher or other purposes. Or use bottled water for drinking and cooking. Be aware, however, that bottled waters are not automatically free of impurities; some contain more than tap water, and some are bottled directly from the tap. To check the purity of a particular brand, contact the National Sanitation Foundation— (800) 673-6275 or www.nsf.org. Avoid distilled waters (from which beneficial minerals, such as fluorides, have been removed).

◆ If you suspect lead in your water, or if testing reveals high levels, changing the plumbing would be the ideal solution, but this is not always feasible. To reduce the levels of lead in the water you drink, use only cold water for drinking and cooking (hot leaches more lead from the pipes), and run the cold-water tap for about five minutes in the morning (as well as anytime the water has been off for six hours or more) before using it. You can tell that lead-free fresh water from the street pipes has reached your faucet when the water has gone from cold to warmer to cold again.

◆ If your water smells and/or tastes like chlorine, boiling it or letting it stand, uncovered, for twenty-four hours will evaporate much of the chemical.

Insecticides. Though some insects, such as gypsy moths, pose a considerable threat to trees and plants, and others, such as roaches and ants, to your aesthetic sensibilities, they rarely pose a health risk to human beings—even pregnant ones. And it's generally safer to live with them than to try to eliminate them through the use of chemical insecticides, some of which have been linked to birth defects. Of course, your neighbors and/or your super (if they don't happen to be pregnant or have small children) may not agree. If your neighborhood is being sprayed, avoid hanging around outside for long periods until the chemical odors

have dissipated—usually about two to three days. When indoors, keep the windows closed. If your building is being sprayed for roaches or other insects, ask that your apartment be skipped. If spraying is absolutely necessary, be sure that all closets and kitchen cabinets are tightly closed to prevent contamination of their contents, and that all food-preparation surfaces are covered. Stay out of the apartment for a day or two if that's possible, and ventilate with open windows for as long as practical. The chemicals are potentially dangerous only as long as the fumes linger. Once the spray has settled, have someone else scrub all the food-preparation surfaces in or near the sprayed area.

Whenever possible, try to take a natural approach to pest control. Pull weeds instead of spraying them. If possible, have someone remove gypsy moth larvae or other insect pests manually from trees and plants, then drop them in a jar of kerosene. Some pests can be eliminated from garden and houseplants by spraying with a forceful stream from the garden hose or with a biodegradable insecticidal soap mixture, though the procedure may need to be repeated several times to be effective. Investing in an infantry of ladybugs or other beneficial predators (available from some garden supply houses) can also wipe out some unfriendly pests.

Inside the house, use "motel" or other types of traps, strategically placed in heavy bug traffic areas, to get rid of roaches and ants; use cedar blocks instead of mothballs in clothes closets; and check an environmentally friendly store or catalog for non-toxic pesticides. If you have young children or pets, keep *all* traps and pesticide products out of their reach. Even "natural" pesticides, including boric acid, can be toxic when ingested or inhaled and can be irritating to the eyes. For more information on natural pest control, contact your regional Cooperative Extension Service (check the blue pages of the phone book) or a local environmental group.

If you have been accidentally exposed to insecticides or herbicides, don't be alarmed. Brief, indirect exposure isn't likely to have done any harm to your baby. What does increase the risk is frequent, long-term exposure, the kind that working daily around such chemicals (as in a factory or heavily sprayed field) would involve.

Paint fumes. In the entire animal kingdom, the period before birth (or egg laying) is spent in hectic preparation for the arrival of the new offspring. Birds feather their nests, squirrels line their tree-trunk homes with leaves and twigs, and human mothers and fathers sift madly through volumes of paint and fabric samples. And almost invariably, plans involve painting the baby's room—which, in the days of lead-based or mercury-added paints, might have posed some threat to the health of the unborn. Today's paints don't contain lead or mercury and therefore probably aren't dangerous. But because you don't know what hazard may turn up in paint next, it's a good idea to consider painting an inappropriate avocation for an expectant mother—even if you're trying desperately to keep busy in those last weeks of waiting. There are also other

THE GREEN SOLUTION

There is no way to eliminate indoor air pollution totally. Furniture, paints, carpets, paneling, all can give off invisible fumes and pollute the air you breathe at home—or at an office or other enclosed space. But don't worry—typical levels of indoor pollution are not harmful to you or your baby, and there are ways of making the air that surrounds you even healthier. You can accomplish this very easily and effectively by filling your home with houseplants. Plants have the ability to absorb noxious fumes in the air while adding oxygen to the indoor environment. Another plus: the joy of seeing these lovely products of nature every day. In making your selections, however, be sure to avoid plants that are toxic when ingested, such as philodendron or English ivy. You won't likely be munching on shrubbery, but the same can't necessarily be said for your baby once he or she begins crawling around the house.

reasons to find someone else to do the task. The repetitive motion of painting can be a strain on back muscles already under pressure from the extra weight of pregnancy. In addition, balancing on ladder tops is precarious, to say the least, and paint odors can bring on an attack of nausea. Enlist the expectant father or someone else to handle this aspect of the preparations.

While the painting is being done, arrange to be out of the house. Whether you're there or not, be sure to keep windows open for ventilation. (If only human nest renovations could always be done as they are for much of the animal kingdom, during the mild days of spring!) Avoid exposure to paint removers entirely, as they are highly toxic,

LET YOUR HOME BREATHE

Though making your home as airtight as possible will cut your fuel bills, it will also increase indoor air pollution. Crack open a window in the winter—and on those beautiful spring days, let the fresh air in.

and steer clear of the paint-removing process (whether chemicals or sanders are used), particularly if the paint that's being removed might be mercury- or lead-based.

AIR POLLUTION

"It seems it isn't even safe to breathe when you're pregnant. Can city air pollution hurt my baby?"

Living in a bus terminal or sleeping nightly in a toll booth on a congested highway might, of course, expose your fetus to excessive pollutants while depriving it of essential oxygen. Ordinary breathing in the big city, however, isn't as risky as you might think. Millions of women live and breathe in major cities across the nation and give birth to millions of healthy babies. Day-to-day breathing, then, will have no detrimental effect on your baby. Even enough carbon monoxide to cause illness in the mother appears not to have deleterious effects on the fetus early in pregnancy (although carbon monoxide poisoning later in pregnancy might). It's common sense, however, to avoid extraordinarily high doses of most air pollutants even when you're not pregnant. Here's how:

♦ Avoid smoke-filled rooms for extended, repeated periods. Keep in mind that cigars and pipes, because they aren't inhaled, release even more smoke into the air than cigarettes do. Since tobacco smoke is one pollutant that's *known* to hurt the fetus (see pages 58–62), ask family, guests in your home, and co-workers not to smoke in your presence.

♦ Have the exhaust system on your car checked to be sure there is no leakage of noxious fumes and that the exhaust pipe isn't rusting away. Never start your car in the garage with the garage door closed; keep the tailgate on a station wagon or minivan closed when the engine is running; keep your car's outside air vent closed when driving in heavy traffic.

♦ If a pollution alert is called in your area, stay indoors as much as you can, with the windows closed and the air conditioner, if you have one, running. Follow any other instructions given by health officials for residents who are at special risk. If you want to work out, go to the gym or go for a long walk at an indoor mall.

♦ Don't run, walk, or bicycle along congested highways, no matter what the weather, since you breathe in more air—and pollution—when you're active. Instead, choose a route through a park or a residential area with little traffic and a lot of trees. Trees, like indoor greenery, help to keep the air clean.

♦ Make sure fireplaces, gas stoves, and wood-burning stoves in your home are vented properly. If they aren't, they can fill the air with carbon monoxide and other possibly hazardous gases. Also, make sure the fireplace flue is open before lighting a fire.

♦ Try the Green Solution (see facing page). Plants, and the air-purification properties they provide, can help you breathe easier inside and out.

♦ If you *do* work in a bus terminal or in a toll booth on a busy highway (or anywhere else where pollution is a problem), consider asking for a temporary transfer to a desk job to eliminate even the hypothetical risk that the pollution might pose to your baby.

OCCUPATIONAL HAZARDS

"You hear a lot about dangers on the job, but how do you know if your workplace is safe?"

Most jobs are completely compatible with the job of feeding and caring for an unborn baby—which is very good news to the millions of expectant mothers who must manage to work full time at both occupations. Though research is ongoing (as you might have already noticed, when it comes to the science of obstetrics, a researcher's job is never done), from what is presently known, it appears that the vast majority of workplaces are perfectly safe for pregnant women and their babies. A few (including chemical factories and X-ray departments) do present some hazards, but these can be avoided with the right precautions or a switch of duties; some others haven't been studied enough yet to establish their safety.

The following is a brief rundown on what's known about the safety of certain jobs during pregnancy:

Office work. Luckily, the computer monitor (also known as a video display terminal or VDT) is not a hazard to pregnant women, as was once believed. This holds true for laptop computers as well. VDTs became the intensely scrutinized focus of media and public attention in the early 1980s, when reports began to link them with pregnancy problems. Of the studies that have been done since then, none has been able to prove a link between the low-level radiation (actually lower than that of sunshine) emitted by VDTs and miscarriages or other pregnancy problems. In addition, in spite of the millions of women exposed to VDTs over the past years, there has been no increase in poor pregnancy outcomes during that time.

Though there isn't any evidence that working (or playing) on a computer can cause poor pregnancy outcomes, there is evidence that it can cause a multitude of physical discomforts, including neck, eye, wrist, arm, and back strain, dizziness, and headaches, all of which can compound the normal discomforts of pregnancy. To reduce these symptoms, try the following:

♦ Take frequent breaks from the sitting position during the day—even a brisk walk to the rest room or to deliver a memo will help.

♦ Do stretching and/or relaxation exercises periodically while sitting at the terminal.

♦ Use a height-adjustable chair with a backrest that supports your lower back. And be sure the monitor is at a comfortable height. The top of it should be level with your eyes and should be about an arm's length away from you. Use an ergonomic keyboard, designed to reduce the risk of carpal tunnel syndrome (see page 241), if possible, and/or a wrist rest. When you put your hands on the keyboard, they should be lower than your elbows and your forearms should be parallel to the floor.

Health care work. Ever since the first doctor cared for the first patient, health

---

ALL WORK AND NO PLAY?

Never mind making a dull mind—all work and no play when you're expecting can make an unhealthy pregnancy. No matter what job you do 9 to 5 (or 6 or 7), make sure you have enough emotional and physical energy left over to do your job of mothering yourself and your fetus. For tips, see page 112.

GETTING ALL THE FACTS

By law, you have the right to know what chemicals you are exposed to on the job; your employer is obliged to tell you. Information on workplace hazards can also be obtained by contacting the National Institute for Occupational Safety and Health (NIOSH), Clearinghouse for Occupational Safety and Health Information, 4676 Columbia Parkway, Cincinnati, OH 45226; (800) 35-NIOSH—(800) 356-4674; www.cdc.gov/niosh/homepage.html; or the Occupational Safety and Health Administration (OSHA), 200 Constitution Avenue NW, Washington, DC 20210; (202) 693-1999; www.osha.gov. NIOSH also makes available a booklet titled *Technical Guidelines for Protecting the Safety and Health of Hospital Workers*. Information about the safety of machinery or other equipment that you operate on the job can often be secured by writing directly to the manufacturer's corporate medical director.

If your job does expose you to hazards, either ask to be transferred temporarily to a safer post or, finances and company policy permitting, begin your maternity leave early.

care workers have taken risks with their own lives in order to save or improve the quality of the lives of others. And while some such risks are an inevitable part of the job, it makes sense for the health care worker, particularly the pregnant one, to protect herself from as many of them as possible. Potential risks include exposure to chemicals (such as ethylene oxide and formaldehyde) used for sterilization of equipment; to some anticancer drugs; to infections, such as hepatitis B and AIDS; and to ionizing radiation (such as that used in diagnosis or treatment of disease). Most technicians working with low-dose diagnostic X rays will not be exposed to dangerous levels of radiation. It is recommended, however, that women of childbearing age working with higher-dose radiation wear a special device that keeps track of daily exposure, to ensure that cumulative annual exposure does not exceed safe levels.

Depending on the particular risk you are exposed to, you might want to either take safety precautions as recommended by NIOSH (see box at left) or switch to safer work for the time being.

Manufacturing work. How safe conditions are in a factory depends on what's being made in it and, to a certain extent, on how principled the people who run it are. The Occupational Safety and Health Administration (OSHA) lists a number of substances that a pregnant woman should avoid on the job.[5] Where proper safety protocols are implemented, exposure to such toxins can be avoided. Your union or other labor organization may be able to help you determine if you are properly protected. You can also get useful information from NIOSH or OSHA (see box).

In-flight work. The rates for pregnancy loss through miscarriage are *slightly* higher than average for women who work aboard airplanes in flight (such as attendants or pilots), especially if they put in very long hours. The exact mechanism for this risk is unclear, but it is believed to be related to exposure to radiation from the sun during high-altitude flights. Radiation is more intense nearer the poles and less so near the equator, so

5. They include acetone, aliphatic acid, alkylating agents, aluminum, aromatic and chlorinated hydrocarbons, arsenic, benzene, carbon monoxide, dimethyl sulfoxide, dioxin, ethylene oxide, lead, lithium, organic mercury compounds, phenols, polychlorinated biphenyls and all organic solvents, trichloroethylene, vinyl chloride, and xylene.

QUIET, PLEASE

Noise is one of the most prevalent of all occupational hazards, and has long been known to cause hearing loss in those exposed to it on a regular basis. Recent studies suggest that regular exposure to excessive noise* during pregnancy may also cause high-frequency hearing loss in the unborn and that it may also be associated with an increased risk of prematurity, intrauterine growth retardation, and low birthweight.

More research needs to be done, but in the meantime expectant mothers who work in an extremely noisy environment—such as a club where loud music is played, in a subway, or in a factory where protective hearing devices are required (you can't put these devices on your fetus)—or who are exposed to

heavy vibrations on the job, should play it safe and seek a temporary transfer or a new job. All expectant mothers should avoid listening to extremely loud music on a regular basis (especially in an enclosed place like a car) and attending rock concerts frequently.

---

*What's excessive noise? Generally, it's safest to avoid more than eight hours of continuous exposure to noises louder than 80 or 90 decibels (such as a lawn mower or truck traffic); more than two hours a day of exposure to noise louder than 100 decibels (such as that from a chain saw, pneumatic drill, or snowmobile); more than fifteen minutes of continuous exposure to sounds louder than 115 decibels (such as that produced by very loud music, auto horns, or sandblasting).

---

flights across the southern United States pose less potential risk than those across the northern states or those that cross either the North or South Pole. Those who ordinarily spend a lot of time flying long distances, particularly at closer proximity to the poles, might want to consider a switch during pregnancy to shorter routes that fly at lower altitudes, or to ground work. If you're concerned about the flying you did before you found out you were pregnant, discuss this with your practitioner—you're more than likely to find reassurance.

Physically strenuous work. Work that involves heavy lifting, physical exertion, long hours, rotating shifts, or continuous standing may somewhat increase a woman's risk for preterm delivery. If you have such a job, you should, by 20 to 28 weeks, request a transfer to a less strenuous position until after delivery and postpartum recovery. (See page 248 for recommendations on how long it is safe

for you to stay at various strenuous jobs during your pregnancy.)

Emotionally stressful work. The stress in some workplaces seems to take its toll on workers in general and on pregnant women in particular. There has been research to suggest that *very* high levels of stress in expectant mothers can result in pregnancy problems (just as extreme stress can cause health problems anytime). So it makes sense to cut down on the stress in your life as much as possible—especially now. One obvious way to do that is to switch to a job that is less stressful, or take early maternity leave. But these approaches aren't feasible for everyone; if the job is financially or professionally critical, you may find yourself even more stressed if you leave it.

You might, instead, consider ways of reducing stress, including daily meditations and exercise and having more fun (seeing a movie instead of working until 10 P.M.). Talking to your employer, explaining that overtime, overwork, and general stress could affect your pregnancy, may help, too. Explain that being allowed to set your own pace at work may make your pregnancy more comfortable (this kind of stress seems to increase the risk of backaches and other painful pregnancy side effects) and help you do a better job. If you're self-employed, cutting back may be even tougher, but it's something you'd be wise to consider.

Other work. Teachers and social workers who deal with young children may come into contact with potentially dangerous infections, such as rubella, fifth disease, and CMV. Animal handlers, meat cutters, and meat inspectors may be exposed to toxoplasmosis (but may well have developed immunity already, in which case their babies would not be at risk), and laundry workers to a variety of infections. If you work where infection is a risk, be sure you're immunized as needed (see page 40) and take appropriate precautions, such as wearing protective gloves, a mask, and so on.

Artists, photographers, chemists, cosmeticians, dry cleaners, those in the leather industry, agricultural and horticultural workers, and others may be exposed to a variety of possibly hazardous chemicals in the course of work. If you work with any suspect substances, you should take appropriate precautions, which in some cases may mean avoiding that part of the job that involves the use of chemicals. But don't be overly concerned about exposure that's already occurred, since in most cases exposure to toxins that isn't massive enough to cause illness in the mother rarely results in damage to the fetus.

What It's Important to Know: PUTTING RISK IN PERSPECTIVE

You want your baby to be born healthy. And you'll do just about anything you can to make sure that's exactly what happens. Give up drinking and smoking. Try to eat well. See your practitioner early and often. Think twice before taking a medication that wasn't prescribed for pregnancy use.

But what about the factors you can't control? The medications or the drinks or the cigarettes you had before you found out you were pregnant? The chemical you were exposed to before you realized it might be dangerous during pregnancy? The virus you caught that gave you a high fever?

Virtually every pregnant woman encounters a teratogen (a substance that is potentially harmful to a developing embryo or fetus) at some point in her pregnancy. Fortunately, the vast majority of these encounters are completely innocuous—they end up having no effect on the pregnancy at all. In figuring out what the chances are that a particular encounter might have been risky, and what that risk is, it helps to consider the following:

How strong is the teratogen? A very few drugs are powerful teratogens. For example, thalidomide, a drug used in Europe in the early 1960s and recently reintroduced in this country for limited use, caused severe deformities in *all* fetuses who were exposed in utero at a particular time in their development. The acne medicine Accutane, a more recently recognized teratogen, causes defects in almost 1 in 5 exposures. At the other extreme are drugs such as the hormone Provera—a progestin—that are believed to cause defects only rarely (an estimated 1 in 1,000 exposed fetuses). Most drugs fall somewhere in between, and, fortunately, few are as potent as thalidomide and Accutane (and Accutane-like compounds). Often it's very difficult to tell whether a drug is teratogenic at all, even when its use appears to be related to the occurrence of certain birth defects. Say, for example, a defect shows up in babies whose mothers took a particular antibiotic for infection with high fever when they were pregnant; the cause of the defect could turn out to be the fever or the infection, not the medication.

Is the fetus genetically susceptible to the teratogen? Just as not everybody exposed to cold germs succumbs, not every fetus that is exposed to a teratogen is affected by it.

When was the fetus exposed to the teratogen? The period of gestation during which most teratogens are capable of doing harm is very brief. For example, thalidomide caused no damage at all when taken after the fifty-second day. Likewise, the rubella virus causes damage in less than 1 percent of fetuses if exposure takes place after the third month. During the six to eight days after conception (before a woman has even missed her period), the fertilized egg, or conceptus, which expands into a ball of cells and travels down the fallopian tubes to the uterus, is largely insensitive to assault from what passes through its mother's system, and rarely suffers malformation. In fact, if it does sustain a minor injury, it has the ability to repair itself. The only risk at this point is that the conceptus will fail to survive because of a genetic mistake or that it will be destroyed by certain external factors, such as a very powerful dose of radiation. The period during which the organs are being formed—from implantation of the conceptus in the uterus around days six to eight through the end of the first trimester—is the interval when the risk of malformation is greatest. After the third month, the risk of this kind of injury is greatly reduced; any damage that does occur usually affects the rate of growth of the fetus or its central nervous or reproductive systems.

How much exposure was there? Most teratogenic effects are dose-related. One brief diagnostic X ray almost certainly won't cause a problem. A series of heavy-dose radiation treatments could. Smoking lightly for the first few months is not likely to harm a fetus; heavy smoking for the entire pregnancy increases certain risks very significantly.

What is the mother's general nutritional status? Just as you will resist a cold virus more effectively if you are well nourished and not run-down, so will your fetus resist teratogens better if he or she is well nourished—through you, of course.

Was the mother affected by the exposure? It's reassuring to know that chemical exposure that isn't toxic enough to cause symptoms in the mother is often not toxic enough to cause problems in the fetus.

Are several factors combining to increase risk? The trio of poor diet, smoking, and alcohol abuse, the duet of smoking and tranquilizers, and other "losing combinations" can greatly increase risk.

Is some unknown protective factor in play? Even when all factors appear identical, not all fetuses are affected in the same way. In experiments with mouse fetuses of identical genetic strains that were exposed to the same teratogens at identical stages in development and at identical dosages, only 1 in 9 was born malformed. No one knows exactly why, though perhaps someday medical science will come up with the solution to this mystery.

WEIGHING RISK VERSUS BENEFIT

Let's face it: Life's full of risks and benefits. Just about everything you do—from crossing the street to taking a cold pill—has some of each attached. Some activities are heavy on the benefits, others are heavy on the risks, still others are pretty evenly balanced. In most cases, there are ways you can reduce the risks without compromising the benefits; in some cases, there aren't.

Weighing risk versus benefit in making life's decisions can make life a lot safer. That's especially true during pregnancy, when so many of the decisions you make affect not just your safety and well-being, but that of your unborn baby. For instance, when you need to decide between pouring wine or sparkling water with your dinner, or making lunch out of fries and a candy bar or eating a sandwich and a piece of fruit instead, or whether or not to light up that cigarette, an assessment of risks and benefits can come in handy. Are the benefits you get from drinking, smoking, or following a junk food diet worth the potential risks to you and your baby?

Most of the time your answer probably will be no. But that doesn't mean that an occasional celebration is off-limits. One small glass of wine, for example, to toast your anniversary: the risk to your baby is nil, and the benefit (a more festive anniversary) is really significant.

Or a big chunk of sugar- and butter-rich cake for your birthday—a lot of empty calories, true. But they won't deprive baby of necessary nutrients over the long run, and after all, it *is* your birthday.

Some risk-versus-benefit decisions are easy. For instance, regular heavy alcohol consumption throughout pregnancy can handicap your child for life (see page 57). Giving up the pleasure you derive from drinking may take considerable effort, but the risks if you don't are clear. Or say you have the flu and you are running a fever that's high enough to pose a threat to your baby. Your doctor won't hesitate to prescribe a safe medication to bring down the fever. In this case, the benefit of using the drug far outweighs its possible harm, if any. On the other hand, if your temperature is only slightly elevated, it poses no threat to your baby and will actually help your body fight the flu virus. So before resorting to medication, your doctor will feel secure in giving your body a chance to cure itself, on the grounds that the possible risk of taking the drug outweighs its potential benefits.

Other decisions are not so clear-cut. What if you have a terrible cold with sinus headaches that have been keeping you up at night? Should you take a cold tablet to help you get some rest? Or should you suffer through sleepless nights, which won't do you or the baby any good? The best way to approach such decisions is:

♦ Determine if there are alternative lower-risk ways of obtaining the benefits you are seeking—perhaps through non-drug approaches (see Appendix, page 547). Try them. If they don't work, continue to evaluate your original option—in this case, cold tablets.

♦ Ask your physician about risks and

benefits. It's important to remember that most drugs have not been tested for use in pregnancy and only a limited number are *known* to cause birth defects. In fact, many have been used safely in pregnancy. New studies are turning up more information on drug safety, or lack of it, daily. Your practitioner has access to this information.

◆ Do some research on your own. For the latest information on the safety of a particular drug during pregnancy, check with the Food and Drug Administration or the March of Dimes. (See Appendix, page 552.)

◆ Determine if there are ways of increasing the benefits and/or decreasing the risks (taking the safest, most effective pain reliever in the smallest effective doses for the shortest possible time), and try to ensure that if you do take this very minimal risk, you will receive the maximum benefit (take your cold tablet before you go to bed, when it will help you get that needed rest).

◆ In consultation with your practitioner (and, when making very complicated decisions, a genetic counselor or maternal-fetal medicine specialist), review all the information you've gathered, weigh risks against benefits—and make your decision.

During pregnancy you will be challenged to make intelligent decisions in dozens of situations, weighing risk against benefit. Keep in mind that an occasional wrong choice isn't likely to affect your pregnancy, though repeated ones might. If you've already made a few not-so-terrific choices and there's no way to undo them, forget them. Just try to make better decisions for the rest of your pregnancy. And always remember, the odds are in your baby's favor!

◆ ◆ ◆

CHAPTER 4

The Pregnancy Diet

There's a tiny new being developing inside of you—a baby in the making. The chances are already excellent that he or she will be born healthy and there's something relatively easy that you can do to make those already excellent chances better still. You already do it at least three times a day. Yes, you guessed it: eating. But the challenge isn't just to eat during pregnancy (though that may be challenge enough during those early months)—it's to eat as well as you can. Think of it this way: Eating well when you're expecting is one of the first and best gifts you can give to your soon-to-arrive bundle of joy—and it's a gift that can keep on giving, bestowing not just a healthier start in life, but a healthier lifetime.

Presenting the Pregnancy Diet—an eating plan dedicated to baby's good health—and yours. What's in it for your baby? Among many other impressive benefits, a better chance for a bouncing birth weight, improved brain development, reduced risk for certain birth defects, and, believe it or not, better eating habits as baby grows to be a potentially picky preschooler (a perk you'll really appreciate when broccoli's on the dinner menu, or when you send sandwiches made with whole wheat bread to school). It may even make it more likely that your child will grow to be a healthier adult.

And your baby's not the only one who's likely to benefit. The Pregnancy Diet can also increase the chances that you'll have a safe pregnancy (some complications, such as anemia and preeclampsia, are more common among women who don't eat well); a comfortable pregnancy (a sensibly selected diet can minimize morning sickness, fatigue, constipation, and a host of other pregnancy symptoms); a balanced emotional state (good nutrition can help temper mood swings); a timely labor and delivery (in general, women on excellent diets are less likely to deliver too early); and a speedier postpartum recovery (a well-nourished body can bounce back faster and more easily, and weight that's been gained at a sensible rate can be shed more quickly). For more on the many benefits of a healthy diet during pregnancy, see *What to Expect: Eating Well When You're Expecting.*

TRY THESE INSTEAD

Looking for more healthy alternatives to your not-so-healthy favorite foods? Here are some ideas to get you started:

Instead of . . .	Try . . .
Potato chips	Soy crisps
A bag of M&M's	Trail mix (nuts, seeds, dried fruit, and maybe a few M&M's)
Before-dinner pretzels	Before-dinner edamame (soybeans, steamed and lightly salted)
Fried chicken	Grilled chicken
Ice cream sundae with sprinkles	Fat-free frozen yogurt with granola
Taco chips dipped in cheese sauce	Veggies dipped in cheese sauce
French fries	Sweet Potato Chips (see page 102)
Anything on white bread	Anything on whole wheat

Luckily, scoring those benefits is a piece of (carrot) cake, especially if you're already eating pretty well, and even if you're not (you'll just have to be a little more selective before bringing fork to mouth). That's because the Pregnancy Diet isn't all that different from the average healthy diet. While a few modifications have been made for the pregnant set (not surprisingly, baby making requires more calories and more of certain nutrients), the foundation is the same: a good, balanced mix of lean sources of protein and calcium, whole grains, fruits, and vegetables. Sound familiar? It should—after all, it's what sensible folks in the nutrition field have been touting for years.

And here's some more good news. Even if you're coming to your pregnancy (and bellying up to the table) with less than ideal eating habits, changing them to follow the Pregnancy Diet won't be that tough—especially if you're committed to making the changes. There are healthy alternatives for almost every unhealthy food and beverage you've ever brought to your lips (see box, above)—which means

there are nourishing ways to have your cake (and cookies, and chips, and even fast food) and eat it, too. Plus, there are countless ways to sneak crucial vitamins and minerals into recipes and favorite dishes—which means that you can eat well when you're expecting without your taste buds being the wiser.

There is a very important point to keep in mind as you embark on making a diet change for the better: What's presented in this chapter is the ideal, the best possible plan for eating well when you're expecting. Something you should strive for, certainly, but nothing you should stress over (especially early in pregnancy, when your appetite for healthy foods may face a smorgasbord of suppressive symptoms—from nausea to food aversions). Hopefully, you'll choose to follow the diet closely, at least most of the time. Or maybe you'll follow it loosely, all of the time. But even if your allegiance remains to burgers and fries, you'll still pick up in the pages that follow at least a few pointers that will help nourish you and your baby better during the next nine months.

NINE BASIC PRINCIPLES FOR NINE MONTHS OF HEALTHY EATING

Bites count. Chew on this: You've got nine months worth of meals and snacks (and nibbles and noshes) ahead of you—each one of them an opportunity to feed your baby well before he or she is even born. So open wide, but think first. Try to make your pregnancy bites count by choosing them (at least most of the time) with baby's needs in mind.

All calories are not created equal. Choose your calories with care, selecting quality over quantity. It may seem obvious—and inherently unfair—but those 200 calories in a plain doughnut are not equal to the 200 calories in a whole-grain raisin-bran muffin. Nor are the 100 calories in ten potato chips equal to the 100 calories in a baked potato served in its skin. Your baby will benefit a lot more from 2,000 nutrient-rich calories daily than from 2,000 mostly empty ones. And your body will show the benefits postpartum as well.

Starve yourself, starve your baby. Just as you wouldn't consider starving your baby after it's born, you shouldn't consider starving it when it's at home in your uterus. A fetus can't thrive by living off your flesh, no matter how ample. It needs regular nourishment at regular intervals—and as the sole caterer of your uterine café, only you can provide it. Even if you're not hungry, your baby is. So don't skip meals. In fact, eating frequently may be the best route to a well-nourished fetus. Research shows that mothers who eat at least five times a day (three meals plus two snacks or six mini meals, for instance) are more likely to carry to term. But what if you've been too busy hugging the toilet to even think

about eating? What if your heartburn has made eating a pain—literally? You'll find plenty of tips on how to eat around these pregnancy inconveniences on pages 116 and 139, as well as in *What to Expect: Eating Well When You're Expecting.*

Efficiency is effective. Think it's impossible to fill each of the Daily Dozen requirements (see page 88) each and every day (let's see . . . six whole grains means one every four hours . . .)? Think again. Worried that even if you do manage to eat it all, you'll end up looking like a pregnant blimp? Worry no more. Instead, become an efficiency expert. Get more nutritional bang for your buck by choosing foods that are lightweights when it comes to calories, heavy hitters when it comes to nutrients. Need an example? Eating a cup of pistachio nuts at 715 calories (about 25 percent of your daily allotment) is a considerably less efficient way of netting a 25-gram protein serving than eating a 4-ounce turkey burger, at 250 calories. Another efficiency case in point: Eating a cup and a half of ice cream (about 500 calories) is a far less efficient way of scoring a 300-milligram calcium serving than eating a cup of nonfat frozen yogurt (about 300 calories). Because fat has more than

---

THE SIX-MEAL SOLUTION

Too bloated, queasy, heartburned, or constipated (or all four) to contemplate a full meal? No matter what tummy troubles are getting you down, you'll find it easier to spread your Daily Dozen into five or six mini meals instead of three squares. And since a grazing approach keeps your blood sugar level, you'll get an energy boost, too (and who couldn't use that?). You'll have fewer headaches, too.

twice as many calories per gram as either proteins or carbohydrates, opting often for lower-fat foods will step up your nutritional efficiency. Choose lean meats over fatty ones; fat-free or low-fat milk and dairy products over full-fat versions; grilled or broiled foods over fried. Spread butter lightly; use a tablespoon of olive oil for sautéing, not a quarter of a cup. Another trick of the efficient-eating trade? Select foods that are overachievers in more than one Daily Dozen category, thus filling two or more requirements at once.

Efficiency is important, too, if you're having trouble gaining enough weight. To start tipping the scale toward a healthier weight gain, choose foods that are dense in nutrients and calories—avocados, nuts, and dried fruits, for instance—that can fill you and your baby out without filling you up too much.

Carbohydrates are a complex issue. Some women, concerned about gaining too much weight during pregnancy, mistakenly drop carbohydrates from their diets like so many hot potatoes. There's no doubt that refined carbohydrates (like white bread, white rice, refined cereals, cakes, cookies, pretzels, sugars, syrups) are nutritionally weak. But unrefined (complex) carbohydrates (whole-grain breads and cereals, brown rice, fresh fruits and vegetables, dried beans and peas, and, of course, hot potatoes—especially in their skins) supply essential B vitamins, trace minerals, protein, and important fiber. Good not only for your baby, but also for you (they'll help keep nausea and constipation in check). And because they are filling and fiber-rich but not fattening, they'll help keep your weight gain in check, too. Recent research suggests yet another bonus for complex carbohydrate consumers: eating plenty of fiber may reduce the risk of developing gestational diabetes. Be careful to move from a low-fiber diet to a high-fiber diet slowly to avoid possible stomach upset.

Sweet nothings are exactly that. Sugar calories are, unfortunately, empty calories. And though empty calories are fine once in a while—even when you're pregnant—they tend to add up a lot more quickly than you'd think, leaving less room in your diet for nutritionally substantial calories. In addition, researchers are finding that sugar may not only be void of value, but in excessive amounts may potentially be harmful. Studies have suggested that in addition to contributing to obesity, sugar may be linked to tooth decay, diabetes, heart disease, and colon cancer. Perhaps sugar's biggest shortcoming, however, is that it is so often found in foods that are, on the whole, nutritionally slight. Sometimes it's just added to improve the flavor of a product whose ingredients aren't naturally up to par—as in a tomato sauce that's made from less-than-ripe tomatoes.

Refined sugar goes by many names on the supermarket shelves, including corn syrup and dehydrated cane juice. Honey, an unrefined sugar, has a nutritional edge because it contains disease-fighting antioxidants. Plus, it is more likely to find its way into more nutritious foods—particularly those whole-grain ones you'd find in the health food sections of your market. Try to limit your intake of all forms of sugar, however, since the calories you save can be spent on foods that pack a much more wholesome punch.

For delicious and nutritious sweetness, substitute fruit (ground dates and raisins, or chopped dried apricots, for example) and fruit juice concentrates (white grape, apple, orange, mango, for example—undiluted, frozen or not) for sugar. They provide the sweetness, but also contain vitamins, trace minerals, and

NO MORE GUILT

Willpower has its place—particularly while you're trying to eat well for two. Still, everyone needs to give in to temptation now and then, without feeling guilty about it. So lose the guilt, hold the deprivation, and allow yourself a treat every once in a while—something that doesn't add appreciably to your nutritional bottom line, but makes your taste buds jump for joy. A blueberry muffin that's probably more sugar than blueberries, but is also off-the-charts yummy. A double scoop of cookies-and-cream (when frozen yogurt just doesn't cut it). The fast-food burger you've been craving all week. And when you say "yes" to that occasional frosted brownie or candy bar, serve it up without a side of remorse.

But when venturing down the path of least nutritious, try to be as selective as you can be—add a slice of banana and some nuts to your ice cream sundae; choose a candy bar that's filled with almonds; order your burger with cheese and tomato. Keeping portions of these foods small is another good strategy—share that serving of onion rings; take a slender slice of pecan pie instead of a hefty slab. And remember to stop before you get too carried away; otherwise, you might just begin to feel that guilt after all.

valuable phytochemicals (plant chemicals that may help the body defend itself against disease and aging), all absent in sugar. Plus, commercially available products sweetened with them are almost invariably made with whole grains and healthy fats and without questionable chemical additives. Buy those or make your own equivalents at home. Some calorie-free sugar substitutes appear to be safe for pregnancy use, particularly Sucralose (Splenda; for more, see page 66).

Good foods remember where they came from. Mother Nature knows a thing or two about nutrition. So it's not surprising that the most nutritious foods are often the ones that haven't strayed far from their natural state. Choose fresh vegetables and fruits when they're in season, or fresh-frozen or unadulterated canned (avoid those that have added sugar, unhealthy or too many fats, or a high sodium content) when fresh are unavailable or you don't have time to prepare them. And speaking of preparation, less is more when it comes to nutri-

ents. Try to eat some raw vegetables and fruit every day, and when you're cooking, opt for steaming or a light stir-fry, so more vitamins and minerals will be retained.

And there's more nutritional know-how in Nature's model. Avoid processed foods (not only have they picked up a lot of chemicals, fat, sugar, and salt on the assembly line, but they're frequently low in nutrition). Choose roasted turkey breast over smoked turkey; macaroni and cheese made with whole-grain macaroni and natural cheese over that bright orange variety; fresh oatmeal made from rolled oats (flavored, if you like, with cinnamon and chopped or dried fruit) over the lower fiber and highly sugared instant varieties.

Healthful eating should be a family affair. If there are subversive elements at home, urging you to bake your famous double chocolate cookies or to add sour-cream-and-onion chips to the shopping list, it's a sure bet that you'll have a harder time eating well. Make other family members your allies by enlisting the whole household to eat healthily with you. Bake Fruity Chocolate Chip Cookies (see page 103) instead of traditional Toll House; shop for baked potato chips (or soy crisps) instead of the greasy varieties. In addition to a healthier baby and a relatively slimmer you, there will be the postpartum bonus of a spouse and older children (if you have any) with improved eating habits. And don't stop after delivery. Research associates a good diet not only with a better pregnancy outcome, but with a lower risk of many diseases, including adult-onset diabetes and cancer. Which means the family that eats well together is more likely to stay healthy together.

Bad habits can sabotage a good diet. The best prenatal diet in the world is easily undermined if the expectant mother doesn't eliminate alcohol, tobacco, and other unsafe drugs from her life. Read about these saboteurs in Chapter 3, and if you haven't done so already, change your habits accordingly.

THE PREGNANCY DAILY DOZEN

Calories. The old adage that a pregnant woman is eating for two is true. But it's important to remember that one of the two is a tiny developing fetus whose caloric needs are significantly lower than yours—a mere 300 a day, more or less. So, if you're of average weight, you need only about 300 calories more than was necessary to maintain your prepregnancy weight.[1] During the first trimester you may need fewer than 300 extra calories daily, unless you're trying to compensate for starting out underweight. As your metabolism speeds up later in pregnancy, you may need somewhat more than 300. Eating more calories than you and your baby need isn't only unnecessary, it's

unwise. Eating too few calories, on the other hand, is not only unwise but also potentially dangerous as pregnancy progresses; women who don't take in enough calories during the second and third trimesters can seriously hamper the development of their babies.

There are four exceptions to this basic formula—and if any apply to you, it's even more important to discuss your caloric needs with your practitioner. If you're overweight, you can possibly do with somewhat fewer calories, as long as you have the right nutritional guidance. If you're seriously underweight, you'll need more calories so you can catch up weight-wise. If you're an adolescent, you're still growing yourself—which means you have unique nutritional needs. And if you're carrying multiples, you'll have to add about 300 calories for each additional baby.

Are those 300 extra calories a license to eat everything in sight? Sad to say, no. You'd be surprised to find how easy it is to spend them. For instance, add four glasses of fat-free milk (or the equivalent in calcium-rich foods that you and baby will be needing) to your daily intake, and you've already outspent them. Do the math and you'll see that you probably should be thinking about cutting down on those high-calorie, low-nutrition treats (hot fudge sundae come to mind?) instead of adding them in.

But while calories count during pregnancy, keep in mind that they don't have to be literally counted. Instead of concerning yourself with complicated

---

1. To determine roughly how many calories you need to maintain your pregnancy weight, multiply that weight by 12 if you're sedentary, 15 if you're moderately active, and up to 22 if you're very active. Because the rate at which calories are burned varies from person to person even during pregnancy, calorie requirements vary, too, so the figure you arrive at is just an estimate.

computations at every meal, step on a reliable scale every once in a while (once a week if you're really curious, once every two to three weeks if you're more scale-phobic) to check your progress. Weigh yourself at the same time of day, either naked or wearing the same clothing (or clothing that weighs about the same), so that your calculations won't be thrown off by a heavy meal one week or a heavy sweater the next. If your weight gain is going according to schedule (an average of about 1 pound a week in the second and third trimesters; see page 170), you're getting the right number of calories. If it's less than that, you're getting too few; if it's more than that, you're getting too many. Maintain or adjust your food intake as necessary, but be certain you never cut out required nutrients along with calories.

Protein: three servings daily. How does your baby grow? Using, among other nutrients, the amino acids (the building blocks of human cells) from the protein you eat each day. Since your baby's cells are multiplying rapidly, protein is an extremely crucial component of your pregnancy diet; aim to have about 75 grams of protein every day. If that sounds like a lot, keep in mind that most Americans (including you, most likely) consume at least that much daily without even trying—and those on high-protein diets pack away a lot more. To get your share of protein, all you have to do is eat a total of three servings of Protein foods from the list that follows. When tallying your Protein servings, don't forget to count the protein found in many high-calcium foods: a glass of milk and an ounce of cheese each provide a third of a Protein serving; a cup of yogurt equals half a serving. Whole grains and legumes contribute protein, too.

Every day have three of the following, or a combination equivalent to three

---

COUNT 'EM ONCE, COUNT 'EM TWICE

Many of your favorite foods fill more than one Daily Dozen requirement in each serving—giving you two for the caloric price of one. Case in point: a slice of cantaloupe nets a Green Leafy and a Vitamin C in one delicious package. One cup of yogurt yields one Calcium serving and half a Protein serving. Use such overlappers as often as you can to save yourself calories and stomach space.

---

servings (a serving contains about 25 grams of protein). Keep in mind that most of the dairy options also fill calcium requirements, which make them especially efficient choices.

24 ounces (three 8-ounce glasses) of milk or buttermilk

1 cup cottage cheese

2 cups yogurt

3 ounces (¾ cup grated) cheese

4 large whole eggs

7 large egg whites

3½ ounces (drained) canned tuna or sardines[2]

4 ounces (drained) canned salmon

4 ounces cooked seafood (shelled shrimp, lobster, clams, etc.)

4 ounces (before cooking) fresh fish

4 ounces (before cooking) chicken, turkey, duck, or other poultry without skin

4 ounces (before cooking) lean beef, lamb, veal, pork, or buffalo

---

2. See pages 147 to 148 for safety tips on eating fish.

VEGETARIAN PROTEINS

Good news for vegans. You don't have to combine to conquer vegetarian proteins, as long as you have some of each type (legumes, grains, and seeds and nuts) every day. To be sure you are getting a full protein serving at each meal, double or choose two half servings listed below. And keep in mind that many of these foods fulfill the requirements for Whole Grains and Legumes as well as Protein.

The following selections are nutritious foods for all pregnant women—you don't have to be a vegetarian to tap into them, and count them in your daily total. In fact, many may be soothing protein alternatives when early-pregnancy queasiness and aversions push meat off the menu.

LEGUMES
(half Protein servings)

¾ cup cooked beans, lentils, split peas, or chickpeas (garbanzos)
½ cup cooked soybeans (edamame)
¾ cup green garden peas
1½ ounces peanuts
3 tablespoons peanut butter
¼ cup miso
4 ounces tofu (bean curd)
3 ounces tempeh
1½ cups soy milk*
3 ounces soy cheese*

½ cup vegetarian "ground beef"*
1 large vegetarian "hot dog" or "burger"*
1 ounce (before cooking) soy pasta

GRAINS
(half Protein servings)

3 ounces (before cooking) whole wheat pasta
⅓ cup wheat germ
¾ cup oat bran
1 cup uncooked (2 cups cooked) oats
2 cups (approximately) whole-grain ready-to-eat cereal*
½ cup uncooked (1½ cups cooked) couscous, bulgur, buckwheat groats
½ cup quinoa
4 slices whole-grain bread
2 whole wheat pitas or English muffins

NUTS AND SEEDS
(half Protein servings)

3 ounces nuts (such as walnuts, pecans, and almonds)
2 ounces sesame, sunflower, or pumpkin seeds
½ cup ground flaxseed

*Protein content varies widely, so check labels for 12 to 15 grams protein per half serving.

Calcium foods: four servings daily. Back in elementary school, you probably learned that growing children need plenty of calcium for strong bones and teeth. Well, so do growing fetuses on their way to becoming growing children. Calcium is also vital for muscle, heart, and nerve development, blood clotting, and enzyme activity. But it's not only your baby who stands to lose when you don't get enough calcium. If incoming supplies are inadequate, your baby-making factory will draw upon the calcium in your own bones to help meet its

quota, setting you up for osteoporosis later in life. So be diligent about getting your four servings of calcium-rich foods a day.

Can't stomach the idea—or the taste—of four glasses of milk each day? Luckily, calcium doesn't have to be served in glasses at all. It can be served up as a cup of yogurt or a piece of cheese. It can be disguised in smoothies, soups, casseroles, cereals, dips, sauces, desserts, and more.

For those who can't tolerate or don't eat dairy products at all, calcium also comes in nondairy form. A glass of calcium-fortified orange juice, for instance, efficiently provides a serving of Calcium and Vitamin C; 4 ounces canned salmon with bones provides both a serving of Calcium and Protein; 1 portion cooked greens yields not only a Green Leafy and a Vitamin C serving, but a bonus of calcium. (See below for more calcium-rich foods.) For women who are vegetarians or lactose-intolerant, or who for other reasons cannot be sure they're getting enough calcium (1,200 mg daily) in their diets, a calcium supplement (one that includes Vitamin D as well) may be recommended.

You should aim for four servings of calcium-rich foods each day, or any combination of them that is equivalent to four servings (so don't forget to count that half cup of yogurt, that sprinkle of cheese!). Each serving listed below contains about 300 milligrams of calcium (you need a total of about 1,200 a day), and many also fill your protein requirements.

¼ cup grated cheese
1 ounce cheese
½ cup pasteurized ricotta cheese
1 cup milk or buttermilk
5 ounces calcium-added milk
    (shake well before serving)

CAN'T FIND YOUR FAVORITE?

Is your favorite fruit, grain, or protein food nowhere to be found on these lists? That doesn't mean it doesn't rate nutrition-wise. For reasons of space, only the more common foods are listed. There are longer food lists in *What to Expect: Eating Well When You're Expecting,* and even longer ones on the USDA National Nutrient Database: www.nal.usda.gov/fnic/foodcomp/search/.

⅓ cup nonfat dry milk
    (enough to make 1 cup liquid)
1 cup yogurt
1½ cups frozen yogurt
1 cup calcium-fortified orange juice
    (shake well before serving)
4 ounces canned salmon with bones
3 ounces canned sardines with bones
3 tablespoons ground sesame seeds
1 cup cooked greens (such as collard or turnip)
1½ cups cooked Chinese cabbage (bok choy)
1½ cups cooked edamame
1¾ tablespoons blackstrap molasses

You'll also score a calcium bonus by eating cottage cheese, tofu, dried figs, almonds, broccoli, spinach, dried beans, and flaxseed.

Vitamin C foods: three servings daily. You and baby both need vitamin C for tissue repair, wound healing, and various other metabolic (nutrient-utilizing) processes. Your baby also needs it for proper growth and for the development of strong bones and teeth. Vitamin C is a nutrient the body can't store, so a fresh supply is needed every day. Lucky for you, vitamin C usually comes from foods that naturally taste good. As you can see from the list of vitamin C foods below, the old standby orange juice (good as it is) is far from the only, or even the best, source of this essential vitamin.

Aim for at least three Vitamin C servings every day. (Fruit fanatic? Help yourself to more.) Your body can't store this vitamin, so try not to skip a day. Keep in mind that many Vitamin C foods also fill the requirement for Green Leafy and Yellow Vegetables and Yellow Fruit.

½ medium-size grapefruit
½ cup grapefruit juice
½ medium-size orange
½ cup orange juice

2 tablespoons orange, white grape, or
    other fortified juice concentrate
¼ cup lemon juice
½ medium-size mango
¼ medium-size papaya
⅛ small cantaloupe or honeydew
    (½ cup cubed)
⅓ cup strawberries
⅔ cup blackberries or raspberries
½ medium-size kiwifruit
½ cup diced fresh pineapple
2 cups diced watermelon
¼ medium-size red, yellow, or
    orange bell pepper
½ medium-size green bell pepper
½ cup raw or cooked broccoli
1 medium-size tomato
¾ cup tomato juice
½ cup vegetable juice
½ cup raw or cooked cauliflower
½ cup cooked kale
1 packed cup raw spinach, or
    ½ cup cooked
¾ cup cooked collard, mustard, or
    turnip greens
2 cups romaine lettuce
¾ cup shredded raw red cabbage
1 sweet potato or baking potato,
    baked in skin
1 cup cooked edamame

**Green leafy and yellow vegetables and
yellow fruits: three to four servings daily.**
These bunny favorites supply the vitamin
A, in the form of beta-carotene, that is vital
for cell growth (your baby's cells are multiplying at a fantastic rate), healthy skin,
bones, and eyes. The green leafies and yellows also deliver doses of other essential
carotenoids and vitamins (vitamin E,
riboflavin, folic acid, and other B vitamins), numerous minerals (many green
leafies provide a good deal of calcium as
well as trace minerals), disease-fighting
phytochemicals, and constipation-fighting
fiber. A bountiful selection of green leafy
and yellow vegetables and yellow fruit can
be found in the list that follows. Folks with

an anti-vegetable bent may be pleasantly
surprised to discover that broccoli and
spinach are not the only sources of vitamin
A and, in fact, that the vitamin comes
packaged in some of nature's most tempting sweet offerings—dried apricots, yellow peaches, cantaloupe, and mangoes,
for example. And those who like to drink
their vegetables may be happy to know
that they can count a glass of vegetable
juice, a bowl of Carrot Buttermilk Soup
(see page 102) or the Breakfast in a Shake
(see page 98) toward their daily Green
Leafy and Yellow allowance.

    Try to eat at least three to four serv-
ings a day. If possible, aim to have some
yellow and some green daily (and eat
some raw for extra fiber). Remember,
many of these foods also fill a vitamin C
requirement.

⅛ cantaloupe, or ½ cup cubed
2 large fresh apricots or 6 dried
    apricot halves
½ medium-size mango
¼ medium-size papaya
1 large nectarine or yellow peach
1 small persimmon
¾ cup pink grapefruit juice
1 pink or ruby red grapefruit
1 clementine
½ carrot, or ¼ cup grated
½ cup raw or cooked broccoli pieces
1 cup coleslaw mix
¼ cup cooked collard greens,
    Swiss chard, or kale
1 packed cup green leafy lettuce
    (such as Romaine, arugula,
    red or green leaf)
1 packed cup raw spinach, or
    ½ cup cooked
¼ cup cooked winter squash
½ small sweet potato or yam
2 medium-size tomatoes
½ medium-size red bell pepper
¼ cup chopped parsley

**Other fruits and vegetables: one to two
servings daily.** In addition to produce

rich in vitamin C and beta-carotene–vitamin A, you need at least one or two "other" types of fruit or vegetable daily. While "Others" were once relegated to a second-class position on the food chain, they're now getting a second look. Turns out they're rich not only in minerals, such as potassium and magnesium, that are vital to good pregnancy health, but also in an impressive host of other up-and-coming trace minerals. Many also have phytochemicals and antioxidants in abundance (particularly those that sport the colors of the rainbow—so pick produce that's brightly hued for the biggest nutritional return). From that apple a day to those headline-making blueberries and pomegranates, "Others" are definitely worthy of a spot in your daily diet.

You're sure to find plenty of "Others" among your favorite fruits and vegetables. Round out your produce picks with one to two from this list daily:

1 medium-size apple
½ cup apple juice or applesauce
½ cup pomegranate juice
2 tablespoons apple juice concentrate
1 medium-size banana
½ cup pitted fresh cherries
¼ cup cooked cranberries
1 medium-size white peach
1 medium-size pear or 2 dried halves
½ cup unsweetened pineapple juice
2 small plums
½ cup blueberries
½ medium-size avocado
½ cup cooked green beans
½ cup fresh raw mushrooms
½ cup cooked okra
½ cup sliced onion
½ cup cooked parsnips
½ cup cooked zucchini
1 small ear cooked sweet corn
1 cup shredded iceberg lettuce
½ cup green garden peas or snow peas

Whole grains and legumes: six or more servings a day. Don't go against the

HOW LOW CAN YOU GO?

Here's the low-down on the low-carb diet fad: When you're expecting, low isn't the way to go. That's because a diet without complex carbohydrates is a diet deficient in vital baby-making nutrients like the ever-important folic acid, among other vitamins and minerals, as well as important-for-you constipation-fighting fiber and B vitamins that help combat morning sickness. Plus, low carb usually means extremely high protein—something that's not good for your developing fetus, either. So put away those diet books (at least until after you deliver) and stay well-balanced for a healthy baby.

grain. Whole grains (whole wheat, oats, rye, barley, corn, rice, millet, wheat berries, buckwheat, bulgur, quinoa, and so on) and legumes (peas, beans, and peanuts) are packed with nutrients, particularly the B vitamins (except for vitamin B_{12}, found only in animal products) that are needed for just about every part of your baby's body. These concentrated complex carbohydrates are also rich in iron and trace minerals, such as zinc, selenium, and magnesium, which have been shown to be very important in pregnancy. An added plus: starchy foods may also help reduce morning sickness. Though these staff-of-life selections have many nutrients in common, each has its own strengths. To get the maximum benefit, include a variety of whole grains and legumes in your diet. Be adventurous: bread your fish or chicken with ground flaxseed or wheat germ seasoned with herbs and Parmesan cheese. Try quinoa as a side dish, or add bulgur or wheat berries to your wild-rice pilaf. Use rolled barley in your favorite oatmeal cookie recipe. Substitute navy beans for limas in your soup. And though you'll probably sometimes eat them, don't count refined grains (breads or cereals made with white flour, for example) towards your requirement on a regular basis. Even if they're "enriched," they are still lacking in fiber, in protein, and in more than a dozen vitamins and trace minerals that are found in the original whole grain.

Try to have six or more from this list every day. Don't forget that whole grains and legumes also contribute towards your protein requirement—often significantly.

1 slice whole wheat, whole rye, or other whole-grain or soy bread
½ whole wheat pita, roll, bagel, 12-inch wrap, tortilla, or English muffin
1 cup cooked whole-grain cereal (such as oatmeal or Wheatena)

1 cup whole-grain ready-to-eat cereal (serving sizes vary, so check labels)
½ cup granola
2 tablespoons wheat germ
½ cup cooked brown or wild rice
½ cup cooked millet, bulgur, couscous, kasha (buckwheat groats), barley, or quinoa
1 ounce (before cooking) whole-grain or soy pasta
½ cup cooked beans, lentils, split peas, or edamame
2 cups air-popped popcorn
1 ounce whole-grain crackers or soy crisps
¼ cup whole-grain or soy flour

Iron-rich foods: some daily. Since large amounts of iron are essential for the developing blood supply of the fetus and for your own expanding blood supply, you'll need to pump up your iron intake during these nine months. Get as much

THE GOOD FAT FACTS

Think all fats are bad news? Some, such as omega-3 polyunsaturated fatty acid DHA (docosahexaenoic acid), are actually making headlines for being healthy. DHA has been shown to lower cholesterol and blood pressure, as well as reduce the risk for heart disease, making it good news for those who are heart health conscious. But the good news about DHA may be even better for pregnant women and new mothers. Because DHA is a major component of the brain and retina, it is essential for proper brain growth and eye development in fetuses and young babies. So getting enough DHA in your diet during pregnancy (especially during the last three months, when your baby's brain grows at a rapid pace) and lactation (the DHA content of a baby's brain triples during the first three months of life) is extremely impor-

tant. And here's another reason to eat your DHA-rich foods: experts suspect that there may be a connection between a low intake of DHA and postpartum depression.

There is no recommended daily requirement for DHA yet, though this is currently being researched. In the meantime, try to regularly eat a variety of foods that contain it. DHA is found in concentrated amounts in oily fish such as salmon (wild is best), trout, herring, anchovies, and sardines as well as in DHA-rich eggs, flaxseed, and walnuts. It's also found in smaller amounts in chicken, regular eggs, crab, and shrimp. Ask your practitioner about pregnancy DHA supplements derived from algae or prenatal vitamin formulas that contain DHA if you're not getting enough of this fabulous fat from your diet.

of your iron as you can from your diet (see the list below). Eating foods rich in vitamin C at the same sitting as iron-rich foods will increase the absorption of the mineral by the body.

Because it's often difficult to fill the pregnancy iron requirement through diet alone, it is recommended that from about the 20th week on, pregnant women take a daily supplement of 30 to 50 milligrams of ferrous iron in addition to their prenatal vitamins. To enhance the absorption of the iron in the supplement, it should be taken between meals with a fruit juice rich in vitamin C (caffeinated beverages, antacids, high-fiber foods, and high-calcium foods can interfere with iron absorption). If routine testing for anemia shows your iron stores are low, your practitioner may prescribe 60 to 120 milligrams.

Small amounts of iron are found in most of the fruits, vegetables, grains, and meats you eat every day. But try to have some of the following higher-iron-content foods daily, along with your supplement. Again, many iron-rich foods also fill other requirements at the same time.

Beef or buffalo
Duck
Cooked clams, oysters, mussels,
    and shrimp
Sardines
Spinach, collards, kale, and
    turnip greens
Seaweed
Pumpkin seeds
Oat bran
Barley
Cooked dried beans
Cooked soybeans (edamame) and
    soy products, such as tofu
Blackstrap molasses
Dried fruit

Fats and high-fat foods: approximately four servings daily (depending on your weight gain). As you're probably all too aware, the requirement for fat is defi-

---

A LITTLE FAT GOES A LONG WAY

Trying to keep those calories down by skipping the dressing on your salad, or the oil in your stir-fry? You'd be getting an "A" for willpower—but less "vitamin A" in your veggies. New research shows that many of the nutrients found in vegetables aren't well absorbed by the body if not accompanied by a side of fat. So make a point of including a little fat (keep in mind that a little goes a long way) with your veggies: enjoy oil with your stir-fry, a side of meat or nuts with your broccoli, dressing with your salad.

---

nitely not only the easiest to fulfill—it's also the easiest to overfill. And though there's no harm—and probably some benefit—in having a couple of extra Green Leafies or Vitamin C foods, excess fat servings, alas, could spell excess pounds. Still, while keeping fat intake moderate is a good idea, eliminating all fat from your diet is a dangerous one. Fat is vital to your developing baby; the essential fatty acids in them are just that—essential. Especially beneficial in the third trimester are omega-3 fatty acids. (See box, facing page.)

Keep track of your fat intake; fill your daily quota but try not to overfill it. And in keeping track, don't forget that the fat used in cooking and preparing foods counts, too. If you've fried your eggs in ½ tablespoon of butter (½ serving) and tossed your cole slaw with a tablespoon of mayonnaise (1 serving), include the 1½ servings in your daily tally.

If you're not gaining enough weight, and increasing your intake of other nutritious foods hasn't done the trick, try adding an extra fat serving each day; the concentrated calories it provides may help you hit your optimum weight-gain stride. If you're gaining too quickly, you can cut back by one or two servings.

The foods in this list are comprised completely (or mostly) of fat. They certainly won't be the only source of fat in your diet (foods such as cream sauces, full-fat cheeses and yogurts, fatty meats, and nuts and seeds are all high in fat), but they're the only ones you need to keep track of. If your weight gain is on target, aim for about four full (about 14 grams each) or eight half servings (about 7 grams each) of fat each day. If not, consider adjusting your fat intake up or down.

1 tablespoon oil (vegetable, olive, canola, sesame)
1 tablespoon regular butter or margarine
1 tablespoon regular mayonnaise
2 tablespoons regular salad dressing
3 tablespoons light cream
2 tablespoons heavy or whipping cream
¼ cup whipped cream
¼ cup sour cream
2 tablespoons cream cheese
2 tablespoons peanut butter

Salty foods: in moderation. At one time, the medical establishment prescribed restricting salt during pregnancy because it contributed to water retention and bloating. Now it is believed that some increase in body fluids in pregnancy is necessary and normal, and that a moderate amount of sodium is needed to maintain adequate fluid levels. In fact, sodium deprivation can be harmful to the fetus. Still, very large quantities of salt and very salty foods (such as those pickles you can't stop eating, soy sauce by the gallon on your stir-fry, and potato chips by the bagful), especially if they're consumed frequently, aren't good for anyone, pregnant or not. High sodium intake is closely linked to high blood

pressure, a condition that can cause a variety of potentially dangerous complications in pregnancy, labor, and delivery. As a general rule, salt only lightly—or don't salt at all—during cooking; salt your food to taste at the table instead. Have a pickle when you crave it, but try to stop at one or two instead of eating half the jar. And, unless your practitioner recommends otherwise (because you are hyperthyroid, for example), use iodized salt to be sure that you meet the increased need for iodine in pregnancy.

Fluids: at least eight 8-ounce glasses daily. You're not only eating for two, you're drinking for two. Your baby's body, like yours, is composed mostly of fluids—as that little body grows, so does its demand for fluids. Your body needs fluids more than ever, too, since pregnancy pumps up fluid volume significantly. What's more, turning on the tap when you're expecting keeps your skin soft, lessens the likelihood of constipation, rids your body of toxins and waste products (and baby's, too), and reduces excessive swelling and the risk of urinary tract infection and preterm labor. If you've always been one of those people who goes through the day with barely a sip, now's the time to tap into fluids. Be sure to get at least 8 cups a day—more if you're retaining a lot of fluid (paradoxically, a plentiful fluid intake can flush out excess fluids), if you're exercising a lot, or if it's very hot. Try not to do your drinking just before meals, though, or you might end up too full to eat.

Of course, not all your fluids have to come from the tap (or from the water cooler). You can count milk (which is two-thirds water), fruit and vegetable juices, soups, decaffeinated coffee or tea (hot or iced), and bottled plain and sparkling waters. Cutting fruit juice with sparkling water (half and half) will keep you from pouring on too many calories.

Fruit and vegetables count, too (five servings of produce net two fluid servings).

Prenatal vitamin supplements: a pregnancy formula taken daily. The theory that a healthy pregnant woman can get virtually all of her nutritional requirements at the kitchen table was held by many medical professionals for a long time. And, indeed, you could—if you lived in a laboratory where your food was prepared to ensure retention of vitamins and minerals and carefully measured to ensure an adequate daily intake; if you never ate on the run or felt too sick to eat; if you knew from day one that you were carrying only one baby; or that your pregnancy wouldn't turn out to be high-risk. But in the real world, a nutritional supplement provides extra health insurance, and women who like to play it safe will feel safer with such insurance.

Still, a supplement is just a supplement. No pill, no matter how complete, can replace a good diet. It's very important that most of your vitamins and minerals come from foods, because that is the way nutrients can be most effectively utilized. Fresh foods contain not only nutrients that we know about and that

---

WHAT'S IN A PILL?

There are no standards set by the FDA, the American College of Obstetricians and Gynecologists, or the National Academy of Sciences specifying exactly what must be in a pill for it to be called a prenatal supplement. Chances are your practitioner will prescribe a supplement, which will take the guesswork out of choosing a formula. (But don't dismiss over-the-counter prenatal vitamins offhand; they often contain the same formula as the prescription vitamins and can cost much less. Check the labels and compare.)

If you are selecting a pregnancy supplement yourself, look for a formula that contains:

◆ No more than 4,000 IU (800 ug) of vitamin A; amounts over 10,000 IU could be toxic. Many manufacturers have reduced the amount of vitamin A in their vitamin supplements or have replaced it with beta-carotene, a much safer source of vitamin A. (*Note:* An *ug* is one-millionth of a gram.)

◆ At least 400 to 600 ug of folic acid (folate)

◆ 250 mg of calcium. If you're not getting enough calcium in your diet, you will need additional supplementation to reach the 1,200 mg needed during pregnancy. Do not take more than 250 mg of calcium (or more than 25 mg of magnesium) *along with* supplementary iron because these minerals interfere with iron absorption. Take any larger doses at least two hours before or after your iron supplement.

◆ 30 mg iron

◆ 50 to 80 mg vitamin C

◆ 15 mg zinc

◆ 2 mg copper

◆ 2 mg vitamin B_6

◆ Not more than 500 ug vitamin D

◆ Approximately the DRI for vitamin E (15 mg), thiamin (1.4 mg), riboflavin (1.4 mg), niacin (18 mg), and vitamin B_{12} (2.6 mg). Most prenatal supplements contain two to three times the DRI of these. There are no known harmful effects from such doses.

◆ Some preparations may also contain magnesium, fluoride, biotin, phosphorus, pantothenic acid, and/or DHA.

can be synthesized in a pill, but probably a great many others that are as yet undiscovered. Half a century ago, a prenatal supplement didn't contain zinc and the other trace minerals we now know to be necessary to good health. But whole-wheat bread has always contained them. Likewise, food supplies fiber and water (fruits and vegetables are loaded with both) and important calories and protein, none of which comes packaged in a pill.

But don't think that because a little is good, a lot is better. Vitamins and minerals at high doses act as drugs in the body and should be treated as drugs, especially by expectant moms; a few, such as vitamins A and D, are toxic at levels not much beyond the recommended dietary allowance (RDAs are now called DRIs, or Dietary Reference Intakes). Any supplementation beyond the DRI should be taken only under medical supervision. The same goes for herbal and other supplements. As for vitamins and minerals you can get from your diet, more isn't less—nor is it considered dangerous. You can't overdo the nutrients by piling up your plate at the salad bar, so no need to hold back when the carrots call or the broccoli beckons.

The Recipes

The recipes that follow are a small sample of the baby-friendly dishes that you can enjoy during your nine months (and beyond, since they're healthy for anyone, pregnant or not). They may look random (a couple of soups, a muffin, a breakfast, a pancake, a cookie, and some drinks), but they illustrate just how easy it is to sneak fruits, vegetables, grains, and other goodness into foods you probably already love—and foods that'll be easy to get down when you're queasy or feeling the burn (heartburn, that is). For many more recipes, see *What to Expect: Eating Well When You're Expecting.*

BREAKFAST IN A SHAKE

Thick and creamy, it's breakfast in a glass.

SERVES 1

½ cup calcium-fortified orange or
    apple juice
1 cup vanilla yogurt
½ cup frozen strawberries
½ ripe mango, sliced

½ ripe banana (frozen ahead of time for
    a thicker shake)
2 tablespoons wheat germ

Place all the ingredients in blender or food processor; blend until smooth, and serve immediately.

NOTE: Shake up the fruit you use in this breakfast shake—almost any combination of fresh or frozen fruit or berries will work. If you're feeling queasy, try substituting calcium-fortified apple juice for the orange, and adding a tablespoon of fresh grated ginger before pureeing.

NUTRITION INFO
1 SERVING YIELDS:

Calcium: 1½ servings

Vitamin C: 2 servings

Green Leafy and Yellow Fruits and Vegetables: 1 serving

Other Vegetables and Fruits: ½ serving

Whole Grains: 1 serving

MORNING MUESLI

The ultimate make-ahead meal (in fact, you can make it the night before). Vary the ingredients to match your mood, your cravings, or the contents of your fridge.

SERVES 1

> ½ cup old-fashioned rolled oats
> ½ cup calcium-fortified apple or
>   orange juice
> 1 cup vanilla yogurt
> 3 dried apricots, chopped
> ¼ cup raisins or chopped dried apple
> ¼ teaspoon ground cinnamon
>   (optional)
> Fruit juice concentrate, Splenda, honey,
>   maple syrup, or brown sugar to taste
>   (optional)
> Fresh fruit of your choice, including any
>   or all of the following: blueberries,
>   sliced bananas, chopped apple, pear,
>   peach, papaya, or mango
> 2 tablespoons chopped toasted walnuts,
>   almonds, or pecans

1. Place the oats, juice, ½ cup of yogurt, apricots, raisins, nuts, and cinnamon, if using, in a sealable container. Stir, then taste for sweetness, and add the sweetener of choice to taste, if desired.

NUTRITION INFO
1 SERVING YIELDS:

Protein: 1 serving

Calcium: 1½ servings

Vitamin C: at least 1 serving (more, depending on the fruit you add)

Green Leafy and Yellow Fruits and Vegetables: at least 1 serving (more, depending on the fruit you add)

Other Vegetables and Fruits: at least 1 serving (depending on the fruit you add)

Whole Grains: 1 serving

---

2. Add the fruit now or if you like it even fresher, add it just before serving; it's delicious either way. Stir to combine, cover, and refrigerate overnight. (You can also make the muesli right before serving.)

3. To serve, top with the remaining ½ cup yogurt and chopped nuts.

NOTE: Don't like your muesli sweet at all? Substitute milk for the juice (the result will also be creamier), omit the cinnamon and sweetener, and use plain yogurt instead of vanilla. Milk can also be used to thin muesli in the morning if it's too thick for your taste.

GINGERBREAD CARROT MUFFINS

These muffins, packed with nutrients, are perfect for those queasy days.

MAKES 12 MUFFINS

> 1 cup whole wheat flour
> ¼ cup ground flaxseed or
>   wheat germ
> ¼ cup old-fashioned rolled oats
> 2 teaspoons ground ginger
> 1 teaspoon ground cinnamon
> ½ teaspoon ground cloves
> 2 teaspoons baking soda
> ⅔ cup finely chopped dried
>   apricots
> ½ cup chopped toasted walnuts or
>   pecans (optional)
> 1 cup white grape juice concentrate
> 2 large eggs, lightly beaten
> ¼ cup canola oil
> 1 teaspoon vanilla extract
> 2 teaspoons minced peeled
>   fresh ginger
> 1 cup grated carrots

1. Preheat the oven to 375°F. Line a standard-size 12-cup muffin tin with paper liners.

2. Place the whole wheat flour, flaxseed or wheat germ, oats, ginger, cinnamon, cloves, and baking soda in a mixing bowl and stir to mix. Add the apricots and nuts, if using, to the bowl and stir to blend.

3. Place the juice concentrate, eggs, oil, vanilla, and fresh ginger in another mixing bowl and whisk to blend. Add the juice mixture to the flour mixture and stir gently just until the batter is smooth and well blended; be careful not to overmix.

4. Gently fold the carrots into the batter. Spoon the batter into the prepared muffin tin, dividing it evenly among the cups.

5. Bake the muffins until a toothpick inserted into the center of a muffin comes out clean, about 20 minutes.

6. Transfer the muffins to a wire rack and let cool completely. The muffins can be stored in an airtight container for 3 days or individually wrapped in plastic wrap (and then in an airtight container or freezer bag) and frozen for up to 1 month.

NOTE: Not a fan of ginger? Leave it out and substitute another teaspoon of cinnamon.

NUTRITION INFO

1 SERVING (TWO MUFFINS) YIELDS:

Protein: 1 serving

Vitamin C: ½ serving

Green Leafy and Yellow Fruits and Vegetables: 1 serving

Whole Grains: 1 serving

Fat: ½ serving

SWEET POTATO PANCAKES

A sweet way to eat your vegetables (and your whole grains).

MAKES 12 PANCAKES; SERVES 4

> 1 cup whole wheat flour
> ¼ cup wheat germ or ground flaxseed
> ⅓ cup chopped toasted walnuts or
>   pecans
> 2 teaspoons baking powder
> 1 teaspoon ground cinnamon
> ½ teaspoon ground ginger (optional)
> ¼ teaspoon ground nutmeg (optional)
> ½ cup milk
> ½ cup white grape or apple juice
>   concentrate
> ¾ cup mashed sweet potato (from about
>   1 medium-size boiled, peeled potato)
> 2 tablespoons canola oil, plus 2
>   teaspoons
> 2 large eggs, lightly beaten
> 1 teaspoon vanilla extract
> ⅔ cup finely chopped dried apricots
>   (optional)

1. Place the flour, wheat germ or flaxseed, walnuts, if using, baking powder, cinnamon, and ginger and nutmeg, if using, in a large mixing bowl and stir to blend.

2. Combine the milk, juice concentrate, sweet potato, 2 tablespoons of oil, eggs, and vanilla in a large bowl and whisk until well blended.

3. Pour the sweet potato mixture into the flour mixture and stir to combine. Fold in the apricots, if using.

4. Heat a little of the remaining canola oil in a large nonstick skillet or griddle over medium heat. Spoon about ¼ cup batter into the skillet, and spread it slightly to flatten. Repeat with more batter, leaving room between the pancakes. Cook until firm and nicely browned, about 3 minutes, then flip the pancakes and brown the second side, about 2 minutes more.

Remove the pancakes to a plate and keep warm while you cook the remaining batter. Add more oil to the skillet as needed.

NUTRITION INFO

1 SERVING (3 PANCAKES) YIELDS:

Vitamin C: 1 serving
(if using fortified juice concentrate)

Green Leafy and Yellow Fruits and Vegetables: 1 serving
(2, if using apricots)

Whole Grains: 1 serving

Fat: ½ serving

TROPICAL FRUIT SOUP

Cool, refreshing, and a soothing way to sip your nutrients.

SERVES 2

> 1 cup frozen strawberries
> 1 ripe mango, peeled, pitted, and sliced
> 1 cup pineapple juice
> 1 tablespoon fresh lime juice,
>   or more, to taste
> 1 tablespoon chopped fresh ginger
> 1 cup vanilla yogurt
> Mint leaves (optional)

l. Place the strawberries, mango, juices, and ginger in a food processor or blender and puree. (You may have to do this in batches.) Add the yogurt and blend well.

NUTRITION INFO

1 SERVING (1 BOWL) YIELDS:

Calcium: ½ serving

Vitamin C: 3 servings

Green Leafy and Yellow Fruits and Vegetables: 1 serving

---

2. Transfer the soup to a container large enough to hold it, cover, and chill for between 1 and 3 hours. Serve the soup in chilled bowls or cups, sprinkled with mint leaves, if desired.

TOMATO AND MOZZARELLA SOUP

Serve up warm, soothing helpings of Vitamin C, Green Leafies, and Calcium in just ten minutes.

SERVES 4

> 1 can (26 ounces) tomato puree
> 1 cup vegetable juice, such as V-8
> 1 cup low-sodium chicken or vegetable
>   broth
> ¼ cup shredded fresh basil, plus 1
>   tablespoon for serving
> 1 teaspoon dried oregano
> 1 cup calcium-fortified milk
> Black pepper, to taste
> 1 cup shredded mozzarella cheese

l. Place the tomato puree, vegetable juice, broth, ¼ cup basil, and oregano in a medium-size saucepan and bring to a boil over high heat. Reduce the heat to low and simmer for 10 minutes to let the flavors blend, stirring occasionally.

2. Add the milk to the soup and stir to combine. Continue simmering (don't boil) until heated through, 2 to 3 minutes. Season to taste with black pepper. Pour the soup into bowls and top each with ¼ cup cheese and a sprinkle of fresh basil.

NUTRITION INFO

1 SERVING (1 BOWL) YIELDS:

Calcium: 1½ servings

Vitamin C: 2 servings

Green Leafy and Yellow Fruits and Vegetables: 2 servings

CARROT BUTTERMILK SOUP

A very creamy way to score a whole day's worth of Green Leafy and Yellows—with a Calcium bonus.

SERVES 2 GENEROUSLY

> 2 cups baby carrots
> 1 small Yukon Gold potato, peeled and coarsely chopped
> ¼ cup peeled and coarsely chopped shallots
> 2 teaspoons butter
> 2 cups low-sodium chicken or vegetable broth
> 2 tablespoons minced fresh dill
> 1 cup buttermilk
> Salt and black pepper

1. Place the carrots, potato, shallots, butter, and broth in a medium-size saucepan and bring to a boil over high heat. Reduce the heat, cover, and simmer until the vegetables are very tender, 20 minutes. Add the dill to the pot, stir to combine, and cook until blended, 1 minute.

2. Add the buttermilk and gently simmer (do not boil) until heated through, 2 to 3 minutes. Season to taste with salt and black pepper, and serve.

NOTE: The soup can also be served chilled with a dollop of plain yogurt.

NUTRITION INFO
1 SERVING (1 BOWL) YIELDS:

Calcium: ½ serving

Green Leafy and Yellow Fruits and Vegetables: 4 servings

SWEET POTATO CHIPS

Get your potato chip fix and a hefty dose of vitamin A in the bargain. Ready in no time and delicious to boot, you won't be able to stop at one.

SERVES 2

> Olive oil cooking spray
> 1 large sweet potato (about ¾ pound)
> 2 teaspoons olive oil
> 1 tablespoon grated Parmesan cheese
> 2 teaspoons chopped fresh flat-leaf parsley

1. Preheat the oven to 425°F. Coat a large rimmed baking sheet with olive oil cooking spray.

2. Peel the sweet potato, then cut it into ¼-inch-thick slices and pat dry with paper towels. Arrange the sweet potato slices on the baking sheet in a single layer and brush the tops with olive oil.

3. Bake the sweet potato slices until the tops brown slightly, 10 to 15 minutes. Turn them over and continue baking until the second side is lightly browned and the potatoes are tender, 10 to 15 minutes more. If you like crisper chips, let them bake a little longer, but watch them carefully so they don't burn.

4. Sprinkle the Parmesan cheese and chopped parsley over the sweet potato chips before serving.

NUTRITION INFO
1 SERVING (8 TO 10 CHIPS) YIELDS:

Green Leafy and Yellow Fruits and Vegetables: 2 servings

FRUITY CHOCOLATE CHIP COOKIES

Chewy with raisins, coconut, and oats; sweet with chocolate chips.

MAKES ABOUT 30 COOKIES

> 2 cups old-fashioned rolled oats
> ¼ cup wheat germ
> ¼ cup ground flaxseed
> ½ cup coconut flakes (preferably unsweetened)
> 1½ teaspoons ground cinnamon
> 6 tablespoons (¾ stick) butter, melted
> ¾ cup white grape juice concentrate
> 1 egg
> 1 cup raisins
> ½ cup chopped toasted almonds, walnuts, or pecans
> ½ cup chocolate chips

1. Preheat the oven to 350°F. Set aside 2 nonstick cookie sheets.

2. Place the oats, wheat germ, flaxseed, coconut, and cinnamon in a large bowl and stir to mix. Add the butter and stir to combine.

3. Combine the juice concentrate, egg, and raisins in a food processor or blender and process until raisins are chopped. Pour the raisin mixture into the oat mixture and stir until well blended. Fold in nuts and chocolate chips.

4. Drop the dough by tablespoons onto the cookie sheets about 1 inch apart, then flatten them with the back of a fork so they form irregular circles.

5. Bake the cookies until they are golden brown and firm, 20 to 25 minutes. Let the cookies rest for 5 minutes, then remove them to wire racks to cool completely before serving. They can be stored in an airtight container at room temperature for 5 days, or frozen for 1 month.

NOTE: Feeling fruity instead of chocolatey? You can substitute ½ cup of chopped dried fruit or dried cherries or blueberries for the chocolate chips.

NUTRITION INFO

1 SERVING (2 TO 3 COOKIES) YIELDS:

Vitamin C: ½ serving	
Other Vegetables and Fruits: ½ serving	
Whole Grains: ½ serving	
Fat: ½ serving	

STRAWBERRY COLADA

A nutritious twist on a tropical favorite. Serve it as a midafternoon smoothie or a very satisfying before-dinner drink.

SERVES 1

> ½ cup pineapple juice
> ½ cup frozen strawberries
> ½ cup low-fat coconut milk
> ½ cup vanilla frozen yogurt

Combine all ingredients in a blender or food processor; blend until smooth, and serve immediately.

NOTE: Banana Coladas are just as yummy. Simply substitute 1 frozen banana for the strawberries. Use both for a Strawberry-Banana Colada.

NUTRITION INFO

1 SERVING YIELDS:

Vitamin C: 2 servings	
Calcium: not quite ½ serving	

No-Tequila Sunrise

A light and refreshing before-dinner drink that's equally tasty at breakfast.

SERVES 1

> Ice cubes
> ¼ cup pomegranate juice
> ½ cup orange juice
> ½ cup sparkling water
> Lime wedge

Fill a tall glass with ice. Pour in the pomegranate juice, followed by the orange juice. Top with sparkling water, and serve with a lime wedge.

NUTRITION INFO
1 SERVING YIELDS:

Vitamin C: 1 serving

Other Vegetables and Fruits: ½ serving

Virgin Mama

This pregnant spin on the Bloody Mary may be missing the vodka, but it still packs a punch.

SERVES 1

> 1 cup vegetable juice, such as V-8
> 2 tablespoons orange juice
> Squeeze of fresh lime or lemon juice
> Worcestershire sauce, to taste
> Tabasco, to taste
> Black pepper, to taste
> Ice cubes
> Lime wedge, for serving
> 1 celery rib, for serving

Pour the vegetable juice into a tall glass. Stir in the orange juice and add a squeeze of lime or lemon juice. Season with Worcestershire sauce and Tabasco to taste, and a sprinkling of black pepper. Fill the glass to the top with ice, and serve with a lime wedge and celery rib.

NUTRITION INFO
1 SERVING YIELDS:

Vitamin C: 2 servings

Green Leafy and Yellow Fruits and Vegetables: 2 servings

Other Vegetables and Fruits: ½ serving

◆ ◆ ◆

Part 2

NINE MONTHS AND COUNTING

From Conception to Delivery

CHAPTER 5

The First Month

Approximately 1 to 4 Weeks

Congratulations—and welcome to your pregnancy! Though you almost certainly don't look pregnant yet, chances are you're already starting to feel it. Whether it's just tender breasts and a little fatigue you're experiencing, or every early pregnancy symptom in the book (and then some), your body is gearing up for the months of baby-making to come. As the weeks pass, you'll notice changes in parts of your body you'd expect (like your belly), as well as places you wouldn't expect (your feet and your eyes). You'll also notice changes in the way you live—and look at—life. But try not to think (or read) too far ahead. For now, just sit back, relax, and enjoy the beginning of one of the most exciting and rewarding adventures of your life.

What You Can Expect at Your First Prenatal Visit

Your first prenatal visit will probably be the longest you'll have during your pregnancy, and definitely will be the most comprehensive one. Not only will there be more tests, procedures[1] (including several that will be performed only at this visit), and data gathering (in the form of a complete medical history), but there will be more time spent on questions (questions you have for the practitioner, questions he or she will have for you) and answers. There will also be plenty of advice to take in—on everything from what you should be eating (and not eating) to what supplements you should be taking to whether (and how) you should be exercising. So be sure to come equipped with a list of the questions and concerns that have already come up, as well as with a pen and notebook (or *What to Expect When You're Expecting Pregnancy Organizer*) to take notes with.

---

1. See Appendix, page 545, for more on the procedures and tests performed.

One practitioner's routine may vary slightly from another's. In general, the examination will include:

Confirmation of your pregnancy. Your practitioner will want to check the following: the pregnancy symptoms you are experiencing; the date of your last normal menstrual period to determine your estimated date of delivery (EDD) or due date (see page 8); your cervix and uterus for signs and approximate age of the pregnancy. A pregnancy test (urine and blood) will most likely be ordered.

A complete history. To give you the best care possible, your practitioner will want to know a great deal about you. Come prepared by checking records at home or calling your primary care doctor to refresh your memory on the following: your personal medical history (chronic illness, previous major illness or surgery, known allergies, including drug allergies); nutritional supplements (vitamins, minerals, herbal, and so on) or medications (over-the-counter, prescription) you are presently taking or have taken since conception; your family medical history (genetic disorders, chronic diseases, unusual pregnancy outcomes); your personal gynecological history (age at first menstrual period, usual length of menstrual cycle, duration and regularity of menstrual periods); your personal obstetrical history (past live births, miscarriages, abortions[2]), as well as the course of past pregnancies, labors, and deliveries. Your practitioner will also ask questions about your social history (such as your age and occupation) and about your

lifestyle habits (how you eat, whether or not you exercise, drink, smoke, or take recreational drugs) and other factors in your personal life that might affect your pregnancy (information about the baby's father, information on your ethnicity).

A complete physical examination. This may include assessment of your general health through examination of heart, lungs, breasts, abdomen; measurement of your blood pressure to serve as a baseline reading for comparison at subsequent visits; notation of your height and your weight (prepregnancy and present); inspection of arms and legs for varicose veins and edema (swelling from excess fluid in tissues) to serve as a baseline for comparison at subsequent visits; examination of external genitalia and of your vagina and cervix (with a speculum in place, as when you get a Pap smear); examination of your pelvic organs bimanually (with one hand in the vagina and one on the abdomen) and also possibly through the rectum and vagina; assessment of the size and shape of the bony pelvis (through which your baby will eventually try to exit).

A battery of tests. Some tests are routine for every pregnant woman; some are routine in some areas of the country or with some practitioners, and not others; some are performed only when circumstances warrant. The most common prenatal tests include:

◆ A blood test to determine blood type and Rh status (see page 29), hCG levels, and to check for anemia (see page 187)

◆ Urinalysis to screen for glucose (sugar), protein, white blood cells, blood, and bacteria

◆ Blood screens to determine antibody titer (levels) and immunity

---

2. Don't be hesitant to mention any and all abortions—they will be important to your practitioner's evaluation of your present pregnancy, and he or she will not stand in judgment of you for making the choice you did. If you wish, you can request that any information about prior abortions not be shared with anyone other than the medical team.

to such diseases as rubella

◆ Tests to disclose the presence of infections such as syphilis, gonorrhea, hepatitis B, chlamydia, and, very often, HIV

◆ Genetic tests for cystic fibrosis, sickle-cell anemia, Tay-Sachs, or other genetic disease, if appropriate (see page 45)

◆ A Pap smear for the detection of cervical cancer

◆ A blood sugar level test to check for any tendency toward diabetes in women with a family history of diabetes and those who have high blood pressure, have previously had an excessively large baby or one with birth defects, or who had gained excessive weight with an earlier pregnancy. (All women receive a glucose screening test for gestational diabetes at around 28 weeks; see page 266.)

An opportunity for discussion. Here's the time to bring out that list of questions and concerns.

What You May Be Feeling

You may experience all of these symptoms at one time or another, or only one or two. What's important to keep in mind from now on is that every woman and every pregnancy is different; few pregnancy symptoms are universal.

PHYSICALLY

◆ Absence of menstruation (though you may stain slightly when your period would have been expected or when the fertilized egg implants in the uterus, around seven to ten days after conception)

◆ Fatigue and sleepiness

◆ Frequent urination

◆ Nausea, with or without vomiting, and/or excessive salivation

◆ Heartburn, indigestion, flatulence, bloating

◆ Food aversions and cravings

◆ Breast changes (most pronounced in women who have breast changes prior to menstruation, and possibly somewhat less pronounced if you've had babies before): fullness, heaviness, tenderness, tingling; darkening of the areola (the pigmented area surrounding the nipple). Sweat glands in the areola become prominent, looking like large goose bumps; a network of bluish lines appears under the skin as blood supply to the breasts increases (though, in some women, these lines may not appear until later).

EMOTIONALLY

◆ Instability comparable to premenstrual syndrome, which may include irritability, mood swings, irrationality, weepiness

◆ Misgivings, fear, joy, elation—any or all of these

A LOOK INSIDE

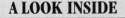

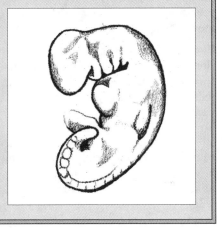

▼ *By the end of the first month of your pregnancy, your baby (who's actually about two weeks old, if you're counting from conception) is a tiny, tadpole-like embryo, much smaller than a grain of rice. Though far from human-looking yet, the embryo has progressed considerably from the shapeless mass of cells it was just a week ago: already there is a head (equipped with a mouth opening), a primitive heart that has begun to pump, and a rudimentary brain. Arm and leg buds will appear soon.*

▲ *There's definitely no way to tell this book by its cover yet. Though you may recognize a few physical changes in yourself—your breasts may be a little fuller, your tummy a tad rounder—no one else is likely to have noticed. Make sure you take a good look at your waist—it may be the last time you'll see it for many months to come.*

What You May Be Concerned About

BREAKING THE NEWS

"When should we tell friends and family that we are expecting?"

This is one question only *you* can answer. Some expectant parents can't wait to tell everyone they know the good news (not to mention a fair number of strangers who happen to pass them in the street or sit next to them on the bus). Others tell only selectively at first, starting with those nearest and dearest (close relatives and friends, perhaps), and waiting until the condition is obvious before making the pregnancy common knowledge. Still others decide they'd rather put off issuing announcements until the third month has passed, just in case of miscarriage (especially if there's been a previous pregnancy loss).

So talk it over, and do what feels most comfortable. Just remember: in spreading the good news, don't forget to take the time to savor it as a twosome.

TELLING THE BOSS

"No one at work knows I'm pregnant yet—and I'm not sure when and how I should tell them, especially my boss. I'm not sure how they'll react."

Since most expectant mothers are also members of the workforce, pregnancy protocol on the job has become an important issue for employees and employers alike. Official leave policies and benefits vary widely from company to company, as do unofficial policies of family-friendliness. In deciding when and how to broach the subject of your pregnancy with the powers that be at your company, you'll need to consider the following:

How you're feeling and whether you're showing. If morning sickness has you spending more time hovering over the toilet than sitting at your desk; if first trimester fatigue has you barely able to lift your head off your pillow in the morning; or if you're already packing a paunch that's too big to blame on your breakfast, you probably won't be able to keep your secret long. In that case, telling sooner makes more sense than waiting until your boss (and everyone else in the office) has come to his or her own conclusions. If, on the other hand, you're feeling fine and still buttoning your waistband with ease, you may be able to hold off on the announcement until later.

What kind of work you do. If you work under conditions or with substances that could be harmful to your pregnancy or your baby (see page 76), you'll need to make your announcement—and ask for a transfer or change of duties—as soon as you find out you're pregnant.

How work is going. A woman announcing her pregnancy at work may unfortunately—and unfairly—raise many red flags, including "Will she still have the stamina to produce while pregnant?" and "Will her mind be on work or on her belly?" and "Will she leave us in the lurch?" You may head off some of those concerns by making your announcement just after finishing a report, scoring a deal, winning a case, coming up with a great idea, or otherwise proving that you can be both pregnant and productive.

Whether reviews are coming up. If you're afraid your announcement might influence the results of an upcoming performance or salary review, wait until the results are in before spilling the beans. Keep in mind that proving you've been passed up for a promotion or raise based solely on the fact that you're expecting (and that you'll soon be a worker and a mother, not necessarily in that order) may be difficult.

Whether you work in a gossip mill. If gossip is one of your company's chief products, be especially wary. Should word-of-mouth of your pregnancy reach your boss's ears before your announcement does, you'll have trust issues to deal with in addition to the pregnancy-related issues. Make sure that your boss is the first to know—or, at least, that those you tell first can be trusted not to squeal.

What the family-friendliness quotient is. Try to gauge your employer's attitude toward pregnancy and family. Ask other women who have been pregnant on the job, if there are any (but keep your inquiries discreet). Check the policies on pregnancy and maternity leave in your copy of the company handbook (if there is one). Or set up a confidential meeting with someone in human resources or the person in charge of benefits. If the company has had a history of being supportive of mothers and mothers-to-be, you may be inclined to make your announcement sooner. Either way, you'll have a

THE PREGNANT WORKER'S RIGHTS

There is much room for improvement in the United States workplace when it comes to families and their needs. Though individual policies vary from company to company, here's what federal law recognizes:

- The Pregnancy Discrimination Act of 1978. This act prohibits discrimination based on pregnancy, childbirth, or related medical conditions. Under this law, employers must treat you as they would treat any employee with a medical disability. However, it does not protect you if you do not produce. If morning sickness brings you in late each day and keeps you from doing a satisfactory job, your employer may be able to fire you or put you on unpaid leave.

   It is, however, considered discriminatory—and illegal—to pass up a woman for a promotion or a job or fire her solely on the basis of her pregnancy. This kind of discrimination, like all kinds of discrimination, can be difficult to prove. Complaints of pregnancy discrimination can be reported to the Equal Employment Opportunities Commission (EEOC), 1801 L Street, NW, Washington, DC 20210; (800) 669-EEOC; www.eeoc.gov. The Wage and Hour Division (look under U.S. Government, Department of Labor, in the telephone book) can offer more information on the Family Medical Leave Act (see below). You can also get help and information from the Women's Bureau of the U.S. Depart-

ment of Labor, Washington, DC 20210; (800) 827-5335; www.dol.gov.

- The Family Medical Leave Act of 1993. All public agencies and private-sector companies that employ at least fifty workers within a seventy-five-mile radius are subject to regulation under this act. If you have worked for such a company for at least a year (and at least 1,250 hours during the year), you are entitled to take twelve weeks of unpaid leave during your pregnancy and for child care each year that you are employed. Barring unforeseen complications or early delivery, you must notify your employer of your leave thirty days in advance. During your leave, you must continue to collect all benefits (including health insurance) usually allowed to employees on disability leave, and when you return you must be restored to an equivalent position with equal pay and benefits. (In some cases, companies may be able to exclude from FMLA women who are considered key employees—those the company can't do without for twelve weeks, and who are in the top 10 percent compensation bracket.)

- State and local laws. Some state and local laws offer additional protection against pregnancy discrimination. A handful of states and some larger companies also offer "temporary disability insurance," which allows for partial wages during time off for medical disabilities, including pregnancy.

better sense of what you'll be facing.

Once you've decided when to make your announcement, you can take some steps to ensure that it's well received:

Know your rights. Pregnant women—and parents in general—have fewer

rights in the United States than in most every other industrialized country. Still, some strides have been made on the federal level through the Pregnancy Discrimination Act and the Family Medical Leave Act (see box above), and many others have been made voluntarily by forward-thinking, family-friendly companies. Become familiar with what the law and your company's policies say you're entitled to, so you'll know what you can and probably can't ask for. For instance, some companies offer paid leave, others unpaid. Still others allow you to use sick days or vacation days as part of your leave. All of this should be detailed in a company handbook, if there is one. Or, set up a confidential meeting with someone in human resources or whoever is in charge of benefits.

Put together a plan. Efficiency is always appreciated on the job, and being prepared invariably impresses people. So

before you go in to make your announcement, have a detailed plan that includes how long you plan to stay on the job (barring any unforeseen medical problems, including premature labor), how long your maternity leave will be, how you plan to finish up business before you leave, and how you propose that any unfinished business be handled by others. If you would like to return part-time at first, now is when you should propose that. Writing up your plan will ensure you won't forget the details.

Set aside the time. Don't try to tell your boss the news when you're in a taxi on the way to a meeting or when she's got

ON-THE-JOB COMFORT AND SAFETY

Even if you don't have any kids at home yet, staying on the job while you're expecting will require that you practice the fine art of juggling work and family (or, at least, a family-to-be). Especially during the first trimester and the last, when the symptoms of pregnancy may be dragging you down and the distractions of pregnancy may be competing for your attention, this juggling act may be exhausting, and sometimes, overwhelming—in other words, good preparation for the years of working and parenting you may have ahead of you. These tips won't make working simultaneously at those two jobs easier, but they may help make them less draining and safer:

◆ Take time for your tummy. Eat three meals a day (at no time in your life was your mother more right about the importance of breakfast), plus at least two snacks, no matter how busy your day is. Scheduling meetings as working meals (and making sure you have some say about what's served) may help. So will keeping a supply of nutritious snacks in your desk and your purse, as well as in the office fridge, if there is one.

◆ Watch your weight. Make sure job stress—or erratic eating—isn't keeping you from gaining enough.

◆ Hang out by the water cooler. Not for the latest gossip, but for frequent refills of your glass. Or keep a refillable water bottle at your desk. Drinking at least 64 ounces of water a day can keep many troublesome pregnancy symptoms at bay, and can help prevent a urinary tract infection (UTI), which has been linked to preterm labor.

◆ Don't hold it in. Emptying your bladder as needed (but at least every two hours) also helps prevent UTIs.

◆ Dress for success and comfort. Avoid tight, restrictive clothing, socks or knee-highs that cut off circulation, as well as heels that are too high or too flat (wide 2-inch heels are best). Wearing support hose designed for pregnancy will help ward off or minimize a variety of symptoms, and may be especially important if you're spending a lot of the day on your feet.

one foot out the door Friday night. Make an appointment to meet, so no one will be rushed or distracted. Try to make it on a day and at a time that is usually less stressful at your office. Postpone the meeting if things suddenly take a turn for the tense.

Accentuate the positive. Don't start your announcement with apologies or misgivings. Instead, let your boss know that you are not only happy about your pregnancy, but confident in your ability and committed in your plan to mix work and family.

Be flexible (but not spineless). Have your plan in place, and open it up to discussion. Then be ready to compromise (make sure there is room for negotiation built into your plan), but not to back down completely. Come up with a realistic bottom line and stick with it.

Set it in writing. Once you've worked out the details of your pregnancy protocol and your maternity leave, confirm it in writing so there won't be any confusion or misunderstanding later (as in "I never said that . . .").

Never underestimate the power of parents. If your company is not as family-friendly as you'd like, consider joining forces to petition for better parental perks. Realize, however, that you and other parents may be met with hostility by childless employees; as family policies

---

◆ Stay off your feet. At least, as much as possible. If your job demands that you stand for long stretches, take plenty of sitting (with your feet up) or walking breaks. If it's feasible, keep one foot on a low stool, knee bent, while you stand, in order to take some of the pressure off your back.

◆ Put your feet up. A stool or box under your desk will help you do this discreetly.

◆ Take a break. Often. Stand up and walk around if you've been sitting; sit down with your feet up if you've been standing. If there's a spare sofa and a slot in your schedule, lie down for a few minutes, on your left side. Do some stretching exercises, especially for your back, legs, and neck.

◆ Watch what you breathe. Stay out of smoke-filled areas; not only is smoke bad for the baby, but it can increase fatigue. Avoid noxious fumes and chemicals (see page 75).

◆ Lift with care. Do any necessary lifting properly, to avoid strain on the back (see page 210).

◆ Pack a toothbrush. Brushing your teeth after meals and snacks is especially important when you're pregnant (see page 181). If you're suffering from morning sickness, supplies with which to freshen your breath (and protect your teeth) between bouts of vomiting will come in particularly handy. Mouthwash can also help dry out a mouth that's full of excess saliva (which is common in the first trimester, and can be embarrassing at work).

◆ Make some adjustments. Two common occupational hazards at the office—carpal tunnel syndrome and backache—are even more common among pregnant workers. See pages 241 and 209 for more.

◆ Take an occasional chill pill. Too much stress isn't good for you or your baby. So try to use breaks to relax as fully as you can: bring headphones so you can listen to music, close your eyes and meditate or indulge in some daydreaming, do some soothing stretches, take a five-minute stroll around the building.

◆ Listen to your body. Slow down your pace if you're feeling tired; go home early if you're exhausted.

become more generous, resentment tends to build among those who can't take advantage of these. Making sure that similar allowances are made for employees who must take time off to care for sick spouses or parents may help unite, rather than divide, the company.

FATIGUE

"I'm tired all the time. I'm worried that I won't be able to continue working."

It would be surprising if you weren't tired. In some ways, your pregnant body is working harder even when you're resting than a nonpregnant body is when mountain-climbing; you're just not aware of the exertion. But it's there. For one thing, your body is manufacturing your baby's life-support system, the placenta, which won't be completed until the end of the first trimester. For another, it's adjusting to the many other physical and emotional demands of pregnancy. Once your body has adjusted and the placenta is complete (around the fourth month), you should have more energy. Until then, you may need to work fewer hours or take a few days off if you're really dragging. But if your pregnancy continues normally, there is absolutely no reason why you shouldn't stay at your job (assuming your practitioner hasn't restricted your activity and/or the work isn't overly strenuous or hazardous; see pages 76 and 248). Most pregnant women are happier and less anxious if they keep busy.

Since your fatigue is legitimate, don't fight it. Consider it a sensible signal from your body that you need more rest. That, of course, is more easily suggested than done. But it's worth the effort:

Baby yourself. If you're a first-time expectant mother, enjoy what will probably be your last chance for a long while to focus on taking care of yourself without feeling guilty. If you already have one or more children at home, you will have to divide your focus. But either way, this is not a time to strive for Supermom-to-Be status. Getting adequate rest is more important than keeping your house white-glove-test clean or serving four-star dinners.

Keep evenings free of unessential activities. Spend them off your feet when you can, reading, watching TV, or scouring baby-name books. If you have older children, read to them, play quiet games with them, or watch classic children's videos with them rather than traipsing off to the playground. If they're old enough to pitch in, enlist them in household chores you normally do. (Fatigue may be more pronounced when there are older children at home, simply because there are so many more physical demands and so much less time to rest. On the other hand, it may be less noticed, since a mother of young children is usually accustomed to exhaustion and/or too busy to pay attention to it.)

And don't wait until nightfall to take it easy. If you can afford the luxury of an afternoon nap, by all means indulge. If you can't sleep, lie down with a good book. A nap at the office isn't a reasonable goal, of course, unless you have a flexible schedule and access to a comfortable sofa, but putting your feet up at your desk or on the sofa in the ladies' room during breaks and lunch hours may be possible. (If you choose to rest at lunch hour, make sure you have a chance to eat, too.) Napping when you're mothering full-time may also be difficult, but if you can time your rest with the children's naptime (if they still nap), you may be able to get away with it—assuming you can tolerate the unwashed dishes and the dust balls under the bed.

Let others baby you. Make sure your spouse is doing his fair share (or preferably more) of household chores, including laundry and marketing. Older children can help out, too. Accept your mother-in-law's offer to vacuum and dust the house when she's visiting. Let your folks take the older kids to the zoo on Sunday. Enlist a friend to baby-sit so you can have a night out occasionally.

Get an hour or two more sleep each night. Skip the eleven o'clock news and turn in earlier; ask your spouse to fix breakfast so you can turn out later.

Be sure that your diet isn't deficient. First-trimester fatigue is often aggravated by a deficiency in iron, protein, or just plain calories. Double-check to make certain you're filling all of your Pregnancy Diet requirements. And no matter how tired you're feeling, don't be tempted to rev up your body with caffeine and candy bars. The energy won't last for long, and after the temporary lift, your blood sugar will plummet, leaving you more fatigued than ever.

Check your environment. Inadequate lighting, poor air circulation or quality ("sick building" syndrome), or excessive noise in your home or workplace can contribute to fatigue. Be alert to these problems and try to get them corrected.

Take a hike. Or a *slow* jog. Or a stroll to the grocery store. Or do a pregnancy exercise or yoga routine. Paradoxically, too much rest and not enough activity can heighten fatigue. But don't overdo the exercise. Stop before that exercise high dissolves into a low, and be sure to follow the precautionary guidelines on page 190.

Though fatigue will probably ease up by month 4, you can expect it to return in the last trimester (could it be nature's way of preparing you for the long sleepless nights you will encounter once the baby has arrived?).

When fatigue is severe, especially if it is accompanied by fainting, pallor, breathlessness, and/or palpitations, it's wise to report it to your practitioner (see Anemia, page 187).

MORNING SICKNESS

"I haven't had any morning sickness. Can I still be pregnant?"

Morning sickness, like a craving for pickles and ice cream, is one of those truisms about pregnancy that ain't necessarily so. Studies show that a little more than one-half of all expectant women experience the nausea and vomiting associated with morning sickness—which means that a little less than one half don't. If you're among those who never suffer from it, or who feel only occasionally or mildly queasy, you can consider yourself not only pregnant but lucky.

"My morning sickness lasts all day. I'm afraid that I'm not keeping down enough food to nourish my baby."

Fortunately, the typical case of morning sickness (a misnamed malady, because it can strike morning, noon, or night—or, as in your case, last all day long) rarely interferes with proper nutrition enough to harm the developing fetus. Even women who actually lose weight during the first few months of pregnancy because they have a hard time keeping any food down are not hurting their baby—as long as they make up for the lost weight in later months. And for most women, the symptoms of morning sickness don't linger much beyond the third month, though an occasional expectant mother will experience them into the second trimester and a few, particularly those expecting a multiple birth, may suffer for a full nine months.

What causes morning sickness? No one knows for sure, but there's no shortage of theories. It is known that the command post for nausea and vomiting is located in the brain stem. A myriad of reasons have been suggested for why this area may be overstimulated during pregnancy, including the high level of the pregnancy hormone hCG in the blood in the first trimester, elevated estrogen levels, the rapid stretching of the uterine muscles, the relative relaxation of muscle tissue in the digestive tract (which makes digestion less efficient), excess acid in the stomach, and the enhanced sense of smell pregnant women develop.

Not all pregnant women experience morning sickness, and among those who do, not all experience it to the same degree. Some have only occasional queasy moments, others feel nauseated round the clock but never vomit, and still others vomit frequently. There are probably several reasons for these variations:

Hormone levels. Higher-than-normal levels (as when a woman is carrying multiple fetuses) can increase morning sickness; lower levels may minimize or eliminate it.

The response of the brain's nausea and vomiting command post to pregnancy hormones and other triggers. This response can affect whether or not a woman experiences morning sickness and to what degree. A woman whose command center is particularly sensitive (for example, she always gets carsick or seasick) is likely to have more severe nausea and vomiting in pregnancy.

Stress levels. It's well known that stress of various kinds can trigger gastrointestinal upset, so it's not surprising that symptoms tend to worsen when stress strikes.

Fatigue. Physical or mental fatigue can also increase the risk of morning sickness and exacerbate symptoms (conversely, severe morning sickness can increase fatigue).

The fact that morning sickness is more common and tends to be more severe in first pregnancies supports the concept that both physical and psychological factors may be involved. Physically, the novice pregnant body is less prepared for the onslaught of hormones and other changes it's experiencing than one that has been through it before. Emotionally, those pregnant for the first time are more likely to be subject to the kinds of anxieties and fears that can turn a stomach; whereas women in subsequent pregnancies may be distracted from their nausea by the demands of caring for older children. (But some women experience more nausea in subsequent pregnancies than they did in their first.)

No matter the cause, the effect of morning sickness is pure misery for the woman who is experiencing it; she needs all the support she can get—from her spouse, family, friends, and practitioner. Unfortunately, there is presently no cure for morning sickness but the passing of time. However, there are ways of alleviating its symptoms while minimizing its effects on your pregnancy.

◆ Eat a diet high in protein and complex carbohydrates, both of which fight nausea. General good nutrition may help, too, so eat as well as you can under the circumstances.

◆ Drink plenty of fluids, especially if you're losing liquid through vomiting. If they are easier to get down than solids when you're feeling green, use them to get your nutrients. Concentrate on any of the following that you can handle: Double-the-Milk Shake (see page 101); fruit or vegetable juices; soups, broths, and bouillons. If you find fluids make you queasier, eat solids with a high water content, such as fresh fruits and vegetables—particularly lettuce, melons, and citrus fruits. Some women find that drinking and eating at the same sitting puts too much strain on their digestive tract; if this is true for you, try taking your fluids between meals.

♦ Take a prenatal vitamin supplement (see page 93) to compensate for nutrients you may not be getting. But take it at a time of day when you are least likely to chuck it back up—possibly with a substantial bedtime snack.

♦ Avoid the sight, smell, and taste of foods that make you queasy. Avoid food smells entirely if they trigger nausea—which they do in many pregnant women, thanks to a more sensitive sense of smell. Don't be a martyr and prepare sausage and eggs for your spouse if the aroma sends you rushing to the bathroom. If odors from the neighbors' apartment are offensive, put some towels under the doors to try to block them; exhaust fans at the windows may also help.

And don't force yourself to eat foods that don't appeal or, worse, make you sick. Instead, with a little nutritional guidance from your conscience, let your eyes, nose, and taste buds be your guides in menu planning. Choose only sweet foods if they're all you can tolerate (get your vitamin A and protein from yellow peaches and cottage cheese at dinner instead of from broccoli and chicken). Or select only savories if they're your ticket to a less tumultuous tummy (have a grilled cheese and tomato sandwich for breakfast instead of cereal and orange juice).

♦ Eat early and often—before you feel hungry. When your stomach is empty, its acids have nothing to digest but its own lining. This can trigger nausea. So can the low blood sugar caused by long stretches between meals. Six small meals are better than three large ones. Carry nutritious snacks (dried fruit, whole-grain crackers or pretzels) with you for snacking.

♦ Eat in bed—for the same reasons you should eat often: to avoid an empty stomach and to keep your blood sugar at an even keel. Before you go to sleep at night, have a snack that is high in protein and complex carbohydrates: a glass of milk and a bran muffin, for example. Twenty minutes before you plan to get out of bed in the morning, have a high-carbohydrate snack: a few whole-wheat crackers or rice cakes, dry cereal, or a handful of raisins. Keep nibbles next to the bed so you don't have to get up for them, in case you wake up hungry in the middle of the night. If you start to associate a particular carbohydrate snack (crackers, for instance) with your nausea, switch to a different snack.

♦ Get some extra sleep and relaxation. Both emotional and physical fatigue can exacerbate nausea.

♦ Greet the morning in slow motion. Don't jump out of bed and dash out the door—rushing tends to aggravate nausea. Instead, stay in bed digesting your snack for twenty minutes, then rise slowly to a leisurely breakfast. If you have older children, let your spouse handle their early morning needs so you can have some quiet time.

♦ Brush your teeth (with a toothpaste that doesn't increase queasiness) or rinse your mouth after each bout of vomiting, as well as after each meal.

(Ask your dentist to recommend a good rinse.) Not only will this help keep your mouth fresh and reduce nausea, it will decrease the risk of damage to teeth or gums that can occur when bacteria feast on regurgitated residue in your mouth.

- Minimize stress. Morning sickness is more common among women who are under a great deal of stress, at work, at home, or both. See page 125 for tips on dealing with stress during pregnancy.

- Try Sea-Bands. The one-inch-wide elastic bands, worn on both wrists, put pressure on acupressure points on the inner wrists and often relieve nausea. They cause no side effects and are widely available at drug and health food stores. Or your practitioner may recommend a more sophisticated form of acupressure: a battery-operated wristband—called the Relief Band—that uses electronic stimulation.

- Try complementary medical approaches (see page 246), such as acupuncture, acupressure, biofeedback, or hypnosis, which often work to lessen nausea. Meditation and visualization can also work for some women.

- Turn to ginger, a spice long known for its tummy-taming properties. Try ginger candies, foods prepared with real ginger, real ginger ale—even the smell of fresh ginger can quell the queasies for some women.

- If nothing else helps, ask your doctor about a prescription of B6 and antihistamines which seems to relieve nausea in some women. Do not take any medication (traditional or herbal) for morning sickness unless it is prescribed by your practitioner.

In an estimated 7 of every 2,000 pregnancies, nausea and vomiting become so severe that medical treatment is needed. If this seems to be the case with you, see page 512.

EXCESS SALIVA

"My mouth seems to fill up with saliva all the time—and swallowing it makes me queasy. What's going on?"

Overproduction of saliva is another common symptom of pregnancy. It's unpleasant but harmless, and typically short-lived, usually disappearing after the first few months. It's more common in women who are also experiencing morning sickness, and it seems to compound the queasiness. There's no sure cure, but brushing your teeth frequently with a minty toothpaste, rinsing with a minty mouthwash, or chewing sugarless gum can help dry things up a bit.

FREQUENT URINATION

"I'm in the bathroom every half hour. Is it normal to be urinating this often?"

Most—though by no means all— pregnant women do make frequent trips to the toilet in both the first and last trimesters. One of the reasons for an initial increase in urinary frequency is the increased volume of body fluids and the improved efficiency of the kidneys, which helps rid the body more quickly of waste products. Another is the pressure of the growing uterus when it is in the pelvis, next to the bladder. This pressure on the bladder is often relieved once the uterus rises into the abdominal cavity, around the fourth month, and doesn't usually return until the third trimester or when the baby "drops" back down into the pelvis in the ninth month. But because the arrangement of internal organs varies slightly from woman to woman, the degree of urinary frequency in pregnancy may also vary. Some women barely notice it; others are bothered by it for most of the nine months.

Leaning forward when you urinate will help ensure that you empty your bladder completely and may reduce trips to the bathroom. If you find that you go frequently during the night, try limiting—but not eliminating—fluids in the hours before bedtime. Don't, however, limit them during the rest of the day.

"How come I'm not urinating frequently?"

No noticeable increase in the frequency of urination may be perfectly normal for you, especially if you ordinarily urinate often. You should, however, be certain you're getting enough fluids (at least eight glasses a day). Not only can insufficient fluid intake be the cause of infrequent urination, it could also lead to urinary tract infection.

BREAST CHANGES

"I hardly recognize my breasts anymore—they're so huge. And they're tender, too. Will they stay that way, and will they sag after I give birth?"

Get used to the chesty look for now; although it may not always be in fashion, it's one of the hallmarks of pregnancy. Your breasts are swollen and tender because of the increased amounts of estrogen and progesterone your body is producing. (The same mechanism operates premenstrually, when many women experience breast changes—but the changes are more pronounced in pregnancy.) These changes are not random; they are aimed at preparing you to feed your baby when it arrives.

In addition to their expanding size, you will probably notice other changes in your breasts. The areola (the pigmented area around the nipple) will darken, spread, and may be spotted with even darker areas. This darkening may fade but not disappear entirely after birth. The little bumps you may notice on the areola are sweat glands, which become more prominent during pregnancy and return to normal afterward. The complex road map of blue veins that traverses the breasts—often quite vivid on a fair-skinned woman—represents a mother-to-baby delivery system for nutrients and fluids. After delivery—or, if you're breastfeeding, sometime after nursing is discontinued—the skin's appearance will return to normal.

What you won't have to get used to, fortunately, is the sometimes agonizing sensitivity of newly pregnant breasts. Though they will continue to grow throughout your pregnancy—possibly increasing as much as three cup sizes—they are not likely to remain tender to the touch past the third or fourth month. As for whether or not they will sag after the baby is born, that is at least partly up to you. Stretching and sagging of the breast tissue result not just from pregnancy itself, but from a lack of support during pregnancy (though the tendency to sag may also be genetic). No matter how firm your breasts are now, protect them for the future by wearing a good support bra. If your breasts are particularly large or have a tendency to sag, it's a good idea to wear a bra even at night. You will probably find a stretchy cotton sports bra most comfortable for sleeping.

If your breasts enlarge early in pregnancy and then suddenly diminish in size (and especially if other pregnancy symptoms also disappear without explanation), contact your practitioner.

"My breasts became very large in my first pregnancy, but they haven't seemed to change at all now that I'm in my second. Could something be wrong?"

Small-chested women who look forward to having their cups running over in pregnancy are sometimes in for a disappointment, at least temporarily, the second or third time around. Though some experience as much enlargement early on as they did in their first pregnancy, others do not—perhaps because the breasts, thanks to their previous experience, don't require as much preparation and respond to the pregnancy hormones less dramatically. In these women, the breasts may gradually enlarge during pregnancy, or may hold off their expansion until after delivery, when milk production begins.

VITAMIN SUPPLEMENTS

"Should I be taking vitamins?"

Virtually no one gets a nutritionally perfect diet every day, especially early in pregnancy, when morning sickness is a common appetite suppressant, or when the little nutrition some women manage to get down often doesn't stay down. While a daily vitamin supplement can't take the place of a good prenatal diet, it can serve as some dietary insurance, guaranteeing that your baby won't be cheated if you don't always hit the nutritional heights you're aiming for. And there are other good reasons to take your vitamins. For one thing, studies have shown that women who take a vitamin supplement containing folic acid during the first months of pregnancy (and even prior to pregnancy) significantly reduce the risk of neural tube defects (such as spina bifida) and possibly other birth defects in their babies. For another, at least one study has shown that taking a supplement containing at least 10 mg of vitamin B_6 before and during early pregnancy can minimize morning sickness.

Good formulations designed especially for expectant mothers are available by prescription or over the counter. (See page 93 for what the supplement should contain.) Do not take any kind of dietary supplements other than such a prenatal formula without your practitioner's approval.

Some women find that taking a vitamin supplement increases nausea, especially early in pregnancy. Switching formulas may help, as may taking your pill with food (unless you usually throw up after eating). A coated pill is likely to be easier to tolerate, as well as easier to swallow. If even that bothers you, you might consider a chewable supplement. But be sure the formula you select approximates the requirements for supplements designed for pregnancy. If your practitioner prescribed your supplement, check with him or her before switching.

In some women, the iron in a prenatal vitamin causes constipation or diarrhea. Again, switching formulas may bring relief. Taking a pregnancy supplement without iron and a separate iron preparation (your doctor can prescribe one that dissolves in the intestines rather than in the more sensitive stomach) may also reduce irritation and relieve symptoms. Discuss the possibilities with your practitioner.

"I eat a lot of cereals and breads that are enriched. If I'm also taking a prenatal supplement, will I be taking in too many vitamins and minerals?"

You can get too much of a good thing, but not usually this way. Taking a prenatal vitamin along with the average diet, which includes plenty of enriched and fortified products, isn't likely to lead to excessive intake of vitamins and minerals. To take in that many nutrients, you'd have to be adding other supplements beyond the prenatal ones—which an expectant mother should never do unless instructed by a physician who knows that she's pregnant. It's wise, however, to be wary of any foods that are fortified with more than the DRI of vitamins A, D, E, and K, since these can be toxic in large amounts. Most other vitamins and minerals are water-soluble, which means any excesses that the body can't use are simply excreted in the urine. Which is, by the way, the reason why supplement-crazy Americans are said to have the most expensive urine in the world.

LOWER ABDOMINAL PRESSURE

"I've been having a nagging feeling of pressure in my lower abdomen. Should I be worried about miscarriage or ectopic pregnancy?"

It sounds like you're very tuned into your body—which can be a good thing (as when it helps you recognize ovulation) or a not-so-good thing (when it makes you worry about the many innocuous aches and pains of pregnancy).

Don't worry. A feeling of pressure (without accompanying pain, bleeding, or other related symptoms) is not a symptom of miscarriage or ectopic pregnancy, and it is common, especially in first pregnancies. Chances are, that sensitive body radar of yours is just picking up some of the many changes that are taking place in your lower abdomen, where your uterus is currently located. What you're feeling may be the sensation of implantation, increased blood flow, the buildup of the uterine lining, or, simply of your uterus beginning to grow.

For further reassurance, ask your practitioner about the feeling (if you're still having it) at your next office visit.

MISCARRIAGE

"Between what I read and what my mother tells me, I'm afraid everything I've done, am doing, and will do might cause a miscarriage."

For many expectant women, the fear of miscarriage keeps their joy guarded in the first trimester. It may even keep them from spreading their happy news until the fourth month, when they begin to feel secure that the pregnancy will indeed continue. And for most of them, it will.

There is still much to be learned about the reasons behind early miscarriage, but several factors are believed *not to cause* the problem. They include:

♦ Previous trouble with an IUD. Scarring of the endometrium (the lining of the uterus) caused by an IUD-triggered infection could prevent a pregnancy from implanting in the uterus, but should not cause miscarriage once implantation is well established. Nor should previous difficulty holding an IUD in place affect a pregnancy.

♦ History of multiple abortions.[3] Scarring of the endometrium from multiple abortions, as from IUD-caused infections, could prevent implantation but should not otherwise be responsible for early miscarriage.

♦ Brief emotional upset—resulting from an argument, or momentary stress at work or at home.

♦ A fall or other minor accidental injury. But *serious* injury could result in miscarriage, so safety precautions—such as wearing a seat belt in the car

---

3. Though not a direct cause of early miscarriage, repeated abortions or other procedures requiring dilation of the cervix may result in a weakened or incompetent cervix—often a cause of late miscarriage (see page 35).

and not climbing on unsteady ladders—should always be observed.

◆ Usual and accustomed physical activity, such as housework; lifting children, groceries, or other moderately heavy objects; hanging curtains; moving light furniture; and moderate and safe exercise.[4]

◆ Sexual intercourse—unless a woman has a history of miscarriage or is otherwise at high risk for pregnancy loss.

There are several factors, however, that *are* believed to somewhat increase the risk of miscarriage. Some factors (poor nutrition; smoking; hormonal insufficiency or imbalance; infection with bacterial vaginosis, chlamydia, or certain other STDs; and certain chronic maternal medical problems, including lupus, congenital heart disease, severe kidney disease, diabetes, thyroid disease), once identified, can usually be eliminated or controlled. Others (infection with rubella or other diseases harmful to the fetus; exposure to large doses of radiation or to drugs harmful to the fetus; a high fever; or an IUD in place at conception) are not easily avoided, but because they are generally onetime events, they are not likely to recur in future pregnancies. A few miscarriage risk factors (such as a malformed uterus, large uterine fibroids, and certain chronic maternal illnesses) are more difficult to overcome, though even these can sometimes be dealt with through surgery or other medical procedures.

Rarely, repeated miscarriages are traced to the mother's immune cells attacking cells in the embryo. Immunotherapy may be helpful in such instances.

4. In a high-risk pregnancy, the physician may limit these activities or even prescribe strict bed rest. But you need limit activity only on direction of your doctor.

When not to worry. It's important to recognize that each cramp, ache, or bit of spotting isn't necessarily a warning of an impending miscarriage. Just about every normal pregnancy will include at least one of these usually innocuous symptoms at one time or another. And though you should report them to your practitioner at your next visit (or sooner if you need some professional reassurance), the following are no cause for concern. *Don't worry* if you have:

◆ Mild cramps, achiness, or a pulling sensation on one or both sides of the abdomen. This is probably caused by the stretching of ligaments that support the uterus. Unless cramping is severe, constant, or accompanied by bleeding, there's no need to worry.

◆ Slight staining a little before or around the time you would have expected your period, about seven to ten days after conception, when the little ball of cells that is going to develop into your baby attaches itself to the uterine wall. Slight bleeding at this time is common and doesn't necessarily indicate a problem with your pregnancy—as long as it isn't accompanied by lower abdominal pain.

◆ Light pink spotting after intercourse. A pregnant woman's cervix becomes more tender and engorged with blood vessels as the pregnancy progresses, and occasionally becomes irritated during intercourse, causing some slight bleeding. This type of bleeding is common and usually doesn't indicate a problem unless the bleeding becomes heavy or is accompanied by cramps. Tell your practitioner about any postintercourse spotting.

POSSIBLE SIGNS OF MISCARRIAGE

When to Call Your Practitioner Immediately, Just in Case

◆ When you experience bleeding with cramps or pain in the center of your lower abdomen. (Severe pain and tenderness on one side in early pregnancy could be triggered by an ectopic pregnancy, and also warrants a call to the practitioner; see page 124.)

◆ When pain is severe or continues unabated for more than one day, even if it isn't accompanied by staining or bleeding.

◆ When bleeding is as heavy as a menstrual period, or light staining continues for more than three days.

◆ When you have a history of miscarriage, and experience either bleeding or cramping or both.

When to Get Emergency Medical Attention

◆ When bleeding is heavy enough to soak several pads in an hour, or when pain is so severe you can't bear it.

◆ When you pass clots or grayish or pink material—which may mean a miscarriage has already begun. If you can't reach your practitioner, go to the nearest emergency room or to the one recommended by his or her office. The doctor may want you to save the material you pass (in a jar, plastic bag, or other clean container) so it can be determined whether or not the miscarriage is simply threatening, is complete, or is incomplete and requires a D & C (dilation and curettage) to complete it.

If you suspect miscarriage. If you experience any of the symptoms listed in the box above, put a call in to your practitioner. If your symptoms are listed under "When to Get Emergency Medical Attention" and your practitioner is not available, leave a message for him or her, and either call 911 or your local EMS (emergency medical service) or head straight to the nearest emergency room.

While waiting for help, lie down if you can, or rest in a chair with your feet up. This may not prevent a miscarriage if it's about to happen, but it should help you to relax. It might also help you to know that most women who have episodes of bleeding in early pregnancy carry to term and deliver healthy babies.

If miscarriage is suspected or diagnosed, see page 492.

"I don't really feel pregnant. Could I have miscarried and not noticed it?"

It's hard to feel pregnant this early in the game, even if you're experiencing such early pregnancy symptoms as morning sickness and fatigue—and especially if you aren't. And it's likely the pregnancy will continue to be an abstract concept for a while, or at least until there's some tangible proof of it—a bulging belly, for instance, or the sound of the baby's heartbeat. But fear of miscarrying without realizing it, while common, is almost always unwarranted. Once a pregnancy is established, the signs that it is aborting are not easily overlooked. Simply "not feeling pregnant" is not, at this point, a reason for concern. For additional reassurance, share your concern with your practitioner at your next visit.

The Condition of Your Baby

"I'm very nervous because I can't really feel my baby. Could it die without my knowing it?"

At this stage, with no noticeable belly swelling and no obvious fetal activity, it's hard to imagine that there's really a living, growing baby inside you. But the death of a fetus or embryo that isn't expelled from the uterus in a miscarriage is *very* rare. When it does happen, a woman eventually loses all signs of pregnancy, including breast tenderness and enlargement, and may develop a brownish discharge, though no actual bleeding. Upon examination, the practitioner will find that the uterus has diminished in size.

If at any time all of your pregnancy symptoms suddenly disappear or you feel as though your uterus isn't growing, call your practitioner. That's a more positive approach than worrying.

Ectopic Pregnancy

"I've been having occasional cramping. Could I have an ectopic pregnancy?"

Very few pregnancies are ectopic, that is, implanted outside the uterus, usually in the fallopian tubes.[5] A good many of these are diagnosed before a woman even realizes she is pregnant. So chances are, if your practitioner has confirmed your pregnancy through a blood test and a physical exam and you've had no signs of ectopic pregnancy, then you can cross this worry off your list.

There are several factors that can make women more susceptible to ectopic pregnancy, including:

5. This usually occurs because some irregularity in the tube blocks the passage of the egg down to the uterus. Rarely, the fertilized egg implants in the ovary, the abdominal cavity, or the cervix.

- A previous ectopic pregnancy
- Previous pelvic inflammatory disease caused by a sexually transmitted disease
- Previous abdominal or fallopian tube surgery with postoperative scarring
- Tubal ligation (surgical sterilization), unsuccessful tubal ligation, or tubal ligation reversal
- An IUD in place when conception occurs (an IUD is more likely to prevent conception in the uterus than outside it—increasing the risk of ectopics in IUD users)
- *Possibly*, multiple induced abortions
- *Possibly*, exposure of the mother to diethylstilbestrol (DES) when she was in the womb, especially if it resulted in significant structural abnormalities of the reproductive tract

Rare as ectopic pregnancy is, every pregnant woman—particularly those at high risk—should be familiar with the symptoms. Occasional cramping, probably the result of implantation, increased blood flow, or ligaments stretching as the uterus grows, is *not* one of them. But any or all of the following might be, and require immediate evaluation by a physician. If you can't reach your physician, go at once to the hospital emergency room.

- Sharp, crampy pain with tenderness, usually in the lower abdomen—on one side initially, though the pain can radiate throughout the abdomen. Pain may worsen on straining of bowels, coughing, or moving. If tubal rupture occurs, pain becomes very sharp and steady for a short time before diffusing throughout the pelvic region.
- Brown vaginal spotting or light bleeding (intermittent or continuous), which may precede pain by several

days or weeks, though sometimes there is no bleeding unless the tube ruptures.

◆ Heavy vaginal bleeding, if the tube ruptures.

◆ Nausea and vomiting—in about 25 percent to 50 percent of women—though this may be difficult to distinguish from morning sickness.

◆ Dizziness or weakness, in some women. If the tube ruptures, weak pulse, clammy skin, and fainting are common.

◆ Shoulder pain (referred from the pelvis), in some women.

◆ Feeling of rectal pressure, in some women.

If an ectopic pregnancy is present, quick medical attention can often save the fallopian tube and the woman's fertility (see page 498 for the treatment of ectopic pregnancies). In fact, studies show that more than half of the women treated for ectopic pregnancy spontaneously conceive and have a normal pregnancy within a year.

STRESS IN YOUR LIFE

"My job is a high-stress one. I wasn't planning to have a baby now, but I got pregnant. Should I quit work?"

Stress has, over the past couple of decades, become an important area for study because of the effect it can have on our lives. Depending on how we handle and respond to it, stress can be good for us (by sparking us to perform better, to function more effectively) or it can be bad for us (when it gets out of control, overwhelming and debilitating us). If the stress at work has you working at top efficiency, has you excited and challenged, then it shouldn't be harmful to your

pregnancy. But if the stress makes you anxious, sleepless, or depressed, if it is causing you to experience physical symptoms (such as headache, backache, or loss of appetite), or if it is exhausting you (see page 114 for tips on handling fatigue), then it could be harmful. In fact, research indicates that *extreme* prenatal maternal stress and the stress hormones it produces may increase the risk of preterm delivery or low birthweight.

Negative reactions to stress can be compounded by the normal mood swings in pregnancy. Since reactions such as appetite loss, bingeing on the wrong foods, or sleeplessness can take a toll on you—and on your baby, if allowed to continue into the second and third trimesters—learning to handle the stress constructively should become a priority now. The following should help:

Talk about it. Allowing your anxieties to surface is the best way of making sure they don't get you down. Maintain open lines of communication with your spouse, spending some time at the end of each day (preferably not too close to bedtime) sharing and talking out concerns and frustrations. Together you may be able to find some relief, some solutions, even some humor, in your respective situations. You may also find it helpful to talk to another family member, your practitioner, a friend, or a member of the clergy—or to join a pregnancy support group, if one is available in your community. If nothing seems to help, consider professional counseling.

Do something about it. Identify sources of stress in your life and determine how they can be modified. If you're clearly trying to do too much, cut back in areas that are not high priority. If you've taken on too many responsibilities at home or at work, decide which can be postponed or delegated to someone else. Learn to say no to new projects or activities before you're overloaded.

Sometimes sitting down with a notepad or electronic organizer and making lists of the hundreds of things you need to get done (at home or at work), and the order in which you're planning to do them, can help you feel more in control of the chaos in your life. Cross items off your list as they're taken care of for a satisfying sense of accomplishment.

Sleep it off. Sleep is the ticket to regeneration—for mind and body. Often feelings of tension and anxiety are prompted by not getting enough shut-eye. If you're having trouble sleeping, see the tips on page 183.

Nourish it. Hectic lifestyles can lead to hectic eating styles. Inadequate nutrition during pregnancy can be a double whammy: it can hamper your ability to handle stress and it can affect your baby's growth and development. So be sure to get three large or six small square meals a day plus plenty of snacks.

Wash it away. A warm bath (but not a hot one) is an excellent way to relieve tension. Try it after a hectic day; it will also help you to sleep better.

Get away from it temporarily. Combat stress with any activity you find relaxing—sports (check first with your practitioner, and observe the guidelines starting on page 190); reading; a good movie; listening to music (consider taking a portable CD player with headphones to work so you can listen to relaxing music during coffee breaks and lunch, or even while you work, if that's feasible); long walks (or short ones during breaks or lunch—but be sure to leave time for eating); meditation (just close your eyes and picture a bucolic scene, or keep them open and gaze at a soothing picture or photo placed strategically in your office); biofeedback; massage (ask your spouse for a back or shoulder rub, or splurge on a professional massage—but make sure the therapist is licensed and knows you're pregnant). Practice relaxation techniques (see box on the facing page), not just because they'll come in handy during childbirth, but because they can help drain the strain anytime.

THE BRIGHT SIDE OF OPTIMISM

It's long been speculated that optimistic people live longer, healthier lives. Now it's been suggested that an expectant mother's optimistic outlook can actually improve the outlook for her unborn baby, too. A recent study found that seeing the bright side reduces the chance of a high-risk woman delivering a preterm or low-birthweight baby.

A lower level of stress in optimistic women definitely plays a part in the lowered risk; high levels of stress, after all, have been implicated in a variety of health problems both in and out of pregnancy. But stress itself doesn't, apparently, tell the whole story. Women who are optimistic are, not surprisingly, more likely to take better care of themselves—eating well, exercising more, avoiding drugs, alcohol, and other harmful substances. And these positive behaviors—fueled by the power of positive thinking—can, of course, have a very positive effect on pregnancy and fetal well-being.

Researchers point out that it's never too late to start reaping the benefits of optimism, even if you're already pregnant. Learning how to expect the best—instead of the worst—can actually help make those expectations come true.

A good reason to start seeing that glass of milk as half full instead of half empty.

RELAXATION MADE EASY

There are many routes to relaxation, including yoga and meditation. You can attend a group course in either of these stress-busters, or learn techniques privately from an instructor. Or, if there's just no time in your busy schedule for either of these options, you can try these simple relaxation techniques, which are easy to learn and to do anywhere, anytime. If you find them helpful, you can do them when anxiety strikes and/or regularly several times a day to try to ward it off.

1. Sit with your eyes closed. Picture a beautiful scene—one that makes you feel peaceful. Then consciously relax your muscles, starting with those in your feet and working up slowly through the legs, torso, neck, and face. Breathe only through the nose (unless it's too stuffy, of course). As you breathe out, repeat the word "one" (or "peace," or any other simple word) to yourself. Continue the repetitions for ten to twenty minutes.

2. Inhale slowly and deeply through your nose, pushing your abdomen out as you do. Count to four. Then, letting your shoulders and neck muscles relax, exhale slowly and comfortably to the count of six. Repeat this sequence four or five times to banish tension.

Get away from it permanently. Maybe the problem isn't worth the stress and anxiety it's generating. For example, if it's your job, consider taking early maternity leave or cutting back to part-time (if either of these options is financially feasible), or temporarily switching positions or delegating at least part of your workload to reduce stress to a manageable level.

Remember, your stress quotient is only going to increase once the baby is born; it makes sense to try to learn how to handle it now.

OVERWHELMING FEAR ABOUT THE BABY'S HEALTH

"I know it's irrational, but I can't sleep or eat or concentrate at work because I'm afraid my baby won't be normal."

Every expectant mother—and father—worries about whether her baby will be normal. Although a moderate dose of worry that doesn't respond to reassurance is an unavoidable side effect of pregnancy, worry that is all-consuming and interferes with functioning needs attention. Talk to your practitioner. Perhaps an ultrasound evaluation of the fetus and/or prenatal screening tests are already on the schedule or can be arranged to help calm your fears. Many practitioners are willing to order these procedures when a patient is extremely anxious, particularly if she feels she has a specific reason to fear for her baby's health (perhaps she spent a lot of time in a hot tub or had a few too many a few too many times before she found out she was pregnant), and even if her concerns seem unfounded or exaggerated. This is because the cost of the procedures is outweighed by the potential price of overwhelming anxiety (especially if it is keeping the mother-to-be from eating and sleeping).

Though these tests can't detect every potential problem, they can, once significant fetal development has taken place, show a great deal. Even the outline on the ultrasound of a normal baby—with all its limbs and organs in place—can offer enormous comfort. That, teamed with other good test results and verbal reassurance from your practitioner (and perhaps from the specialist who has evaluated the ultrasound), can help you get on with the vital business at hand: caring for yourself and nourishing your baby. You might find comfort, too, talking to other expectant mothers—perhaps in an early pregnancy class or chat room; after all, just hearing that everyone else has the same concerns can be reassuring.

If nothing seems to calm you down, professional counseling may be needed to reduce anxiety.

DEPRESSION

"I know I should feel happy about my pregnancy, but I seem to be suffering from postpartum depression prematurely."

You may be mistaking depression for the very normal mood swings of pregnancy—experienced by about 7 in 10 expectant mothers. These swings may be more pronounced in the first trimester and, in general, in women who ordinarily suffer from emotional ups and downs before their periods. Feelings of ambivalence about the pregnancy once it's confirmed, which are common even when a pregnancy is planned, may exaggerate the swings still more. Though there's no cure for mood swings, avoiding sugar, chocolate, and caffeine (all of which can push a low even lower), following the Pregnancy Diet, getting a good balance of rest and exercise, and talking your feelings out can help to keep those mood swings on the upside as much as possible.

If your lows are consistent or frequent, you may be one of the 10 percent to 20 percent of pregnant women who battle mild to moderate depression during pregnancy. Depression during pregnancy can increase risks for compli-

cations—much as depression can affect the body when you're not pregnant. Some of the factors that can put a woman at risk for such depression are:

◆ A personal or family history of mood disorder

◆ Financial or marital stress

◆ Lack of emotional support from and communication with the baby's father

◆ Hospitalization or bed rest because of pregnancy complications

◆ Anxiety about her own health, especially if she has a chronic medical condition or has previously experienced complications or illness during pregnancy

◆ Anxiety about her baby's health, especially if there is a personal or family history of miscarriage, neonatal loss, birth defects or other problems

The most common symptoms of true depression, in addition to feeling sad, empty, and emotionally lethargic,

FOR THE OTHER PREGNANT HALF

There isn't a page in this book that isn't intended for both expectant mothers and fathers. As a father-to-be, you'll gain plenty of insight into the pregnancy experience (as well as make some sense out of those crazy symptoms your spouse has been complaining about) by reading along with her, month by month. But because you're likely to have some questions and concerns that are uniquely yours, there's a chapter dedicated to you—the other pregnant half. See Chapter 17: *Fathers Are Expectant, Too.*

include: sleep disturbances (you get too much or too little); changed eating habits (not eating at all or eating continually); prolonged or unusual fatigue and/or excessive agitation or restlessness; extended loss of interest in work, play, and other activities or pleasures; reduced ability to concentrate and think; exaggerated mood swings; and even self-destructive thoughts. There may also be unexplained aches and pains. If that sounds like what you're experiencing, start by trying those tips for dealing with postpartum depression that seem applicable to your life now (see page 412).

If the symptoms continue for longer than two weeks, speak to your practitioner about your depression or ask for a referral to a therapist who can offer supportive psychotherapy.[6] Getting the right help is important, because depression can keep you from taking optimum care of yourself and your baby, now and after delivery. Deciding whether antidepressant medication will be part of the treatment plan will require sitting down with your practitioner (and therapist) to weigh possible risks against possible benefits. While SSRIs (selective serotonin reuptake inhibitors) such as Prozac and Zoloft can be used late in pregnancy, there is the chance they can cause very brief jitteriness and shakiness in a baby just after birth. Consultation with your practitioner will be necessary before beginning or continuing these or other antidepressants during your pregnancy.

Consult your practitioner, too, before turning to any alternative treatments. Over-the-counter supplements, such as SAM-e and St. John's Wort, touted for their mood-elevating properties, have not been studied enough to consider them safe for use in pregnancy. But bright light therapy (which increases levels of the mood-regulating hormone serotonin in the brain) has been shown to cut depressive symptoms during pregnancy in half. And eating fish and seafood rich in fatty acids has been shown to lower the risk of depression during pregnancy and after.

Being depressed during pregnancy does put you at somewhat greater risk of postpartum depression. The good news is that getting the right treatment during pregnancy—and/or right after delivery—can help prevent postpartum depression. Ask your practitioner about this.

PICKING UP OLDER CHILDREN

"Should I be picking up my two-year-old now that I'm pregnant again? She's pretty heavy."

You'll have to come up with a better excuse to get her to walk on her own two feet. Unless your practitioner has instructed you otherwise, carrying moderately heavy loads (even a strapping preschooler) is okay, though you should avoid exerting yourself to the point of exhaustion (see page 210 for tips on avoiding back strain when lifting). And, in fact, blaming your child's as yet unborn sibling for your reluctance to carry her can needlessly set up feelings of rivalry and resentment toward the baby even before the pint-size competition arrives on the scene.

As your pregnancy progresses, however, your back may not be amenable to the strain of toting both a fetus and a toddler, and in that case, you should keep the lifting to a minimum. But be sure you blame your back, and not the baby, for this slowdown in pickups, and compensate for it with plenty of holding and hugging from a sitting position.

---

6. Because depression can also be a symptom of a thyroid condition (which requires prompt treatment during pregnancy), a blood test should rule that possibility out first if it hasn't already.

WHEN TO CALL THE PRACTITIONER

It's best to set up a protocol for emergency with your practitioner before an emergency strikes. If you haven't, and you are experiencing a symptom that requires immediate medical attention, try the following: First call the practitioner's office. If he or she isn't available and doesn't call back within a few minutes, call again and leave a message saying what your problem is and where you are headed. Then go directly to the nearest emergency room or dial 911 or your local EMS (emergency medical service).

When you report any of the following, be sure to mention any other symptoms you may be experiencing, no matter how unrelated they may seem to the immediate problem. Also be specific, mentioning when you first noticed each symptom, how frequently it recurs, what seems to relieve or exacerbate it, and how severe it is.

CALL IMMEDIATELY FOR ANY OF THE FOLLOWING:

◆ Severe lower abdominal pain, on one or both sides, that doesn't subside and is accompanied by bleeding, or nausea and vomiting

◆ Severe upper-midabdominal pain, with or without nausea, and swelling of hands and face

◆ Heavy vaginal bleeding (especially when combined with abdominal or back pain)

◆ Coughing up of blood

◆ A gush or steady leaking of fluid from the vagina

◆ A sudden increase in thirst, accompanied by reduced urination, or no urination at all for an entire day

◆ Painful or burning urination, if accompanied by chills and fever over 102°F and/or backache

◆ Very sudden and severe swelling or puffiness of hands, face, and eyes, accompanied by headache, vision difficulties, or sudden significant weight gain (more than two pounds) not related to overeating

◆ Vision disturbances (blurring, dimming, double vision) that persist for two hours or more

◆ Extremely severe vomiting accompanied by pain and/or fever

What It's Important to Know: GETTING REGULAR MEDICAL CARE

In the past few decades, the self-care health movement has instructed Americans—through books, videos, television, newsletters, and, more recently, the Internet—in everything, from taking their own blood pressure and pulse, to home-treating muscle strains, to preventing an infection. The impact this education has had on the effectiveness of our health care has been unquestionably positive, cutting down on the number of trips we have to make to our doctors and making us better patients when we do go. Best of all, it's made us aware of the responsibility we each have for our own health, and it has the potential of making us a lot healthier in the years to come.

Even in pregnancy, there are countless steps you can take to make your own nine months safer and more comfortable, your labor and delivery easier, and

- Frequent (more than three times a day) diarrhea, particularly if it's bloody or mucousy

- Fewer than ten fetal movements per hour (see page 242) after 28 weeks

CALL YOUR PRACTITIONER THE SAME DAY (OR THE NEXT MORNING, IF IT'S THE MIDDLE OF THE NIGHT) FOR THE FOLLOWING:

- Severe lower abdominal pain, on one or both sides, that doesn't subside

- Vaginal spotting (though slight staining a week to ten days after conception or light pink spotting after intercourse in late pregnancy is *not* cause for concern)

- Bleeding from nipples or rectum, or blood in your urine

- Swelling or puffiness of hands, face, eyes

- Severe headache that persists for more than two or three hours

- Sudden weight gain of more than two pounds not related to overeating

- Painful or burning urination

- Fainting or dizziness

- Chills and fever over 100° F (in the absence of cold or flu symptoms), call the same day; fever over 102°F, call right away. (Either way, start bringing down any fever over 100°F promptly by taking acetaminophen.)

- Severe nausea and vomiting; vomiting more often than two or three times a day in the first trimester; vomiting later in pregnancy when you didn't earlier

- Allover itching, with or without dark urine, pale stools, or jaundice (yellowing of skin and whites of the eye)

- Absence of noticeable fetal movement for more than twenty-four hours after the 20th week

Your practitioner may want you to call for different reasons or within different parameters. So show this list to your practitioner, and if there is anything to add or change, write it down here.

_____

_____

_____

_____

_____

your expected end product healthier. But to try to go it alone, even for a few months, is to abuse the concept of self-care—which is built on the foundation of a cooperative partnership between patient and health professional, each providing different skills and know-how. Not surprisingly, getting regular medical care in the form of prenatal visits makes a difference. Women who see a practitioner regularly during pregnancy have bigger, healthier babies, and are less likely to deliver prematurely and to have other serious pregnancy-related problems.

A SCHEDULE OF PRENATAL VISITS

Ideally, a first visit to a physician or nurse-midwife should take place during the preconception period, while baby is still in the planning stages. That's an ideal many women, especially those whose pregnancies are unplanned, can't always manage to achieve. Second best, and still very good, is a visit as soon as you suspect you have conceived.[7] An internal exam will help to confirm your

7. Some practitioners schedule the first visit at six weeks.

pregnancy, and a physical and health history will uncover any conditions or problems that may need monitoring. After that, the schedule of visits will vary depending on the predilection of the practitioner you've chosen as well as on your obstetrical and medical profile. In an uneventful low-risk pregnancy you can probably expect to see your practitioner monthly (in some practices, visits may be scheduled less often) until the end of the 32nd week. After that you may begin going every two weeks until the last month, when weekly visits are customary.[8]

For what you can expect at each prenatal visit, see the monthly chapters.

TAKING CARE OF THE REST OF YOU

You're understandably preoccupied with prenatal matters during pregnancy. But though your health care should begin with your belly, it shouldn't end there. And don't just wait for problems to drop into your lap. Pay a visit to your dentist; most dental work, particularly the preventive kind, can be done safely during pregnancy (see page 181). See your allergist, if necessary. You probably won't begin a course of allergy shots now, but if your allergies are severe, he or

---

8. Studies suggest that healthy, well-educated women do well with as few as nine scheduled pregnancy visits. Still, most women are comfortable with more.

WHEN IN DOUBT

Sometimes the body's signals that something is wrong aren't clear. You feel unusually exhausted, achy, not quite right, but you have none of the symptoms listed on pages 130–131. If a good night's sleep and some extra relaxation don't team up to make you feel better in a day or two, check with your practitioner. Chances are what you're feeling is normal—par for the pregnancy course. But it is also possible that you've become anemic or you're fighting an infection of some kind. Certain conditions—cystitis, a urinary tract infection, for example— can do their dirty work without causing any clear-cut symptoms. So when in doubt, check it out.

she may want to monitor your condition. Your family doctor or a specialist should also be monitoring any chronic illnesses or other medical problems that don't fall under the purview of the obstetrician; if you're seeing a nurse-midwife for pregnancy, you should see an ob/gyn or your family physician for *all* major medical conditions.

If new medical problems come up while you're pregnant, don't ignore them. Even if you've noticed symptoms that seem relatively innocuous, it's more important than ever to consult with your physician promptly. Your baby needs a *wholly* healthy mother.

◆ ◆ ◆

The Second Month

Approximately 5 to 8 Weeks

Perhaps you planned your pregnancy practically to the moment of conception, and for weeks you've known that you're expecting. Or maybe pregnancy sneaked up on you and you didn't find out about it until well into the second month. Either way, you're probably still getting used to the idea that a new life is developing inside you. It's likely you're also still getting used to the demands of pregnancy—from the physical (so that's why I'm tired!) to the logistical (the shortest route to the bathroom is . . .) to the dietary (make it a double skim latte, hold the caffeine).

What You Can Expect at This Month's Checkup

If this is your first prenatal visit, see page 106. If this is your second exam, you'll find that it will be a much shorter visit. And since those initial tests were taken care of, you probably won't be subjected to much poking and prodding this time. You can expect your practitioner to check the following, though there may be variations depending upon your particular needs and your practitioner's style of practice.[1]

◆ Weight and blood pressure

◆ Urine, for sugar and protein

◆ Hands and feet for edema (swelling), and legs for varicose veins

◆ Symptoms you have been experiencing, especially unusual ones

◆ Questions or problems you want to discuss—have a list ready

1. See Appendix, page 545, for more on the procedures and tests performed.

A LOOK INSIDE

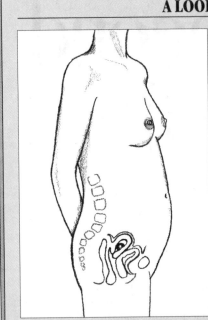

▼ *Though only an inch long, the embryo looks much more like a baby now. Gone is the tail, and by the end of the second month, arms and feet (complete with fingers and toes!) have formed, along with eyes (eyelids sealed shut), ears, a nose tip, and a tongue. All major body organs and systems are present, but still have a great deal of developing to do. The embryo makes spontaneous movements, though it will be many weeks before they will be strong enough to be felt. The placenta, which will serve as baby's life support system, is busily being built.*

▲ *Even though you still won't look like you're pregnant to those around you, you might notice your clothes are getting a little tighter around the waist. You might also need a larger bra now. By the end of this month, your uterus, usually the size of a fist, has grown to the size of a large grapefruit.*

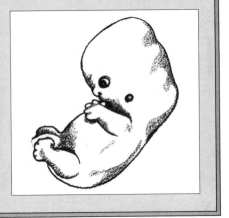

What You May Be Feeling

As always, remember that every pregnancy and every woman is different. You may experience all of these symptoms at one time or another, or only one or two. Some may have continued from last month, others may be new. You may also have other, less common, symptoms. Don't be surprised, no matter what your symptoms, if you don't "feel" pregnant yet.

PHYSICALLY

◆ Fatigue and sleepiness

◆ A need to urinate frequently

◆ Nausea, with or without vomiting, and/or excessive salivation

◆ Constipation

◆ Heartburn, indigestion, flatulence, bloating

- Food aversions and cravings
- Breast changes: fullness, heaviness, tenderness, tingling; darkening of the areola (the pigmented area around the nipple); sweat glands in the areola become prominent, like large goose bumps; a network of bluish lines appear under the skin as blood supply to the breasts increases
- Increased or slight whitish vaginal discharge (leukorrhea)
- Occasional headaches (similar to the headaches in women taking birth control pills)

- Occasional faintness or dizziness
- Tightness of clothing around waist and breasts; abdomen may appear enlarged, probably due to bowel distention rather than uterine growth

EMOTIONALLY

- Instability comparable to premenstrual syndrome (but probably more pronounced), which may include irritability, mood swings, irrationality, weepiness
- Misgivings, fear, joy, elation—any or all of these

What You May Be Concerned About

VENOUS CHANGES

"I have unsightly blue lines under the skin, on my breasts and abdomen. Is that normal?"

Not only are these veins (which can make your entire chest and belly look like a road map) normal and nothing to worry about, they are a sign that your body is doing what it should. They're part of the network of veins that has expanded to carry the increased blood supply of pregnancy—which will be nourishing your baby. They may show up earliest and be much more prominent in very slim or light-complexioned women. In some women, particularly those who are overweight or dark-skinned, the veins may be less visible or not noticeable at all, or may not become obvious until later in pregnancy.

"Since I became pregnant I've got awful-looking spidery purplish-red lines on my thighs. Are they varicose veins?"

They aren't pretty, but they aren't varicose veins. They are probably spider nevi, commonly dubbed "spider veins," for obvious reasons. Spider veins can result from the hormone changes of pregnancy, although some women are also genetically predisposed to developing them (eating enough vitamin C foods and getting into the habit of not crossing your legs may help minimize the number of spider veins you end up with). They usually fade and disappear after delivery; if they don't, they can be treated by a dermatologist—either with saline injections or the use of a laser. Both treatments destroy the blood vessels, causing them to collapse and eventually disappear.

"My mother and grandmother both had varicose veins during pregnancy and had trouble with them ever after. Is there anything I can do to prevent the problem in my own pregnancy?"

Because this particular problem often runs in families, you're wise to think about prevention now—especially since varicose veins tend to worsen with subsequent pregnancies.

Normal, healthy veins carry blood from the extremities back to the heart. Because they must work against gravity, they are designed with a series of valves that prevent backflow. When these valves are missing or faulty, as they are in some people, blood tends to pool in the veins where the pressure of gravity is greatest (usually in the legs, but sometimes in the rectum, as hemorrhoids, or in the vulva), resulting in bulging. Veins that are easily distended, or distensible, can further contribute to the condition. The problem is more common in people who are overweight, and occurs four times more often in women than in men. In women who are susceptible, the condition often surfaces for the first time during pregnancy. There are several reasons for this: increased pressure from the uterus on the pelvic veins; increasing pressure on leg veins; expanded blood volume; and pregnancy-hormone-induced relaxation of the muscle tissue in the veins.

The symptoms of varicose veins aren't difficult to recognize, but they vary a great deal in severity. There may be a mild achiness or severe pain in the legs, or a sensation of heaviness, or swelling—or none of these. A faint outline of bluish veins may be visible, or serpentine veins may bulge from ankle to upper thigh or vulva. In severe cases the skin overlying the veins becomes swollen, dry, and irritated (consult your practitioner about moisturizing). Occasionally, thrombophlebitis (inflammation of a vein due to a blood clot) may develop at the site of a varicosity (see page 510), so always check with your practitioner about symptoms of varicose veins.

Fortunately, varicose veins during pregnancy often can be prevented, or the symptoms minimized, by taking measures to eliminate unnecessary pressure on the leg veins. Here's how:

◆ Avoid excessive weight gain.

◆ Avoid long periods of standing or sitting. When sitting, avoid crossing legs and elevate them when possible. Periodically flex your ankles when standing or sitting. When lying down, raise your legs by placing a pillow under your feet. When resting or sleeping, try to lie on your left side.

◆ Avoid heavy lifting.

◆ Avoid straining during bowel movements. Taking steps to avoid constipation (see page 156) will help.

◆ Wear support panty hose (light support hose seem to work well without being uncomfortable) or elastic stockings, putting them on before getting out of bed in the morning (before blood pools in your legs) and removing them at night before getting into bed. Check with your practitioner about size and style.

◆ Don't wear restrictive clothing. Avoid tight belts or pants; stockings and socks with elastic tops; and snug shoes. Also avoid high heels, favoring flats or medium chunky heels instead.

◆ Get some exercise, such as a brisk twenty- to thirty-minute walk or swim every day. But, if you are experiencing pain, avoid high-impact aerobics, jogging, cycling, and weight training (see page 190).

◆ Be sure to get enough vitamin C (from foods, not supplements), which helps to keep veins healthy and elastic.

Surgical removal of varicose veins isn't recommended during pregnancy, although it can certainly be considered a few months after delivery.[2] In most cases,

2. Surgery or sclerotherapy to remove varicose veins is primarily cosmetic, and the problem can recur after treatment.

however, the problem will clear up or improve spontaneously after delivery, usually by the time prepregnancy weight is reached.

COMPLEXION PROBLEMS

"My skin is breaking out the way it did when I was a teenager."

The glow of pregnancy that some women are lucky enough to radiate isn't just a result of their joy over impending motherhood, but of the increased secretion of oils brought about by hormonal changes. And so, alas, are the less-than-glowing breakouts of pregnancy that some not-so-lucky women experience (particularly those whose skin ordinarily breaks out monthly before their periods). Though such eruptions are hard to eliminate entirely, the following suggestions may help keep them to a minimum:

◆ Be faithful to the Pregnancy Diet—it's good for your skin as well as for your baby.

◆ Don't pass a tap without filling your glass. Drinking water helps keep your skin moist and clear.

◆ Wash your face two or three times a day with a gentle cleanser.

◆ Use an oil-free moisturizer to keep skin hydrated. Sometimes skin that is overly dried by harsh acne soaps and other products is actually more prone to break out.

◆ Choose skin-care products and make-up labeled "noncomedogenic"—which means they won't clog pores. If you use foundation and powder, make sure they're oil-free.

If your practitioner approves, take a vitamin B$_6$ supplement (no more than 25 to 50 mg). This vitamin is sometimes suggested in treating hormonally induced skin problems (and may also help minimize morning sickness; see page 117).

If your skin problems are severe enough to warrant your consulting a dermatologist, be sure to let him or her know you are expecting. Some drugs used for acne, particularly Accutane and Retin-A, should *not* be used by pregnant women because they can be harmful to the fetus. Ask your dermatologist about other preparations that are considered safe during pregnancy.

For some pregnant women, dry, often itchy, skin is a problem. Moisturizers may be helpful. (For optimum absorption, they should be applied while the skin is still damp after a bath or shower.) So are drinking plenty of fluids and keeping rooms well humidified (see page 457) in the heating season. Bathing too frequently, particularly with soap, tends to increase dryness. So cut down on bathing (take short showers instead) if your skin is dry, and try using a mild soapless cleanser, such as Cetaphil or Aquanil.

For some women who suffer from eczema, pregnancy exacerbates the condition. Low-dose cortisone creams are safe to use during pregnancy in moderate amounts. Ask your practitioner or dermatologist which ones he or she recommends.

WAISTLINE EXPANSION

"Why does my waist seem to be expanding already? I thought I wouldn't 'show' until the third month at least."

Your expanding waistline may very well be a legitimate by-product of pregnancy, especially if you started out slender, with little excess flesh for your growing uterus to hide behind. Or it may be the result of bowel distention, thanks to excess gas and constipation, both very common in early pregnancy. On the other hand, it's also quite possible that your "show" may be an indication that you're gaining weight too quickly. If you've gained more than 3 pounds so far, analyze your diet—you may be consuming too many calories, possibly empty ones. Review the Pregnancy Diet, and read about weight gain on page 169.

LOSING YOUR FIGURE

"Will my figure ever be the same after I have a baby?"

The 2 to 4 permanent pounds the average woman puts on with each pregnancy, and the flab that often accompanies them, are not an inevitable result of being pregnant. They're the result of gaining too much weight, eating the wrong foods, and/or not getting enough exercise during those nine months and afterward.

The weight gain of pregnancy has just two legitimate purposes: to nourish the developing fetus now, and to store up reserves for breastfeeding the baby after delivery. If a woman gains only enough weight to serve those purposes and she keeps physically fit, her figure will generally return to prepregnancy form (or close) within about six months after her baby is born, especially if she is using up fat stores by breastfeeding.[3] So stop worrying and start taking action.

With attention to diet and exercise now, you can look better than ever after pregnancy, because you will have learned how to take optimum care of your body. If your spouse joins you in

pursuit of a healthier lifestyle (you'll both benefit from the company), he can look better, too.

MEASURING TOO SMALL (OR TOO BIG)

"At my last prenatal visit, my midwife told me my uterus is measuring a little small. Does this mean the baby's not growing right?"

Parents rarely wait until their babies are born to begin worrying about their size. But—just as is usually the case after birth—there's rarely anything to worry about. After all, trying to size up your uterus from the outside isn't an exact science anytime in pregnancy, and especially not this early in the game. Calculating what that size should be isn't easy either (unless you're certain about which day you conceived), since the date of your pregnancy may be off by as much as several weeks on either side. Chances are your midwife is planning to schedule an ultrasound to pinpoint more precisely the size of your uterus and the date of your pregnancy and to see if there are any discrepancies, which there most likely aren't.

"I was told my uterus is measuring 12 weeks, but according to my dates I'm only 9 weeks pregnant. Why is my uterus so large?"

There's a good chance that your uterus is bigger than it's supposed to be because you're farther along than you think. Probably you and your practitioner originally miscalculated the date or the size (again, external observations of uterine size are not an exact science). In order to check this out, and because there are other, much less likely explanations (for example, that you might be carrying twins, have uterine fibroids, or

---

3. Some nursing mothers find they shed very little weight while breastfeeding, but usually are able to return to prepregnancy weight soon after weaning their babies. If they don't, it is usually because they are consuming too many calories and burning too few. Bottle-feeding mothers will have to lose weight postpartum through diet and exercise.

excess amniotic fluid), your practitioner will likely order an ultrasound.

A TILTED UTERUS

"My doctor said my uterus is tilted. Is this a problem?"

Probably not. About 1 in 5 women has a tilted (or retroverted) uterus, in which the fundus (or top) of the uterus is tilted toward the back instead of the front. In most cases, the uterus rights itself by the end of the first trimester.

In the unlikely event that your uterus doesn't right itself, you may experience symptoms, including feeling a heaviness on your bladder, as though a brick (your uterus) were lying on it; an inability to empty your bladder completely; and long periods without voiding (four or more hours). If you experience these symptoms, call your practitioner as soon as you can to avoid having the problem escalate to a serious urinary tract infection. (Also see page 435.)

HEARTBURN AND INDIGESTION

"I have indigestion and heartburn all the time. Will this affect my baby?"

While you are painfully aware of your gastrointestinal discomfort, your baby is blissfully oblivious to and unaffected by it—as long as it isn't interfering with your eating the right foods.

Though indigestion can have the same cause (usually overindulgence) during pregnancy as when you're not pregnant, there are additional reasons why it may be plaguing you now. Early in pregnancy, your body produces large amounts of the hormones progesterone and relaxin, which tend to relax smooth muscle tissue everywhere in the body, including the gastrointestinal (GI) tract. As a result, food sometimes moves more slowly through your system, resulting in bloating and indigestion. This may be uncomfortable for you, but it is beneficial for your baby because this alimentary slowdown allows better absorption of nutrients into your bloodstream and subsequently through the placenta and into your baby.

Heartburn results when the ring of muscle that separates the esophagus from the stomach relaxes, allowing food and harsh digestive juices to back up from the stomach to the esophagus. These stomach acids irritate the sensitive esophageal lining, causing a burning sensation right around where the heart is—thus the term heartburn—though the problem has nothing to do with your heart. During the last two trimesters the problem can be compounded by your blossoming uterus as it presses up on your stomach.

It's nearly impossible to have an indigestion-free nine months; it's just one of the less pleasant facts of pregnancy. There are, however, some pretty effective ways of avoiding heartburn and indigestion most of the time, and of minimizing the discomfort when it strikes:

◆ Avoid gaining too much weight; excess weight puts excess pressure on the stomach.

◆ Don't wear clothing that is tight around your abdomen or waist.

◆ Eat six small meals rather than three big ones.

◆ Eat slowly, taking small mouthfuls and chewing thoroughly.

◆ Stay upright for several hours after eating. Don't eat a big meal right before bed.

◆ Eliminate from your diet any food that you notice causes GI discomfort. The most common offenders are hot and highly seasoned foods; fried or fatty foods; processed meats; chocolate, coffee, alcohol, carbonated beverages; spearmint and peppermint.

♦ Chew sugarless gum for a half hour after meals. It can reduce excess acid.

♦ Don't smoke.

♦ Avoid bending over at the waist; bend instead with your knees.

♦ Sleep with your head elevated about six inches. Lying on your left side may also help.

♦ Relax (see page 127). Also try some complementary or alternative medical (CAM) approaches (see page 246), such as meditation, visualization, biofeedback, or hypnosis.

♦ Ask your practitioner to recommend an antacid or other over-the-counter medication that is safe for use in pregnancy. If you're having trouble getting your calcium requirements, you may want to take a calcium-containing antacid such as Tums or Rolaids. But avoid preparations containing sodium or sodium bicarbonate.

FOOD AVERSIONS AND CRAVINGS

"Certain foods, particularly green vegetables, that I've always liked taste strange now. Instead, I have cravings for foods that are less nutritious."

The pregnancy cliché of a harried husband running out in the middle of the night, raincoat over his pajamas, for a pint of ice cream and a jar of pickles to satisfy his wife's cravings is probably played out more often in the heads of cartoonists than in real life. Not many pregnant women's cravings carry them—or their spouses—that far.

Still, most of us do find that our tastes in food change somewhat in pregnancy.

Studies show that up to 90 percent of expectant mothers experience a craving for at least one food (most often ice cream—though usually without the pickles—or fruit), and between 50 and 85 percent have at least one food aversion. To a certain extent, these sudden gastronomic eccentricities can be blamed on hormonal havoc, which probably explains why food aversions and cravings are most common in the first trimester of first pregnancies, when that havoc is at its height.

Hormones, however, don't offer the only explanation for pregnancy food aversions and cravings. The long-favored theory that these are sensible signals from our bodies—that when we develop a distaste for something, it's usually bad for us, and that when we crave something, it's usually something we need—has some merit. Such a signal comes when the black coffee that used to be the mainstay of your workday becomes totally unappealing. Or the cocktail before dinner seems too strong even when it's weak. Or you suddenly can't get enough grapefruit. On the other hand, when you can't stand the sight of fish, or broccoli suddenly tastes bitter, or you crave ice-cream sundaes, you certainly can't credit your body with sending accurate signals.

The fact is that body signals relating to food are notoriously unreliable, probably because we've departed so significantly from nature's food chain that we can no longer interpret these signals correctly. Before ice-cream sundaes were invented, when food came from nature, a craving for carbohydrates and calcium would have steered us toward fruits and milk or cheese. With the wide variety of tempting (but often unwholesome) options available today, it's no wonder our bodies are confused.

It wouldn't be reasonable to expect you to totally ignore cravings and aversions. But you can respond to them without putting your baby's nutritional needs in jeopardy. If you crave something that you know you'd probably be better off without, then seek a substitute that satisfies the craving at least somewhat, but without filling you up on empty calories: chocolate frozen yogurt instead of a frozen chocolate bar; a bag of trail mix instead of jelly beans; baked taco chips instead of the kind that turn your fingers orange. If substitutes don't satisfy, sublimation may be helpful. When unwholesome urges strike, try something else you like: taking a brisk walk, reading a good book, visiting an on-line pregnancy chat room, playing computer games. And, of course, occasionally giving in to less nutritious cravings is fine, as long as they don't include something risky (such as an alcoholic beverage) and as long as your indulgence doesn't take the place of nutritious foods in your diet.

If you experience a sudden aversion to coffee or alcohol or chocolate ice cream, great. It will make giving them up for the duration all the easier. If it's chicken or lettuce or milk you can't tolerate, you don't have to force-feed yourself, but you do have to find compensating sources of the nutrients they supply. (See the Pregnancy Diet, Chapter 4, for appropriate substitutions.)

Most cravings and aversions disappear or weaken by the fourth month. Cravings that hang in there longer may be triggered by emotional needs—the need for a little extra attention, for example. If both you and your spouse are aware of this need, it should be easy to satisfy. You might, instead of requesting a middle-of-the-night pint of Rocky Road (with or without the kosher dill), settle for an oatmeal cookie or two and some quiet cuddling or a romantic bath for two.

Some women find themselves craving, even eating, such peculiar substances as clay, ashes, and laundry starch. Since this habit, known as pica, can be dangerous and may be a sign of nutritional deficiency, particularly of iron, it should be reported to your practitioner.

MILK AVERSION OR INTOLERANCE

"I can't tolerate milk, and drinking four cups a day would really make me uncomfortable. But will my baby suffer if I don't drink milk?"

It's not milk your baby needs, it's calcium. Since milk is the most convenient source of calcium in the American diet, it's the one most often recommended for filling the greatly increased requirement during pregnancy. But there are many substitutes that fill the nutritional bill just as well.

Many people who are lactose-intolerant (they can't digest the milk

---

PASTEURIZED, PLEASE

When it was invented by French scientist Louis Pasteur in the mid-1800s, pasteurization was the greatest thing to happen to dairy products since cows. And it still is, particularly as far as pregnant women are concerned. To protect yourself and your baby from infection with hazardous bacteria, such as listeria, make sure that all the milk you drink is pasteurized, and that all the cheeses and other dairy products you eat are made from pasteurized milk ("raw milk" cheeses are not). Juice, which can contain *E. coli* and other dangerous bacteria, should also *always* be pasteurized. Even eggs now come pasteurized (which eliminates the risk of salmonella, apparently without changing taste or nutrition), though they are not widely available yet.

ARE YOU REALLY LACTOSE-INTOLERANT?

Many people incorrectly blame digestive distress on lactose intolerance. To see if you can tolerate dairy products in moderate amounts, have a family member give you a smoothie with regular nonfat milk for several days and then a smoothie with lactose-free nonfat milk for several more—without telling you which is which. If you have symptoms only with the regular milk, you are probably lactose-intolerant.

sugar lactose) can tolerate some kinds of dairy products, such as hard cheeses, fully processed yogurts, and lactose-free or lactose-reduced milk and cottage cheese, in which 70 to 100 percent of the lactose has been converted to a more easily digested form. (Another advantage of using lactose-free milk products: some are fortified with calcium. Check labels and choose one that is.) Taking a lactase tablet before ingesting milk or milk products, or adding lactase drops or tablets to your milk, can also minimize or eliminate dairy-induced tummy troubles.

Even if you've been lactose-intolerant for years, you may discover that you are able to handle some dairy products during the second and third trimesters, when fetal needs for calcium are the greatest. If that's so, don't overdo it; try to stick primarily to products that are less likely to provoke a reaction. No reason to provoke digestive unrest, after all.

If you can't tolerate *any* dairy products or are allergic to them, you can still get all the calcium your baby requires by drinking calcium-fortified juices and eating the nondairy foods listed under Calcium-Rich Foods on page 95.

If your problem with milk isn't physiological but just a matter of distaste, try some of the dairy or nondairy calcium-rich alternatives. There are bound to be plenty that don't offend your taste buds. Or you can try to fool your taste buds with milk that comes to your table incognito (in oatmeal, soups, muffins, sauces, shakes, frozen desserts, puddings, and so on).

If, in spite of all your best efforts, you can't seem to get enough calcium into your diet, ask your practitioner to recommend a calcium supplement. You'll also need to be sure that you're getting enough vitamin D (which is added to cow's milk); check your prenatal vitamin.

CHOLESTEROL

"My husband and I are very careful about our diets, and we limit our cholesterol and fat intake. Should I continue to do this while I'm pregnant?"

Pregnant women, and to a lesser extent nonpregnant women of childbearing age, are in an enviable position as far as bacon, egg, and steak lovers are concerned: they are protected to a certain degree against the artery-clogging effects of cholesterol. In fact, cholesterol is necessary for fetal development, so much so that the mother's body automatically increases its production, raising blood cholesterol levels by anywhere from 25 to 40 percent. Though you don't have to eat a high-cholesterol diet to help your body step up production, you can feel free to indulge a bit.[4]

---

4. Women who have hypercholesteremia, a familial type of high blood cholesterol, are exceptions to the loosening of the cholesterol reins in pregnancy. These women should continue to follow their doctors' advice about diet.

Have an egg every day if you like (though not uncooked or even under-cooked, unless the eggs are pasteurized), use cheese (preferably low- or reduced-fat) to meet your calcium requirement, and enjoy an occasional steak, all without guilt. But don't overdo, because many high-cholesterol foods are high in fat and calories, and an excess of them could send the numbers on your scale soaring. Too much fat could also put you over your fat quota. And remember that many foods high in cholesterol are also high in animal fats that may be contaminated by undesirable chemicals—another good reason to limit them.

But while you don't necessarily have to hold the mayo (and the butter, and the egg yolks, and the lamb chops) all of the time, everyone else in your household (except for under-two-year-olds)[5] should, most of the time. That goes most emphatically for adult men, both those with borderline-to-high cholesterol counts and those who just want to avoid developing such a problem. Because serving two sets of breakfasts, lunches, and dinners—one cholesterol-lenient and one cholesterol-trimmed—is not only a strain on the cook but also unfair to those being denied, it's wise to continue, or to institute, a healthy heart regimen for family meals. Lean toward lean meats, poultry without the skin, low-fat dairy products, cholesterol-combating oils (such as olive and canola), and the white of the egg rather than the yolk. (Or use the new DHA—see page 91—omega-3-rich eggs, which come from hens that are fed a heart-healthy diet.) Enjoy your cholesterol splurges on the sly, when you know no one else is around to drool.

---

5. Babies under two need fat and cholesterol for proper growth and brain development, and should never be placed on a fat- and cholesterol-restricted diet except under medical supervision.

A MEATLESS DIET

"I eat chicken and fish but no red meat. Can I supply my baby with all the nutrients he needs without meat?"

Your baby can be just as happy and healthy as any beef-eating mother's offspring. Fish and poultry, in fact, give you more protein and less fat for your calories than beef, pork, lamb, and organ meats. A red-meatless diet also usually contains less cholesterol, which may not make a big difference to you while you're pregnant, but represents a plus for your spouse and other family members over the age of two.

A VEGETARIAN DIET

"I'm a vegetarian and in perfect health. But everyone says that I have to eat meat, fish, eggs, and milk products to have a healthy baby. Is this true?"

Vegetarians of every variety can have healthy babies without compromising their dietary principles. But they have to be even more careful in planning their diets than meat-eating mothers-to-be, being particularly sure to get all of the following:

Adequate protein. For the ovo-lacto vegetarian, who eats eggs and milk products, adequate protein intake can be ensured if you get ample quantities of both. A vegan (a strict vegetarian who eats neither milk nor eggs) has to depend on vegetable proteins to meet her four-serving protein allowance (one more than the nonvegetarian needs; see Vegetarian Proteins, page 95). Some meat substitutes are good protein sources; others are low in protein and high in fat and calories. Read the labels carefully, keeping in mind that 20 to 25 mg of protein equals one serving.

Adequate calcium. This is no problem for the vegetarian who eats dairy products, but adroit maneuvering is needed for those who don't. Many soy products are fairly high in calcium, but beware of soy milks loaded with sucrose (sugar, corn syrup, honey); look for a pure soybean product instead and check calcium content as listed on the label (about 300 mg equals one serving). For tofu to be counted as a calcium food, it must have been coagulated with calcium (most are; check labels). Some brands of stone-ground corn tortillas are good nondairy sources of calcium, providing as much as half a calcium serving per tortilla (again, check the labels). Another easy-to-take nondairy source of calcium is calcium-added juice. For yet others, see the Calcium-Rich Foods list on page 95. For added insurance, it is recommended that vegans also take a calcium supplement (vegetarian formulas are available).

Vitamin B₁₂. While B_{12} deficiencies are rare, vegetarians, particularly vegans, often don't get enough of this vitamin because it is found primarily in animal foods. So they should be certain to take a vitamin supplement that includes B_{12}, as well as folic acid and iron.

Vitamin D. This important vitamin occurs naturally only in fish liver oils. It is also produced by our skin when we are exposed to sunlight, though because of the vagaries of weather, cover-up clothing, and the dangers of spending too much time in the sun, this is an unreliable source of the vitamin for most women, especially those who are dark-skinned. To ensure adequate intake of vitamin D, federal law requires that milk be fortified with 400 mg of vitamin D per quart. If you don't drink cow's milk, be sure that there is vitamin D added to the soy milk you drink or in the pregnancy supplement you are taking. Be careful, however, not to take vitamin D in doses beyond pregnancy requirements, since it can be toxic in excessive amounts.

LOW-CARBOHYDRATE DIETS

"I've been on a low-carb/high-protein diet to lose weight. Can I continue the diet while I'm pregnant?"

The only kind of diet that's appropriate during pregnancy is a well-balanced one—which is why the Pregnancy Diet is high in protein *and* carbohydrates. Diets that limit carbohydrates (including fruits, vegetables, and grains) limit the nutrients that growing fetuses (and their growing mothers) need, and are inherently unwise. In fact, such programs have been linked to low birthweight. Also an important point: expectant mothers should never diet for weight loss. There will be plenty of time for that after the baby's born—when, hopefully, the weight-loss diet you choose will be well balanced, too. Which brings up another important point: hype may make a diet popular, but it doesn't make it healthy.

JUNK-FOOD JUNKIE

"I'm addicted to junk foods— doughnuts, chips, burgers, and fries. I know I should be eating healthier, but I'm not sure I can change my habits."

There's never been a better time to make that change. Before you became pregnant, your dietary indiscretions could affect only you; now they can affect your baby as well. Make a daily diet of doughnuts and fast-food burgers, and you'll be denying your baby adequate nourishment during the most important nine months of his or her life.

Eat junk food on top of a balanced diet, and your baby won't be the only one growing.

Happily, any addiction can be broken—even one to junk food. Here are several ways to make your withdrawal almost as painless as it is worthwhile:

Change the locale of your meals. If you're used to breakfasting on a Danish at your desk, have a better breakfast at home instead. If you usually lunch at the local burger place and you know you can't resist the quarter-pounder and fries, order in a nutritious sandwich from the local deli—or go to restaurants that don't serve burgers.

Stop thinking of eating as a catch-as-catch-can proposition. Rather than settling for what's easiest or nearest, select what's best for your baby. Plan meals and snacks ahead of time to be sure you get all of your Daily Dozen.

Don't give temptation a tumble. Keep candy, chips, sugary cookies, and sugar-sweetened soft drinks out of the house (other family members will survive without them, and in fact will benefit from their absence). When the treat-laden coffee wagon bell chimes at work, don't answer it. Stock home and workplace with wholesome snacks such as fresh and dried fruit, nuts, whole-grain baked goods, bread sticks and crackers, juices, hard-cooked eggs, and string cheese (the last two will need refrigeration at work, or an ice pack to keep them company in your lunch box).

Substitute. Can't imagine lunch without a burger? Make it a veggie burger or a turkey burger, now available at more and more restaurants and takeouts—for less fat and fewer calories. (Add cheese, lettuce, tomato, pickles, and all the rest of your favorite burger fixings, and you may not even wonder where the beef is.)

Crave a doughnut with your morning coffee? Dunk a whole-grain muffin instead. The midnight munchies have you searching for the taco chips? Settle for the baked, low-fat variety, dipped in salsa for more flavor and a healthy helping of vitamin C.

Don't use lack of time as an excuse for sloppy eating. It takes no more time to make a roast turkey and cheese, lettuce, and tomato sandwich to take to work, or to prepare a container of fruit and yogurt, than it does to stand in line for a burger.

If the prospect of preparing a real dinner every night seems overwhelming, cook enough for two or three dinners at one time and give yourself alternate nights off. And keep it simple: elaborate dishes in general, in addition to being labor intensive, are often high in fat and calories and low in nutrition. For a quickie meal, broil a fish fillet and top it with your favorite jarred salsa, a little chopped avocado, and a squeeze of fresh lime juice. Layer tomato sauce and low-fat mozzarella cheese on a cooked boneless chicken breast, then run it under the broiler. Or scramble some eggs and wrap them in a corn tortilla along with shredded low-fat Cheddar and some microwave-steamed vegetables. When you don't have time to start from scratch (when do you ever?), don't hesitate to use canned beans, low-sodium soups, frozen or packaged ready-to-prepare healthy main courses[6] (your local health food market's sure to have a wide selection, and many supermarkets do, too), plain frozen vegetables, or the fresh, pre-washed cut-up vegetables and salads sold loose or bagged in supermarket produce sections.

---

6. Check the nutrition label to be sure there are no unhealthy additives, that protein content is adequate, and that sodium is not excessive.

ADDITIVES ASSESSED

The additives in our foods are approved for use by the FDA, but there are many consumer advocates who question the approval process and the safety of some of these additives. The Center for Science in the Public Interest (CSPI), a watchdog agency, rates the following common (but not necessarily pronounceable) additives this way:

CONSIDERED SAFE (except for the occasional individual who may be allergic to one of these). Feel free to use products that contain: alginate; alpha tocopherol (vitamin E); ascorbic acid (vitamin C); beta-carotene; calcium propionate; calcium stearoyl lactylate; carrageenan; casein; citric acid; EDTA; erythorbic acid; ferrous gluconate; fumaric acid; gelatin; glycerin (glycerol); gums: arabic, furcelleran, ghatti, guar, karaya, locust bean, xanthan; lactic acid; lecithin; mono- and diglycerides; phosphate salts; phosphoric acid; plant sterol esters; polysorbate 60, 65, 80; potassium sorbate; propylene glycol alginate; sodium ascorbate; sodium benzoate; sodium carboxymethylcellulose (cmc); sodium caseinate; sodium citrate; sodium propionate; sodium stearoyl lactylate; sorbic acid; sorbitan monostearate; starch; modified starch; Sucralose; thiamin mononitrate; vanillin, ethyl vanillin; vegetable oil; sterol esters.

NOT TOXIC, but large amounts may be unsafe or promote bad nutrition. Cut back on: caffeine; corn syrup; dextrose (corn sugar, glucose); high-fructose corn syrup; hydrogenated starch hydrolysate; hydrogenated vegetable oil; invert sugar; maltitol; mannitol; salatrim; salt; sorbitol; sugar.

CAUTION ADVISED; these additives may pose a risk and need to be better tested. Try to avoid: artificial colorings; citrus red 2 and red 40; aspartame (NutraSweet; Equal); brominated vegetable oil (BVO); butylated hydroxyanisole (BHA); butylated hydroxytoluene (BHT); heptyl paraben; quinine.

CAUTION ADVISED for those with allergies, sensitivities, or other negative reactions. If you have such a reaction, avoid: artificial coloring; yellow 5; artificial and natural flavoring; aspartame (NutraSweet; Equal); beta-carotene; caffeine; carmine; cochineal; casein; gum tragacanth; HVP (hydrolyzed vegetable protein); lactose; MSG (monosodium glutamate); quinine; sodium bisulfite; sulfites; sulfur dioxide.

UNSAFE in the amounts typically consumed or very poorly tested. Avoid: acesulfame potassium; artificial colorings (blue 1; blue 2; green 3; red 3; yellow 6); cyclamate; Olestra (Olean); potassium bromate; propyl gallate; saccharin; sodium nitrite; sodium nitrate.

Don't use a tight budget as an excuse for eating junk food. A glass of orange juice or milk costs no more than a can of cola. A homemade broiled chicken breast and baked potato costs less than a fast-food chicken sandwich and fries.

Quit cold turkey. If you find one always leads to another and then another, don't fool yourself by thinking you can have just one Coke or just one doughnut. Instead, tell yourself that junk food is out—at least until you deliver. You may be surprised to find, once the baby's born, that your new good eating habits are as hard to break as your old bad ones—which will make setting a good dietary example for your child all the easier.

Follow the Pregnancy Diet. Try to make it part of your life.

Fast Food

"I go out with friends for fast food after a movie about once a month. Do I have to skip this for the rest of my pregnancy?"

In the past few years, most of the major fast-food chains have at least attempted to provide more options for health-conscious consumers. Unfortunately, many of these options have since been pulled from menus because they didn't sell. (Surprise! It seems those who frequent fast-food restaurants don't go there looking for health food.) Still, if you pick and choose with care, you can walk out of most fast-food restaurants without doing too much dietary damage, as long as you don't walk *in* to them too frequently. Checking the nutrition information that's posted or available on request will help guide those selections. See page 232 for more.

Chemicals in Foods

"With additives in packaged foods, pesticides on vegetables, PCBs in fish, antibiotics in meat, and nitrates in hot dogs, is there anything I can safely eat during pregnancy?"

Reports of hazardous chemicals in just about every item in the American diet are enough to scare the appetite out of anyone, and especially a pregnant woman afraid not only for her own health but for that of her unborn child. Thanks to the media, "chemical" has become synonymous with "dangerous," and "natural" with "safe." But neither generalization is true. Everything we eat is made up of chemicals. Some chemicals are harmful, some are not; some are even beneficial. And although "natural" is often better than artificial or unnatural, natural things, too, can be harmful. A "natural" mushroom can be poisonous; "natural" eggs, butter, and animal fats are associated with heart disease; and too much "natural" sugar and honey are linked to diabetes.

That's not to say that you have to give up eating entirely in order to protect your baby from food hazards. In spite of anything you might have heard, no food or additive presently in use has been absolutely proven to cause birth defects. And in fact, most expectant American women fill their shopping carts and their stomachs without giving food safety a second thought and have perfectly healthy babies. Clearly, from what we know presently, the danger to a developing fetus from the chemical additives in food is remote.

Still, if you want to try to eliminate even this remote risk, use the following as a guide to help you decide what to drop into your shopping cart and what to pass up.

◆ Use the Pregnancy Diet as the foundation for food selection. Because it steers away from processed foods, it steers you clear of many potential perils. It also supplies Green Leafies and Yellows, rich in protective beta-carotene, as well as other fruits and vegetables rich in phytochemicals, which may counteract the negative effects of toxins in our food.

◆ Use most sugar substitutes sparingly. See page 65 for the reasons why.

◆ Whenever possible, cook from scratch with fresh ingredients or use frozen or packaged organic ready-to-eat foods. You'll avoid many questionable additives found in processed foods, and your meals will be more nutritious, too.

◆ Stick to fish that is considered safe, keeping in mind that pregnant women (as well as nursing moms and young children) should play it safer than the general population. According to the

Environmental Protection Agency (EPA) guidelines, you should avoid shark, swordfish, king mackerel, and tilefish. These large fish contain high levels of methyl mercury, a chemical that can harm the fetus's developing nervous system. (This is true of regular consumption, so don't worry if you've already eaten some of these fish.) You should also limit your consumption of tuna (chunk light tuna contains less mercury) and fresh water fish caught by family and friends to an average of 6 ounces (cooked weight) per week; commercially caught fish usually has lower levels of contaminants, so you can safely eat more. Beware, too, of eating any fish from waters that are contaminated (with sewage or industrial runoff, for example) or tropical fish, such as grouper, amberjack, and mahimahi (which sometimes contain toxins). Fortunately, that leaves plenty of fish in the sea to enjoy safely and often (an average of 12 ounces of cooked fish per week is considered safe according to government guidelines). Choose from salmon (wild caught is best), sole, flounder, haddock, tilapia, halibut, ocean perch, pollack, cod, and trout, as well as other smaller ocean fish and seafood of all kinds. Remember, *all* fish and seafood should be well cooked.[7]

◆ Generally avoid foods preserved with nitrates and nitrites (or sodium nitrates), including frankfurters, salami, luncheon meats, and smoked fish and meats. Look for those brands that do not include these preservatives. (Keep in mind, however, that all ready-to-eat meats should be heated until steaming; see page 151.)

◆ Whenever you have a choice between a product with artificial colorings, flavorings, preservatives, and other additives and one without, opt for the one that's additive free. Some artificial additives are questionable (see box, page 146) and are used to enhance foods that aren't very nutritious to start with.

◆ In cooking, don't use MSG or flavor enhancers that contain it. In Chinese restaurants, request no MSG when ordering.[8]

◆ Choose lean cuts of meat and remove visible fat before cooking, since chemicals that livestock ingest tend to concentrate in the fat of the animal. With poultry, remove both the fat and the skin to minimize chemical intake. And don't eat organ meats (such as liver and kidneys) very often, for the same reason. When it's available and your budget permits, buy poultry and meat that has been raised organically, without hormones or antibiotics. Free-range chickens are not only less likely to be contaminated with these chemicals, they are also less likely to carry such infections as salmonella because the birds are not kept in cramped, disease-breeding quarters.

◆ As a precaution, give all vegetables and fruits a bath. Thoroughly rinse all produce under running water.[9] Scrub

---

7. For the latest information on fish safety, contact the FDA at (888) SAFE-FOOD (723-3366) or www.cfsan.fda.gov or the EPA at (800) 490-9198 or www.epa.gov/ost/fish.

8. MSG is considered safe to use during pregnancy, but some people do have negative reactions to it, such as headaches and stomach upset.

9. You may wish to use dish detergent on produce; however, there is some disagreement about its safety. Some experts say it's fine, others say that the detergent might be absorbed by the produce, which might present its own set of problems. A produce wash product may be safer, although these have not been tested by the FDA. If you do use detergent or produce wash, be sure to rinse very thoroughly.

skins when possible and practical to remove surface chemical residues, especially when a vegetable has a waxy coating (as cucumbers and sometimes tomatoes, apples, peppers, and eggplant do). Peel skins that still seem "coated" after washing.

◆ Beware of picture-perfect produce. Fruits and vegetables that appear to have been embalmed, so unblemished are they, may very well have been protected by heavy levels of pesticides in the fields or may have been coated in preservatives to ensure good looks that will endure even after a long trip to the market. The less pretty produce may be the healthier bet.

◆ Buy organic produce when possible and practical. Produce that is certified organic usually is as close as possible to being free of all chemical residues. Transitional produce may still contain some residues from soil contamination, but should be safer than conventionally grown produce. If organic produce is available locally and you can afford the premium price, make it your choice. If it isn't available, ask the produce manager at your favorite market to order it. It's worth a shot. He might listen, especially if you're a good customer. The more demand there is for organic produce, the lower prices will drop.

◆ Favor domestic produce. Imported produce (and foods made from such produce) often contain higher levels of pesticides than that grown in the U.S., since pesticide regulation in other countries is often lax or nonexistent. Bananas, all of which are imported, are safe, however; government monitoring sources have found them virtually free of pesticides.

◆ Vary your diet. Variety ensures not only a more interesting gastronomic experience and better nutrition, but also better chances of avoiding excessive exposure to any one potentially toxic substance. Switch between broccoli, kale, and carrots, for instance; melon, peaches, and strawberries; salmon, halibut, and sole; cereals made from whole wheat, corn, and oats.

◆ Don't be fanatic. Though it's smart to try to avoid theoretical hazards in food, making your life stressful in order to do so isn't necessary.

SUSHI SAFETY

"Sushi is my favorite food, but I heard you're not supposed to eat it while you're pregnant. Is that true?"

Sorry to say, sushi and sashimi will have to go the way of sake (the Japanese wine often served with them) during pregnancy—which is to say, they're off-limits. Same holds true for raw oysters and clams, "seared" tuna or salmon, fish tartars or carpaccios, and other raw or barely cooked fish and shellfish. But that doesn't mean you have to steer clear of your favorite Japanese restaurants. Plenty of other options exist there—even at the sushi bar. Rolls that contain thoroughly cooked fish or seafood and/or vegetables are, in fact, healthy options—just make sure you reach for the low-sodium soy sauce. (Don't, however, worry about any raw fish you've eaten up to this point.)

HOT STUFF

"I love spicy food—the hotter, the better. Is it safe to eat it while I'm pregnant?"

Hot mamas-to-be can continue to challenge their taste buds with four-alarm chilis, salsas, and stir-fries—as long as you can tolerate the almost

EATING SAFE

A more immediate—and proven—threat than the chemicals in your food are the little organisms—bacteria and parasites— that can contaminate it. These nasty villains can cause anything from mild stomach upset to severe illness. To make sure that the worst thing you'll pick up from your next meal is a little heartburn, shop, prepare, and eat with care:

♦ When in doubt, throw it out. Make this your mantra of safe eating. It applies to any food you even *suspect* might be spoiled. Read and abide by freshness dates on food packages.

♦ When food shopping, avoid fish, meat, and eggs that are not well refrigerated or kept on ice. Steer clear of jars that are leaky or don't "pop" when you open them, and cans that are rusty or seem swollen or otherwise misshapen.

♦ Wash your hands *before* food is handled and *after* touching raw meat, fish, or eggs. If you have a cut or infection on your hand, wear rubber or plastic gloves while you prepare food, and remember, they need to be washed as often as your bare hands.

♦ Keep kitchen counters and sinks clean. Use nonporous surfaces (such as glass, stainless steel, and Formica) rather than porous ones (wood or plastic with dirt-collecting gashes) for food preparation, and keep these scrupulously clean (wash with soap and hot water or in the dishwasher). Wash dishcloths frequently and keep sponges clean (replace them often, too); they can harbor bacteria.

♦ Serve hot foods hot, cold foods cold. Leftovers should be refrigerated quickly and heated until steaming before reusing. (Perishable foods that have been left out for more than two hours should be tossed.) Don't eat frozen foods that have been thawed and then refrozen.

♦ Thaw foods in the refrigerator, time permitting. (Measure the interior temperature with a refrigerator thermometer and be sure it stays at 41°F or less. Ideally, the freezer should be at 0°F, though many freezers are not designed to meet that requirement; don't worry if yours isn't.) If you're in a rush, thaw in the microwave or in a watertight plastic bag submerged in cold water (and change it

---

inevitable heartburn and indigestion that follow. There's no risk to the pregnancy or the fetus from spicy foods and, in fact, since peppers of all kinds (including hot ones) are packed with vitamin C, many of these foods are extra-nutritious. So enjoy, but don't forget to take along the antacid.

SPOILED FOOD

"I ate a container of yogurt this morning without realizing that it had expired a week ago. It didn't taste spoiled, but now I'm concerned that I've hurt the baby."

No need to cry over spoiled milk . . . or yogurt. Though eating dairy products that have recently "expired" is never a particularly good idea, it's rarely a dangerous one. If you haven't shown any ill effects from your postdate snack (symptoms of food poisoning usually occur within eight hours), there's obviously no harm done. Besides, food poisoning is an unlikely possibility if the yogurt had been refrigerated continuously. In the future, however, check dates more carefully before you buy or eat perishables, and, of course, never eat foods that appear to have developed mold. For more on food safety, see the above box.

every thirty minutes). Never thaw foods at room temperature.

♦ Marinate meat, fish, or poultry in the refrigerator, not on the counter. Discard the marinade after use, since it contains potentially hazardous bacteria. If you'd like to use the marinade as a dip or sauce, or to baste with, reserve a portion for that purpose before you add the meat, poultry, or fish.

♦ Never eat raw or undercooked meats, poultry, fish, or shellfish while you're expecting. Always cook meats and fish (to 160°F) and poultry (to 180°F) thoroughly. In general, the thermometer should be placed in the thickest part of the food, away from bone, fat, or gristle. In poultry, it should be placed in the dark meat.

♦ Don't eat eggs that are runny (prefer well-scrambled to sunny-side up), and if you're mixing a batter that contains raw eggs, resist the urge to lick the spoon (or your fingers!). The exception to this rule: eggs that are pasteurized, since this process effectively eliminates the risk of salmonella poisoning.

♦ Wash raw vegetables thoroughly (especially if they won't be cooked thoroughly before eating).

♦ Avoid alfalfa and other sprouts, which are often contaminated with bacteria.

♦ Stick to pasteurized dairy products, and make sure those that you use have been refrigerated continuously. Soft cheeses, such as feta, brie, blue cheeses, and soft Mexican-style cheese made from unpasteurized milk (also called "raw milk"), can be contaminated with listeria (see page 460) and are particularly dangerous for pregnant women.

♦ Hot dogs and cold cuts (such as salami, bologna, corned beef, and liverwurst) can also be contaminated with listeria. As a precaution, even ready-cooked meats like these should be heated to 165°F before you eat them.

♦ Juice should be pasteurized, too. Avoid unpasteurized juice or cider, whether it's bought at a health food store or a roadside stand. If you're not sure whether a juice is pasteurized, don't drink it.

♦ When eating out, avoid establishments that seem to ignore basic sanitation rules. Some signs are pretty obvious: Perishable foods are kept at room temperature; kitchen workers and waiters handle food directly with their hands; the bathrooms are unclean; and so on.

"I got food poisoning from something I ate last night, and I've been throwing up. Will that hurt my baby?"

You're much more likely to suffer from the food poisoning than your baby is. The major risk—for you and your baby—is that you'll become dehydrated from vomiting and diarrhea. So make sure you get plenty of fluids (which are more important in the short term than solids) to replace those that you're losing. And contact your practitioner if your diarrhea is severe and/or your stools are bloody or mucousy. See page 459 for more.

READING LABELS

"I'm eager to eat well, but it's difficult to figure out what's in the products I buy."

Labels aren't designed to help you as much as to sell you. Keep this in mind when food shopping, and learn to read the small print, especially the ingredients list and the nutrition label (which is designed to help you).

The ingredients listing will tell you, in order of predominance (with the first ingredient the most plentiful and the last the least), exactly what is in the product. A quick perusal will tell you whether the

YOU CAN'T TELL A FRUIT BY ITS COVER

When it comes to nutrition, the darker the color of *most* fruits and vegetables, the more vitamins and minerals (especially vitamin A) you'll be able to harvest from them. But keep in mind that it's the color inside—not outside—that signals good nutrition. So while cucumbers (dark on the outside, pale on the inside) are lightweights in that department, cantaloupes (pale on the outside, dark on the inside) are standouts (see page 89 for more).

major ingredient in a cereal is refined grain or a whole grain. It will also tell you when a product is high in sugar, salt, fat, or additives. For example, when sugar is listed near the top of the ingredients list or when it appears in several different forms on a list (corn syrup, honey, and sugar), you know the product is high in sugar. Checking the grams of sugar on the label will not be useful until the FDA orders that the grams of "added sugar" be separated from the grams of "naturally occurring sugar"—in fruits, for example. Though the number of grams of sugar on the present label may be the same on a container of orange juice and a container of fruit drink, they are not equivalent, since one comes from nutritious fruit juice and one from added sugar.

Nutrition labels, which appear on most packaged products on your grocer's shelves, can be particularly valuable for a pregnant woman counting her protein and watching her calories, as they provide the grams of the former and the number of the latter in each serving. The listing of percentages of the government's recommended dietary allowance (now called DRIs—Dietary Reference Intakes), however, is less useful, because the DRI for pregnant women is different from the DRI used on package labels. Still, a food that scores high in a wide variety of nutrients is a good product to purchase.

While it's important to pay attention to the small print, it's sometimes just as important to ignore the large print. When a box of English muffins trumpets boldly, "Made with whole wheat, bran, and honey," reading the small print may reveal that that the major ingredient (first on the list) is white, not whole-wheat, flour, that the muffins contain precious little bran (it's near the bottom of the ingredients list), and that there's a lot more white sugar (it's high on the list) than honey (it's low).

"Enriched" and "fortified" are also banners to be wary of. Adding a few vitamins to a poor food doesn't make it a good food. You'd be much better off with a bowl of oatmeal, which comes by its vitamins honestly, than with a refined cereal with 12 grams of added sugar and a few pennies' worth of vitamins and minerals added.

What It's Important to Know: PLAYING IT SAFE

The home. The highway. The back-yard. The most significant risks faced by pregnant women are not from pregnancy complications, but from accidents.

Accidents often seem "accidental," that is, a chance happening, yet most are the direct result of carelessness—often on the part of the victim herself—and many can be avoided with a little extra caution and common sense. There's a wide variety of steps you can take to play it safe while you're expecting:

- Recognize that you're not as graceful as you were prepregnancy. As your abdomen grows, your center of gravity will shift, making it easier for you to lose your balance. You will also find it increasingly difficult to see your feet. These changes can contribute to your becoming accident-prone.

- Always fasten your seat belt—and keep it fastened—in autos and on air-planes. If you are sitting in the front passenger seat in a car with an air bag, be sure your seat is as far back as possible. If you are driving a car with an air bag in the steering wheel, tilt the wheel toward your chest, away from your tummy, and sit at least ten inches from the steering wheel if pos-sible. Keep objects off your lap and off the dashboard, since they can be-come projectiles. When you can, ride in the backseat.

- Never climb on a shaky chair or lad-der, or better still, don't climb at all.

- Don't wear high spiky heels, smooth-soled shoes, sloppy slippers, or thongs that can snap, all of which encourage falls and twisted ankles. And don't walk in socks or stockings on a slippery floor.

- Be careful getting in and out of the tub; be sure your tub and shower are equipped with nonskid surfaces. Sturdy grab bars make the bathing experience even safer as you get bulkier and less graceful.

- Check your house and backyard for hazards: rugs without skid-proof bot-toms, especially at the top of stairs; toys or junk on stairways; poorly lit stairs and hallways; wires strung across the floor; overwaxed floors; icy sidewalks and steps.

- Keep night-lights on to light your way during those nocturnal visits to the bathroom and back. Also make sure there are no stumbling blocks lying on your path to the toilet.

- Observe the safety rules of whatever sport you play; follow all the tips for safe exercise and activity on page 190.

- Don't overdo it, and make sure you get enough sleep. Fatigue is a major contributor to accidents.

◆ ◆ ◆

The Third Month

Approximately 9 to 13 Weeks

This is the last month of your first trimester, and early pregnancy symptoms may still be going strong. Which means you're probably not sure whether you're tired from first-trimester fatigue, or because you woke up three times to go to the bathroom. But there are better days ahead. If you've been suffering from nausea and vomiting, there's likely a light at the end of the morning sickness tunnel. As energy levels pick up, you'll soon have more get-up-and-go—and as urinary urges ease, you may have to get up and go less often. Even better, you may hear the amazing sound of your baby's heartbeat at this month's checkup—which might make all those uncomfortable symptoms seem worthwhile.

What You Can Expect at This Month's Checkup

This month you can expect your practitioner to check the following, though there may be variations depending upon your particular needs and your practitioner's style of practice:[1]

♦ Weight and blood pressure

♦ Urine, for sugar and protein

♦ Fetal heartbeat

1. See Appendix, page 545, for an explanation of the procedures and tests performed.

♦ Size of uterus, by external palpation (feeling from the outside), to see how it correlates to estimated date of delivery (EDD), or due date

♦ Height of fundus (the top of the uterus)

♦ Hands and feet for edema (swelling), and legs for varicose veins

♦ Questions or problems you want to discuss—have a list ready

What You May Be Feeling

As always, remember that every pregnancy and every woman is different. You may experience all of these symptoms at one time or another, or only a few of them. Some may have continued from last month, others may be new. Still others may hardly be noticed because you've become so used to them. You may also have other, less common, symptoms.

PHYSICALLY

♦ Fatigue and sleepiness

♦ A need to urinate frequently

♦ Slight increase in vaginal discharge

♦ Nausea, with or without vomiting, and/or excessive salivation

♦ Constipation

A LOOK INSIDE

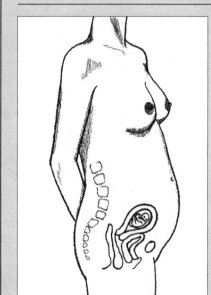

of an apple. The head—which sits on a neck now instead of flat on the shoulders—is still disproportionately large, taking up half of baby's crown-to-rump length; the whorl of a hair pattern is discernible on the scalp. The fetus's eyes are moving closer together and its ears are positioning themselves on the sides of the head—making it look more human. Fingers and toes have soft nails covering them now, and the hands have become more functional. Inside the fetus's mouth, taste buds have developed, as has the sucking reflex, and twenty buds that will one day become baby teeth have formed. Baby is making urine now, and excreting it in the amniotic fluid. The external genitalia are now well developed enough so that the sex of the baby can be detected, and the heartbeat can be heard with a Doppler.

▲ This month, your uterus is a little bigger than a grapefruit and your waist may start to thicken. By the end of the month, your uterus can be felt right above your pubic bone in the lower abdomen.

► Your baby is a fetus now—and a fast-growing one, reaching 2½ to 3 inches in length and weighing 1½ ounces by the end of the month. It is about the size

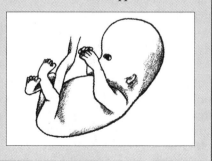

- Heartburn, indigestion, flatulence, bloating

- Food aversions and cravings

- Breast changes: fullness, heaviness, tenderness, tingling; darkening of the areola (the pigmented area surrounding the nipple); sweat glands in the areola becoming prominent, like large goose bumps; expanding network of bluish lines under the skin

- Additional veins visible elsewhere, as blood supply to abdomen and legs also increases

- Occasional headaches

- Occasional faintness or dizziness

- Tightness of clothing around waist and bust, if it wasn't tight already; abdomen may appear enlarged by end of month

- Increasing appetite

EMOTIONALLY

- Instability comparable to premenstrual syndrome (but probably more pronounced), which may include irritability, mood swings, irrationality, weepiness

- Misgivings, fear, joy, elation—any or all

- A new sense of calmness

What You May Be Concerned About

CONSTIPATION

"I've been terribly constipated for the past few weeks. Is this common?"

Very common. And there are good reasons why. For one, high levels of certain hormones circulating during pregnancy cause the muscles of the bowel to relax, making elimination sluggish. For another, the growing uterus puts pressure on the bowel, cramping its normal activity.

But you don't have to accept constipation as inevitable just because you're pregnant. Irregularity can be overcome by taking the following measures, which can also help head off hemorrhoids, a common result of irregularity:

Fight back with fiber. Avoid refined foods (such as white rice and white bread), which are often constipating, and focus on such fiber-rich selections as fresh fruit and vegetables (raw or lightly cooked, with skin left on when possible);

whole-grain cereals; whole-grain breads, cakes, and other baked goods; legumes (beans and peas); and dried fruit (raisins, prunes, apricots, figs). You need about 25 to 35 grams of fiber daily.[2] If you've never been a big fiber fan, add these foods to your diet gradually or you may find your digestive tract protesting loudly. (But since flatulence is a common complaint of pregnancy as well as a frequent, but usually temporary, side effect of a newly fiber-infused diet, you may find your digestive tract protesting for a while anyway.) Spreading your daily fare out over six small meals rather than trying to squeeze the works into three overly filling ones may make you less uncomfortable.

---

2. Nutrition labels on packaged foods specify the grams of fiber in a serving; use them to help you be sure you're getting enough. But remember, there can also be plenty of fiber in foods, such as produce, that don't come packaged with nutrition labels.

If your constipation doesn't seem to respond to such dietary manipulation, combined with the other tactics below, add high-powered fiber in the form of wheat bran or psyllium (follow package directions) to your diet, starting with a sprinkle and working up to a couple of tablespoons. But avoid larger quantities of these ultra-high-fiber items; as they move speedily through your system, they can carry away important nutrients before they've had a chance to be absorbed. No matter how uncomfortable you are, don't resort to herbal remedies, castor oil, or other stimulant laxatives. Though some may combat constipation, their side effects can be very uncomfortable—and after long-term use, even harmful. In fact, don't take any medication for constipation (over-the-counter, prescribed, or herbal) without your practitioner's okay.

Drown your opponent. Constipation doesn't stand a chance against an ample fluid intake. Most fluids—particularly water and fruit and vegetable juices—are effective in softening stool and keeping food moving along the digestive tract. Some people find drinking hot water flavored with lemon especially helpful. If constipation is severe, prune juice may do the trick.

When you gotta go, go. Holding in bowel movements regularly can weaken muscles that control them and lead to constipation. Timing can help avoid this problem. For example, have your high-fiber breakfast a little earlier than usual, so it will have a chance to kick in before you have to dash off to work.

Check your supplements and medications. Constipation can sometimes be traced to calcium or iron supplements, to antacids containing calcium or aluminum, or to other medications (over-the-counter or prescribed). If you

suspect that is the case with you, discuss with your practitioner whether you should change the supplement formula or the medication you take.

Start an exercise campaign. An active body encourages active bowels, so fit a brisk walk of about half an hour into your daily routine (some people find even a ten-minute walk works); supplement it with any exercise you enjoy that is safe during pregnancy (see Exercise During Pregnancy, starting on page 190).

If your efforts don't seem to be productive, consult with your practitioner. He or she may prescribe a bulk-forming stool softener for occasional use.

"All my pregnant friends seem to have problems with constipation. I don't; in fact, I've remained very regular. Is my system working right?"

Pregnant women are so programmed by mothers, friends, books, even doctors, to expect constipation that those who do become constipated accept it as normal and inevitable, and those who don't worry that there's something wrong.

But from the sound of things, your system couldn't be working better. Chances are your new digestive efficiency is attributable to your lifestyle—one that you've been enjoying for a long while or one you've adopted since you learned you were expecting. Stepping up your consumption of fiber-rich foods and fluids, and exercising regularly, are bound to counteract the natural digestive slowdown of pregnancy and keep things moving smoothly. If this dietary style is new to you, the productivity of your digestive tract may decrease a little (and flatulence, which often temporarily accompanies such dietary changes, may ease up) as your system gets used to the rough stuff, but you will probably continue to be "regular."

ANOTHER REASON FOR BEING TIRED, MOODY, AND CONSTIPATED

Have you been tired, moody, and constipated lately? Welcome to the pregnancy club. Surging gestational hormones, of course, trigger those pesky symptoms in most pregnant women. However, a shortage of another hormone, thyroxine, can mimic these common pregnancy complaints, as well as many others—weight gain, skin problems of all kinds, muscle aches and cramps, a decrease in libido, memory loss, swelling (especially of hands and feet), even carpal tunnel syndrome. (Another common symptom, an increased sensitivity to cold, is more clear-cut during pregnancy, since expectant moms tend to be warmer rather than chillier.) Consequently, hypothyroidism (a deficiency of thyroid hormone due to an underactive thyroid gland) may be easy for physicians to miss in an expectant mom. Yet the condition, which affects 1 in 50 women, can have an adverse affect on pregnancy (also wreaking havoc in the postpartum period; see page 417), so proper diagnosis and treatment are vital.

Hyperthyroidism (when too much thyroid hormone is produced by an overactive gland) is seen less often in pregnancy, but can also cause complications if left untreated. Symptoms of hyperthyroidism—many of which may also be hard to distinguish from pregnancy symptoms—include fatigue, insomnia, irritability, warm skin and sensitivity to heat, rapid heartbeat, and weight loss (or trouble gaining weight).

If you have ever been diagnosed with thyroid problems in the past (even if they have since cleared up) or if you currently take medication for a thyroid condition, it's very important to let your practitioner know. Since the body must produce more thyroid hormone during pregnancy to keep up with fetal demands, it's possible you may need medication again or may need your current medication adjusted.

If you have never been diagnosed with a thyroid condition, but you're experiencing some or all of the symptoms of hypo- or hyperthyroidism (and especially if you have a family history of thyroid disease, since the genetic link is very strong), check with your doctor. A simple blood test can determine whether you have a problem or not. Be sure it measures both the level of thyroid hormone in the blood (T4) and the amount of TSH (thyroid-stimulating hormone; abnormal levels mean that the body is working hard to compensate for an underactive or overactive gland). When a TSH is too high or too low, it can spell trouble even when actual thyroid levels are within the normal range.

"I'm not at all constipated. In fact, for the last couple of weeks I've had loose stools—almost diarrhea. Is this normal or something to worry about?"

When it comes to pregnancy symptoms, normal is often what's normal for you. And in your case, more frequent stools may be just that. Every body reacts differently to pregnancy hormones—yours may be reacting by stepping up, not slowing down, on production of bowel movements. It's also possible that this increased bowel activity is due to a positive change in your diet and exercise habits.

You can try cutting back on bowel-stimulating foods, such as dried fruits (particularly prunes), and adding bulking foods (such as bananas) until your stool becomes more firm. To compensate for the fluids you're losing through loose stools, make sure you're drinking enough.

If your stools are very frequent (more than three a day) or watery, bloody, or mucousy, check with your practitioner. Severe diarrhea requires prompt intervention during pregnancy.

FLATULENCE (GAS)

"I'm very bloated from gas and worry that the pressure, which is so uncomfortable for me, might also be hurting the baby."

Snug and safe in a uterine cocoon, protected on all sides by impact-absorbing amniotic fluid, your baby is impervious to your intestinal distress. If anything, he or she probably is soothed by the bubbling and gurgling of your gastric Muzak.

Baby won't be happy, though, if bloating—which often worsens late in the day—prevents you from eating regularly and properly. To avoid this risk (and to minimize your own discomfort), take the following measures:

Stay regular. Constipation is a common cause of gas and bloating.

Graze, don't gorge. Large meals just add to that bloated feeling. They also overload your digestive system, which isn't at its most efficient anyway in pregnancy. Instead of three large meals a day, eat six small ones or three moderate-size meals plus a couple of snacks.

Don't gulp. When you rush through meals or eat on the run, you're bound to swallow as much air as food. This captured air forms painful pockets of gas in your gut.

Keep calm. Particularly during meals: Tension and anxiety can cause you to swallow air, which in turn can lead to gassiness. Taking a few deep breaths before meals may help to relax you.

Steer clear of gas-producers. Your stomach will tell you what they are—they vary from person to person. Common offenders include onions, cabbage, fried foods, rich sauces, sugary sweets, and, of course, the notorious beans.

WEIGHT GAIN

"I'm concerned that I didn't gain any weight in my first trimester."

Many women have trouble putting on an ounce in the early weeks; some even lose a few pounds, usually courtesy of morning sickness. Fortunately, nature offers some protection for the babies of mothers who are too queasy to eat well during the first trimester: the fetus's need for calories and certain nutrients during this time is not as great as it will be later, so not gaining early on isn't likely to have an effect. But not gaining weight from here on in *can* have an effect—a significant one—because calories and nutrients will be more and more in demand as your baby-making factory picks up steam.

So don't worry, but do eat. And start watching your weight carefully to make sure it begins to move upward at a satisfactory rate (an average of about 1 pound a week through the eighth month). If you continue to have trouble gaining weight, try packing more of a nutritional wallop with the calories you take in, through efficient eating (see page 85). Try, too, to eat a little more food each day, by not skipping meals and by adding more frequent snacks. If you can't eat a lot at one sitting, have four to six small meals daily instead of three big ones. Save salads and soups and fill-you-up beverages for after your main course to avoid putting a damper on your appetite. Enjoy foods high in good fats (nuts, fatty fish, avocados, olive oil). But don't try to add pounds by adding junk food to your diet—that kind of weight gain will round out your hips and thighs, not your baby.

"I was shocked to find out that I'd already gained 13 pounds in the first trimester. What should I do now?"

You can't turn back the scales. That weight is there to stay for now, at least until some time after delivery. And you can't apply the extra pounds toward next trimester's gain, either. Your fetus needs a steady supply of calories and nutrients, particularly during the months to come, so you can't cut back on calories now, expecting your baby to get sufficient nourishment from the excess weight you've already accumulated. Dieting to lose or maintain weight is never appropriate during pregnancy, and it is an especially dangerous game during the second and third trimesters, when fetal growth is dramatically swift and significant.

But while you can't do anything about the weight you've gained so far, there's plenty you can do to ensure that you don't continue putting on pounds at an excessive rate. Some women experience an early weight-gain blitz because they overindulge in the kinds of starchy sweets they find comforting to their morning-sick tummies. If that was your problem, it should be less and less so as queasiness tapers off and an appetite for a more varied diet returns. Other women gain too much in the first trimester because they've bought into the misconception that no-holds-barred eating is a pregnant woman's right and responsibility. Review the Pregnancy Diet (see Chapter 4 and *What to Eat When You're Expecting*) to find out why it isn't, and to learn how you can eat for your baby's health without munching your way to a 60-pound weight gain. Gaining efficiently, on the highest-quality foods possible, will not only accomplish that goal but will make the weight you do gain easier to shed in the postpartum period.

HEADACHES

"I find that I'm getting a lot more headaches than ever before. Do I have to suffer with them?"

That women are more susceptible to headaches during the time they're supposed to stay away from certain pain relievers is one of the ironies of pregnancy. It's an irony you'll have to live with, but it's not necessarily one you'll have to suffer with excessively. Prevention, teamed with the right home remedies (see below)—and if those fail, acetaminophen (Tylenol)—can offer some relief from the recurrent headaches of pregnancy.

The best way to prevent and treat the headache depends on the cause or causes. Pregnancy headaches are most commonly the result of hormonal changes (which are responsible for the increased frequency and severity of many types of headaches, including sinus headaches), fatigue, tension, hunger, physical or emotional stress, or any combination of these.

With many of the following ways of overcoming and preventing headaches, you can fit the possible cure to the probable cause:

Relax. Pregnancy can be a time of high anxiety, with tension headaches a common result. Some women find relief through meditation and yoga. You can take a course or read a book on these or other relaxation techniques, or try those on page 127.

Of course, relaxation exercises don't work for everyone; some women find that they increase tension instead of alleviating it. For them, lying down in a dark, quiet room, or stretching out on the sofa or with their feet up at their desk for ten or fifteen minutes is a better foil for tension and tension headaches.

Get enough rest. Pregnancy can also be a time of extreme fatigue, particularly in the first and last trimesters, and often for the full nine months for women who work long hours at a job and/or have other children to care for. Sleep can be elusive once the belly starts swelling ("How will I ever get comfortable?") and the mind starts racing ("How will I ever get everything done before the baby comes?"), which compounds fatigue. Making a conscious effort to get more rest, day and night, can help keep headaches at bay. But be careful not to sleep *too much,* as excess sleep can also give you a headache.

Eat regularly. To avoid hunger headaches triggered by low blood sugar, be sure not to miss meals. Carry high-energy snacks (such as whole-grain crackers, granola bars, dried fruit) with you in your purse, stash them in the glove compartment of your car and in your office desk drawer, and always keep a supply on hand at home.

Seek some peace and quiet. If you're "allergic" to noise, stay away from it whenever possible. Avoid loud music, noisy restaurants, packed parties, and crowded department stores. At home, lower the volume on the telephone's ringer, the TV, and the radio.

Don't get stuffy. If an overheated, smoke-filled, unventilated room touches off headaches, avoid such locations entirely when possible or at least leave them for a stroll outdoors now and then. Dress in layers when you know you're going somewhere stuffy, and keep comfortable by removing layers as needed. If your workplace is poorly ventilated, move to a better-ventilated office or area if that's possible; take frequent breaks if it isn't.

Switch lighting. Some women find that other environmental factors, such as lighting, can trigger headaches. For example, a windowless work space lit by fluorescent bulbs might be a culprit. Switching to incandescent lighting and/or a room with windows may help.

Try alternatives. Some alternative and complementary medical approaches—including acupuncture, biofeedback, and massage—can bring headache relief (see page 246).

Go hot and cold. For relief of sinus headaches, apply hot and cold compresses to the aching area, alternating thirty seconds of each for a total of ten minutes, four times a day. For tension headaches, try ice applied to the back of the neck for twenty minutes while you close your eyes and relax. (Use an ordinary ice pack or a special neck pillow that holds a gel-based cold pack.)

Straighten up. Slouching or looking down to read or do other close work for long stretches of time can also cause headaches, so watch your posture.

If an unexplained headache persists for more than a few hours, returns very often, is the result of fever, or is accompanied by visual disturbances or puffiness of the hands and face, notify your practitioner at once.

"I suffer from migraine headaches. I heard they are more common in pregnancy. Is this true?"

Some women find their migraines strike more frequently during pregnancy; others find they are less frequent. It isn't known why this should be so, or even why some people have recurrent migraines and others never have a single one.

Migraines are headaches that are in a class by themselves. Their development is related to constriction, or narrowing, of the blood vessels in the head, followed by their sudden dilation, or opening.

This interferes with blood flow and causes pain and other symptoms. Though symptoms vary from person to person, a migraine is usually preceded by fatigue. The fatigue may then be followed by nausea with or without vomiting and diarrhea, sensitivity to light, and possibly a misting over or a zigzagging pattern in one or, occasionally, both eyes. When the headache finally arrives, anywhere from minutes to hours after the first warning symptom, the pain, which is intense and throbbing, is usually localized on one side, but it can spread to the other side. Some people also experience tingling or numbness in one arm or side of the body, dizziness, ringing in the ears, runny nose, runny and/or bloodshot eyes, and temporary mental confusion.

If you've had migraines in the past, be prepared for dealing with them during pregnancy, preferably through prevention. If you know what brings on an attack, you can try to avoid the culprit. Stress is a common one (see page 125 for tips on handling it), as are chocolate, cheese, coffee, and red wine. Try to determine what, if anything, can stave off a full-blown attack once the warning signs appear. Many people are helped by one or more of the following: splashing the face with cold water or applying a cold cloth or ice pack; avoiding noise, light, and odors by lying down in a darkened room for two or three hours, eyes covered (napping, meditating, or listening to music, but not reading or watching TV); trying biofeedback (see page 246). If these don't help, discuss with your physician which migraine medications are safe to take during pregnancy, and which of these might be most effective.

If you experience for the first time what seems like a migraine, call your practitioner immediately. The same symptoms could also be indicative of a pregnancy complication. As with any unexplained headache that persists for more than a few hours, returns very often, is the result of fever, or is accompanied by visual disturbances or puffiness of the hands and face, it's important to notify your practitioner at once.

STRETCH MARKS

"I'm afraid I'm going to get stretch marks. Can they be prevented?"

For many women—especially those who favor bikinis—stretch marks are dreaded more than cellulite. Nevertheless, 90 percent of all women will develop these pink or reddish, slightly indented, sometimes itchy streaks on their breasts, hips, and/or abdomen sometime during pregnancy.

As their name implies, stretch marks are caused by the skin stretching, generally due to a large and/or rapid increase in weight. Expectant mothers who have good, elastic skin tone (because they either inherited it or earned it through years of excellent nutrition and exercise) may slip through several pregnancies without a single telltale striation. Others may be able to minimize, if not prevent, stretch marks by keeping weight gain steady, gradual, and moderate. Promoting elasticity in your skin by nourishing it with a good diet may also help. Though there's no medical proof that creams really help prevent stretch marks, some women claim they do. If nothing else, it may be fun for your spouse to rub them on your tummy. An added plus: using a moisturizer may help prevent your skin from becoming dry and itchy.

If you do develop stretch marks, you can console yourself with the knowledge that they will gradually fade to a silvery sheen some months after delivery. You can also discuss with a dermatologist the possibility of reducing their visibility *postpartum* with laser therapy or Retin-A.

Baby's Heartbeat

"My friend heard her baby's heartbeat at ten weeks. I'm a week ahead of her and my practitioner hasn't picked up my baby's yet."

The ordinary stethoscope, once used routinely for detecting the fetal heartbeat, isn't powerful enough to pick up the beat until the 17th or 18th week at the earliest. Today the heartbeat can be heard as early as the 10th or 12th week with a Doppler, a handheld ultrasound device that amplifies the sound. Even with a Doppler, the heartbeat may not be audible this early because of the baby's position, the location of the placenta, the position of the uterus, or excess layers of maternal fat. It's also possible that a slightly miscalculated due date may be causing the delay. Wait until next month. By your 14th week, the miraculous sound of your baby's heartbeat is certain to be available for your listening pleasure. If it isn't, or if you are very anxious, your practitioner may order an ultrasound, which will pick up a heartbeat that, for some reason, was difficult to hear with the Doppler. (Frequent use of the Doppler, by the way, is considered perfectly safe.)

Sexual Desire

"All of my pregnant friends say that they had an increased desire for sex early in pregnancy—some had orgasms and multiple orgasms for the first time. How come I feel so unsexy?"

Pregnancy is a time of change in many aspects of your life, not the least of them sexual. Some women who have never had either an orgasm or much of a taste for sex suddenly experience both for the first time when pregnant. Other women, accustomed to having a voracious appetite for sex and to being easily orgasmic, suddenly find that they are completely lacking in desire and are difficult to arouse. These changes in sexuality can be disconcerting, guilt-provoking, wonderful, or a confusing combination of all three. And they are all perfectly normal.

As you'll see when you read Making Love During Pregnancy (page 233), there are many logical explanations for such changes and for the feelings that they may provoke. Some of these factors may be strongest early in pregnancy: nausea and fatigue may make you feel understandably unsexy; or being able to make love without worrying about trying to get (or trying not to get) pregnant may free you of inhibitions and make you sexier than ever; or feeling sexy may result in guilt because you think you should be feeling motherly instead. Other physical and emotional factors that may make orgasm easier to achieve, more powerful, or more elusive continue throughout gestation.

Most important is recognizing that your sexual feelings during pregnancy—and your partner's as well—may be more erratic than erotic; you may feel sexy one day and not the next. Mutual understanding and open communication will see you through, as will a sense of humor.

Oral Sex

"I've heard that oral sex is dangerous during pregnancy. Is this true?"

Cunnilingus (oral stimulation of the female genitalia) is safe throughout pregnancy as long as your partner is careful not to blow any air into your vagina. Doing this could force air into your bloodstream and cause an embolism, which could obstruct a blood vessel and could prove deadly to both mother and baby.

Fellatio (oral stimulation of the penis) is always safe during pregnancy and for some couples is a very satisfactory substitute when intercourse isn't permitted. For more information on what's safe and what's not when it comes to sex and the pregnant couple, see page 233.

CRAMP AFTER ORGASM

"I get an abdominal cramp after orgasm. Is this a sign that sex is hurting my baby? Will it cause a miscarriage?"

Cramping—both during and after orgasm, and sometimes accompanied by backache—is very common and harmless during a normal, low-risk pregnancy. Its cause can be physical: a combination of the normal increased blood flow to the pelvic area during pregnancy, the equally normal congestion of the sexual organs during arousal and orgasm, and the normal contractions of the uterus following orgasm. Or it can be psychological: a result of the common, but unfounded, fear of hurting the baby during intercourse. Or it can be a combination of physical and psychological factors, since the mind-body connection is so strong when it comes to sex.

The cramping is not a sign that sex is hurting the fetus. Most experts agree that sexual relations and orgasm during a normal, low-risk pregnancy are perfectly safe and are not a cause of miscarriage. If the cramps bother you, ask your partner for a gentle low back rub. It may relieve not only the cramps but any tension that might be triggering them, as well. Some women also experience cramps in the legs after intercourse. See page 243 for tips on relieving the discomfort. (Also see Making Love During Pregnancy, page 233.)

TWINS AND MORE

"I'm already very big. Could I be carrying twins?"

It's more likely that you're just carrying a little extra weight because you gained more than your share in the first trimester. Or that you're small-boned to begin with and uterine expansion is noticeable earlier on you than it would be on someone with a bigger frame. A relatively large abdomen in and of itself is not generally considered a sign that an expectant mother is carrying multiple fetuses; in making the diagnosis, a practitioner will look at other factors, including the following:

A large-for-date uterus. The size of the uterus, not of the abdomen, is what counts in the diagnosis of multiple fetuses. If your uterus seems to be growing more rapidly than expected for your due date, a multiple pregnancy would be suspected. Other possible explanations for a large-for-date uterus include a miscalculated due date, an excessive amount of amniotic fluid, or fibroids.

Exaggerated pregnancy symptoms. When twins are being carried, the typical troubles of pregnancy (morning sickness, indigestion, edema, and so on) can be doubled, or at least seem that way. But all of these can also be exaggerated in a singleton (one-fetus) pregnancy.

More than one heartbeat. Depending on the position of the babies, a practitioner may be able to hear two (or more) distinctly separate heartbeats. But because the heartbeat of a single fetus may be heard at several locations, the locating of two (or more) confirms twins (or more) only if the heartbeats are different in rate. So twins aren't often diagnosed this way.

Predisposition. Though there are no factors that increase the chances of hav-

TWINS

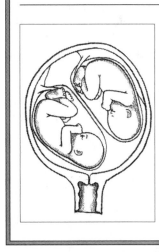

◄ *Fraternal twins, which result from two eggs being fertilized at the same time, each have their own placenta.*

► *Identical twins, which come from one fertilized egg that splits and then develops into two separate embryos, may share a placenta or—depending on when the egg splits— they may each have their own placenta.*

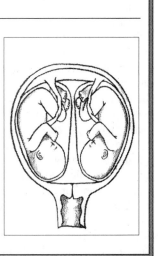

ing identical twins, there are several that make a woman more likely to have nonidentical twins. These include nonidentical twins in the mother's family, advanced age (women over thirty-five more frequently release more than one egg), the use of fertility drugs to stimulate ovulation, and in vitro fertilization. Twins are also more common among black women than white, but are less common among Asian and Hispanic women.

If one or more of these factors lead the practitioner to the conclusion that there's a possibility of more than one fetus, an ultrasound exam will be ordered. In virtually every case (except in the rare instance where one camera-shy fetus remains stubbornly hidden behind the other), this technique will accurately diagnose a multiple pregnancy.

"We'd barely adjusted to the fact that I was pregnant when we found out I'm carrying twins. Are there any extra risks for them—or for me?"

Multiple births are multiplying at a fantastic rate; 1 out of every 33 sets of parents can expect to see double (or triple, or more) in the delivery room, up from 1 in 100 a generation or two ago. And although some multiple births are still conceived the old-fashioned way—as a result of random throws of nature's dice or because of an inherited predisposition—scientists point to several new factors in explaining the current baby-baby boom. One is the increase in older mothers: women over thirty-five, because their ovulation tends to be erratic (with greater chances of more than one egg being released at a time), are more likely to conceive a multiple birth. Another is the use of fertility drugs which increase the likelihood of multiple births by increasing the release of multiple eggs. Still another is the use of in vitro fertilization, a procedure where eggs fertilized in a test tube are implanted into the uterus, which, since several ova are involved, also yields an increased risk of multiple births. And finally, some research has linked folic acid supplementation, which is recommended for all women of childbearing age, with an increased chance for twins.

But if today's mother is more likely to conceive twins, she is also much more likely to deliver those twins in good condition. Much of this success is attributable to the advance-warning capabilities of ultrasound; rare is the couple nowadays that is taken by surprise by twins in the delivery room. Advance warning makes not only for fewer practical and logistical complications after birth (having to dash to the store at the last minute for an extra crib and layette), but also for fewer medical complications during pregnancy and at delivery. Armed with the knowledge that you are carrying more than one baby, you and your practitioner can take many precautions that can reduce your risk of certain pregnancy complications (hypertension, anemia, and abruptio placenta—when the placenta separates from the uterus prematurely—are more common in multiple pregnancies) and improve your chances of carrying the babies to term and delivering them in top-notch condition:

Extra medical care. Much of the higher risk a multiple pregnancy carries can be reduced with expert medical monitoring by an obstetrician (like other high-risk pregnancies, a twin pregnancy should not be overseen by a midwife). You will be scheduled for more frequent appointments than will the woman carrying a single fetus—often seeing the doctor every other week after the 20th week and weekly after the 30th. And you will be watched more closely for signs of complications so that if one develops, it can be treated quickly. Be aware of when it is important to call the doctor; see page 130.

Extra nutrition. Eating for three (or more) is at least double the responsibility of eating for two. On top of all the other good things it can do for all babies, excellent nutrition can have a dramatic impact on one of the most common problems of multiple pregnancies: low birthweight. Instead of being born at 5 pounds and less (once the standard in multiple births), twins who are nourished on a superior diet can weigh in at a much healthier 6 to 7 pounds or more.

Many dietary requirements are multiplied with each fetus you're carrying. Specifically, that translates to approximately 300 additional calories, one additional Protein serving, one additional Calcium serving, and one additional Whole Grains serving for each additional fetus. Because that's a lot of food to fit into a stomach cramped by a rapidly growing uterus, and because prenatal gastrointestinal discomforts, such as morning sickness and indigestion, are often multiplied in multiple pregnancies, the quality of the food you eat will be particularly important. Avoiding foods low on the nutrition ladder will help ensure that you'll have room for the good stuff. Eating efficiently and spreading your requirements out over at least six small meals and many snacks, rather than trying to get your Daily Dozen and then some in at three sittings, should help, too. And since an additional fetus also means an increased need for such nutrients as iron, folic acid, zinc, copper, calcium, vitamin B_6, vitamin C, and vitamin D, make sure you're taking your prenatal supplement regularly, as well as an iron supplement if one is prescribed by your practitioner.

Extra weight gain. An additional baby means additional weight gain—not just because of the baby itself, but because of the extra baby by-products (often including an extra placenta and additional amniotic fluid). Your physician will probably advise a carefully monitored weight gain of at least 35 to 45 pounds above your prepregnancy weight (unless you're very overweight), or almost 50 percent more than is recommended in a singleton pregnancy. That means about 1 pound a week in the first half of pregnancy and 1½ pounds a week in the second. Particularly if this weight is gained on an excellent diet, it will go a long way toward producing healthier, heavier babies.

Extra rest. Your body will be working twice as hard at baby building, so it's going to need twice as much rest for its efforts. It's your job to make sure it gets it when it needs it. Make time for a nap or a rest with your feet up by depending more on others for help around the house and with errands, and by taking shortcuts (for example, use frozen vegetables and prewashed salad greens). And, if at all possible, work fewer hours at your job, or even stop work early if fatigue is really knocking you out. Your doctor may also limit exercise and other activities.

Extra help for the extra symptoms of multiple pregnancies. Since the common discomforts of pregnancy (including morning sickness, indigestion, backache, constipation, hemorrhoids, edema, varicose veins, shortness of breath, and fatigue) are likely to be exaggerated in a mom carrying more than one fetus, she needs to be aware of the various routes to relief. Though relief may be more elusive in a twin pregnancy, the suggestions in this book for dealing with these complaints apply to all mothers, whether they are expecting one baby or more than one. Consult with your doctor for additional advice or if symptoms seem particularly severe.

An extremely uncommon complaint that occasionally complicates a multiple pregnancy in the later months is separation of the lower joint of the pelvic bone. This separation, caused by the additional weight of two or more fetuses, can cause limited mobility and severe localized pain in the pelvic area; contact your obstetrician if you experience either of these symptoms.

Extra caution. Depending on how your pregnancy is going, the doctor may prescribe taking an early leave from work (as early as the 24th week in some cases), getting help with the housework, and, if serious complications threaten, complete bed rest at home. Hospital bed rest during the last months of pregnancy is usually reserved for very complicated multiple pregnancies. Following your doctor's orders to the letter, no matter how difficult that might be, is one of the best ways you can help your babies go to term. (Keep in mind, however, that "term" in a multiple pregnancy is shorter than "term" in a singleton pregnancy. Recent research suggests that the ideal time for delivery of twins and triplets is about 37 weeks, rather than the usual 40 weeks.) But, just in case, it may be a good idea to take your childbirth classes during your second trimester, and to know the signs of impending early labor (see page 273).

"Everybody thinks it's so exciting that we're going to have twins—except us. We're disappointed and scared. What's wrong with us?"

Absolutely nothing. Our prenatal daydreams rarely involve two cribs, two high chairs, two strollers, or two babies. We prepare ourselves psychologically, as well as physically, for the arrival of one baby; when we hear that we're going to have two, feelings of disappointment are not unusual. Neither is fear. The impending responsibilities of caring for one new infant are daunting enough without having them doubled.

So accept the fact that you are ambivalent about the dual arrivals, and don't burden yourself with guilt. Instead, use this time before delivery to get used to the idea of twins. Talk to each other and to anyone you know who has twins. Your practitioner may also be able to provide the name of a local parents-of-twins support group or the name of a mother of twins in your area. Sharing your feelings, and recognizing that you're not the first expectant parents to experience them, will help you feel more accepting of, and in time even excited about, this pregnancy. Twins may be double the effort at first, but they're almost always double the pleasure down the road.

A CORPUS LUTEUM CYST

"My doctor said that I have a corpus luteum cyst on my ovary. She said that it won't be a problem, but I'm concerned."

Every month of a woman's reproductive life, a small yellowish body of cells forms after ovulation. Called a corpus luteum (literally "yellow body"), it occupies the space in the follicle formerly occupied by the ovum, or egg. The corpus luteum produces progesterone and estrogen, and is programmed by nature to disintegrate in about fourteen days. When it does, diminishing hormone levels trigger menstruation. In pregnancy the corpus luteum, sustained by the hormone hCG (human Chorionic Gonadotropin), which is generated by the cells that develop into the placenta (the trophoblast), continues to grow and produce progesterone and estrogen to nourish and support the new pregnancy until the placenta takes over. In most cases, the corpus luteum starts to shrink about six or seven weeks after the last menstrual period and ceases to function at about 10 weeks, when its work of pro-

viding bed and board for the baby is done.

In an estimated 1 in 10 pregnancies, however, the corpus luteum fails to regress at the expected time and develops into a corpus luteum cyst. Usually, as your doctor has already assured you, the cyst won't present a problem. But just as a precaution, the physician will monitor its size and condition regularly via ultrasound and, if it becomes unusually large or if it threatens to twist or rupture, will consider removing it surgically. Such intervention is necessary with only about 1 percent of all corpus luteum cysts, and after the 12th week, the surgery rarely threatens the pregnancy.

INABILITY TO URINATE

"The last few nights I've been unable to urinate, even though my bladder seems very full."

It sounds like you have a stubbornly tilted uterus that has refused to right itself and is now pressing on your urethra, the tube leading from the bladder. The pressure of this increasingly heavy load can make urination impossible. There may also be urinary leakage when the bladder becomes very overloaded.

Sometimes actually manipulating the uterus by hand to move it off the urethra and into the proper position can solve the problem. Other times catheterization (removing the urine through a tube) is also necessary. Speak to your practitioner about what would be best in your case.

STREP THROAT

"My oldest child came down with strep throat. If I catch it, is there a risk to the baby?"

If there's one thing kids are good at sharing, it's their germs. Consequently, the more kids you have at home (particularly of the school-going variety), the greater your chances of coming down with colds and other infections while you're expecting.

So step up preventive measures (not sharing drinks, resisting the temptation to finish that germ-filled sandwich, washing your hands frequently) and boost your immune system (which is lowered during pregnancy anyway) by eating well and getting enough rest.

If you do suspect that you've succumbed to strep, go to your practitioner for a throat culture right away. The infection will not harm the baby, as long as it is treated promptly with the right type of antibiotic. Your practitioner will prescribe one that is effective against strep and is perfectly safe for use during pregnancy. *Never* take medication prescribed for your children or someone else in the family.

What It's Important to Know:
WEIGHT GAIN DURING PREGNANCY

Put two pregnant women together anywhere—in a doctor's waiting room, on a bus, at a business meeting—and the questions are certain to start flying. "When are you due?" "Have you felt the baby kicking yet?" "Have you been feeling sick?" And perhaps the most commonly posed of all: "How much weight have you gained?"

The comparisons are inevitable, and sometimes a little disturbing. Women who started off with a bang, enthusiastically eating their way to 10-pound first-trimester gains, wonder "How much is too much?" Others, their appetites daunted by bouts of morning sickness, end up with net gains that barely register on the practitioner's scale (perhaps even with a slight weight loss) and wonder "What's too little?" All wonder "How much is just right?"

Total increase. Though it was once in medical vogue to limit a woman's pregnancy weight gain to 15 pounds, it is now recognized that this kind of weight gain was insufficient. Babies whose mothers gain under 20 pounds are more likely to be premature, small for their gestational age, and to suffer growth restriction in the uterus.

Not as hazardous, but also risky, was the next vogue, which urged women to eat to their hearts' and souls' content and gain any amount of weight. There are some potential problems with gaining too much weight: assessment and measurement of the fetus become more difficult; excess weight can result in extra back-

MORE WEIGHTY ISSUES

Need yet another reason to keep an eye on the scale? Researchers have found that women who gained more than the recommended 25 to 35 pounds during pregnancy were nearly 75 percent more likely to have difficulty breastfeeding. The more extra weight, the harder time they had.

aches, leg pain, increased fatigue, and varicose veins; the baby may become so large that a vaginal delivery becomes difficult or impossible; if surgery, such as cesarean section, is needed, it becomes more difficult, and postoperative complications more common; and after pregnancy the excess weight may be hard to shed.

Though there's a good chance that a woman with an enormous weight gain may have an oversized baby, the mother's weight gain and the weight of her infant don't always correlate. It's possible to gain 40 pounds and deliver a 6-pound baby, and to gain 25 and have an 8-pounder. The quality of the food that contributes to the weight gain is even more significant than the quantity.

The sensible and safe pregnancy weight gain for the average woman is between 25 and 35 pounds. A petite, small-boned woman's gain is likely to be at the lower end of the range and a larger, big-boned woman's gain is likely to be at the high end. That gain allows about 6 to 8 pounds for baby and 14 to 24 pounds for placenta, breasts, fluids, and other by-products (see box on the facing page). It also ensures a speedier return to prepregnancy weight for mom.

The formula changes for women with special needs. Women who begin pregnancy extremely underweight should try to gain enough weight during the first trimester so that they start the second trimester at or close to their ideal weight; then they should aim to gain the requisite 25 to 35 pounds on top of that. Women who start pregnancy 10 to 20 percent or more overweight can safely gain somewhat less weight, though not less than 15 pounds, and only on the best-quality food and under careful medical supervision. Pregnancy is never a time for weight loss or maintenance, because a fetus can't survive on a mother's fat stores alone; they provide calories but no nutrients.

Women who are carrying more than one fetus also need to have their weight-gain goal adjusted by their physicians. Though it doesn't double for twins or triple for triplets, it does increase significantly—to 35 to 45 pounds for twins, higher still when there are more than two fetuses.

Rate of increase. The average-weight woman should gain approximately 3 to 4 pounds total during the first trimester, and about a pound a week, for a total of about 12 to 14 pounds, during the second trimester. Weight gain should continue at a rate of about 1 pound a week during the 7th and 8th months, and in the 9th month drop off to a pound or two—or even none at all—for a total of 8 to 10 pounds during the third trimester.

Rare is the woman who can tailor her weight gain precisely to the ideal formula. And it's fine to fluctuate a little— ½ pound one week, 1½ pounds the next. But the goal of every pregnant woman should be to keep weight gain as steady as possible, without any sudden jumps or drops. If you gain more than 3 pounds

WEIGHT INSURANCE

A recent study found that underweight women could improve the weight of their babies by taking a vitamin supplement formulated for pregnancy that contains 25 mg of zinc. If you are underweight, make sure your supplement includes that amount of zinc.

BREAKDOWN OF YOUR WEIGHT GAIN
(All weights are approximate)

Baby	7½ pounds
Placenta	1½ pounds
Amniotic fluid	2 pounds
Uterine enlargement	2 pounds
Maternal breast tissue	2 pounds
Maternal blood volume	4 pounds
Fluids in maternal tissue	4 pounds
Maternal fat stores	7 pounds
Total average	30 pounds overall weight gain

in any one week in the second trimester, or if you gain more than 2 pounds in any week in the third trimester, especially if it doesn't seem to be related to overeating or excessive intake of sodium, check with your practitioner. Check, too, if you gain no weight for more than two weeks in a row during the 4th to 8th months.

If you find that your weight gain has strayed significantly from what you planned (for instance, that you gained 14 pounds in the first trimester instead of 3 or 4, or that you gained 20 pounds in the second trimester instead of 12), take action to see that it gets back on a sensible track, but don't try to stop it in its tracks. With your practitioner, readjust your goal to include the excess you've already gained and the weight you still have to gain. Keep in mind that your baby requires a steady daily shipment of nutrients throughout the pregnancy, which can only come through what you eat. Monitor your weight from the beginning, and you'll never be tempted to put your baby on a diet to keep yourself from getting fat.

◆ ◆ ◆

CHAPTER 8

The Fourth Month

Approximately 14 to 17 Weeks

Finally, the beginning of the second trimester, which is, for many pregnant women, the most comfortable of the three. And with the arrival of this milestone come some welcome changes. For one, most of the more pesky early pregnancy symptoms may be gradually easing up or even disappear-

ing. You can look forward to feeling (hopefully) less queasy, if you don't already, and more energetic. Another change for the better: by the end of this month, the bulge in your lower abdomen may be looking less like the remains of a large lunch and more like the beginnings of a pregnant belly.

What You Can Expect at This Month's Checkup

This month you can expect your practitioner to check the following, though there may be variations depending upon your particular needs and upon your practitioner's style of practice:[1]

◆ Weight and blood pressure

◆ Urine, for sugar and protein

◆ Fetal heartbeat

◆ Size of uterus, by external palpation (feeling from the outside)

◆ Height of fundus (top of the uterus)

◆ Hands and feet for edema (swelling), and legs for varicose veins

◆ Symptoms you've been experiencing, especially unusual ones

◆ Questions or problems you want to discuss—have a list ready

1. See Appendix, page 545, for an explanation of the procedures and tests performed.

A LOOK INSIDE

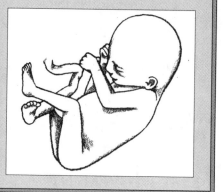

ounces), with the body now growing faster than the head, reaching more human proportions. Fingerprints and toe prints have developed, and temporary hair, called lanugo, has appeared on the body. Baby can suck his or her thumb, swallow amniotic fluid and pass it as urine, and make practice breathing movements. The placenta is fully functional, serving as baby's source of nourishment and oxygen; in a baby girl the uterus is formed and the ovaries equipped with primitive egg cells. Baby's bones are getting harder and its arms and legs are moving (you might even begin to feel those first kicks soon!).

▲ *Your uterus is now about the size of a small melon, and can be felt around 1½ inches below your belly button by the end of the month. If you haven't done so already, you'll probably begin to outgrow your regular clothes.*

▶ *Your baby is getting longer and heavier (about 5 inches and as many*

What You May Be Feeling

A s always, remember that every pregnancy and every woman is different. You may experience all of these symptoms at one time or another, or only a few of them. Some may have continued from last month, others may be new. Still others may hardly be noticed because you've become so used to them. You may also have other, less common, symptoms.

PHYSICALLY

- ◆ Fatigue

- ◆ Decreased urinary frequency

- ◆ An end to, or a decrease in, nausea and vomiting (in a few women, "morning sickness" will continue; in a very few it is just beginning)

- ◆ Constipation

- Heartburn, indigestion, flatulence, bloating

- Continued breast enlargement, but usually decreased tenderness

- Occasional headaches

- Occasional faintness or dizziness, particularly with sudden change of position

- Nasal congestion and occasional nosebleeds; ear stuffiness

- "Pink toothbrush" from bleeding gums

- Increase in appetite

- Mild swelling of ankles and feet, and occasionally of hands and face

- Varicose veins of legs and/or hemorrhoids

- Slight whitish vaginal discharge

- Fetal movement near the end of the month (but usually not this early unless you are very slender or if this is not your first pregnancy)

EMOTIONALLY

- Instability comparable to premenstrual syndrome, which may include irritability, mood swings, irrationality, weepiness

- Joy and/or apprehension—if you have started to feel and look pregnant at last

- Frustration at being "in-between"—your regular wardrobe doesn't fit anymore, but you're not looking pregnant enough for maternity clothes

- A feeling you're not quite together —you're scattered, forgetful, drop things, have trouble concentrating

What You May Be Concerned About

FETAL MOVEMENT

"I haven't felt the baby moving yet; could something be wrong? Or could I just not be recognizing the kicking?"

Fetal movement may be the greatest source of joy in your pregnancy. More than a positive pregnancy test, an expanding belly, or even the sound of the fetal heartbeat, those little kicks and flutters affirm that you've got a new life growing inside you.

However, few expectant moms, particularly first-timers, feel their first kick in the fourth month. Though the embryo begins to make spontaneous movements by the 7th week, these movements, made by very tiny arms and legs, do not become apparent to the mother until much later. That first momentous sensation of life, or "quickening," can occur anywhere between the 14th and 26th weeks, but generally closer to the average of the 18th to 22nd week. Variations on that average are common. A woman who's had a baby before is likely to recognize movement earlier (because she knows what to expect and because her uterine muscles are more lax, making it easier to feel a kick) than one who is expecting her first child. A very slender woman may notice very early, weak movements, whereas an overweight woman may not be aware of movements until they've become more vigorous.

Sometimes, fetal movements aren't noticed when expected because of a miscalculated due date. Other times, the kicks and flutters are there but a woman fails to recognize them. Often early movements are mistaken for gas or ordinary twitches in the digestive tract.

Nobody can tell a first-time mother-to-be exactly what she can expect to feel; a hundred pregnant women may describe that first movement in a hundred different ways. Perhaps the most common descriptions are "a fluttering in the abdomen" and "butterflies in the stomach." But early fetal movements have also been described as "a bumping or nudging," "a twitch," "a growling stomach," "someone hitting my stomach," "a bubble bursting," "the squirmies," "like being turned upside-down on an amusement park ride."

Although it isn't unusual to be unaware of fetal movements until the 20th week or later, your practitioner may order an ultrasound to check on the baby's condition if you haven't felt anything—and he or she hasn't been able to elicit fetal response by prodding—by the 22nd week. If the fetal heartbeat is strong, however, and everything else seems to be progressing normally, the practitioner may hold off testing even longer.

APPEARANCE

"I get depressed when I look in the mirror or step on a scale—I look so fat."

In a society as obsessed with slenderness as ours, where those who can "pinch an inch" despair, the weight gain of pregnancy can easily become a source of depression. It shouldn't. There's an important difference between pounds added for no good reason (just willpower gone astray) and pounds gained for the best and most beautiful of reasons: your

A PREGNANT POSE

If you've been dodging the camera lately ("no need to put yet *another* 10 pounds on me!"), consider striking a pregnant pose. Though you may prefer to forget what you look like pregnant, your child-to-be will definitely relish seeing his or her first "baby" pictures one day—and so will you, eventually. To preserve your pregnant progress for posterity, have someone take a photo of your profile each month. Dress in a leotard for more dramatic documentation of your silhouette, and compile your photos in a pregnancy album, alongside the ultrasound shot, if you have one.

child and its support system are growing inside you.

In the eyes of many beholders, a pregnant woman isn't just beautiful inside but outside as well. Many women and their spouses consider the rounded pregnant silhouette the most lovely—and sensuous—of feminine shapes.

As long as you're eating right and not exceeding the recommended limits for pregnancy weight gain (see page 169), you needn't feel "fat"—just pregnant. The added inches you're seeing are all legitimate by-products of pregnancy and will disappear soon enough after the baby is born. If you *are* exceeding the limits, self-defeating depression won't keep you from getting fatter (and may even fuel your appetite), but careful scrutiny of your eating habits might. Remember, however, that dieting to lose or keep from gaining weight during pregnancy is extremely unsafe. Never cut back on the Pregnancy Diet requirements because you're afraid of putting on too much weight; just become more efficient in filling them.

Watching your weight gain isn't the only way to give your appearance an edge. Wearing clothes that flatter your changing figure will also help; instead of trying to squeeze into your old wardrobe, choose from the growing selection of creative maternity styles available that celebrate the pregnant shape, rather than attempt to hide it (see below). You'll like your mirror image better, too, if you get an easy-care hairstyle, pamper your complexion, and take the time to apply makeup if you ordinarily wear it.

MATERNITY CLOTHES

"I can't squeeze into my baggy jeans anymore, but I dread buying maternity clothes."

There's never been a more fashionable time to be pregnant. Gone are the days when pregnancy wardrobes were limited to dowdy smocks and overblouses. Not only are today's maternity clothes a lot more interesting to look at and practical to wear, but pregnant women can supplement and mix-and-match these specialized purchases with a variety of other items that they can continue to wear even after they get their shape back.

Consider the following when preparing to make your pregnancy fashion statement:

- You still have a long way to grow. Don't embark on a whirlwind spending spree on the first day you can't button your jeans. Maternity clothes can be costly, especially when you consider the relatively short period of time they can be worn. So buy as you grow, and then buy only as much as you need (once you've checked what you can use that's already in your closet, you may end up needing a lot less than you'd figured). Though the pregnancy pillows available in try-on rooms in maternity stores can give a good indication of how things will fit later, they can't predict how you will carry (high, low, big, small) and which outfits will end up being the most comfortable when you need comfort most.

- You're not limited to maternity clothes. If it fits, wear it, even if it isn't from the maternity department. Buying nonmaternity clothing for maternity use (or using items you already own) is, of course, the best way of avoiding throwing away a fortune on clothes you'll only wear briefly. And depending on what the designers are showing in a particular season, anywhere from a few to many of the fashions on the regular racks may be suitable for pregnant shapes. But be wary of spending a lot on such purchases. Though you may love the clothes now, you may love them considerably less after you've worn them throughout your pregnancy; postpartum, you may have a strong impulse to pack them away like so many maternity clothes.

- Your personal sense of style counts when you're pregnant, too. If you normally dress in tailored, casual, or decidedly fashion-forward clothes, don't try to talk yourself into flowered, hyper-feminine maternity dresses. Though the novelty of looking the part of the lady-in-waiting may carry you contentedly through a month or two, it's doomed to fizzle out long before you're able to relinquish the maternity clothes, leaving you to face the rest of your pregnancy in clothes you despise.

- Don't hide it, flaunt it. Many of today's maternity fashions celebrate the pregnant belly with clingy fabrics and styles. And that's something to celebrate—since belly-accentuating maternity wear actually slims your silhouette down, rather than "fattening" you up. Another great option: Low-cut jeans and pants that are stylish *and* comfortable, since they can be worn under your belly.

◆ Among your most important accessories are the ones the public never sees. A well-fitting, supportive bra is vital during pregnancy, when breast expansion generally makes your old bras useless. Bypass the sale racks and put yourself in the hands of an experienced fitter at a well-stocked lingerie department or shop. With any luck, she will be able to tell you approximately how much extra room and support you need and which kind of bra will provide it. But don't stock up. Buy just a couple (one to wear and one to wash), and then go back for another fitting when you start growing out of them.

Special maternity underwear isn't usually necessary and, unless you're used to high-waisted briefs, won't be terribly comfortable. A nice alternative is bikini underwear, bought in a larger than usual size (if necessary), that you can wear *under* your belly. Buy them in favorite colors and/or sexy fabrics to give your spirits a lift (but make sure the crotches are cotton).

◆ A pregnant woman's best friend can be her spouse's closet. It's all there for the taking (though it's probably a good idea to ask first): oversized T-shirts and regular shirts that look great over pants or leggings, sweatpants that accommodate more inches than yours do, running shorts that will keep up with your waistline for at least a couple more months, belts with the few extra notches you need.

◆ Both a borrower and a lender be. Accept all offers of used maternity clothes, even if the offerings don't precisely suit your usual style. In a pinch, any extra dress, jumper, or pair of slacks may do—you can make any borrowed item more "yours" with accessories (a fabulous scarf or a flashy pair of sneakers, for example).

When your term is over, offer to lend those maternity outfits you bought and can't or don't want to wear postpartum to newly pregnant friends; between you and your friends, you'll be getting your money's worth from your maternity clothes.

◆ Cool is in. Hot stuff (fabrics that don't breathe, such as nylon and other synthetics) isn't so hot when you're pregnant. Since your metabolic rate is higher than usual, making you warmer, you'll feel more comfortable in cottons. Knee-highs or thigh-highs will also be more comfortable than pantyhose, but avoid those that have a narrow constrictive band at the top. Light colors, mesh weaves, and loose garments will also help you keep your cool in warm weather. When the weather turns cold, dressing in layers is ideal, since you can selectively peel off as you heat up or when you go indoors.

HAIR DYES, RELAXERS, AND PERMANENTS

"My hair has started to lose all its body—it's flat and limp. Is it safe for me to get a permanent?"

Though the pregnant belly is the most obvious physical effect a gestating fetus has on its mother, it's by no means the only one. The changes are evident everywhere—from the palms of the hands (which may temporarily turn a ruddy red) to the inside of the mouth (gums may swell and bleed). The hair is no exception. It can take a turn for the better (when lackluster hair suddenly sports a brilliant shine) or for the worse (when once bouncy hair goes limp).

Ordinarily, a permanent or a body wave might be the obvious answer to hair that has taken a wrong turn, but it isn't during pregnancy. For one thing, hair responds unpredictably under the influence of pregnancy hormones; a permanent might not take at all, or might result in an unflattering frizz instead of bouncy waves. For another thing, the chemical solutions used in permanents are absorbed through the scalp into the bloodstream, so there are questions about the safety of their use during pregnancy. So far, studies of the effects of such chemicals on the fetus have been extremely reassuring: no link has been found between the use of permanents and the development of birth defects. But since more study will be necessary before these substances are completely exonerated, the very cautious may wish to stay "straight" until after delivery. Don't be concerned, however, about a permanent you've already had—the risk is only theoretical, and certainly not worth worrying about.

Excellent nutrition may help revive some of your hair's luster; "extra volume" shampoos, conditioners, and styling products (and your trusty curling iron) may help restore the bounce. But by and large, your hair will probably continue to limp its way through your pregnancy. So, it might make sense to switch to a style that doesn't depend on fullness, such as a very short cut, or one that builds volume in, such as a layered cut.

"I get my hair relaxed regularly, but is that safe to keep doing while I'm expecting?"

Just one more sacrifice you'll have to make for your baby-to-be. Though there's no evidence that hair relaxers are dangerous during pregnancy, there's no proof that they're completely safe, either. And since they contain strong chemicals that can be absorbed through the skin— and because your hair may react differently and strangely to the chemicals now that you're pregnant—it's probably safest to let your hair do what comes naturally. You can relax, however, about any relaxing you've already done.

"I was about to go for my coloring appointment, when I heard from a friend that hair dyes can cause birth defects. Is this true?"

Though some extra-prudent practitioners still advise their patients to stay away from hair dyes when they're expecting, studies have not linked these products to birth defects. Apparently, so little of the chemicals in the dyes is absorbed through the skin, it's not likely that it would have any adverse affect.

But, while you may not have to worry about the impact on your baby if you continue coloring your hair, you may have to worry about the impact on your appearance. For hormonal reasons, your hair may react differently when you're expecting—leaving you with a color you may not have expected.

REALITY OF PREGNANCY

"Now that my abdomen is swelling, the fact that I'm really pregnant has finally sunk in. Even though we planned this pregnancy, we suddenly feel scared, trapped by the baby— even antagonistic toward it."

Even the most eager of expectant couples may be surprised to find themselves with second thoughts as their pregnancy starts to become a reality. But actually it's not surprising when you think about it. After all, an unseen little intruder is suddenly turning your lives upside-down, depriving you of freedoms you'd always taken for granted and making unexpected demands on you—both physically and emotionally. Every aspect of the lifestyle you've become accustomed to—from how you spend your evenings to what you eat and drink to how often you make love—is being altered by this child even before its birth. And the knowledge that these changes will become still more imposing after delivery compounds these mixed feelings, deepening your apprehension.

Studies show that a little prenatal ambivalence, a little fear, even a little antagonism, is not only normal, it's healthy—as long as these feelings are acknowledged and confronted. And now is the best time to do that. Work out any resentments now (over not being able to stay out as late on Saturday nights, or pick up and go on a weekend trip when the spirit moves you, to work at your typical pace, or to spend your money the way you please), and you won't find yourself struggling with them after delivery. Sharing your feelings with your partner is the best way to do this— and encourage him to do likewise. You may both find some reassurance, too, by talking to friends who have already made the transition to parenthood.

Although the lifestyle changes may be greater or lesser, depending on how you and your spouse decide to order your priorities, it's true that your life is never going to be exactly the same again once your "two" becomes "three." But as some parts of your world become more constricted, others will open up. You may find yourself reborn with your baby's birth. And this new life may turn out to be the best yet.

UNWANTED ADVICE

"Now that it's obvious I'm expecting, everyone—from my mother-in-law to strangers on the elevator—has advice for me. It drives me crazy."

Short of taking up a reclusive existence on a desert island, there's no way for a pregnant woman to escape the unsolicited advice of those around her. There's just something about a bulging belly that brings out the "expert" in everyone. Take your morning jog around the park and someone is sure to chide:

"You shouldn't be running in your condition!" Lug home two bags of groceries from the supermarket and you're bound to hear: "Do you think you ought to be carrying such heavy bundles?" Or reach up for a subway strap and you may even be warned: "If you stretch that way the umbilical cord will wrap around your baby's neck!"

Between such gratuitous advice and the inevitable predictions about the sex of the baby, what's an expectant mother to do? First of all, keep in mind that most of what you hear is probably nonsense. Old wives' tales that *do* have foundation in fact have been scientifically substantiated and have become part of standard medical practice. Those that do not, though still tightly woven into the tapestry of pregnancy mythology, can be confidently dismissed. Those recommendations that leave you with a nagging doubt ("What if they're right?") are best checked with your doctor, nurse-midwife, or childbirth educator.

Whether it's possibly plausible or obviously ridiculous, however, don't let unwanted advice get your dander up. Neither you nor your baby will profit from the added tension. Instead, keeping your sense of humor handy, you can take one of two approaches: Politely inform the well-meaning stranger, friend, or relative that you have a trusted practitioner who counsels you on your pregnancy and that you can't accept advice from anyone else. Or, just as politely, smile, say thank you, and go on your way, letting their comments go in one ear and out the other—without making any stops in between.

But no matter how you choose to handle unwanted advice, you'd also do well to get used to it. If there's anyone who attracts a crowd of advice-givers faster than a pregnant woman, it's a woman with a new baby.

"Now that my pregnant belly is showing, friends, colleagues, even strangers come up to me and touch it—without even asking. I'm uncomfortable with that."

They're round, they're cute, and they're filled with something even cuter—let's face it, pregnant bellies just scream out to be touched. Still, though touching a pregnant belly may be an irresistible impulse, it's also an inappropriate one—particularly without the owner's permission.

Some women don't mind being the center of so much touching attention; others actually enjoy it. But if all this uninvited rubbing is rubbing you the wrong way, don't hesitate to say so. You can do this bluntly (though politely): "I know you find my belly tempting to touch, but I'd really rather you didn't." Or you can try a little belly turning, rubbing the rubber right back ("How do *you* like it?"). Which just might make him or her think twice next time before reaching out and touching a pregnant belly without permission.

FORGETFULNESS

"Last week I left the house without my wallet; this morning I completely forgot an important business meeting. I can't focus on anything, and I'm beginning to think I'm losing my mind."

You're not alone. Many pregnant women begin to feel that as they're gaining pounds, they're losing brain cells. Even women who pride themselves on their organizational skills, their capacity to deal with complicated issues, and their ability to maintain their composure suddenly find themselves forgetting appointments, having trouble concentrating, and losing their cool. Fortunately, the scatterbrain syndrome (similar to but more pronounced than that which many women experience premenstrually) is only temporary. Like numerous other symptoms, it's caused by the hormonal changes of pregnancy.

Feeling tense about this intellectual fogginess will only compound it. Recognizing that it is normal (and not "in your head"), even accepting it with a sense of humor, may help to ease it. Reducing the stresses in your life as much as possible will also help. It just may not be feasible to do as much as efficiently as you did before you took on the added job of baby-making. Taking informal inventory or keeping written checklists at home and at work (and referring to them before leaving home or work) can help contain the mental chaos as well as keep you from making potentially dangerous mistakes (such as forgetting to lock the door or turn off the burner under the teakettle before leaving the house). Relying on an electronic organizer can help, too, assuming you don't misplace it.

Although ginkgo biloba has been touted for its memory-boosting properties, it is not considered safe for use during pregnancy—so you'll have to forget about using this herbal preparation in your battle against pregnancy-induced forgetfulness.

And you might as well get used to working at a little below peak efficiency. The fog may well continue through the early weeks after your baby's arrival (due to fatigue, not hormones) and perhaps may not lift completely until baby is sleeping through the night.

BREATHLESSNESS

"Sometimes I feel a little breathless. Is this normal?"

Take a deep breath (if you can!) and relax. Mild breathlessness is normal, and many pregnant women experience it beginning in the second trimester. And, once again, you can blame your pregnancy hormones. These hormones stimulate the respiratory center to increase the frequency and depth of the breaths, giving you the feeling you're "breathing hard." They also swell the capillaries of the respiratory tract and other capillaries in the body, and relax the muscles of the lungs, bronchial tubes, and other muscles. As pregnancy progresses, that deep breath becomes even harder to take as the growing uterus pushes up against the diaphragm, crowding the lungs and making it difficult for them to expand fully.

Severe breathlessness, on the other hand, is not normal. Especially when breathing is rapid, lips or fingertips seem to be turning bluish, and/or there is chest pain and rapid pulse, severe breathlessness could be a sign of trouble and requires an immediate call to the doctor or trip to the emergency room.

DENTAL PROBLEMS

"My mouth has suddenly become a disaster area. My gums bleed every time I brush, and I think I have a cavity. But I'm afraid to go to the dentist because of the anesthesia."

With so much of your attention centered on your abdomen during pregnancy, it's easy to overlook your mouth—until it screams for equal time, which it frequently does because of the heavy toll a normal pregnancy can take on the gums. The gums, like the mucous membranes of the nose, become swollen, inflamed, and tend to bleed easily because of pregnancy hormones. These hormones also make gums more susceptible to plaque and bacteria, which can soon make matters worse. Red, tender, bleeding gums could signal gingivitis, which, if left untreated, can develop into periodontitis. Studies show that this serious form of gum disease during pregnancy

increases a woman's risk of having a premature or low-birthweight baby and having preeclampsia—a particularly compelling argument for proper dental hygiene. Another is the tendency for uncared-for teeth to loosen in their sockets during pregnancy (which explains the old wives' tale that a woman loses a tooth for each baby). Fortunately, these potential problems are completely avoidable. Following a program of preventive dental care throughout pregnancy—and preferably throughout life—will avert most tooth and gum problems:

♦ Watch what you eat, particularly between meals. Save sweets (particularly sticky ones) for times when you can brush soon after. If you do indulge between meals and can't get to a toothbrush, see tips below for other tooth-cleaning options. Consume plenty of foods high in vitamin C; vitamin C strengthens gums, reducing the possibility of bleeding. Also be sure to fill your calcium requirements daily (see page 94). Calcium is needed throughout life to keep teeth strong and healthy.

♦ Floss and brush regularly, according to your dentist's or dental hygienist's directions.

♦ To further reduce bacteria in the mouth, brush your tongue when you brush your teeth. This will also help keep your breath fresh.

♦ When you can't brush after eating, chew a stick of sugarless gum or nibble on a chunk of cheese or a handful of peanuts (unless allergies are an issue; see page 188). All seem to have antibacterial cleansing capabilities.

♦ Whether or not you're experiencing dental discomfort, be sure to make an appointment with your dentist at least once during the nine months for a checkup and cleaning. The cleaning is important to remove plaque, which can not only increase the risk of cavities but also make your gum problems worse. Avoid X rays unless they are absolutely necessary, and then take the special precautions suggested on page 70. If some routine repair work requires anesthesia, postpone it if you can. Problems that will get worse if left untreated should be taken care of promptly. If you've had gum problems in the past, you should also see your periodontist during your pregnancy.

It's best not to wait until your mouth is hollering for help—which is why the best dental treatment is prevention. But if you suspect a cavity or other incipient trouble, make an appointment with your dentist or periodontist right away; putting off necessary dental work is usually far riskier than having it done. For example, badly decayed teeth that are not taken care of can be a source of infection that spreads throughout the system, putting both mother and fetus in danger. Impacted wisdom teeth that are either infected or causing severe pain should also be attended to promptly.

However, it is true that special precautions must be taken when major dental work is done during pregnancy. In most procedures, a local anesthetic will suffice. If a general anesthetic is absolutely required, then it should be administered by an experienced anesthesiologist to ensure that the supply of oxygen to the fetus isn't compromised and that the anesthetic used is safe during pregnancy. Discuss the anesthesia with both your dentist and your physician beforehand to ensure safety. Check with your physician to find out whether he or she thinks an antibiotic will be needed prior to the time of and/or after dental work.

If the dental work leaves you with chipmunk cheeks and you can't chew solids, you're going to have to make some dietary alterations. If you are put on a fluid-only diet, you can obtain adequate nutrients temporarily by sipping milkshakes (see Double-the-Milk Shake, page 101). Supplement the shakes with citrus juices (if they don't burn your gums), other fruit and vegetable juices, and homemade "creamed" soups made from ready-to-eat vegetable soups (canned or instant) pureed with cottage cheese, yogurt, or skim milk. Once you can manage soft foods, add pureed vegetables, fish, or tofu; scrambled eggs; unsweetened yogurt; applesauce or other cooked fruit; mashed bananas or potatoes; and creamy hot cereals enriched with nonfat dry milk.

"Can I use teeth-whitening products while I'm pregnant?"

It's probably safer to dazzle people with your personality than with "whitened" teeth while you're expecting. There have yet to be any major studies done on the effects, if any, of using a professional or at-home tooth-whitening system (such as those that employ peroxide or ultraviolet light). For now, the general consensus among dentists and physicians falls into the old better-safe-than-sorry category: Until more is known, pregnant women should not bleach or otherwise whiten their teeth. (Don't worry if you've already done some whitening; again, there are no proven risks.)

"I found a nodule on the side of my gum that bleeds every time I brush my teeth."

If it's not one thing in pregnancy, it's another. But not to worry. What you discovered this time is probably a pyogenic granuloma, which can appear on the gum or elsewhere on the body. And though it bleeds easily and is also known by the ominous-sounding term "pregnancy tumor," it is perfectly harmless. It usually regresses on its own after delivery. If it becomes very annoying before that, it can be removed surgically.

TROUBLE SLEEPING

"I've never had a sleep problem in my life—until now. I can't seem to settle down at night."

Your mind is racing, your belly burgeoning—it's no wonder you can't settle in for a good night's sleep. You could write this insomnia off as good preparation for the sleepless nights that likely lie ahead in the first months of your baby's life, or you could try the following tips for getting more sleep:

◆ Get enough exercise. A body that gets a workout by day (see page 190 for guidelines) will be a sleepier body at night. But don't exercise too close to bedtime, since the exercise-induced high could keep you from crashing when your head hits the pillow.

◆ Don't nap in the daytime (though naps are okay for those who don't have trouble sleeping at night). Rest breaks are fine, though.

◆ Set a leisurely pace at dinner. Don't gobble your meals in front of the TV; partake at the table, with your spouse, another family member, or a friend, and help yourself to a healthy helping of relaxing conversation. But don't eat a heavy meal too close to bedtime.

◆ Develop a bedtime routine and stick to it. After dinner, maintain the easy pace, focusing on activities that relax you. Indulge in light reading (but nothing you can't put down) or television (avoid violent or emotionally wrenching dramas, as well as the news), soothing music, some stretching or yoga, relaxation exercises (see page 127), a warm bath, a backrub, or some lovemaking.

◆ Have a light snack before you turn in. Too much food or none at all before bedtime can interfere with sleep. The old sleepy-time standard, a glass of warm milk, may be especially effective—not only because it may remind you of being tucked in with your teddy bear, but because milk contains the amino acid L-tryptophan, which raises the level of serotonin in the brain, inducing sleepiness. Other foods that contain L-tryptophan include turkey (which is why Thanksgiving dinner often sends people to the sofa for a nap) and eggs. If such savories don't appeal to you so late in the day, try sweeter soporific snacks: oatmeal cookies or a muffin and milk; fruit and cheese; yogurt and raisins.

◆ Get comfortable. Be sure your bedroom is neither too hot nor too cold, that your mattress is firm and your pillows supportive. See page 208 for suggestions on comfortable sleep positions; the sooner in pregnancy you learn to sleep comfortably on your left side, the easier it will be for you to do it later on.

◆ Get some air. A stuffy environment is not a good sleeping environment. So open a window in all but the coldest or hottest weather (when a fan or air-conditioning can help circulate the air). And don't sleep with the covers over your head. This will decrease the oxygen and increase the carbon dioxide you breathe in, which can cause headaches.

◆ Stay out of your bed except to sleep (or make love). Associating the bed with reading, TV watching, sorting the mail, or other activities interferes with sleep for some people.

♦ If frequent trips to the bathroom are interfering with your sleep, limit fluids after 6 P.M.[2] and stand as little as possible during the day, since excessive standing increases nighttime urination.

♦ Clear your mind. If you've been losing sleep over problems at work or at home, try to solve them during the day, or at least talk about them with your spouse or someone else early in the evening. If you have no one to talk to, write down your concerns and then try to come up with a solution for at least one of them. But try to put any worries out of your mind as bedtime approaches.

♦ Don't use such crutches as medications (traditional or herbal) or alcohol to assist you in falling asleep. These could be harmful in pregnancy, and they don't help in the long run anyway. Avoid caffeine (in tea, coffee, soft drinks) and/or large quantities of chocolate after noon since they can interfere with sleep in the short run.

♦ Don't go to sleep until you're tired. You may need less sleep than you think you do. Putting off your bedtime may, paradoxically, help you sleep better.

♦ Don't lie in bed for hours tossing and turning. If you're not sleeping, get out of bed and do something. That may tire you enough so that you can get back to bed and actually fall asleep.

♦ Judge the adequacy of your sleep by how you feel, not by how many hours you stay in bed. Keep in mind that many people who believe they have sleep problems actually get more sleep than they think. You're getting enough rest if you're not chronically tired (beyond the normal fatigue of pregnancy).

♦ Try to get up at the same time each day, even on weekends and holidays. Eventually, this will help regulate your sleep pattern.

♦ Don't worry about your insomnia. It won't hurt you or your baby. When you can't sleep, get up and read, go on-line, or watch TV until you get drowsy. Worrying about not sleeping will certainly be more stressful than lack of sleep itself.

SNORING

"My husband tells me that I've been snoring lately—which I've never done before. Is that something to worry about?"

Snoring can disrupt a good night's sleep both for the snorer and her bedmate (and since there will be plenty of disruptions to your sleep once baby's born, you should try to avoid as many as possible now). It may simply be triggered by normal pregnancy stuffiness, in which case sleeping with a humidifier on and with your head well elevated may help. But snoring can also be a sign of sleep apnea, a condition in which breathing stops briefly during sleep, temporarily reducing the amount of oxygen that's taken in. Since a continuous flow of oxygen is especially important when you're breathing for two, it's probably a good idea for pregnant women who snore to be monitored for sleep apnea, and treated if necessary. Extra weight can contribute to snoring and sleep apnea, so make sure you aren't gaining too much. Ask your practitioner about sleep apnea at your next visit.

---

2. But be sure to get your full quota of fluids each day (at least eight glasses) before that cut-off time.

VAGINAL DISCHARGE

"I've noticed a slight vaginal discharge that's thin and whitish. Does this mean I have an infection?"

A thin, milky, mild-smelling discharge (leukorrhea) is normal throughout pregnancy. It's much like the discharge many women have prior to their menstrual periods. Since it increases until term and may become quite heavy, some women are more comfortable wearing panty liners during the last months of pregnancy. Do not use tampons, which could introduce unwanted germs into the vagina.

Aside from offending your esthetic sensibilities (and possibly your partner's, during oral sex), this discharge should be of no concern. Keeping yourself clean, fresh, and dry will help, of course; see tips for how to accomplish this in the next question. *Do not* douche. Douching upsets the normal balance of microorganisms in the vagina and can lead to bacterial vaginosis (BV), a serious vaginal infection, and even preterm birth. It can also force air into the vagina, which can be dangerous during pregnancy.

"I think I have a vaginal infection. Should I go get some of the medication I usually use, or do I need to see the doctor?"

Pregnancy is never a time for self-diagnosis or treatment—not even when it comes to something as seemingly simple as a vaginal infection. Even if you've had vaginal infections a hundred times before, even if you know the symptoms backward and forward (a yellowish, greenish, or thick and cheesy discharge that has a foul odor, accompanied by burning, itching, redness, or soreness), even if you've treated yourself successfully with over-the-counter preparations in the past—this time around, call your practitioner.

How you will be treated will depend on what kind of infection you have. If you have a yeast infection, which could be passed on to your baby during delivery (in the form of thrush, an innocuous, easily treated yeast infection of the mouth), your practitioner may prescribe vaginal suppositories or gels, ointments or creams that are inserted with an applicator. (Unfortunately, medication may banish a yeast infection only temporarily. The infection often returns off and on until after delivery, and may require repeated treatment.) If the cause of your symptoms turns out to be bacterial vaginosis, prompt treatment with oral medication, which is most effective, is essential. Untreated, BV can increase the risk of preterm delivery.

You may be able to hasten your recovery and prevent reinfection by keeping the genital area clean and dry. Do this by practicing meticulous hygiene, especially after going to the bathroom (always wipe from front to back); rinsing the vaginal area thoroughly after soaping during a bath or shower; avoiding exposure to irritating deodorant soaps, bubble baths, and perfumes; wearing cotton underwear and avoiding tight slacks, exercise pants, or leotards (especially those that aren't cotton).

Eating 1 cup of yogurt containing live lactobacillus acidophilus cultures (check the label—most yogurts do) daily can also dramatically reduce the risk of vaginal infections. *Do not douche;* see the preceding question for an explanation of why douching is unsafe.

If the infection turns out to be a sexually transmitted one, avoiding intercourse (and any other sexual contact that includes your genitals) until both you and your partner are infection-free is generally recommended. Condoms may be suggested for the remainder of the pregnancy or for six months after the condition has cleared. To prevent reinfection, care should be exercised to avoid transferring germs from anus to vagina (with fingers, penis, or tongue).

ELEVATED BLOOD PRESSURE

"My blood pressure was up a little bit at my last visit. Should I be worried?"

Worrying about your blood pressure will only send the readings higher. Besides, a slight increase at one visit is probably nothing to worry about. Perhaps you were stressed because you were caught in traffic on the way to your appointment, or because you had a pile of papers to finish back at work. Maybe you were just nervous—you were afraid you'd gained too much weight or not enough; you had some worrisome symptoms to report; you were anxious to hear the baby's heartbeat. Or maybe medical settings just make you edgy—giving you what is known as "white coat hypertension."

An hour later, when you were relaxed, your pressure might very well have been perfectly normal. But because it is often difficult to determine the cause of an isolated elevated reading, your practitioner may advise you to take a few blood-pressure-lowering precautions until the next visit. These may include taking it easy, avoiding excessive sodium and fat in your diet, and increasing your intake of fruits and vegetables. In some cases, your blood pressure may also be monitored over a twenty-four-hour period as you go about your normal routine to see if it really is elevated.

If your blood pressure remains *slightly* elevated, however, you may be among the 1 to 2 percent of pregnant women who develop transient high blood pressure during pregnancy. This type of hypertension is perfectly harmless and disappears after delivery.

What is considered normal blood pressure in pregnancy varies somewhat over the course of nine months. A baseline reading (what is normal for you) is obtained at the first prenatal visit. Generally blood pressure drops a little over the next several months. But somewhere around the seventh month, it usually begins to rise a bit.

During the first or second trimester, if systolic pressure (the upper number) is over 130 or rises by 30 over the baseline reading or the diastolic pressure (the lower number) is over 85 or rises by 15 over the baseline reading and stays up for at least two readings taken at least six hours apart, close observation, and possibly treatment, is warranted. In the third trimester, treatment is usually begun only if the rise is greater than that.

If such an increase in blood pressure is accompanied by sudden weight gain (more than 2 pounds not related to overeating), severe edema (swelling due to water retention), particularly of hands and face, as well as ankles, and/or protein in the urine, the problem may turn out to be preeclampsia (also called pregnancy-induced hypertension—PIH). In women who receive regular medical care, this condition is generally diagnosed before it progresses to more serious symptoms, which include blurred vision, headaches, irritability, and gastric pain. If you should experience any of the symptoms of preeclampsia (page 248 and page 500), call your doctor immediately.

SUGAR IN THE URINE

"At my last office visit the practitioner said that there was sugar in my urine. She said not to worry, but I'm convinced I have diabetes."

Take your doctor's advice—don't worry. A small amount of sugar in the urine on one occasion during pregnancy does not a diabetic make. Your body is probably doing just what it's supposed to do: making sure that your fetus, which depends on you for its fuel supply, is getting enough glucose (sugar).

Since it is insulin that regulates the level of glucose in your blood and ensures that enough is taken in by your body cells for nourishment, pregnancy triggers *anti*-insulin mechanisms to make sure enough sugar remains circulating in your bloodstream to nourish your fetus. It's a perfect idea that doesn't always work perfectly. Sometimes the anti-insulin effect is so strong that it leaves more than enough sugar in the blood to meet the needs of both mother and child—more than can be handled by the kidneys. The excess is "spilled" into the urine. Thus "sugar in the urine"—a not uncommon occurrence in pregnancy, especially in the second trimester, when the anti-insulin effect increases. In fact, roughly half of all pregnant women show some sugar in the urine at some point in their pregnancies.

In most women, the body responds to an increase in blood sugar with an increased production of insulin, which will usually eliminate the excess sugar by the next office visit. This may well be the case with you. But some women, especially those who are diabetic or have tendencies toward diabetes (because of a family history of the condition, or because of their age or weight), may be unable to produce enough insulin at one time to handle the increase in blood sugar, or they may be unable to use the insulin they do produce efficiently. Either way, these women continue to show high levels of sugar in both blood and urine. In those who were not previously diabetic, this is known as gestational diabetes.

All pregnant women are given a glucose screening test around the 28th week to check for gestational diabetes (see page 266); women at higher risk may be screened earlier.

ANEMIA

"A friend of mine became anemic during pregnancy. How can I tell if I am, and can I prevent it?"

A blood test for anemia is administered at the first prenatal visit, but few women turn out to be iron-deficient then. Some may have come into pregnancy low on iron, thanks to monthly menstrual blood loss. But when menstruation stops with conception, iron stores, if dietary intake is adequate, are quickly replenished. It isn't until around the 20th week, when the blood volume has expanded significantly, that the amount of iron needed for producing red blood cells increases, depleting those stores again. Because not all pregnant women get the iron they need to keep up with their bodies' demands, many develop iron-deficiency anemia by the third trimester.

When the iron deficiency is mild, there may be no symptoms; but as oxygen-carrying red blood cells are further depleted, the anemic mother-to-be begins to exhibit such symptoms as pallor, extreme fatigue, weakness, palpitations, breathlessness, and even fainting spells. This may be one of the few instances where the fetus's nutritional needs are met before the mother's, since babies are rarely iron-deficient at birth.

While all pregnant women are susceptible to iron-deficiency anemia, certain groups are at particularly high risk: those who have had several babies in quick succession, those who are carrying more than one fetus, those who have been vomiting a lot or eating little because of morning sickness, and those who came to pregnancy undernourished and/or have been eating poorly since they conceived.

To prevent iron-deficiency anemia, it is generally recommended that expectant mothers eat a diet rich in iron (see Iron-Rich Foods list, page 97). Just be careful what you chase your iron down with. Taking caffeinated beverages along with high-iron foods (or iron supplements) will reduce the amount of iron absorbed. On the other hand, taking vitamin C–rich foods along with the iron will increase absorption. But since it is close to impossible to get enough iron from food alone, daily iron supplementation of 30 to 50 mg (in addition to your prenatal vitamin) is also usually prescribed for pregnant women. And another 30 mg may be recommended when iron-deficiency anemia is diagnosed.

The vast majority of anemia cases in pregnancy can be traced to an inadequate intake of iron. When iron deficiency is ruled out, testing may be needed to check for other causes.

NOSEBLEEDS AND NASAL STUFFINESS

"My nose has been congested a lot, and sometimes it bleeds for no apparent reason. Should I be concerned?"

No, but you should stock up on tissues. Nasal stuffiness, often with accompanying nosebleeds, is a common complaint in pregnancy. That's because the high levels of estrogen and progesterone circulating in the body bring increased blood flow to the mucous membranes of the nose, causing them to soften and swell—much as the cervix does in preparation for childbirth.

You can expect the stuffiness to get worse before it gets better—which won't be until after delivery. You may also develop sinus congestion and a postnasal drip, which can occasionally lead to nighttime coughing or gagging. Don't use medication or medicated nasal sprays to clear things up, unless they are prescribed by your practitioner. Saline (salt) sprays are, however, completely safe and can be surprisingly effective.

Congestion and bleeding are more common in winter, when heating systems force hot, dry air into the house, drying delicate nasal passages. Using a humidifier may help overcome this dryness. You might also try lubricating each nostril with a dab of petroleum jelly, applied gently with a cotton swab. Some people find nasal strips, available at drug stores, helpful in alleviating stuffiness. Since they are not medicated, they are also safe to use.

Taking an extra 250 mg of vitamin C (with your practitioner's approval), in addition to your required vitamin C foods, may help to strengthen your capillaries and reduce the chance of bleeding. (But don't take megadoses of the vitamin unless prescribed.)

Sometimes a nosebleed will follow overly energetic nose-blowing, so easy does it. Correct nose-blowing is an art, which you would do well to master: first gently close one nostril with your thumb, and then carefully blow out the opposite side. Repeat with the other nostril, continuing to alternate until you can breathe through your nose.

To stem a nosebleed, sit or stand leaning slightly forward, rather than lying down or leaning backward. Using your thumb and forefinger, pinch the area just above your nostrils and below the bridge of your nose, and hold for five minutes; repeat if the bleeding continues. If the bleeding isn't controlled after three tries, or if the bleeding is frequent and heavy, call your doctor.

ALLERGIES

"My allergies seem to have worsened since my pregnancy began. My nose is runny and my eyes tear all the time."

You may be mistaking the normal nasal stuffiness of pregnancy for allergies. Or pregnancy may have indeed aggravated your allergies, though some

NO PEANUTS FOR YOUR LITTLE PEANUT?

It's long been known that parents who have or have had allergies may pass allergic tendencies—though not necessarily the specific allergies—to their unborn child. Some research suggests that allergic mothers (or mothers who have had allergies in the past) who eat highly allergenic foods (such as peanuts and dairy products) while they're pregnant or nursing may be more likely to pass on allergies to those foods in their offspring. If you have ever suffered from allergies, speak to your practitioner and an allergist about whether and how you should consider restricting your diet during pregnancy (and postpartum, if you'll be breastfeeding).

fortunate women actually find temporary relief during this time. Since it sounds like you are not so fortunate, check with your practitioner to see what you can safely use to relieve any severe symptoms. Some antihistamines and other medications are safe for use in pregnancy (your usual medication may or may not be one of these).[3]

In general, however, the best approach to dealing with allergies in pregnancy is preventive—avoiding the offending substance or substances, assuming you know what they are:

◆ If pollens or other outdoor allergens trouble you, stay indoors in an air-conditioned and air-filtered environment as much as you can during

your susceptible season. Wash your hands and face to remove pollen when you come indoors, and wear large curved sunglasses to keep pollens from floating into your eyes when outdoors.

◆ If dust is a culprit, make sure someone else does the dusting and sweeping. A vacuum cleaner, damp mop, or a damp cloth-covered broom kicks up less dust than an ordinary broom, and an absorbent cloth (look for one specifically designed to pick up dust) will do better than a traditional feather duster. Stay away from musty places like attics and libraries full of old books.

◆ If you're allergic to certain foods, stay away from them, even if they are good foods for pregnancy. Consult the Pregnancy Diet for substitutes.

◆ If animals bring on allergy attacks, let friends know of the problem in advance so that they can rid a room of both pets and their dander before you visit. And of course, if your own pet is suddenly triggering an allergic response, try to keep one or more areas

GET YOUR FLU SHOTS

The Centers for Disease Control recommends that every woman who will be pregnant during flu season (generally October through March) be given the flu shot. The shot will not affect the fetus, and the side effects to the mother are practically nil. The worst that can happen is you'll develop a mild fever and feel more tired than usual for a few days. Pregnant women should not get Flumist, the nasal spray flu vaccine. Flumist, unlike the flu shot, is made from live flu virus, and could actually give you a mild case of the flu.

3. If your nose is very runny, the secretions are thick, or you're sneezing a lot, increase your fluid intake to compensate for any loss and to thin the secretions.

in your home (particularly your bedroom) pet-free.

- Tobacco smoke allergy is easier to control these days, since fewer people smoke and more smokers oblige if they are asked to refrain. To ease your allergy, as well as for the benefit of your baby, you should avoid exposure to cigarette, pipe, and cigar smoke. Don't be embarrassed to say, "Yes, I mind very much if you smoke."

What It's Important to Know: EXERCISE DURING PREGNANCY

Executives do it. Senior citizens do it. Doctors, lawyers, and construction workers do it. If they do it, pregnant women wonder, shouldn't we?

"It," of course, is exercise. And the answer for most women with good health and normal pregnancies is a resounding yes. The concept of pregnancy as an illness, and an image of the pregnant woman as a delicate creature too frail to climb a flight of stairs or carry a bag of groceries, are dated. Moderate physical activity (thirty minutes a day) is now considered not only thoroughly safe, but also extremely beneficial for most expectant mothers and their babies. In fact, recent studies show that even vigorous exercise appears safe—and does not increase the risk of preterm delivery.

As anxious as you might be to hit the jogging trail, however, there is one vitally important stop you must make first—at your practitioner's office. Even if you're feeling terrific, you must obtain a practitioner's okay before suiting up in oversized sweatpants. Pregnant women who are in a high-risk category may have to curb exercise or even eliminate it entirely for now. But if yours is among the great majority of normal pregnancies, and your practitioner has given you the go-ahead, suit up and read on.

THE BENEFITS OF EXERCISE

It appears that women who don't get any exercise during pregnancy become progressively less fit as the months pass by—mostly because they are becoming heavier and heavier. A good exercise program (which can be built right into your daily lifestyle) can counteract this trend toward decreasing fitness. It can also give you more energy (surprised?); help you feel better both physically and mentally; improve your sleeping (as long as you don't exercise right before bedtime); strengthen muscles and increase endurance; help you handle the imbalance of an enlarging abdomen; reduce backaches, constipation, bloating, and swelling (of hands and feet, for example); and help you get back into prepregnancy shape sooner after delivery. Strengthening your body and your endurance may even help you cope better with labor.

The following categories of exercise can be particularly useful during pregnancy:

Aerobics. These are rhythmic, repetitive activities strenuous enough to demand increased oxygen to the muscles, but not

SHOULDER AND LEG STRETCHES

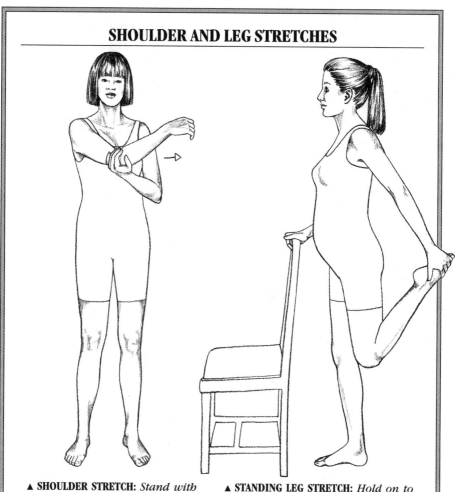

▲ **SHOULDER STRETCH:** *Stand with feet shoulder width apart and knees slightly bent. Hold your arm just below the elbow with your opposite hand. Pull your elbow toward the opposite shoulder as you exhale. Try to hold each stretch for five to ten seconds.*

▲ **STANDING LEG STRETCH:** *Hold on to the back of a heavy chair or other stable object for support. Grasp your foot behind you with the same side hand. Pull the heel to the buttocks while extending your upper leg backward from the hip joint. Keep your back straight. Repeat on the opposite side; hold each stretch for ten to thirty seconds.*

so strenuous that demand exceeds supply. Aerobic activities include walking, jogging, bicycling, and swimming. Exercise too strenuous to be sustained for the twenty to thirty minutes necessary to reach this "training effect" (such as sprinting) is not considered aerobic.

Aerobic exercises stimulate the heart and lungs as well as muscle and joint activity, producing beneficial overall body changes, including an increase in the ability to process and utilize oxygen, which is an important plus for you and your baby. It improves circulation (enhancing the transport of oxygen and nutrients to your fetus while decreasing the risk of varicose veins, hemorrhoids, and fluid retention for you); increases muscle tone and strength (often preventing or relieving backache and constipation, making it easier to carry the extra weight of pregnancy, and facilitating delivery); builds endurance (making you better able to cope with a lengthy labor); may help control blood sugar; burns calories (allowing you to eat more of the good food you and your baby need without gaining excessive weight, and promising a better postpartum figure); lessens

---

STAYING FIT AND HEALTHY

Does exercise help or hurt the immune system? It depends on how hard the workout is. Studies have shown that exercising to the point of exhaustion, such as you might if you were training for a marathon, can wear down the immune system and lead to more frequent illnesses. So clearly, overdoing the workouts isn't smart—especially when you're trying to stay healthy for two.

On the other hand, engaging in moderate exercise, such as daily brisk walks or swims, can boost the immune system, leading to fewer colds and other illnesses. And light activity, such as walking (but not heavy exercise), can reduce the severity and duration of a cold, should one strike. But while it's fine to continue walking when your nose is running, if you have a fever, a cough, the flu, or another illness, you need to rest. Take a break from exercise until you're feeling better.

---

fatigue and promotes good sleep; imparts a feeling of well-being and confidence; and in general heightens your ability to cope with the physical and emotional challenges of childbearing.

Calisthenics. These are rhythmic, light gymnastic movements that tone and develop muscles and can improve posture. Calisthenics especially designed for pregnant women can be very useful in relieving backache, in improving physical and mental well-being, and in preparing your body for the arduous task of childbirth. Calisthenics designed for the general population, however, may be unsafe.

Weight training. This type of exercise can increase your muscle tone. But it is important to avoid heavy weights (over 25 pounds), or those that require grunting or breath holding, which may compromise blood flow to the uterus. Use light weights with multiple repetitions instead.

Water workouts. One of the most comfortable and effective ways to exercise during pregnancy is to take to the water. Water workouts—including swimming, water aerobics and calisthenics, strength training, and flexibility exercises—will not only get you into, or keep you in, shape, they may also lift your mood. And they will be less wearing on your body. Thanks to the support of the water, you weigh only one-tenth of your normal weight in the pool (a definite plus as your abdomen grows), so you can work harder and longer with less exertion. Water exercises are less stressful on your joints, too, so they are unlikely to cause injury. Another plus: workouts in the water won't cause overheating, unless the water is too warm. Since water workouts are so safe, you can continue them—assuming no pregnancy complications—until you go into labor. Just watch out for slippery poolsides, avoid diving, and don't swim in water that is over your head. Keep

BASIC POSITION (THROUGH FOURTH MONTH) AND KEGEL EXERCISES

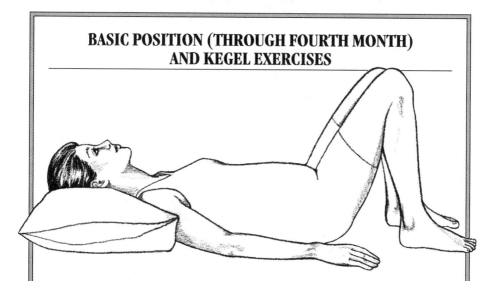

Lie on your back, knees bent, feet about twelve inches apart, soles flat on the floor. Your head and shoulders should be supported by cushions, and your arms resting flat at your sides. Note: The Basic Position should be used only through the fourth month. After that time exercising flat on one's back is not recommended.

To do Kegels, firmly tense the muscles around your vagina and anus.* Hold for as long as you can (working up to eight to ten seconds), then slowly re-lease the muscles and relax. Work up to three sets of ten to twenty during the day. Also do three sets of quick Kegels: count rapidly to ten or twenty, contracting or relaxing the pelvic muscles at each count. Kegels can be done anytime during or after pregnancy, in a standing or sitting position.

---

* To be sure you are using the right muscles, try to stop the flow of urine midstream when you're on the toilet. If you stop it, those are the right muscles.

in mind, too, that exercises done in the water should be especially designed for water use. Using "land" exercises in the water is much less effective.

Yoga. Yoga's emphasis on breathing, relaxation, posture, and body awareness makes it a perfect choice while you're expecting. Choose a yoga class or program that's specifically designed for the pregnant woman; some traditional positions are not appropriate and need to be modified depending on what stage of pregnancy you're in. Physically, yoga can build strength, increase endurance, improve posture and alignment (encouraging grace at a time when grace is especially elusive), promote better circulation and more efficient respiration, and reduce pregnancy aches and pains, especially those in the lower back and legs. Certain positions are even purported to minimize indigestion and nausea. Psychologically, yoga can release tension and anxiety and promote relaxation. By helping a woman learn to visualize, stay focused, and isolate and relax individual body parts, yoga serves as excellent childbirth preparation as well.

Relaxation techniques. Breathing and concentration exercises relax mind and body, help conserve energy for when it's needed, enhance the ability to focus on a task, and increase body awareness—all of which can help a woman better meet the challenges of childbirth. Relaxation techniques (see page 127) are valuable in combination with more physical routines, or alone—especially in high-risk pregnancies, when more active exercise is prohibited.

Pelvic toning. Kegels (see page 193) are simple movements designed to tone the muscles in the vaginal and perineal area, strengthening them in preparation for delivery. Doing them faithfully may help you avoid an episiotomy or a bad tear. Kegels will also aid recovery postpartum (making sex more enjoyable, and helping to prevent incontinence). This exercise is one virtually every pregnant woman can perform and benefit from, anytime, anywhere.

Developing a Good Exercise Program

Get started. The best time to start getting fit is before you get pregnant. But it's never too late to start exercising—even if you're already pushing nine months. First, though, make sure you have the go-ahead from your practitioner.

Get off to a slow start. Once you've decided to begin a fitness program, it's tempting to start off with a bang, running three miles the first morning or working out twice the first afternoon. Unfortunately, such enthusiastic beginnings lead not to fitness but to sore muscles, sagging resolve, and abrupt endings. They can also be dangerous.

Of course, if you followed an exercise program before pregnancy, you can

PELVIC TILT

Assume the Basic Position. Exhale as you press the small of your back against the floor. Then inhale and relax your spine. Repeat this several times. The tilt can also be done standing up straight, with your back against a wall (inhale while pressing the small of your back into the wall). The standing version is an excellent way to improve your posture. After the fourth month, do Pelvic Tilts standing up only, or use this variation: while kneeling on all fours or standing up, rock your pelvis back and forth, keeping your back straight. This version of the Pelvic Tilt is also helpful in combating sciatica pain.

NECK RELAXER

and the rest of you. Sit in a comfortable position on a straight-backed chair with your eyes closed. 1. Gently tilt your head to one side, bringing your ear toward your shoulder as far as you can comfortably go (but don't raise your shoulder toward your ear) and inhaling as you do. Hold the position three to six seconds. Exhale and relax. Then repeat to other side. Repeat three or four times, alternating the direction of the tilt and relaxing between tilts. Do this exercise several times a day. 2. Slowly bend your head forward, bringing your chin toward your chest as far as you can comfortably go. Then slowly roll your cheek to the right toward your shoulder as far as you can comfortably go (don't raise your shoulder toward your cheek). Hold three to six seconds. Exhale and relax. Repeat the stretch on the left. Repeat set three or four times several times a day.

The neck is often a focus of tension, tightening under stress. This exercise can help to relax both your neck

probably continue it—though possibly in a modified form (see Playing It Safe, page 199). If you're a fledgling athlete, however, build up slowly. Start with ten minutes of warm-ups followed by five minutes of more strenuous workout and a five-minute cool-down. Stop strenuous exercise sooner if you begin to tire. After a few days, if your body has adjusted well, increase the period of strenuous activity by about five minutes a week until you are up to twenty to thirty minutes or more, if you feel comfortable.

Get off to a slow start every time you start. Warm-ups can be tedious when you're eager to get your workout started (and over with). But as every athlete knows, they're an essential part of any exercise program. They ensure that the heart and circulation aren't taxed suddenly, and reduce the chances of injury to muscles and joints, which are more vulnerable when cold—and particularly vulnerable during pregnancy. So walk before you run, swim slowly or jog slowly in place in the pool before you start your laps.

CHOOSING THE RIGHT PREGNANCY EXERCISE

Select the type of exercise that's right for you. Though you can probably continue a sport or activity you are already proficient at, it's not advisable to take up a new one during pregnancy.

Exercises that even a novice can do during pregnancy include:

◆ Walking at a brisk pace

◆ Swimming in shallow water that is neither too hot nor too cold*

◆ Water workouts designed especially for pregnancy*

◆ Cycling on a stationary bike at a comfortable tension and speed*

◆ A step machine, at a comfortable tension, or stair climbing

◆ Rowing machine, at a comfortable tension and speed

◆ Calisthenics designed for pregnancy

◆ Yoga designed for pregnancy

◆ Pelvic toning (Kegel exercises)*

◆ Relaxation routines*

Exercises that only a well-trained, experienced athlete should engage in during pregnancy:

◆ Jogging, up to two miles per day, preferably on a treadmill or on even terrain[†]

◆ Doubles tennis (but not singles, which can be too strenuous)

◆ Cross-country skiing

◆ *Light* weight lifting (breathe out on lifting; avoid holding your breath and straining)

◆ Cycling (with extreme caution and with a helmet)

◆ Ice skating (with extreme caution; but not once your belly becomes large enough to interfere with proper balance)

Stretch it out. After a brief warm-up, try a few stretches. Hold each stretch for ten to twenty seconds and don't overstretch or bounce. (Because your joints are probably looser than usual, you may also be more prone to injury.)

Finish as slowly as you start. Collapse seems like the logical conclusion to a workout, but it isn't physiologically sound. Stopping abruptly traps blood in the muscles, reducing blood supply to other parts of your body and to your baby. Dizziness, faintness, extra heartbeats, or nausea may result. So finish your exercise with exercise: about five minutes of walking after running, easy paddling after a vigorous swim, light stretching exercises after almost any activity. Stretches after exercise can be held for twenty to thirty seconds, but don't

bounce. Top off your cool-down with a few minutes of relaxation.

You can help avoid dizziness (and a possible fall) if you get up slowly when you've been exercising on the floor. Do your stretches after aerobics, and be sure not to stretch to your limit, since this can damage joints that have been loosened by pregnancy.

Watch the clock. Too little exercise won't be effective; too much can be debilitating. A full workout, from warm-up to cool-down, can take anywhere from thirty minutes to an hour or even more. If you had been working out prepregnancy and you have your practitioner's okay, you can continue the same schedule—as long as the exercises you choose are safe (see the box above). But keep the level of exertion mild to moderate. If you haven't exer-

- Hiking (but not on uneven terrain or at high altitude)

- Volleyball (with caution)

- Pilates, Alexander technique, tai chi (adapted for pregnancy, and as long as the woman remains comfortable with the positions)

- Kick-boxing (as pregnancy progresses, many women find they can't kick as high or move as quickly)

- Dance workouts (as long as is comfortable)

Exercises that even an experienced athlete should avoid, because of their greater risks, include:

- Jogging more than two miles per day[†]

- Horseback riding

- Waterskiing

- Diving or jumping into pools

- Scuba diving (diving gear may restrict circulation; decompression sickness is hazardous to the fetus)

- Softball, football, and other contact sports

- Sprinting (too much oxygen is demanded too quickly)

- Downhill skiing (risky because of the possibility of a serious fall)

- Cross-country skiing above 10,000 feet (the high altitude deprives both mother and fetus of oxygen)

- Bicycling on wet pavement or winding paths (where falls are likely), and cycling leaning forward in racing posture (can cause backache)

- Calisthenics not designed for pregnancy

*These are non-weight-bearing exercises, the easiest to continue throughout pregnancy.

[†]A few very fit women can continue more rigorous exercise programs with no apparent ill effects. Check with your practitioner before doing so yourself.

cised regularly in the past, working up to half an hour (including warming up and cooling down) three times a week or more is a realistic and safe goal. If time is limited, try brisk walking for ten-minute periods three times a day.

Keep it up. Exercising erratically (four times one week and none the next) won't get you in shape. Exercising regularly (three or four times a week, every week) will. If you're too tired for a strenuous workout, don't push yourself, but do try to do the warm-ups so that your muscles will stay limber and your discipline won't dissolve. Many women find they feel better if they do some exercise—though not necessarily their full workout—every day.

Work exercise into your schedule. The best way to be sure of doing your exer-cise is to allot a specific time for it: before getting into your work for the day; during a coffee or lunch break; or before dinner. If you have no regular block of free time for an exercise session, you can build exercise into your existing schedule. Walk to work, if you can, or park your car or get off the bus or subway a mile or so from your job and walk the rest of the way. Pick a parking spot as far as possible from the market or department store. Or walk an older child to school (or to a friend's) instead of driving. Climb stairs instead of using elevators or escalators. Spend Saturday afternoon strolling in a favorite museum—you won't even realize you've been walking for an hour or two. Instead of flopping down in front of the TV with your spouse after the dinner dishes are done, ask him to join you for a walk. No

DROMEDARY DROOP

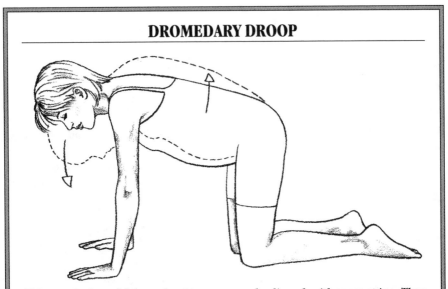

This exercise is useful throughout pregnancy and into labor, to relieve the pressure of the enlarged uterus on your spine. Get down on your hands and knees, with your back in a naturally relaxed position (don't let your spine sag). Keep your head straight, your *neck aligned with your spine. Then hump your back, tightening your abdomen and buttocks, and allow your head to drop all the way down. Gradually release your back and raise your head to the original position. Repeat several times.*

matter how busy your day, if there's the will, there's always a way to fit in some form of exercise.

Compensate for the calories you burn. Perhaps the most fun part of a pregnancy exercise program is the extra eating you'll have to do. As always, make those calories count. Take this opportunity to add even *more* good-for-baby nutrients to your diet. You'll have to consume about 100 to 200 additional calories for every half hour of strenuous exercising. If you believe you're consuming enough calories but you still are not gaining weight, you may be exercising too much.

Replace the fluids you use up. For every half hour of strenuous activity, you will need at least a full glass of extra liquid to

compensate for fluids lost through perspiration. You will need more in warm weather, or when you are perspiring profusely: drink before, during, and after exercising—but no more than 16 ounces at a time. The scale can give you a clue about how much extra fluid you need to drink: two 8-ounce glasses for each pound lost through perspiration during exercise (weigh yourself before and after a typical workout, and you'll find out how many pounds you usually lose). It's a good idea to start your fluid intake thirty to forty-five minutes before your planned workout.

Choose the right group. If you prefer a group approach to exercise, take an exercise class that is specifically designed for pregnant women. Since not everyone who claims to be an expert is one, ask for the instructor's credentials before enrolling. For some women, classes are better than solo exercising (particularly when self-discipline is lacking) and provide support and feedback. The best programs maintain moderate intensity; meet at least three times weekly; individualize to each woman's capabilities; don't use music that's too fast, which may push participants into working too hard; and have a network of medical and exercise specialists available for questions.

Make it fun. Any workout, group or otherwise, should be an experience you look forward to rather than dread, one you think of as fun, not as torture. So select exercises you enjoy and, if you like, take along a companion when you can. Exer-cising with a mate or a friend has, incidentally, been shown to increase the odds of sticking with a program. So instead of meeting a friend for a coffee and scone, meet for a walk.

PLAYING IT SAFE

Don't work out on an empty stomach. Mother's rule about not swimming after a meal had some validity. But exercising on an empty stomach isn't wise, either. If you haven't eaten for hours, it's a good idea to have a light snack and a drink fifteen to thirty minutes before beginning your warm-ups. Best are items high in potassium, such as a banana or orange juice. If you're uncomfortable eating that close to exercising, have your snack an hour before.

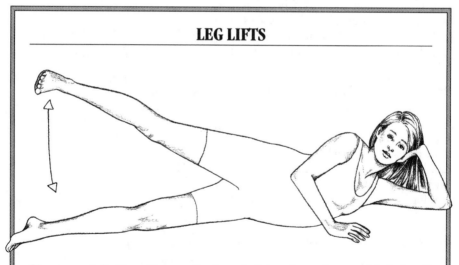

LEG LIFTS

Lie on your left side, with your shoulders, hips, and knees in a straight line. Place your right hand on the floor in front of your chest and support your head with your left. Relax and inhale; then exhale while slowly raising your right leg as high as you can, keeping your foot flexed (pointing toward your belly) and your inner ankle facing directly down. Inhale while slowly lowering your leg. Repeat ten times, then turn and repeat ten times on the other side. This exercise can be done with the leg either straight or bent at the knee.

Dress for the occasion. Wear clothes that are loose or that stretch when you move. Right down to your underwear (which should be cotton), fabrics should let your body breathe. Your bra or sports bra should be comfortable and give plenty of support. Well-fitting athletic shoes will help protect your feet and joints. And the shoes should be designed for the appropriate activity. Running shoes, for example, won't do for walking workouts—and in fact may lead to a fall.

Select the right surface. Indoors, a wood floor or a tightly carpeted surface is better than tile or concrete for your workouts. (If the surface is slippery, don't exercise in socks or footed tights.) Outdoors, soft running tracks and grassy or dirt trails are better than hard-surfaced roads or sidewalks; level surfaces are better than uneven ones. If you run, avoid running downhill, which can be rougher on your joints and muscles than an uphill run. In the last trimester an uphill run may be too exhausting and should also be avoided.

Divide your time. Divide your exercise schedule, if possible, into two or three brief sessions, rather than doing one long session a day. This tones muscles better. Also, do exercises slowly and don't do a rapid series of repetitions. Instead, rest briefly between movements (the muscle buildup occurs then, not while you're in motion).

Do everything in moderation. *Never* exercise to the point of exhaustion, especially when you're pregnant; the chemical by-products of overexertion are not good for the fetus. (Even if you're a trained athlete, you still shouldn't exercise to your fullest capacity, whether it exhausts you or not.) There are several ways of checking to see whether you're overdoing it. First, if it feels good, it's probably okay. If there's any pain or

strain, it's not. A little perspiration is fine; a drenching sweat is a sign to slow down. So is being unable to carry on a conversation as you go. A pulse that still is over 100 beats per minute five minutes after completing a workout means you've worked too hard. So does needing a nap when you're finished. You should feel exhilarated, not drained, after exercising.

Know when to stop. Your body will signal when it's time by saying, "Hey, I'm tired." Take the hint right away, and throw in the towel. More serious signals suggest a call to the doctor: pain anywhere (hip, back, pelvis, chest, head, and so on); a cramp or stitch that doesn't go away immediately when you stop; uterine contractions and chest pain; lightheadedness or dizziness; very rapid heartbeat (tachycardia); severe breathlessness; dif-

---

EXERCISE RED FLAGS IN PREGNANCY

Certain traditional exercise activities are very risky in pregnancy. These include any that put you flat on your back after the fourth month; that pull on the abdomen (such as full sit-ups or double leg lifts); that might force air into the vagina (such as upside-down "bicycling," shoulder stands, or exercises where you bring knee to chest while kneeling on all fours); that stretch the inner thigh muscles (such as sitting on the floor with the soles of the feet together and pressing down on or bouncing your knees); that cause the small of the back to curve inward; that require "bridging" (bending over backward) or other contortions; or that involve deep flexion or extension of joints (such as deep knee bends), jumping, bouncing, sudden changes in direction, or jerky motions.

TAILOR SIT, TAILOR STRETCH

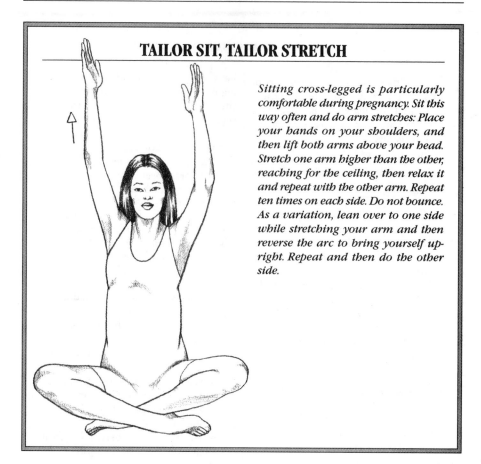

Sitting cross-legged is particularly comfortable during pregnancy. Sit this way often and do arm stretches: Place your hands on your shoulders, and then lift both arms above your head. Stretch one arm higher than the other, reaching for the ceiling, then relax it and repeat with the other arm. Repeat ten times on each side. Do not bounce. As a variation, lean over to one side while stretching your arm and then reverse the arc to bring yourself upright. Repeat and then do the other side.

ficulty walking or loss of muscle control; sudden headache; increased swelling of your hands, feet, ankles, or face; amniotic fluid leakage or vaginal bleeding; or, after the 28th week, a slowing down or total absence of fetal movement. In the second and third trimesters, you may notice a gradual decrease in your performance and efficiency. This is normal and another signal to take it easier.

Stay cool. Until research shows otherwise, exercise or environments that raise a pregnant woman's temperature more than 1½ to 2°F should be avoided (blood is shunted away from the uterus to the skin as the body attempts to cool off). So stay out of saunas, steam rooms, or hot tubs, and don't exercise outdoors in very hot or humid weather, or indoors in a stuffy, overheated room. If you generally walk outdoors, try an air-conditioned mall instead when the temperature soars.

Make sure your workout clothes are cool, too. Wear light clothes in summer, and underdress for outdoor exercise in winter (you should feel slightly chilly when you first go out). Or wear layers, so you can remove one or two as you heat up. And don't wait for your body to tell you when you're overheated—stop before you reach that point.

Proceed with caution. Even the most skilled sportswoman can lack grace when she's pregnant. As the center of gravity

DO TRY THESE AT HOME

Make these simple exercises part of your workout—or just use them periodically during your busy day (even during breaks at work) to keep your circulation going.

Breathing exercise. This deep-breathing exercise can help you learn how to breathe during labor, as well as strengthen one of the muscles you'll need during labor. Sit on the floor with your back against a wall or on a chair with a supportive back. Place your hands on your belly and take a deep breath in (your belly will expand outward). Exhale and contract (or tighten) your transverse abdominal muscle (the muscle you use to hold in your stomach). Do ten repetitions. (Don't worry—you can't squish the baby.) This exercise will help your back feel better, keep your abdominals strong, and prepare you for pushing out the baby.

Waist twists. While sitting or standing, turn from side to side, slowly twisting at the waist. Look over one shoulder, then the other. Your arms should swing freely and with each repetition.

Hip flexors. Stand perpendicular to the back of a heavy chair with one hand resting on it for balance. Extend the opposite leg out in front with your knee bent slightly. Slowly straighten your leg while raising it to hip position (or as high as is comfortable). Exhale as you straighten your leg. Inhale and lower your leg back to the floor. Repeat with your other leg.

Chest stretches. Place your hands on either side of an open door or doorway. They should be at shoulder level with your elbows bent. Lean forward until you feel the stretch in your chest. Hold for ten to twenty seconds. Repeat five times.

Squat. Stand with your feet flat and shoulder width apart. Slowly lower into a squat position, keeping your heels flat on the floor and keeping your back straight. If your heels begin to rise, slightly widen your foot placement. Hold the squat for ten to thirty seconds, resting your arms on your knees. Slowly stand back up by placing your hands on your knees and pushing up with your arms. Repeat five times. This exercise is especially helpful if you plan on laboring or delivering in the squatting position.

---

shifts forward with the uterus, a fall becomes an ever-increasing possibility. Be aware, and be careful. Late in pregnancy, avoid sports that require sudden moves or a lot of balance.

Be aware of the added risk of injury. For a variety of reasons (an altered center of balance, lax joints, absentmindedness), women are more subject to injury when they are expecting. So don't take chances.

Stay off your back, and don't point your toes. After the fourth month, don't exercise flat on your back, as the weight of your enlarging uterus could compress major

blood vessels, restricting circulation. Pointing, or extending, your toes—at any time in pregnancy—could lead to cramping in your calves. Flex your feet instead, turning them up toward your face.

Taper off in the last trimester. Though everyone has heard stories of pregnant athletes who have stayed in the pool or on the jogging trails right up until delivery, for most women it is wise to slack off somewhat during the last three months. Cutting back is particularly wise in the ninth month, when mild stretching routines and brisk walking or water workouts should provide adequate exercise. Serious athletic pursuits can be resumed at about six weeks postpartum (see page 426).

Even when you're not working out . . . don't just sit there. Sitting for an extended period without a break causes blood to pool in your leg veins, can cause your feet to swell, and could lead to other problems. If your work entails a lot of sitting, or if you watch TV for hours at a time or travel long distances frequently, be sure to break up every hour or so of sitting with five or ten minutes of walking. And while at your seat, periodically do some exercises that enhance circulation, such as taking a few deep breaths; extending your lower legs, flexing your feet, and wiggling your toes. Also try contracting the muscles in your abdomen and buttocks (a sort of sitting pelvic tilt). If your hands tend to swell, periodically stretch your arms above your head, opening and closing your fists several times as you do.

IF YOU DON'T EXERCISE

Exercising during pregnancy can certainly do you a lot of good. But sitting it out (whether by choice or on doctor's orders), getting most of your exercise from opening and closing your car door, won't hurt, either. In fact, if you're abstaining from exercise on doctor's orders, you're helping your baby and yourself. Your doctor will almost certainly restrict exercise if you have a history of three or more miscarriages or of premature labor, or if you have an incompetent cervix, bleeding or persistent spotting in the second or third trimester, more than one fetus, heart disease, or a diagnosis of placenta previa or pregnancy-induced hypertension (preeclampsia). Your activity may also be limited if you have high blood pressure, diabetes, thyroid disease, anemia or other blood disorders, or a fetus that isn't thriving; are seriously over- or underweight; or have had an extremely sedentary lifestyle up until now. A history of precipitous (very brief) labor or of a fetus that didn't thrive in a previous pregnancy might also be a reason for a red light (or at least a yellow one) on exercise.

In some cases arm-only exercises or water workouts designed for pregnancy may be okayed when other exercises are taboo. Check with your doctor.

◆ ◆ ◆

The Fifth Month

Approximately 18 to 22 Weeks

What was once completely abstract is fast becoming palpable—literally. Chances are that sometime near the end of this month or the beginning of the next, you will feel your baby's movements for the first time. That miraculous sensation, along with the serious rounding of your abdomen, will finally make the pregnancy feel more like a reality. Though your baby is far from ready to make a personal appearance in the nursery, it's really nice to know there's actually someone in there.

What You Can Expect at This Month's Checkup

Yet another checkup—and by this time you probably know the drill. This month, you can expect your practitioner to check the following, though there may be variations depending upon your particular needs and upon your practitioner's style of practice:[1]

◆ Weight and blood pressure

◆ Urine, for sugar and protein

◆ Fetal heartbeat

◆ Size and shape of uterus, by external palpation (feeling from the outside)

◆ Height of fundus (top of uterus)

◆ Feet and hands, for edema (swelling), and legs for varicose veins

◆ Symptoms you have been experiencing, especially unusual ones

◆ Questions or problems you want to discuss—have a list ready

1. See Appendix, page 545, for an explanation of the procedures and tests performed.

What You May Be Feeling

As always, remember that every pregnancy and every woman is different. You may experience all of these symptoms at one time or another, or only a few of them. Some may have continued from last month, others may be new. Still others may hardly be noticed because you've become so used to them. You may also have other, less common, symptoms.

PHYSICALLY

♦ Fetal movement

♦ Increasing whitish vaginal discharge (leukorrhea)

A LOOK INSIDE

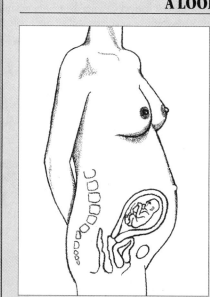

▲ You're halfway through your pregnancy now—and your uterus will hit your belly button sometime around the 20th week. By this point, there is no hiding the fact that you're pregnant.

▶ At the end of the month, your fetus is 7 to 9 inches long (which means that it is almost halfway to birth length) and weighs nearly a pound. As muscles strengthen, nerve networks expand, and the skeleton continues to harden, the fetus is much more active and coordinated—capable of numerous gymnastic feats (including somersaults) that help baby grow and develop motor skills. These movements are also—finally!—strong enough for you to feel. Ears are well developed now, and can start to recognize sound; baby also has regular periods of wakefulness and sleep, and can make a variety of faces, including frowns and grimaces. Eyebrows and head hair are visible. The skin is wrinkled, pink, and translucent, and is covered with a greasy white substance called vernix, which provides protection against the amniotic fluid and will make baby slippery (and thus easier to deliver) at birth. A baby boy's testicles have started their descent from the abdominal cavity into the scrotum.

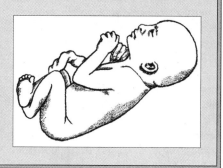

- Achiness in the lower abdomen and along the sides (from stretching of the ligaments supporting the uterus)

- Constipation

- Heartburn, indigestion, flatulence, bloating

- Occasional headaches, faintness, or dizziness

- Nasal congestion and occasional nosebleeds; ear stuffiness

- "Pink toothbrush" from bleeding gums

- Hearty appetite

- Leg cramps

- Mild swelling of ankles and feet, and occasionally of hands and face

- Varicose veins of legs and/or hemorrhoids

- Faster pulse (heart rate)

- Easier—or more difficult—orgasm

- Backache

- Skin color changes on abdomen and/or face

- A protruding navel

EMOTIONALLY

- A growing sense of reality about the pregnancy

- Fewer mood swings, but occasional weepiness and irritability may still occur

- Continued absentmindedness

What You May Be Concerned About

FATIGUE

"I get tired when I am exercising or doing heavy cleaning; should I stop?"

Not only should you stop when you get tired, you should stop before then, if possible. Exerting yourself to the point of exhaustion is never a good idea. During pregnancy it's a particularly bad one, since overwork takes its toll not only on you but on your baby as well. Pay careful attention to your body's signals. If you become breathless when you're jogging, or find the vacuum suddenly feels as if it weighs a ton, take a break.

Instead of marathon activity sessions, pace yourself. Work or exercise a bit, rest a bit. Ultimately, the work, or the workout, gets done, and you won't feel drained afterward. If occasionally something doesn't get done, consider it good training for the days when the

demands of parenthood will often keep you from finishing what you start. See page 114 for tips on dealing with fatigue.

FAINTNESS AND DIZZINESS

"I feel dizzy when I get up from a sitting or lying-down position. And yesterday I nearly fainted while I was shopping. Am I okay? Can this hurt my baby?"

On soap operas, a fainting spell is considered one of the most reliable indicators of pregnancy. Scriptwriters, however, are off the mark. Fainting is not a common symptom of pregnancy.

Dizziness and lightheadedness, however, *are* fairly common among pregnant women, for a variety of reasons. In the first trimester, dizziness may occur

HOT AND COLD: HANDLING TEMPERATURE EXTREMES WHEN YOU'RE EXPECTING

Whether you live in a particularly warm or cold climate year-round or you just happen to be carrying baby through the hottest summer or coldest winter on record, there are plenty of ways to stay safe and comfortable when the thermometer is going to extremes.

Beating the heat. With your metabolism working overtime, it's easy to overheat when you're pregnant. To keep your cool, dress lightly in breathable fabrics, like cotton. Avoid exercising outside in the heat of the day; take your strolls before breakfast or after dinner instead, or attend exercise classes in an air-conditioned fitness center—and always quit before you feel overheated. Stay out of the sun as much as possible, particularly on very hot days, and when you must go out, be sure to apply plenty of sunscreen (sun will intensify the normal skin color changes some women experience). Take a tepid bath or shower to cool off. Or go for a swim, if that's practical. Stay air-conditioned when possible. If you have no air-conditioning at home, spend time at the library, a museum, or mall. Fans alone won't help you keep your cool when the temperature is over 90°F.

Most important of all: drink, drink, drink. Stay hydrated (which will help keep you from feeling weak and dizzy on a warm day, minimize the miseries of many other pregnancy symptoms, and help prevent urinary tract infections and preterm labor) by downing at least eight glasses of water a day, more if you're exercising and/or perspiring a lot. Carrying a water bottle with you wherever you go will help get you, and keep you, in the hydration habit. Avoid caffeine and alcohol, which can dehydrate you, as well as sugary drinks and full-strength fruit juices, which keep fluid in your digestive tract instead of letting it circulate around your body.

Curbing the cold. Though expectant moms are more likely to stay warm through the winter than nonpregnant citizens are, there are certain cold weather precautions you're wise to take. Lower temperatures may reduce blood flow to the placenta, which can reduce the amount of nutrients reaching the fetus. Dressing warmly in the winter months (and don't forget your hat, since heat is most likely to escape through an unprotected head) can help avoid this problem. But make sure you use layers; that way you can peel them off inside if you start to heat up.

because there's not yet an adequate blood supply to fill the rapidly expanding circulatory system; in the second trimester, it may be caused by the pressure of an expanding uterus on the mother's blood vessels. Dizziness can also strike anytime you get up too quickly from sitting or lying down. This is caused by a sudden shifting of blood away from the brain as you change positions. The cure is simple: Always get up very gradually. Jumping up in a hurry to answer the phone is likely to land you right back on the sofa.

You might also feel dizzy when your blood sugar is low. This kind of dizziness can be avoided by getting some protein (which helps maintain even blood sugar levels) at every meal and by eating more frequent, smaller meals or snacking between your usual mealtimes. Carry a box of raisins, a piece of fruit, or some whole-wheat crackers or breadsticks in your bag for quick blood sugar lifts. Dizziness can also be a sign of dehydration, so be sure you're getting your full quota of fluids—at least eight cups a day, more if it's hot or if you've been exercising.

A dizzy spell can also be triggered by indoor stuffiness—in an overheated store, office, or bus—especially if you're overdressed. In that case, getting some fresh air by going outside or opening a window may bring relief. Taking off your coat and loosening your clothes—especially around the neck and waist—should help, too.

If you feel lightheaded and/or think you are going to faint, try to increase circulation to your brain by lying down, if possible, with your feet (not your head) elevated, or by sitting down with your head between your knees, until the dizziness subsides.[2] If there's no place to lie or sit, kneel on one knee and bend forward as though you were trying to tie your shoelace. Actual fainting is rare, but if you do faint, there is no need for concern—although the flow of blood to your brain is temporarily reduced, this will not affect your baby.

Tell your practitioner about the dizzy spells at your next visit; actual fainting should be reported right away. Frequent dizziness or fainting could be a sign of anemia, and needs to be evaluated.

FETAL MOVEMENT PATTERNS

"I felt little movements every day last week, but I haven't felt anything at all today. What's wrong?"

Anxiety over when the first movement will be felt is often replaced by anxiety that fetal movements don't seem frequent enough, or that they haven't been noticed for a while. At this stage of pregnancy, however, these anxieties, while understandable, are usually unnecessary. The frequency of noticeable movements at this point varies a great deal; patterns of movement are erratic at best. Though the fetus

is stirring almost continuously, only some of these movements are strong enough for you to feel. Others may be missed because of the fetal position (facing and kicking inward, for instance, instead of outward). Or because of your own activity—when you're walking or moving about a lot, your fetus may be rocked to sleep; or it may be awake, but you may be too busy to notice its movements. It's also possible that you're sleeping right through your baby's most active period; for many babies that is in the middle of the night. (Even at this stage, babies are most likely to act up when their moms are lying down.)

One way to elicit fetal movement if you haven't noticed any all day is to lie down for an hour or two in the evening, preferably after a glass of milk, orange juice, or other snack. The combination of your inactivity and the jolt of food energy may be able to get your fetus going. If that doesn't work, try again in a few hours, but don't worry. Many mothers find they don't notice movement for a day or two at a time, or even three or four days, before the 20th week. After that time, though there's still no need to panic, it's probably a good idea to call your practitioner for reassurance if twenty-four hours go by without perceptible fetal activity (assuming, of course, that you've already started feeling movement).

After the 28th week, fetal movements become more consistent, and it's a good idea for mothers to get into the habit of checking fetal activity daily (see page 243).

SLEEPING POSITION

"I've always slept on my stomach. Now I'm afraid to. And I just can't seem to get comfortable any other way."

Giving up your favorite sleeping position during pregnancy can be as traumatic as giving up your teddy bear was

---

2. First aid for mothers-to-be who've actually fainted is the same as the preventive measures.

when you were six. You're bound to lose some sleep over it—but only until you get used to the new position. And the time to get used to it is now, before your expanding belly makes it even more difficult to get comfortable.

Two common favorite sleeping positions—on the belly and on the back—are not the best choices during pregnancy. The belly position for obvious reasons: as your stomach grows, it's like sleeping on a watermelon. The back position, though more comfortable, rests the entire weight of your pregnant uterus on your back, your intestines, and two major blood vessels: the aorta (the vein responsible for bringing blood from the heart to the rest of your body) and the inferior vena cava (the vein responsible for returning blood from the lower body to the heart). This can aggravate backaches and hemorrhoids, make digestion less efficient, interfere with breathing and circulation, and possibly cause hypotension, or low blood pressure.

This doesn't mean you have to sleep standing up. Curling up or stretching out on your side—preferably the left side—with one leg crossed over the other and

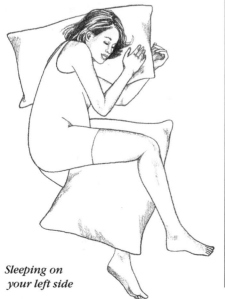

*Sleeping on
your left side*

with a pillow between them (see illustration), is best for both you and your fetus. It not only allows maximum flow of blood and nutrients to the placenta but also enhances efficient kidney function, which means better elimination of waste products and fluids and less swelling (edema) of ankles, feet, and hands.

Very few people, however, manage to stay in one position through the night. Don't worry if you wake up and find yourself on your back or abdomen. No harm done; just turn back to your side. You may feel uncomfortable for a few nights, but your body will soon adjust to the new position. A "body pillow," at least five feet long, or a wedge-shaped pillow can offer support, making side sleeping much more comfortable and staying on your side much easier. If you don't have either of these, you can improvise with any extra pillows, placing them against your body in different positions until you find that perfect combination for catching z's.

BACKACHE

"I'm having a lot of backaches. I'm afraid I won't be able to stand up at all by the ninth month."

The aches and discomforts of pregnancy are not designed to make you miserable—though that's often the upshot. They are the side effects of the preparations your body is making for that momentous moment when your baby is born. Backache is no exception. During pregnancy, the usually stable joints of the pelvis begin to loosen up to allow easier passage for the baby at delivery. This, along with your oversized abdomen, throws your body off balance. To compensate, you tend to bring your shoulders back and arch your neck. Standing with your belly thrust forward—to be sure that no one who passes fails to notice you're pregnant—compounds the problem. The result: a deeply curved lower back, strained back muscles, and pain.

Even pain with a purpose hurts. But without defeating the purpose, you can conquer (or at least subdue) the pain. The best approach, as usual, is prevention: coming into pregnancy with strong abdominal muscles, good posture, and graceful body mechanics. But it's not too late to learn body mechanics that will minimize pregnancy backache. To align your body properly, practice the Pelvic Tilt (see page 194). The following should also help:

◆ Try to keep weight gain within the recommended parameters (see page 169). Excess pounds will only add to the load your back is struggling under.

◆ Don't wear very high heels, or even very flat ones without proper support. Some practitioners recommend wide two-inch heels to help keep the body properly aligned. There are shoes and shoe inserts designed especially to help alleviate leg and back problems during pregnancy; ask your practitioner or a salesperson at a good shoe store about these options.

◆ Learn the proper way to lift heavy loads (packages, children, laundry, books). Don't lift abruptly. Stabilize your body first by assuming a wide stance (feet shoulder-width apart) and tucking your buttocks in. Bend at the knees, not at the waist, and lift with your arms and legs rather than your back. (See illustration.) If backache is a problem, try to limit the carrying you do. If you're forced to carry a heavy load of groceries, divide them between two shopping bags and carry one in each arm, rather than carrying it all in front of you.

◆ Try not to stand for long periods. If you must, keep one foot up on a stool with your knee bent to prevent strain on your lower back. When you're standing on a hard-surfaced floor—in the kitchen while cooking or washing dishes, for example—put a small skid-proof rug underfoot to ease the pressure.

Bend at the knees when you lift

◆ Sit smart. Sitting puts more stress on your spine than almost any other activity, so it pays to do it right. That means sitting, when possible, in a chair that offers adequate support, preferably one with a straight back, arms (use them for assistance when you rise from the chair), and a firm cushion that doesn't allow you to sink down into it. Avoid backless stools and benches. And wherever you're sitting, try to avoid crossing your legs. Not only can leg crossing promote circulation problems (making varicose veins, spider veins, and edema more likely), it can cause you to tilt your pelvis too far forward, aggravating backache. Whenever possible, sit with your legs slightly elevated (see illustration).

◆ Sitting for long periods can be as bad for your back as sitting the wrong way. Try not to sit for more than an hour without taking a walking/stretching break; setting a half-hour limit would be even better.

◆ Sleep on a firm mattress, or put a board under an overly soft one. A comfortable sleeping position aided by a body pillow (one that's at least five feet long) will help minimize aches and pains when you're awake. When getting out of bed in the morning, swing your legs over the side of the bed to the floor, rather than twisting to get up.

◆ Ask your practitioner if a pregnancy crisscross support sling for your belly will be helpful in lessening the strain on your lower back.

◆ Avoid reaching far above your head, which puts a strain on back muscles. Instead of stretching to put away dishes, hang a painting, or adjust the curtains, use a low, steady footstool (or a tall friend).

◆ Alternate cold and heat to temporarily relieve sore muscles. Use an ice pack for fifteen minutes, followed by heating pad for fifteen minutes or a warm (but not hot) bath. Wrap both cold pack and heating pad in a towel or cloth.

◆ Learn to relax. Many back problems are aggravated by stress. If you think yours might be, try some relaxation exercises when pain strikes. Also follow the suggestions beginning on page 125 for dealing with stress in your life.

◆ Do simple exercises that strengthen your abdominal muscles, such as the Dromedary Droop (page 198) and the Pelvic Tilt (page 194). Join a pregnancy yoga or water gymnastics class, or consider water therapy if you can find a medically (and pregnancy-) savvy water therapist.

◆ Consider visiting a chiropractor or a physical therapist who specializes in

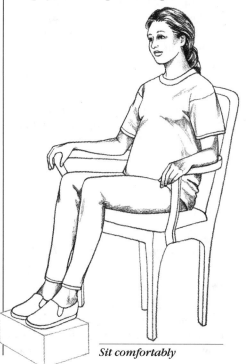

Sit comfortably

pregnancy—or try some alternative therapy like acupuncture or biofeedback (see page 246).

CARRYING OLDER CHILDREN

"I have a three-and-a-half-year-old who always wants to be carried up the stairs. But my back is breaking from her weight."

It would be a good idea to break her habit rather than continue breaking your back; the strain of carrying a growing fetus is enough without adding some 30 or 40 pounds of preschooler. But be careful not to blame her sibling-to-be for the change in parental policy—blame your back instead. Singing a special up-the-stairs song ("Here we go walking up the stairs, up the stairs, up the stairs, Here we go walking up the stairs, And having lots of fun" to the tune of "Here We Go 'Round the Mulberry Bush") or challenging her to a race to the top may make stair climbing more fun. And don't forget to make much ado about her efforts when she does agree to walk on her own.

Of course, there will be times when your child won't take "walk" for an answer. So learn the proper way to lift (see page 210), and be assured that this lifting in no way compromises your unborn baby, unless your practitioner has restricted such activities.

FOOT PROBLEMS

"My shoes are all beginning to feel uncomfortably tight. Could my feet be growing, too?"

The belly isn't the only part of the pregnant body that's prone to expansion. And your shoes may be pinching for a number of reasons. First of all, your feet may be swollen, thanks to the normal fluid retention of pregnancy. They may also be carrying a little extra fat if your weight gain has been on the high side. On top of all that, they may be spreading; though they play no part in childbirth, the joints in your feet (along with all your other joints) are loosened up by hormones preparing for delivery. The swelling in your feet will go down after delivery and the weight will probably be lost. But though the joints will tighten up, it's possible that your feet will be permanently larger—by as much as a full shoe size. Good news for those who love shoe shopping; not so good for those who dread it.

In the meantime, try the tips for reducing excessive swelling (see page 263) if that seems to be your problem, and get a couple of pairs of shoes that fit you comfortably now and will meet your "growing" needs (so you won't end up barefoot and pregnant). Both should have heels no more than two inches high, nonskid soles, and plenty of space for your feet to spread out (shop for them at the end of the day, when your feet are the most swollen); and both should be made of leather or canvas so your feet can breathe. If you choose carefully, you can find not just walking and workout shoes, but work and dress shoes that meet these requirements.

There are shoes and orthotic inserts specially designed to correct the distorted center of gravity of pregnancy. They not only can make your feet more comfortable but can reduce back and leg pain as well. They are available in two different designs, one to take you through the first six months of pregnancy and the other to take you through the final trimester. Ask your practitioner for a recommendation.

Elasticized slippers worn for several hours a day may also be useful in reducing fatigue and achiness in feet and lower legs, though they don't seem to reduce swelling. If your legs are aching and tired at the end of the day, wearing such slippers while you're at home may help.

FAST-GROWING HAIR AND NAILS

"It seems to me that my hair and nails have never grown so fast before."

The bounteous circulation and increased metabolism caused by pregnancy hormones are nourishing your skin cells well. Happy effects of this increased nourishment are nails that grow faster than you can manicure them, and hair that grows before you can secure appointments with your stylist (and if you're really lucky, is thicker and more lustrous now).

The extra nourishment can, however, also have less happy effects. It can cause hair to grow in places you would rather it didn't. Facial areas (lips, chin, and cheeks) are most commonly plagued with this pregnancy-induced hirsutism, but arms, legs, back, and belly can be affected, too. Much of the excess hair disappears within six months postpartum, though some may linger longer.

Though there's no known risk, it's probably not a good idea to use depilatories or bleach cream once you find out you're pregnant. Your skin may not react well to the chemicals, and it's even possible that they may be absorbed into your bloodstream. Electrolysis is also not recommended during pregnancy, though no adverse affects due to electrolysis have been documented; the same holds true for laser hair removal. Don't worry about any electrolysis or laser treatments you've already had, since any risk is purely theoretical. Plucking and shaving, of course, present no problem.

A SPA TREAT

"A friend gave me a gift certificate to a day spa for my birthday. It includes a lot of fun things like aromatherapy treatments and a massage. Are these safe while I'm pregnant?"

No one deserves—and needs!—a day of pampering more than an expectant mother. (With the exception of a new mother—but once you have the baby, you're not likely to find the time for spa treatments.) So feel free to indulge now, but with the following suggestions:

Share the news. First, with your practitioner to be sure there are no specific caveats in your particular situation. Then, when you call to make your appointment, tell the receptionist that you are pregnant. Discuss with him or her the restrictions you will have, so that you can tailor treatments to fit your needs. Also be sure to inform any esthetician or therapist who will be working on you that you're pregnant.

Massage with caution. There's nothing like a massage to rub away the aches and pains of pregnancy, as well as the stress and strain. But make sure that your massage therapist is trained in prenatal massage and follows the guidelines on page 214.

Avoid plant oils and herbals. Because the effects of most plant oils in pregnancy are unknown and some may be harmful, be wary of any massage or treatment that uses aromatherapy. Pregnant women should particularly avoid the following oils: basil, cedarwood, clary sage, fennel, juniper, marjoram, myrrh, rosemary, sage, and thyme. These oils can stimulate uterine contractions.

Relax, in the right position. Especially after the fourth month, it's best to avoid spending a lot of time flat on your back. Ask your massage therapist to use a table that's equipped with a cutout for your belly or special pillows designed for pregnancy use, or to position you on your left

GETTING RUBBED THE RIGHT WAY

Aching for some relief from that nagging backache—or from that anxiety that's keeping you up at night? Massage can rub those pregnancy pains, strains, and stresses away—plus help you get a better night's sleep. To make sure that your pregnancy massages are not only relaxing but also safe, follow these tips:

◆ Avoid massage during the first trimester, since it may trigger dizziness and add to morning sickness.

◆ Be sure the masseuse you use is licensed by the state you live in; if your state does not license massage therapists, then accreditation by a national massage therapy organization (such as the American Massage Therapy Association) will do.

◆ Seek a therapist who is fully familiar with the dos and don'ts of massage during pregnancy. For example: *Do* use a special table with an opening through which your expanded belly can fit, so you can comfortably lie face-down and the therapist can get to your back. *Don't* massage the abdomen, or at least limit it to a very light touch. *Don't* massage the feet and ankles or the webbing between the thumb and index finger, since it is believed that certain spots in those areas can trigger contractions; *don't* use aromatherapy oils (see page 213).

Once you're sure you're in good hands—relax and enjoy!

---

side. Facials, manicures, pedicures, and other treatments should be done either in a sitting or semi-reclining position or while you're lying on your left side.

Get the glow. But be in the know about which facial and body treatments—such as glycolic peels—might be especially irritating to skin made more super-sensitive by pregnancy hormones. Discuss with the esthetician which preparations are least likely to provoke a reaction. And steer clear of botox, too.

Keep cool. Soaking in a hot tub or using a sauna definitely should *not* be a part of the treatment plan (because they might raise your body temperature excessively). Herbal wraps are also out while you're expecting. But a *warm* bath as part of hydrotherapy is safe and relaxing.

Watch what you breathe. If a manicure or pedicure is on the agenda, make sure it's done in a well-ventilated space. Inhaling those strong chemical smells is never a good idea, but especially not when you're breathing for two.

SKIN DISCOLORATION

"I have a dark line down the center of my abdomen and dark spots on my face. Is this discoloration normal, and will it remain after pregnancy?"

Blame it on those pesky (but practical) pregnancy hormones. Just as they caused the hyperpigmentation, or darkening, of the areolas around your nipples, they are now responsible for the darkening of the linea alba—the white line you probably never noticed, which runs down the center of your abdomen to the top of your pubic bone. During pregnancy, it's renamed the linea nigra, or black line. It may be more noticeable in dark-skinned women than those who are fair-skinned.

Some women, more often those with darker complexions, also develop discolorations—in a masklike configuration or a confettilike appearance—on foreheads, noses, and cheeks. The patches are dark in light-skinned women and light in dark-skinned women. This "mask of pregnancy," or chloasma, will gradually fade after delivery. In the meantime, bleaching probably won't lighten chloasma (and is not a good idea anyway), though cover-up makeup may camouflage it.

Many women also find that freckles and moles become darker and more noticeable and that darkening of the skin occurs in high-friction areas, such as between the thighs. All this hyperpigmentation will fade after delivery.

Sun can intensify the discoloration, so when you are outdoors in sunny weather, use a sunblock with a sun protection factor (SPF) of 15 or more on all exposed skin and avoid spending long hours in the sun (even with sunblock). A hat that completely shades your face and long sleeves to protect your arms (if you can take the heat) can also help. Since there is some evidence that the excess pigmentation may be related to folic acid deficiency, be sure you're taking a vitamin supplement that contains folic acid and that you are eating green leafy vegetables, oranges, and whole-wheat bread or cereal daily.

"If I can't work on my tan while I'm pregnant, can I at least use sunless tanner?"

Apparently, sunless tanners haven't been a priority for researchers, who have yet to do a major study on the safety of these cosmetic products during pregnancy. So while there's no evidence that they're harmful while you're expecting—it's likely that they aren't, since (according to the sunless tanner industry) the active chemical that produces that tan is absorbed only by the first three layers of the skin—there's no evidence that they're completely safe, either.

Check with your practitioner if this lack of information leaves you unsure how to proceed. Some okay the use of sunless tanners after the first trimester; others feel it's more prudent to stay pale the whole nine months. Either way, don't worry about any sunless tanners you've used so far.

In making your decision, you may also want to consider a strictly logistical factor: once your belly starts getting in the way, there's not much chance you'd be able to apply the tanner evenly—a challenge, let's face it, even when you *can* reach your legs easily.

OTHER STRANGE SKIN SYMPTOMS

"My palms seem to be red all the time. Is it my imagination?"

No, and it isn't your dishwashing liquid, either. It's your hormones again. Increased levels of pregnancy hormones cause red, itchy palms (and sometimes red, itchy soles of the feet) in two-thirds of white and one-third of black pregnant women. The dishpan look will disappear soon after delivery.

Your nails may not escape pregnancy unscathed, either. You may find they are more brittle or soft, and have developed grooves. Nail polish may make them worse. If they show signs of infection, ask your practitioner about treatment. And be sure you are getting your four Calcium servings daily (see page 94).

"My legs and feet turn bluish and blotchy sometimes. Is something wrong with my circulation?"

Due to stepped-up estrogen production, many expectant women experience this kind of transitory, mottled

NINE MONTHS AND COUNTING

discoloration when they're chilly. It's insignificant, and will disappear postpartum.

"I've developed a tiny, floppy growth of skin under my arm. I'm worried that it could be skin cancer."

What you're describing is probably a skin tag, another benign skin problem common in pregnant women and often found in high-friction areas, such as under the arms. Skin tags frequently develop in the second and third trimesters and may regress after delivery. If they don't, they can be easily removed by your physician.

To be sure of the diagnosis, show the tag to your practitioner at your next visit.

"I seem to have broken out in a heat rash. I thought only babies got that."

Actually, anyone can develop a heat rash. But it is particularly common in pregnant women because of the increase in eccrine perspiration, the kind that comes from sweat glands distributed over the entire body surface and is involved in heat regulation. Patting on some cornstarch after your shower and trying to keep as cool as possible will help minimize discomfort and recurrence.

On the plus side, apocrine perspiration, the kind produced by glands under the arms, under the breasts, and in the genital area, diminishes in pregnancy. So though you may have heat rash, you are less likely to have body odor. If you itch *all over* but have no rash, call your practitioner.

VISION

"My eyesight seems to be deteriorating since I got pregnant. And my contacts don't seem to fit anymore. Am I imagining it?"

No, chances are you really aren't seeing as well as you were prepregnancy. Your eyes are just another of the seemingly unrelated body parts that can fall prey to pregnancy hormones. Not only can your vision seem less sharp, but hard contact lenses, if you wear them, may suddenly no longer feel comfortable. Fluid retention, which changes the curvature of the eye, may be at least partially to blame for these annoying changes. Eye dryness, which is caused by a hormone-induced decrease in tear production, can also contribute to irritation and discomfort. And if that's not enough, fluid increases that change the cornea's shape can actually cause some pregnant women to become more near- or farsighted.

Your vision should clear up and your eyes return to normal after delivery. Since being refitted for new hard lenses during pregnancy doesn't make financial sense, you might consider switching to glasses or soft contacts, if that's possible, until you deliver.

Also, now isn't the time to consider corrective laser eye surgery. While the procedure won't harm the baby, it could overcorrect your vision and take longer to heal, possibly requiring a second corrective surgery later on. Ophthalmologists recommend avoiding the surgery during pregnancy, in the six months preconception, and for at least six months postpartum.

Though a slight deterioration in visual acuity is not unusual in pregnancy, other symptoms could signal a problem. If you experience blurring or dimming vision or often see spots or floaters, or have double vision that persists for more than two or three hours, don't wait further for it to pass; call your practitioner at once. Briefly seeing spots after you have been standing for a while or when you get up suddenly from a sitting position is fairly common and nothing to worry about—though you should report it to the doctor.

ROUTINE ULTRASOUND

"I'm having a perfectly normal pregnancy, with no problems at all. But my practitioner is still recommending that I have an ultrasound this month. Is it really necessary?"

These days, ultrasounds aren't reserved for problem pregnancies. In fact, most practitioners order a detailed (Level 2) ultrasound routinely at 20 to 22 weeks—mostly as reassurance that everything is going exactly the way it should be (though it can also be performed for diagnostic reasons; see page 49). And because it is noninvasive and can't harm the fetus or the pregnancy, it's a risk-free way to obtain that reassurance.

Also on the plus side for parents, it's fun to get a sneak peek at your baby—and to take home a souvenir photo to start the album with. Just make sure you check with your practitioner before signing up at one of those store-front ultrasound studios popular in malls. Though the detailed 3-D photos they provide may be suitable for framing, technicians may not be adequately trained—and may even give you inaccurate information about your baby.

"I'm going for my 20-week ultrasound, and I'm not sure whether to find out the baby's sex or not."

This is one pregnancy decision only a mother and father can make. Unless there is a medical reason why that information is vital, it's entirely optional. And there are no right or wrong decisions. Some parents opt to know for practical reasons: it makes layette shopping, nursery painting, and name selection (only one to pick!) a lot simpler. Others opt to know because they simply can't stand the suspense. But many parents still prefer the guessing game, and decide to find out the old-fashioned way, when baby's lower half finally makes its way out into the world. The choice is yours.

If you do decide to find out now, keep in mind that determining the sex of a baby through ultrasound is not an exact science (unlike amniocentesis, which determines the sex of the baby through chromosomal analysis). Many parents have been told by the sonographer they are expecting a girl only to have the practitioner announce, "It's a boy!" (or vice-versa) upon delivery. So if you do choose to find out if it's a girl or a boy when you go for your ultrasound, remember that it's only a guess, however educated it may be.

A LOW-LYING PLACENTA

"The doctor said my ultrasound showed that the placenta was down near the cervix. She said that it was too early to worry about it; but of course I started worrying."

Like a fetus, a placenta can do a lot of moving around during pregnancy. It doesn't actually pick up and relocate, but it does appear to migrate upward as the lower segment of the uterus stretches and grows. Though an estimated 20 to 30 percent of placentas are in the lower segment in the second trimester (and an even larger percentage before 20 weeks), the vast majority move into the upper segment by the time delivery nears. If this doesn't happen and the placenta remains low in the uterus, a diagnosis of "placenta previa" is made. This complication occurs in very few full-term pregnancies. And in only 1 out of 4 of these very few cases is the placenta located low enough—partially or completely covering the cervix, or mouth of the uterus—to cause a serious problem.

In other words, your doctor is right. It's too early to worry—and statistically speaking, the chances are slim that you'll ever have to worry.

WEARING A SEAT BELT

"Is it safe to fasten my seat belt in the car? What about in airplanes?"

The most common way for a woman of childbearing age to lose her life is in a car crash. And the best way to avoid such a fatality—as well as serious injury to you and your unborn child—is to always buckle up. Statistics prove conclusively that it is a lot safer to fasten your seat belt than not to fasten it.

For maximum safety and minimum discomfort, fasten the belt below your belly, across your pelvis and upper thighs. If there is a shoulder harness, wear it over your shoulder (not under your arm), diagonally between your breasts and to the side of your belly. And don't worry that the pressure of an abrupt stop will hurt the fetus; it is well cushioned by amniotic fluid and uterine muscle, among the world's best shock-absorbing materials.

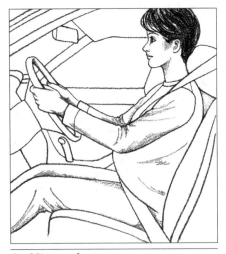

Buckling up for two

Fastening your seat belt on airplanes when the seat belt sign is illuminated isn't only required by the FAA, it's your best protection against being thrown from your seat during turbulence. So buckle up in the air, too.

OUTSIDE INFLUENCES ON THE WOMB

"I have a friend who insists that taking her unborn baby to concerts will make him a music lover, and another one whose husband reads to her tummy every night to give their baby a love of literature. Isn't this all nonsense?"

In the study of the unborn, there's certainly no shortage of nonsense. Incredibly, however, scientists are starting to find that some of these apparently over-the-top theories may actually have a basis in fact. Still, much more research needs to be done before anyone can answer your question with certainty.

Because the ability to hear is quite well developed in the fetus by the end of the second trimester or the beginning of the third, it's true that your friends' babies are hearing the music and the readings. What that will mean in the long run isn't really clear. Some researchers in the field believe that it is actually possible to stimulate the fetus prior to birth to produce, in a sense, a "superbaby." There are methods that claim to turn out babies who can speak at six months and read at a year and a half, by exposing the fetus to increasingly complex rhythmic imitations of a mother's heartbeat.

Though there are no proven benefits to prenatal manipulation of a baby's intellectual development, there are theoretical risks. For one thing, fetuses, like newborns, have natural patterns of sleep and wakefulness—patterns that parents might unwittingly disrupt in their well-

CARRYING BABY, FIFTH MONTH

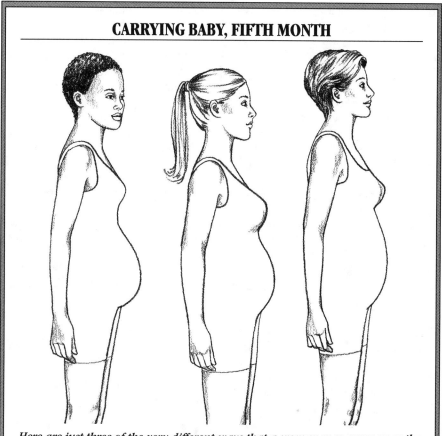

Here are just three of the very different ways that a woman may carry near the end of her fifth month. The variations on these are endless. Depending on your size, your shape, the amount of weight you've gained, and the position of your uterus, you may be carrying higher, lower, bigger, smaller, wider, or more compactly.

meant attempts to make the womb a classroom. These stimulating disruptions could actually hamper development, rather than nurture it (much as waking a napping newborn for a game of flash cards might). For another thing, fetuses, like newborns, have individual patterns of development that need to be respected; tampering with these patterns could be harmful in the long run. Most important, there's always the danger that in the pursuit of intellectual excellence, parents might lose sight of what all babies and children need—and benefit from—most: unconditional love.

That isn't to say that attempting to make contact with your baby before birth, and even reading to it or playing music for it, is either harmful or a waste of time. Any kind of prenatal communication may give you a head start on the long process of parent-baby bonding. This may not necessarily translate into more closeness as your baby gets older, but it may make those earliest days easier.

Of course, if you feel silly talking to

your bloated abdomen, there's no reason to worry that your baby will miss out on getting to know you. He or she is getting used to the sound of your voice—and Dad's, too—every time you talk to each other or someone else. That's why infants seem to recognize and respond to their parents' voices at birth.

Your voice, because it is heard not only from outside but from inside, is especially familiar, and appears to be comforting, too. Research shows that a fetus's heart rate slows in response to its mother's voice, suggesting that babies are soothed by their moms even before birth.

Your fetus can also hear other sounds from the outside world, and may become familiar with those that are common in your surroundings. Whereas a newborn who had little prenatal exposure to a barking dog may startle and cry at first hearing the sound, one who's heard a lot of barking won't even blink.

Exposure to music may also affect the fetus. Research has shown that some fetuses demonstrate a preference (by a change in their movements) for certain types of music—usually the gentler kind. There's even evidence that babies may remember music they've listened to in utero. In one study, a piece by Debussy was played over and over for pregnant women when both they and their fetuses were tranquil. After birth, the same piece of music appeared to have a soothing effect on the babies, calming and quieting them down. Whether this early music appreciation has any lasting impact isn't documented. But most experts would agree that exposing a baby to good music after he or she is born is probably a lot more significant in the creation of a music lover than exposing a fetus in utero.

It's also been suggested that, since the sense of touch is also already developed in the uterus, stroking your abdomen and "playing" with a little knee or bottom when it's pushed up may also help

parent-child bonding—and whether this is true or not, there's certainly no harm in trying. Of course, it's unlikely that you'll need to make a conscious effort to touch your baby more; even strangers can hardly keep their hands off a pregnant belly—as you've probably noticed.

There's one thing for sure: whether or not your in-utero interactions will be ultimately enriching to your baby, they can be rewarding for you now, making the little one in your uterus seem more real, and bringing you (and your spouse) closer to your child before he or she is even born. So enjoy making baby contact now, but don't worry about teaching facts or imparting information—there's plenty of time for that later. As you'll discover, children grow up all too soon anyway. There's no need to rush the process, particularly before birth.

PARENTHOOD

"I keep wondering if I will be happy with my baby once it's born."

Most people approach any major change in their lives—marriage, a new career, or an impending birth—wondering whether it will be a change they'll be happy with. And it's always much more likely to be a happy change if expectations about it are realistic.

If you have images of bringing a cooing, smiling, advertisement-ready baby home from the hospital, you may want to read up on what newborns are really like. Not only won't your newborn be smiling or cooing for many weeks, he or she may hardly communicate with you at all, except to cry—and this will almost invariably be when you're sitting down to dinner or starting to get romantic, have to go to the bathroom, or are so tired you can't move.

And if your visions of parenthood consist of nothing but leisurely morning

PREGNANT WOMEN ARE DELICIOUS

If mosquitoes seem to love snacking on you more than ever now that you're pregnant, it's not just your imagination. Scientists have found that pregnant women attract twice as many mosquitoes as nonpregnant women do, possibly because those pesky bugs are fond of carbon dioxide and pregnant women tend to take more frequent breaths, thereby releasing more of this mosquito-friendly gas. Another reason why mosquitos make a beeline for expectant mothers: they're heat-seeking, and expectant mothers generally have higher body temperatures, what with all that baby-making going on. So if you live in or travel to an area where mosquitoes are a problem (especially if they pose a health risk), take proper precautions. You can avoid their bites by staying indoors in heavily mosquito-infested areas, by using tight-fitting screens on windows, and by using a non-DEET-based insect repellent.

walks through the park, sunny days at the zoo, and hours coordinating a wardrobe of miniature, sparkling clean clothes, another reality check is probably in order. There'll be many mornings that turn into evenings before you and your baby ever have the time to see the light of day; many sunny days that will be spent largely in the laundry room; very few tiny outfits that will escape unstained by spit-up, pureed bananas, and baby vitamins.

What you *can* expect realistically, however, are some of the most wondrous, miraculous experiences of your life. The fulfillment you will feel when cuddling a warm, sleeping bundle of baby (even if that cherub was a colicky devil moments before) is incomparable. That—along with that first toothless smile meant just for you—will be well worth all the sleepless nights, delayed dinners, mountains of laundry, and frustrated romance.

Can you expect to be happy with your baby? Yes, as long as you're expecting a real one.

ABDOMINAL PAIN

"I'm very worried about the pains I've been getting on the lower sides of my abdomen."

What you are probably feeling is the pregnancy equivalent of growing pains: the stretching of muscles and ligaments supporting the enlarging uterus. Most pregnant women experience these pains, which may be crampy or sharp and stabbing, and often are most noticeable when you are getting up from a bed or chair, or when you cough. The pain may be brief, or may last for several hours. As long as it is occasional and not persistent—and is not accompanied by fever, chills, bleeding, increased vaginal discharge, faintness, or other unusual symptoms—there's no cause for concern. Getting off your feet and resting in a comfortable position should bring some relief. You should, of course, mention the pain to your practitioner at your next visit, so that he or she can reassure you that this is just another normal, if annoying, part of pregnancy.

LATE MISCARRIAGE

"I know they say that once you pass the third month, you don't have to worry about miscarriage. But I know someone who lost her baby in the fifth month."

While it's essentially true that there's little reason to worry about miscarriage after the first trimester, it does occasionally happen that a fetus is lost between the 12th and 22nd weeks. This is known as a late miscarriage and it is *rare* in a healthy woman with an uneventful, low-risk pregnancy. After the 22nd week, when the fetus usually weighs over 500 grams (17½ ounces) and there is the possibility that it can survive with specialized care, its delivery is considered a premature birth and not a miscarriage.

Unlike the causes of early miscarriages, which are frequently related to the fetus, the causes of second-trimester miscarriages are usually related to either the placenta or the mother. The placenta may separate prematurely from the uterus, be implanted abnormally, or fail to produce adequate hormones to maintain the pregnancy. The mother may have had surgery that affected her ability to hold a pregnancy. Or she may suffer from serious infection, uncontrolled chronic illness, severe malnutrition, an abnormally shaped uterus, an incompetent cervix or PPROM (see page 507). Serious physical trauma, such as that sustained in an accident, rarely triggers miscarriage at any stage in pregnancy.

Early symptoms of a midtrimester miscarriage include a pink vaginal discharge for several days, or a scant brown discharge for several weeks. Should you experience such a discharge, don't panic—it could be nothing serious. But do call your practitioner the day you first notice it. If you have heavy bleeding with or without cramping, call your practitioner immediately or go to the hospital emergency room. (See page 496, if this happens, for treatment of threatened miscarriage and prevention of future miscarriages.)

JETTISONING JET LAG

Add jet lag to the normal fatigue of pregnancy and you're likely to want to end your trip before it begins. So it makes sense to try to minimize—if you can't completely eliminate—the physically draining effects of travel across time zones. Here's how:

Start switching time zones before you leave. Ease yourself into the time zone you're headed for by setting your watch—and your schedule—gradually back or forward. If you're heading east, start getting up a little earlier and going to bed a little earlier a few days before your departure. If you're heading west, go to bed a little later and get up a little later (if you can). On your plane ride, try to sleep if it's an appropriate sleeping time at your destination, or stay awake if it's not.

Live on local time. Once you arrive at your destination, start living on local time full-time. If you arrive at your Paris hotel room at 7 A.M., exhausted from an overnight flight, resist the urge to nap until noon. Instead, sustain yourself with a hearty breakfast and step out for a slow-paced day of sightseeing. Don't push yourself—take frequent breaks to sit down with your feet up—but do try hard to stay out of the prone position. If you lie down, sleep will almost undoubtedly overcome you. Dine, too, according to the local clock and not your internal one (snack if you're hungry, but hold off on a full meal until the clock strikes "eat"), and strive to stay awake until as close to your usual bedtime (local time) as possible. This should help you sleep through the local night. Avoid sleeping in, too, which could make going to bed at a normal time the next night more difficult. Ask for a wake-up, even if you think you won't need it.

TRAVEL

"Is it safe for me to go ahead with the vacation my spouse and I had planned for this month?"

For most pregnant women, travel during the second trimester is not only safe and comfortable but the perfect chance to get away with their spouses for a last fling (at least for a while) as a twosome. And with no diapers, no bottles, no jars of messy baby food to worry about, it'll certainly never be as easy to vacation with your baby again. This is also the ideal time to schedule a business trip or two.

Of course you will need your practitioner's permission; if you have high blood pressure, diabetes, or other medical or obstetrical problems, you may not get the green light. (That doesn't mean you can't vacation at all. If you can't travel, pick a hotel or resort within an hour's drive of your doctor's office—and

enjoy!) Even in a low-risk pregnancy, traveling a great distance isn't a terrific idea in the first trimester when your body is still making its initial physical and emotional adjustment to pregnancy. Likewise, long-distance travel is not recommended in the last trimester, for obvious reasons: should you go into labor early, you'd be stranded far from your practitioner.

Once you have your practitioner's permission, you will only need to do a little planning and take a few precautions to ensure a safe and pleasant voyage for you and your baby:

Choose a suitable destination. Traveling to a hot, humid climate may be uncomfortable because of your increased metabolism; if you do choose such a locale, make sure your hotel and transportation are air-conditioned and that you stay hydrated and out of the sun. Travel to areas at high altitude (over 7,000 feet above sea

---

Seek out sun. Getting some sunlight will help you reset your biological clock, so be sure to spend some time outdoors on your first day at your new destination. If there's no sun to be found, at least spend some time outdoors in the daylight. If you've gone west to east, the best sun to seek is morning sun; if you've gone east to west, take to the outdoors in the late afternoon.

Eat, drink, and be less jet-lagged. Anyone who travels frequently knows how dehydrating air travel can be. And dehydration can make jet lag symptoms more severe (not to mention put you at risk for pregnancy complications). So drink plenty of water on the plane, and continue drinking once you have arrived. Take time to eat regularly, too. Concentrate on foods that are high in long-term energy boosters, such as protein and complex carbohydrates. Getting some exercise (nothing strenuous; a walk in a park or a few laps in the hotel

pool are just right) will also help you feel less fatigued.

Don't look for a miracle. Don't use *any* over-the-counter, prescription, or herbal preparation for jet lag (or any purpose) without your practitioner's approval. Even an herbal remedy like melatonin, which some believe can prevent or cure jet lag (though the jury is still out), is not safe to use during pregnancy.

Give it time. You should start to feel less tired and more in sync with the local schedule within a couple of days.

You may find sleep problems—and the fatigue that inevitably accompanies them—continuing to plague you during the entire trip. But, let's face it, that may have less to do with jet lag and more to do with the fact that you're carrying around a lot of extra baggage—the kind you can't ask a skycap or bellman to help you with.

level) may be dangerous, since adjusting to the decrease in oxygen may be too taxing for both you and your baby. If you *must* make such a trip, you should try to ascend gradually, if possible (if you're driving, for example, try to go up 2,000 feet a day, rather than going up 8,000 feet all at once). To minimize the risk of developing acute mountain sickness (AMS),[3] also plan on limiting exertion for a few days after your arrival, drink lots of fluids, eat frequent small meals instead of three large ones, avoid rich and heavy food, and seek sleeping accommodations, if feasible, at a somewhat lower altitude. If you're in your last trimester, your doctor may recommend you have a nonstress test on each of the first three days of your stay, and then further tests semiweekly. Any signs of fetal distress will probably warrant the administration of oxygen and return to lower altitude.

Other inappropriate destinations are developing regions of the world for which vaccinations would be necessary, since some vaccines may be hazardous during pregnancy (check with your practitioner). Not insignificantly, these same locales may be hotbeds of certain potentially dangerous infections for which there are no vaccines—another reason to avoid them when you're expecting.

Plan a trip that's relaxing. A single destination is preferable to a grand tour or business trip that takes you to six cities in six days. A vacation for which *you* set the pace is a lot better than one where a group tour guide sets it for you. A few hours of sightseeing or shopping (or meetings) should be alternated with time spent reading, relaxing, seeing a film or concert, or napping.

Insure yourself. Get travel insurance, in case a pregnancy complication should require you to change your plans and stick close to home. Consider medical evacuation insurance as well if you're traveling overseas, in case you need to return home quickly and under medical supervision. Medical travel insurance may also be useful if your home insurance plan does not include foreign medical care.

Carry a medical history. It is always wise, but particularly when you're pregnant, to travel with a medical information card listing your blood type, medications you're taking and/or are allergic to, and any other pertinent medical data, along with your practitioner's name, address, and telephone number. Keep all medications in your carry-on luggage and tuck an extra prescription for each Rx medication you are taking into your purse or passport folder, in case your bags and medication are lost, temporarily or permanently, en route. You may have to have a prescription you've brought from home cosigned by a local doctor; often a doctor at a hospital emergency room will agree to do the honors. An extra pair of glasses—or at least a prescription for glasses—may also be useful.

Pack a pregnancy survival it. Make sure you take enough vitamins to last the trip; packets of dry skim milk if you think you won't be able to find pasteurized fresh milk (but only reconstitute it with safe water; see below); some whole-grain crackers and other favorite nonperishable snacks; Sea Bands (see page 118) if you are susceptible to motion sickness and medication for traveler's stomach okayed by your practitioner;[4] comfortable shoes roomy

---

3. Symptoms of AMS include: lack of appetite, nausea, vomiting, flatulence, restlessness, headache, lassitude, shortness of breath, scanty urine, and psychological changes.

4. If you do come down with diarrhea, it will also be important to replace electrolytes and fluids. You can do this by eating salted crackers and drinking bottled juices mixed half and half with bottled water. Or ask your practitioner about taking along a rehydration product that replaces electrolytes.

TRAVELER'S TUMMY

If, in spite of your best efforts, you come down with travel-related tummy problems, taking the medication recommended by your practitioner (which, hopefully, you remembered to take with you) may help. If it doesn't, or if you have more than three loose movements in eight hours or also have nausea and vomiting, chills, or fever, you should see a doctor.

enough to accommodate feet swelled by long hours of sightseeing or work; and this book for reference. You may also want to carry a thermometer, alcohol swabs, sunblock, some Band-Aids, an antibiotic ointment, witch hazel pads if hemorrhoids are a problem, cream for itching, and antibacterial spray or wipes for disinfecting public toilets.

Have the name of a local obstetrician handy, just in case. Your doctor may be able to provide you with one. If not, contact the local medical association in the city you're traveling to or the International Association for Medical Assistance to Travelers (IAMAT, 417 Center Street, Lewiston, NY 14092; [716] 754-4883), which will, for a small donation, provide you with a directory of English-speaking physicians throughout the world. Some major hotel chains can also provide you with this kind of information. If for any reason you find yourself in need of a doctor in a hurry when you're overseas and your hotel can't provide you with one, you can call the American embassy, an American military base, or the nearest teaching hospital. Or you can head for the hospital's emergency room. If you have medical travel insurance, you should have a number to call for help.

Take your Pregnancy Diet with you. You may be on vacation, but your baby is working as hard as ever at growing and developing, and has the same nutritional requirements he or she always has. Self-sacrifice isn't required at mealtimes, but prudence is. Order thoughtfully and you will be able to savor the local cuisine while also fulfilling your baby's requirements. Don't skip breakfast or lunch in order to save up for a lavish dinner.

Don't drink the water (or even brush your teeth with it) unless you're certain it's safe. If the purity of the water is questionable at your destination, plan to use bottled water for drinking and brushing, or bring along a water pot or an immersion heater that can heat local water to a rolling boil; these are available in travel stores and from travel catalogs. (Iodine, often used to disinfect water, may not be safe for pregnant women.) You can also substitute fruit juices to get your daily fluids. Avoid ice, too, unless you are certain it was made from bottled or boiled water.

Don't swim in the water, either. In some areas, lakes and oceans may be polluted. Check with the CDC (Centers for Disease Control) about the waters at your destination to be sure of safety before taking a dip. Beware, too, of pools that are not properly chlorinated.

Eat selectively. In some regions, it may not be safe to eat raw unpeeled fruits or vegetables or salads. (Peel fruit yourself, washing the fruit first and your hands after peeling to avoid transferring germs to the fruit; bananas and oranges tend to be safer than other fruits, because of their thick skins.) In all regions, avoid lukewarm or room-temperature cooked foods, raw or undercooked meat, fish, and poultry, as well as unpasteurized or unrefrigerated dairy products and food sold by street vendors—even if it's hot. For complete information on such restrictions, on other foreign health hazards, and on immunizations for travel, contact the Centers for Disease Control and Prevention's Traveler's Hotline at (877) FYI-TRIP (394-8747) or on-line at www. cdc.gov/travel. Travel warnings are also available from the State Department at (202) 647-5225 or on-line at www.travel.state.gov.

Head off traveler's irregularity. Changes in schedule and diet can compound constipation problems. So make sure you get plenty of the three most effective constipation combaters: fiber, fluids, and exercise (see Constipation, page 156). It may also help to eat breakfast (or at least part of it) a little early, so you'll have time to use the bathroom before you set out for the day.

When you've gotta go, go. Don't encourage a urinary tract infection or constipation by postponing trips to the bathroom. Go as soon as you feel the urge (and can find a public restroom).

Get the support you need. Support hose, that is. Particularly if you already suffer from varicose veins—but even if you only suspect you may be predisposed to them—wear support hose when you'll be doing a lot of sitting (in cars, planes, or trains, for example) and when you'll be doing a lot of standing (in museums, on airport lines). They'll also help minimize swelling in your feet and ankles.

Don't be stationary while on the move. Sitting for long periods can restrict the circulation in your legs, so be sure to shift in your seat frequently, and stretch, flex, wiggle, and massage your legs often—and avoid crossing your legs. If possible, take your shoes off and elevate your feet a bit. Get up at least every hour or two to walk the aisles when you are on a plane or train. When traveling by car, don't go for more than two hours without stopping for a stretch and a stroll. While

you're sitting, do the simple exercises described on page 203.

If you're traveling by plane: Check with the airline in advance to see if it has special regulations concerning pregnant women (many airlines do). Arrange ahead of time for a seat in the bulkhead (preferably on the aisle, so you can get up and stretch or use the restroom as needed), or if seating is not reserved, ask for preboarding. *Do not fly in an unpressurized cabin.* All commercial jets are pressurized, but small private or feeder airline planes may not be, and pressure changes at high altitudes may rob you—and your baby—of oxygen.

When booking your flight, ask whether any meal will be served or available for purchase—more and more often, the "friendly skies" are also the "go hungry skies." If the pickings will be slim (snack mix and an apple) or nonexistent, bring along a meal of your own (a sandwich or salad, for instance). Even if you will be scoring a meal, keep in mind that it may be (a) tiny (b) inedible (c) a long time in coming, due to flight delays, or (d) all of the above. Pack snacks accordingly: crackers or breadsticks, cheese sticks or wedges, raw vegetables, fresh fruit, trail mix, some healthy chips. And don't forget to drink plenty of bottled water (don't drink airplane tap water), milk and juice to counter the dehydration caused by air travel. (This will also encourage trips to the bathroom, which will ensure your legs get stretched periodically.)

Wear your seat belt comfortably fastened below your abdomen. If you're traveling to a different time zone, take jet lag (see box, page 222) into account. Rest up in advance, and plan on taking it easy for a few days once you arrive.

If you're traveling by car: Keep a bagful of nutritious snacks and a thermos of juice or milk handy for when hunger strikes.

For long trips, be sure the seat you will occupy is comfortable; if it isn't, consider buying or borrowing a special cushion for back support, available in auto supply stores and through some catalogs. A pillow for neck support may also add to your comfort. If you aren't behind the wheel, set your seat as far back as possible to give your legs maximum stretching room and to put more space between you and the passenger-side air bag, if there is one. If you are the driver, sit as far back as you can and tilt the steering wheel up and away from your belly. And of course, keep your seat belt fastened at all times.

If you're traveling by train: Check to be sure there's a dining car with a full menu. If not, bring adequate meals and snacks along. If you're traveling overnight, arrange for a sleeper car. You don't want to start your trip exhausted.

EATING OUT

"I try hard to stay on a healthy diet, but with a business lunch nearly every day, it seems impossible."

For most pregnant women it isn't substituting mineral water for martinis that poses a challenge at business lunches (or when dining out after hours); it's trying to put together a meal that's nutritionally sound from a menu of buttery sauces, elegant but empty starches, and tempting sweets. But with the following suggestions, it is possible to take the Pregnancy Diet out to lunch or dinner.

♦ Look for whole-grain options before you leap into the bread basket. If there aren't any in the basket, ask if there are any in the kitchen—at the very least, there may be whole-wheat sandwich bread. If not, try not to fill up on the white stuff. Go easy, too, on the butter you spread on your bread

and rolls, as well as the olive oil you dip them into. There will probably be plenty of other sources of fat in your restaurant meal—dressing on the salad, butter or olive oil on the vegetables—and, as always, fat adds up quickly.

♦ Order a green salad as a first course, and ask for the dressing (or plain oil and vinegar) on the side so you can stay within the guidelines for fat intake. Other good first-course choices include shrimp cocktail, steamed seafood, grilled portobello mushrooms, and other grilled vegetables.

♦ If you're ordering soup, opt for a clear consommé or broth, lentil or bean soups (a large bowl may serve as a meal, especially when liberally sprinkled with grated cheese), or vegetable soups (particularly sweet potato, carrot, or winter squash varieties, as well as tomato-based ones). Generally steer clear of cream soups and chowders (unless you know they're made with milk or yogurt, not cream).

♦ Select a high-protein, low-fat main course. Fish, seafood, chicken, and veal are usually the best bets, as long as they're not fried or bathed in butter, oil, or rich sauces. If everything comes with a sauce, ask for yours on the side. Often chefs will accommodate a request for fish or chicken broiled, grilled, or roasted with little or no fat. If you're a vegetarian, scan the menu for tofu, beans and peas, cheeses, and combinations of these. Vegetable lasagna, for example, might be a good choice in an Italian restaurant, bean curd and vegetables in a Chinese one.

♦ As side dishes, look for white or sweet potatoes (in any form but fried, heavily buttered, or candied), brown rice, kasha or groats, pasta, legumes (dried beans and peas), and lightly cooked fresh vegetables. Salad bars can be great as long as you fill your plate with undressed greens and trimmings (which you can top with cheese and a light dressing or just a bit of a full-fat dressing) and avoid the choices already swimming in oil or mayonnaise. Also, avoid salad bars that don't look well tended, refrigerated, and clean, or don't come equipped with a "sneeze guard."

◆ If you're eating out daily, try to stick (at least most of the time) to unsweetened and unliqueured fresh or cooked fruits and berries (with a spoonful of whipped cream, if you like). If your sweet tooth demands more, fruit sorbet, frozen yogurt, or an occasional scoop of regular ice cream are fine, too. If you're craving serious sweets, join the "two spoons" club and share a decadent dessert with the table.

BEST BETS IN RESTAURANTS

It's not always possible to pick your restaurant, particularly if you're not picking up the tab. When you do have the choice, keep in mind that there are some cuisines that suit the expectant diner better than others and that there is a growing group of enlightened restaurateurs who try to provide healthy food no matter what the cuisine of origin. When you can't choose, don't despair. You can eat well in almost any restaurant if you order wisely.

In restaurants that specialize in a certain type of cuisine, it helps to know what to look for and what to avoid. Use the following as a *general* guide, recognizing that cooking styles vary, even within a particular cuisine.

Seafood, steak house, American. In these, broiled, grilled, or roasted fresh seafood, poultry, and meats (select lean choices, when possible), all good first choices, are the specialties of the house, and are often served with baked potatoes, fresh vegetables, and salads. Some offer a bountiful salad bar with a variety of "undressed" vegetables and fruit, which, when chosen judiciously, can help you fill a lot of requirements at one sitting. *Tips:* Though a shift toward the use of whole grains is slowly taking place in such establishments, most still provide only refined breads in their baskets, so be prepared to fill your grain requirements at other meals or with wild rice or legumes (beans, peas) as side dishes, if they're available. *Vegetarians:* Though some of these restaurants have a vegetarian special on their menu daily (such as a pasta or a legume dish), others will only serve up a platter of vegetables— so plan to compensate later on for the protein you're missing.

Italian. The Mediterranean diet has a well-deserved reputation for being healthy. Enjoy grilled and roasted fish, chicken, veal, or lean beef entrees; fresh cooked greens (such as spinach, broccoli, and broccoli rabe); salads (especially those with nutritious dark greens, such as romaine and arugula); and pizza with tomato sauce, cheese, and fresh vegetables (such as peppers and broccoli); pasta tossed with fish, seafood, chicken, or cheese. Choose marinara or other tomato-based or vegetable-based sauces over cream sauces, and whole-wheat pizza and pasta, when available. *Tip:* Avoid anything breaded, deep or pan fried, or blanketed in a rich sauce. Take advantage when a restaurant offers a reduced-fat cheese option on pizza or other dishes. *Vegetarians:* Pizza, pasta, and vegetable-cheese dishes (vegetable lasagna, eggplant Parmesan) are good options for those who eat dairy products.

A couple of heaping spoonfuls of Parmesan cheese will add additional protein and calcium to any pasta dish. Vegans can opt for dishes with beans when available, or vegetarian pasta dishes, along with salads and greens, although protein may be hard to come by.

French. Avoid classic French cuisine, which is often high in animal fat, and select the lighter contemporary dishes. Concentrate on fish, poultry, and meats that have been roasted, braised, stewed, grilled, or poached, and skip the rich sauces, pastry shells ("en croûte"), pâtés (they're held together with fat), sausages and duck confit (also prime sources of fat), organ meats, and rare or raw beef (steak tartare). Certain bistro favorites, such as roasted chicken with vegetables or stews made with meat or poultry and vegetables or beans are fine, too. *Tips:* Order a salad or vegetable-based soup as a first course to take the edge off your appetite and to be sure you get enough vegetable servings. Ask for rich sauces on the side if you want to "taste." *Vegetarians:* Protein choices may be limited, so check the menu in advance.

Chinese. Well-prepared Chinese food features fish, meats, poultry, and vegetables that are quickly stir-fried and at the peak of nutrition. True, Chinese food can be high in sodium (thanks to soy sauce), high in fat (thanks to often generous use of oils), and may contain MSG (see page 148). But these days most Chinese restaurants will honor a request to prepare food with no MSG, with little or no oil, and with "light" soy sauce. In many you can request brown rice. Soups and steamed dumplings are good starters. Order dishes that have plenty of fish, shellfish, poultry, meat, or bean curd (tofu) rather than those that are just garnished with protein foods; try steamed preparations; don't add soy sauce at the table (unless you've requested none in the prepara-tion, in which case, add to taste). *Tips:* Steer clear of fried ("crispy") foods, including egg rolls; high-sugar sweet-and-sour dishes; and spareribs. Limit the quantity of white rice and white noodles. If spicy foods tend to bring on heartburn, order yours "not spicy." *Vegetarians:* Easy pickings for vegans since bean curd (tofu) and often "mock" meats (made from soy or wheat) are available and nutritiously prepared. Nutritious vegetables, like broccoli, are also plentiful.

Japanese. Avoid fried dishes (agemono, katsu, agedashi, tempura) as well as those that contain raw fish or seafood (sushi, sashimi; see page 149). Go for simmered (nimono), broiled, or grilled (yakitori) dishes; miso soups, vegetable sushi rolls; soybean dishes; stews (domburi), stir-fries (sukiyaki), and noodles (choose buckwheat soba). Edamame (steamed soybeans) makes a tasty and nutritious first course. Dipping sauces usually contain no fat, though some may be high in sugar and salt. *Tips:* If you crave tempura, "steal" a few pieces from your dinner companion's plate; but don't even taste the raw fish or seafood. *Vegetarians:* Choices may be limited. Before getting seated, check to be sure there is a dish made with tofu or soybeans or you may end up with a bowl of noodles.

Thai. As with most Asian food, Thai dishes tend to have both good choices and not so good ones. Look for baked or grilled fish or poultry. Also good: stir-fries, hotpot dishes, and soups—just make sure there's plenty of fish, poultry, meat, seafood, or tofu in these. *Tips:* Ask for stir-fries to be light on the oil and avoid deep-fried foods, curries, and other dishes made with coconut milk or cream, as well as those with sweet sauces (too much sugar). *Vegetarians:* Look for dishes made with tofu; some establishments also have "mock" meats.

Indian. If the spices don't upset your digestive tract, Indian restaurants can feed you well. They can provide protein-rich baked and roasted (tandoori) fish or chicken (often marinated in yogurt), as well as nutritious salads, soups, and vegetable dishes, and whole-grain Indian breads (roti, chapati, and paratha). *Tip:* Skip the fried dishes and ask for brown rice, when available. *Vegetarians:* Lentil, pea, chickpea, cheese, and vegetable dishes are always available, making this cuisine an ideal choice.

Mexican, Spanish, and Tex-Mex. Again, favor eateries that feature lighter cuisine, use vegetable oil rather than lard, and include plenty of vegetables on their menu. Even better are those that also offer low-fat cheeses, whole-wheat tortillas, and brown rice. Good menu choices: gazpacho and black bean soups, asada (grilled chicken and seafood), Veracruz-style dishes (made with tomato sauce), salsas, and picante sauces. Paella (a Spanish chicken-seafood stew) usually has plenty of protein, but also can fill you up with a lot of nonnutritious white rice. *Tips:* If the salad comes in a fried taco shell, ask to have the taco omitted. If there's no salad, you can drink one in the form of gazpacho. Stay away from the fried foods and limit white rice, taco chips, and refried beans (the latter may be laced heavily with lard), and order plain beans, if available, for a side dish. *Vegetarians:* If the restaurant uses vegetable oil instead of lard, bean and cheese enchiladas, burritos, and quesadillas are great choices, if they're not fried; some restaurants even offer soy cheeses, fake bacon, and tofu "sour cream" for vegans.

Cajun or Louisiana style. Cajun food can be delicious but can also be very heavy on the fat. Stick with boiled, steamed, broiled, and grilled fish or seafood and hearty seafood/poultry/vegetable stews such as jambalayas and gumbos.

Tips: Eschew fatty pork chops and fried dishes and go easy on the white rice. *Vegetarians:* Choices may be limited, so check ahead; beans are usually an option, if they're not prepared with animal fat.

Southern; soul food. In most such restaurants, food is fried or otherwise fat laden. Even the healthy greens, such as turnip and collards, may be prepared with excessive fat or bacon drippings. If you're lucky, you'll be able to find a cook who'll broil, bake, barbecue, or grill you a serving of fish or chicken. If all you can get is fried chicken, ask for a breast and peel off the crust and/or the skin before eating. Side dishes are almost certain to be tricky. Hush puppies are fried, as are onion rings. Potatoes are usually either fried or mashed with hefty amounts of butter. Most other starches—biscuits, corn bread (unless it's made with nondegerminated cornmeal), dumplings, and stuffings—are nutritionally weak. *Tips:* Order yams or sweet potatoes (at least you'll get some beta-carotene). Ask if the greens on the menu can be steamed or sautéed and served without a lot of fat (if not, greens traditionally prepared are still better than none at all). Just make up for the extra fat you're taking in by being a little more careful for the next day or two. *Vegetarians:* Again, probably slim pickings. Check the menu before sitting down.

Greek and Middle Eastern. Like other Mediterranean cuisines, these are high on the list of good bets. Favor baked, grilled, and roasted fish, poultry, and lean meats (including shish kebab); dishes that combine vegetables with fish or meat and/or feta cheese; lentil, broad bean, and chickpea dishes; yogurt-based soups; sautéed greens (horta); vegetable salads; and cooked whole grains, such as bulgur. *Tips:* Ask for whole-wheat pita, with hummus or olive oil instead of butter. Avoid white rice and rice-stuffed dishes, and fried and phyllo-wrapped specialties. *Vegetarians:*

These restaurants are often good choices, including dishes with beans, lentils, polenta, bulgur, and cheese.

German, Russian, and Middle European. These cooking styles are traditionally heavy on breadings, dumplings, noodles, and high-nitrate, high-fat sausages and wursts, and light on nutritiously cooked vegetables and broiled fish and meats. Some more contemporary eateries will offer simply broiled or roasted fish and poultry. When they don't, scan the menu for anything broiled or grilled (chops, chicken, steak) or for a meat-and-vegetable stew like goulash. Kasha or potatoes makes a good side dish. *Tips:* Try to get the good along with the "wurst" by filling up on a salad or a vegetable side dish, if available. *Vegetarians:* Options may be few.

Pizzerias. Two slices of the typical thin-crusted cheese pizza generally provide more than a full protein serving, two calcium servings, and a variety of vitamins and trace minerals, for a not unreasonable 400 to 500 calories. A whole-wheat pizza adds a couple of whole-grain servings as well. But pizza can also quickly fill your fat allowance for the day, especially if you add extra cheese, pepperoni, or sausage, so order accordingly. *Tips:* Choose a vegetable topping (peppers and/or broccoli are ideal) and ask for reduced or nonfat cheese, if available. Add a salad and you've got a nutritious meal. *Vegetarians:* Cheese pizza can be a good choice for those who eat dairy products, but a pizza with just sauce and vegetables doesn't supply adequate protein for vegans, who should look for a pizzeria that offers the option of soy cheese or even soy pepperoni.

Coffee shops and diners. More contemporary eateries offer a wide range of healthful specials (omelettes made with egg whites, oat bran waffles, veggie burgers, turkey burgers), excellent breads (multigrain), and freshly cooked vegetables. Almost all offer such traditional favorites as broiled fish and roasted chicken, salads (no-bacon Cobb, chef, Niçoise), and sandwiches (sliced chicken, turkey, Swiss cheese, sliced egg, tuna with light mayo) on whole wheat with lettuce and tomato and a side of salad or vegetables. *Tips:* Avoid slaw if it's heavy on the mayo. Skip the fries (both French and home-style). Get salad dressings on the side. Substitute mustard for mayo, when possible. And don't eat more than one pickle—they're very high in sodium. *Vegetarians:* Eggs, cheese sandwiches, salads, and veggie burgers are good choices.

Delis. Hold the pickles and sauerkraut (too salty), fatty and often nitrate-preserved fish, meats, and cold cuts such as smoked salmon, white fish, pastrami, corned beef, frankfurters, salami, bologna, ham, and tongue. Instead order sliced fresh turkey or chicken (not the processed variety); broiled or roasted chicken or fish; tuna, egg, or chicken salad; or Swiss cheese on whole wheat. Add side orders of cole slaw (vinegar-based slaws are lower in fat and calories than mayo-based) and sliced tomato and lettuce. *Tips:* Also hold the added mayo (the fat calories add up quickly); ask for mustard instead. Order a salad, if available (dressing on the side) or ask for melon or fruit salad to compensate for the usual dearth of healthy vegetable side dishes. *Vegetarians:* Egg and cheese dishes are usually available, but for vegans, choices may be limited, though some delis offer vegetarian soups with beans or lentils and even veggie burgers.

Jewish-style or kosher delis or restaurants. As with other delis (see above), avoid processed meats and fish and order the usually abundant roasted or broiled poultry and fish choices for your main course. *Tips:* Avoid fatty meats and limit your intake of fried potato pancakes, oily potato puddings, highly sweetened noodle puddings (kugels) and blintzes, and stuffed derma (kishke) to a few bites. And don't overdo the salty kosher pickles. *Vegetarians:* In a kosher restaurant that serves meat, there may be little to nothing for the vegetarian, except perhaps salads and vegetables. In one that serves dairy exclusively, there will probably be good options, at least for the ovo-lacto vegetarian. Keep in mind that at both dairy and meat restaurants, many of the vegetarian dishes aren't that nutritious.

Health food and vegetarian restaurants. These are, not surprisingly, top-notch nutritionally. To fill your protein requirement, choose from dishes made with cheese, yogurt, tofu, legumes (beans, lentils, peas), fish or poultry, or fake meats (veggie burgers, hot dogs, and so on). Enjoy the whole grains and the fresh vegetables. *Tips:* Desserts may contain lots of sugar, but as long as they are made with fresh fruits and/or whole grains, they'll also provide nutrition. *Vegetarians:* This type of restaurant is ideal, whether you're vegan or ovo-lacto.

Fast-food restaurants. Obviously, you're not going to find health food at a fast-food restaurant (unless it's one of the small but growing number of healthy-food fast-food establishments that specialize in smoothies, wraps, and other nutritious offerings). But you can find some items that are better than others, including: grilled, broiled, or roasted chicken; grilled or barbecued chicken sandwiches (order with lettuce and tomato, without mayo, and add a slice of cheese if you're in need of calcium); turkey or chicken or cheese subs (pick the "wheat" bread over the white, and ask for extra tomato); bean-and-cheese or chicken burritos or soft tacos; single cheeseburgers (preferably with lettuce and tomato); thin-crust cheese pizza with vegetable toppings (skip the pepperoni); pita sandwiches; baked potatoes (avoid high-fat toppings); salads (grilled chicken or chef, but ask for fat-reduced dressing); and soups. Veggie burgers are increasingly available, too; add cheese to yours. Salad bars are fine as long as they look clean and well maintained. Concentrate on fresh vegetables, cheese, and eggs, and top them with a fat-reduced dressing. *Tips:* Steer clear of double or bigger burgers, and fried chicken or fish, any of which may contain at least half a day's calorie allotment; try not to order your own fries (sneak just a few from a meal mate); avoid shakes (they generally have too many calories and very little, if any, milk). One major chain offers frozen yogurt for dessert, a decent way to appease your sweet tooth and take in a little calcium. When in doubt, ask to see the nutrition information on the various offerings and select a main dish with no more than 500 calories for 20 grams of protein. (Calorie count should be lower if protein total is lower.) *Vegetarians:* Unless you're in a healthy-food fast-food restaurant, your options will be limited. Pizza, cheese-and-veggie subs, cheese quesadillas and burritos, and baked potatoes with cheese and broccoli can work for those who eat dairy, but others may be out of luck, unless veggie burgers are offered.

What It's Important to Know:
MAKING LOVE DURING PREGNANCY

Religious and medical miracles aside, every pregnancy begins with sex. So why is it that what got you into this situation in the first place may now have become one of your biggest problems?

Whether sex becomes virtually nonexistent, just a little uncomfortable, or better than ever, almost every expectant couple finds that their sexual relationship undergoes some kind of change during the nine months of pregnancy.

Variations in sexual appetite and response before conception are wide to begin with. What constitutes a satisfying sex life to one couple—"obligatory" relations once a week, for instance—would be completely unsatisfactory for another, for whom once a day might not always be enough. After conception, such variations may be even more exaggerated. And sexual, physical, and emotional upheaval sometimes leaves the once-a-day couple less in the mood for love than the once-a-week couple, and vice versa.

Though there are variations from couple to couple, a general down-up-down pattern of sexual interest for the three trimesters of pregnancy is common. It's not surprising that a diminution of sexual interest may occur early in pregnancy (in one survey, 54 percent of women reported reduced libido in the first trimester). After all, fatigue, nausea, vomiting, and painfully tender breasts make less than ideal bedfellows. In women with comfortable first trimesters, however, sexual desire may remain more or less the same. And a sizable minority of expectant women find it increases significantly—often because the hormonal changes of early pregnancy leave the vulva engorged and ultrasensitive, and/or because the heightened breast sensitivity is pleasurable for them. These women may experience orgasms or multiple orgasms for the first time.

Interest often—though not always —picks up during the midtrimester, when the couple is physically and psychologically better adjusted to the pregnancy. As delivery nears, libido usually wanes again, even more drastically than in the first trimester—for obvious reasons: first, the bulk of the abdomen is more and more difficult to get around; second, the aches and discomforts of advancing pregnancy are capable of cooling the hottest passion; and third, late in the trimester it's hard to concentrate on anything but that eagerly and anxiously awaited event.

Sexual pleasure, like sexual interest, seems to diminish in some, but certainly not all, couples. A study found that in one group of women, 21 percent received little or no pleasure from sex before conception. The percentage of these women finding sex not pleasurable rose to 41 percent at 12 weeks of gestation, and to 59 percent going into the ninth month. The same study found that at 12 weeks, about 1 in 10 couples were not having sex at all; by the ninth month, more than a third were abstaining. But the study also found that more than 4 in 10 women were still enjoying sex at this point— more than half of these with *no* problems.

In other words, sex during pregnancy is different for every couple. You may find it's the best you've ever had. Or something you wish you could enjoy but can't. Or it may become an uncomfortable obligation. You may even abandon it altogether. Normalcy in pregnancy lovemaking, as in so many other aspects of pregnancy, is what is right for you.

UNDERSTANDING SEXUALITY DURING PREGNANCY

Unfortunately, some practitioners are as inhibited about sexuality as some of the rest of us. Often they don't tell expectant couples what to expect, or not to expect, in the intimate part of their relationship. And that leaves many couples uncertain how to proceed.

Understanding why making love during pregnancy is different than it is at other times can help ease fears and worries, and can make having intercourse (or not having it) more acceptable and more pleasurable.

First of all, there are many physical changes that affect desire and actual sexual pleasure both positively and negatively. Some negative factors can be dealt with to minimize their interference in your sex life; others you may just have to learn to live with—and love with.

Nausea and vomiting. If your morning sickness stays with you day and night, you may just have to wait out its symptoms. (In most cases, queasiness will start letting up by the end of the first trimester.) If it strikes just at certain hours, keep your schedules flexible, and put the good times to good use. Don't pressure yourself to feel sexy when you're feeling lousy; morning sickness can be aggravated by emotional stress. (See page 115 for tips on minimizing morning sickness.)

Fatigue. This, too, should pass by the fourth month (though it will probably return in the last trimester). Until then, make love while the sun shines (when the opportunity presents itself), instead

of trying to force yourself to stay up late for romance. If your weekend afternoons are free, cap off lovemaking with a nap, or the other way around.

The changing shape. Making love can be both awkward and uncomfortable when a bulging belly seems to loom as large and forbidding as a Himalayan mountain. As pregnancy progresses, the gymnastics required to scale that growing abdomen may not seem, to some couples, worth the effort. (But there are ways to get around the mountain; read on for more.) In addition, the woman's full-figured silhouette may turn off one or both partners. You may be able to psych yourself out of this socially conditioned reflex by thinking: big (in pregnancy) is beautiful.

The engorgement of genitals. Increased blood flow to the pelvic area, caused by hormonal changes of pregnancy, can heighten sexual response in some women. But it can also make sex less satisfying (especially later in pregnancy) if a residual fullness persists after orgasm, leaving a woman feeling as though she didn't quite make it. For the male, too, the engorgement of the pregnant woman's genitalia may increase pleasure (if he feels pleasantly and snugly caressed) or decrease it (if the fit is so tight he loses his erection).

Leakage of colostrum. Late in pregnancy, some women begin producing the premilk called colostrum. Colostrum can leak from the breasts during sexual stimulation, and it can be disconcerting in the middle of foreplay. It's nothing to worry about, of course, but if it bothers you or your partner, you can refrain from breast play.

Breast tenderness. Some fortunate couples revel throughout pregnancy in the fun of full-and-firm-for-the-first-time breasts. But many find that in early pregnancy, the breasts may have to be neglected during love play because they are painfully tender. (Be sure you communicate your discomfort to your partner, rather than suffering, and resenting, his touch in silence.) For many, tenderness diminishes toward the end of the first trimester, but the continued sensitivity and enlargement of the breasts enhances sex for some couples.

Alterations in vaginal secretions. Normal vaginal secretions increase in volume and change in consistency, odor, and taste during pregnancy. The increased lubrication may make intercourse more enjoyable for a couple if the woman's vagina has always been dry and/or uncomfortably narrow. Or it might make the vaginal canal so wet and slippery that a man may have trouble reaching orgasm. (A little extra foreplay for him may help him out in that department.) The heavier scent and taste of the secretions may also make oral sex unpleasant to some. Massaging scented creams into the pubic area or the inner thighs (but not the vagina) may help.

Bleeding caused by the sensitivity of the cervix. The mouth of the uterus also becomes engorged during pregnancy—crisscrossed with many additional blood vessels to accommodate increased blood flow—and much softer than before pregnancy. This means that deep penetration can occasionally cause bleeding, particularly late in pregnancy when the cervix begins to ripen for delivery. If this occurs (and your practitioner assures you that the bleeding is not due to any potential complication that requires abstinence from intercourse), simply avoid deep penetration.

There is a full complement of psychological hang-ups that can interfere with sexual enjoyment during pregnancy. These, too, can be minimized.

Fear of hurting the fetus or causing a miscarriage. In normal pregnancies, sexual intercourse will do neither. The fetus is well cushioned and protected inside the amniotic sac and uterus, and the uterus is securely sealed off from the outside world by a mucous plug in the mouth of the cervix.

Fear that having an orgasm will stimulate miscarriage or early labor. Although the uterus does contract following orgasm—and these contractions can be quite pronounced in some women, lasting as long as half an hour after intercourse—such contractions are not a sign of labor and pose no danger in a normal pregnancy. In fact, studies show that couples who are sexually active during pregnancy have lower rates of premature labor than those who abstain (possibly because a close physical relationship often means a couple is staying close emotionally, which has a positive effect on pregnancy outcome). However, orgasm, particularly the more intense kind that may be triggered by masturbation, may be prohibited in pregnancies at high risk for miscarriage or premature labor.

Fear that the fetus is "watching" or "aware." Though your baby may enjoy the gentle rocking of uterine contractions during orgasm, he or she can't see what you're doing, has no idea what is happening, and will certainly have no memory of it. Fetal reactions (slowed movement during intercourse, then furious kicking and squirming and speeded-up heartbeat after orgasm) are responses solely to hormonal and uterine activity.

Fear that the introduction of the penis into the vagina will cause infection. As long as the male does not have a sexually transmittable disease, there is no danger of infection to either mother or fetus through intercourse during the first seven or eight months—in the amniotic sac, the baby is safe from both semen and infectious organisms. Most practitioners believe that this is true even during the ninth month—as long as the sac remains intact (the membranes haven't ruptured). But because they could rupture at any time, some suggest that a condom be worn during intercourse in the last 4 to 8 weeks of pregnancy, as added insurance against infection.

Anxiety over the coming attraction. Both the mother- and father-to-be are subject to mixed feelings over the upcoming blessed event. Thoughts about the responsibilities and lifestyle changes and the financial and emotional cost of bringing up baby can inhibit relaxed lovemaking. This ambivalence, which many expectant parents experience, should be confronted and talked through openly rather than being brought to bed.

The changing relationship. A couple may have trouble adjusting to the idea that they will no longer be just lovers, or husband and wife, but mother and father as well. After all, many of us still avoid associating our own parents with sex, though we are living proof that such an association exists. On the other hand, some couples may discover that the new dimension in their relationship brings a new intimacy to lovemaking—and with it, a new excitement.

Subconscious hostility—of the expectant father toward the expectant mother, because he is jealous that she has become the center of attention; or of mom-to-be toward dad-to-be because she feels she is doing all the suffering (particularly if the pregnancy has been a rough one) for the baby they both want and will both enjoy. Such feelings are important to talk out, but again, not in bed.

Belief that intercourse during the last six weeks of pregnancy will cause labor to begin. It *is* true that the uterine contractions triggered by orgasm become stronger as pregnancy proceeds. But unless the cervix is "ripe," these contractions do not appear to bring on labor—as many hopeful and eager overdue couples can attest. However, since no one knows exactly what mechanism initiates labor, abstinence is often prescribed for women who seem to have a tendency toward preterm delivery. Some practitioners feel that using a condom for such women will decrease the contractions that occur due to the avoidance of the prostaglandins in the semen.

Fear of "hitting" the baby once the head is engaged in the pelvis. Even couples who were relaxed about having intercourse earlier can tighten up toward the end of pregnancy because the baby is too close for comfort. Many practitioners suggest that though deep penetration can't hurt the baby, if it's uncomfortable at this time, it should be avoided.

Psychological factors can also affect sexual relations for the better:

Switching from procreational to recreational sex. Some couples who worked hard at becoming pregnant may be delighted at being able to have sex for its own sake—free of ovulation predictor kits, charts, calendars, and anxiety. For them, sex becomes really enjoyable for the first time in months, or even years.

Though sexual intercourse during pregnancy may be different from what you've experienced before, it is in most cases perfectly safe. In fact, it can be good for you, both physically and emotionally: it can keep you and your spouse close; it can help you get in shape, preparing your pelvic muscles for delivery; and it's relaxing—which is beneficial for everyone concerned, baby included.

WHEN SEXUAL RELATIONS MAY BE LIMITED

Since lovemaking has so much to offer the expectant couple, it would be ideal if every couple could take advantage of it throughout pregnancy. Alas, for some this isn't possible. In high-risk pregnancies, intercourse may be restricted at certain times, or even for nine months. Or, intercourse may be permitted without orgasm for the woman, or foreplay may be allowed as long as penetration is avoided or a condom is used. Knowing precisely *what* is safe and *when* is essential; if your practitioner instructs you to abstain, ask why and whether he or she is referring to intercourse, orgasm, or both, and whether the restrictions are temporary or apply for the entire pregnancy.

Intercourse will probably be restricted under the following circumstances:

♦ Anytime unexplained bleeding occurs

♦ During the first trimester if a woman has a history of miscarriages or threatened miscarriage, or shows signs of a threatened miscarriage

♦ During the last 8 to 12 weeks if a woman has a history of premature or threatened premature labor, or is experiencing signs of early labor

♦ If the amniotic membranes (the bag of waters) have ruptured

♦ When placenta previa is known to exist (the placenta is located near or over the cervix, where it could be prematurely dislodged during intercourse, causing bleeding and threatening mother and baby)

♦ In the last trimester, if twins are being

EXERCISE THAT'S ACTUALLY A PLEASURE

There's no better way to mix business with pleasure than performing Kegels during sex. These exercises tone the perineal area in preparation for childbirth, reducing the likelihood that you'll need an episiotomy, as well as minimizing the risk of a tear. Doing Kegels often will also speed postpartum recovery in the area. And though you can perform Kegels anywhere, anytime (see page 193 for how) doing them during intercourse can increase pleasure for you both. Exercise was never this much fun!

---

carried, or even in the second trimester if more than two fetuses are present

ENJOYING IT MORE, EVEN IF YOU'RE DOING IT LESS

Good, lasting sexual relationships—like good, lasting marriages—are rarely built in a day (or even a really terrific night). They grow with practice, patience, understanding, and love. This is true, too, of an already established sexual relationship that undergoes the emotional and physical assaults of pregnancy. Here are a few ways to "stay on top":

♦ Never allow how frequently or infrequently you have intercourse to interfere with other aspects of your relationship. The quality of lovemaking is always more important than the quantity—and never more so than during pregnancy.

♦ Recognize the possible strains that expectant parenthood may have placed

GETTING COMFORTABLE

When you're making love at this point in your pregnancy (and later on, too), position matters. Side-lying positions (front-to-front or front-to-back) are often most comfortable, because they keep you off your back. Ditto woman on top (which allows you more control over penetra- tion). Rear entry can work well, too. Man on top is fine for quickies (as long as he keeps his weight off of you by supporting himself with his arms), but after the fourth month it's not a good idea to spend too much time flat on your back.

on your relationship, and acknowledge any changes in the intensity of sexual desire that either or both of you may be feeling. Discuss any problems openly; don't sweep them under the bedcovers. If any problems seem too big to handle by yourselves, seek professional help.

◆ Think positive: making love is good physical preparation for labor and delivery—especially if you remember to do your Kegels during intercourse; see box, page 193. (Not many athletes have this much fun in training.)

◆ Think of having to try new positions during pregnancy as an adventure. But give yourselves time to adjust to each position you try. (You might even consider a "dry run"—trying out a new position fully clothed first, so that it'll be more familiar when you try it for real.) See the box above for ideas.

◆ Keep your expectations within reality's reach. Though some women achieve orgasm for the first time during pregnancy, at least one study showed that most women are less likely to achieve orgasm *regularly* during pregnancy than before con- ception—particularly in the last trimester, when only 1 out of 4 women reaches climax consistently. Your goal doesn't always have to be orgasm; sometimes just physical closeness can satisfy.

◆ If the doctor has ruled out sexual intercourse during any period of your pregnancy, ask if orgasm—via mutual masturbation—is okay. If it's taboo for you, you might still get pleasure out of pleasuring your partner in this way.

◆ If the doctor has prohibited orgasm for you but not coitus, you might still be able to make love without your reaching climax. Though this may not be completely satisfying for you, it can provide a sense of intimacy while providing pleasure for your partner. Another possibility: intercourse between the thighs, with no penetration.

Even if the quality, or quantity, of your sexual relations isn't quite what it once was, understanding the dynamics of sexuality during pregnancy can keep the relationship strong—even strengthen it—without spectacular or frequent intercourse.

◆ ◆ ◆

The Sixth Month

Approximately 23 to 27 Weeks

Those little arms and legs are starting to pack quite a punch now,
and as these calisthenics—and
sometimes bouts of hiccups—become
visible from the outside, they may even
entertain those around you. Baby's grown
quite a bit, but is still a relatively light
load compared to what he or she will be
in a couple of months. Assuming all's well
and your practitioner approves, now is a
great time to try some calisthenics—and
other physical activities—yourself.

What You Can Expect at This Month's Checkup

It will probably be business pretty
much as usual at this month's
checkup. As you end your second
trimester, you can expect your practitioner to check the following, though
there may be variations depending upon
your particular needs and on your practitioner's style of practice:[1]

♦ Weight and blood pressure

♦ Urine, for sugar and protein

♦ Fetal heartbeat

♦ Height of fundus (top of uterus)

♦ Size of uterus and position of fetus,
by external palpation (feeling from
the outside)

♦ Feet and hands for edema
(swelling), and legs for varicose
veins

♦ Symptoms you may have been
experiencing, especially unusual
ones

♦ Questions and problems you want
to discuss—have a list ready

1. See Appendix, page 545, for an explanation of
the procedures and tests performed.

A LOOK INSIDE

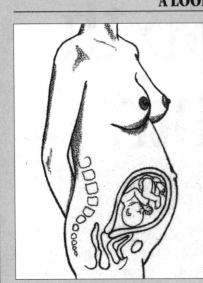

▲ *At the beginning of this month, your uterus is around 1½ inches above your belly button. By the end of the month, your uterus has grown an inch higher and can be felt approximately 2½ inches above your belly button. The uterus is the size of a basketball now— and you might even look like that's what you're carrying around in your belly!*

▶ *Your baby is over a foot long and weighs close to 2 pounds. Still quite ac-tive, the fetus is even more coordinated in its movements (pedaling its feet and pushing them up against the uterine wall, perhaps to practice walking), and has developed a strong grip (which it may use to grasp on to the umbilical cord). Fortunately, the um-bilical cord, which is baby's lifeline, is designed to withstand all of this activ-ity; its tough, spiral composition helps prevent kinks or knots. Baby's eyes can open and close and react to light (a fetus may even use its hands to shield its eyes if a very bright light is shone at its mother's belly). Vocal cords are functioning, although baby won't make a sound until that first after-birth cry. Hiccups, however, are com-mon and may shake baby's uterine home often. A baby born now can sur-vive with intensive care.*

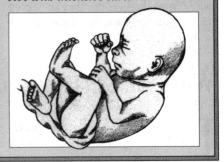

What You May Be Feeling

As always, remember that every pregnancy and every woman is different. You may experience all of these symptoms at one time or an-other, or only a few of them. Some symp-toms may have continued from last month, others may be new. Still others may hardly be noticed because you've become so used to them. You may also have other, less common, symptoms.

PHYSICALLY

◆ More definite fetal activity

◆ Whitish vaginal discharge (leukorrhea)

◆ Achiness in the lower abdomen and along the sides (from stretching of ligaments supporting the uterus)

◆ Constipation

- Heartburn, indigestion, flatulence, bloating
- Occasional headaches, faintness, or dizziness
- Nasal congestion and occasional nosebleeds; ear stuffiness
- "Pink toothbrush" from bleeding gums
- Hearty appetite
- Leg cramps
- Mild swelling of ankles and feet, and occasionally of hands and face
- Varicose veins of the legs and/or hemorrhoids

- Itchy abdomen
- A protruding navel
- Backache
- Skin pigmentation changes on abdomen and/or face
- Enlarged breasts

EMOTIONALLY

- Fewer mood swings
- Continued absentmindedness
- A beginning of boredom with the pregnancy ("Can't anyone think about anything else?")
- Some anxiety about the future

What You May Be Concerned About

PAIN AND NUMBNESS IN THE HANDS

"I keep waking up in the middle of the night because some of the fingers on my right hand are numb; sometimes they even hurt. Is that related to my pregnancy?"

Numbness and tingling in the fingers and toes is normal in pregnancy and is thought to be due to swelling tissues pressing on nerves. Pain, however, is not the norm. If the numbness and pain are confined to your thumb, index finger, middle finger, and half of your ring finger, you probably have carpal tunnel syndrome (CTS). Though this condition is most common in people who regularly perform tasks that require repetitive motions of the hand (such as piano playing or typing), it is also common in pregnant women. That's because the carpal tunnel in the wrist, through which the nerve to the affected fingers runs, becomes

swollen during pregnancy (as do so many other tissues in the body), with the resultant pressure causing numbness, tingling, burning, and pain. The symptoms can also affect the hand and wrist, and can radiate up the arm.

The swelling and accompanying symptoms may be more severe at night. That's because fluids that accumulate in your lower extremities during the day are redistributed to the rest of your body (including your hands) when you're lying down. Sleeping on your hands can make the problem worse, so try elevating them on a separate pillow at bedtime. When numbness occurs, shaking your hands may relieve the problem. If it doesn't, and the numbness (with or without pain) is interfering with your sleep, discuss the problem with your practitioner. Often wearing a wrist splint is helpful. So is avoiding tobacco (which should be avoided anyway) and caffeine. Some people have found that acupuncture brings relief. If you think the problem is related to your work habits as well as your pregnancy, then you should be sure to do the following: take frequent breaks while working with your hands; stop when you feel pain; lift objects with your whole hand; and type with a soft touch, making sure your wrists are straight and that your hands are lower than your elbows.

The nonsteroidal anti-inflammatory drugs and steroids usually prescribed for carpal tunnel syndrome may not be recommended during pregnancy. Check with your practitioner. The pain from pregnancy-related carpal tunnel syndrome usually goes away two to three weeks postpartum.

PINS AND NEEDLES

"I frequently get a tingling sensation in my hands and feet. Does this indicate a problem with my circulation?"

As if it weren't enough to be on tenterhooks during pregnancy, some women occasionally experience the disconcerting tingling sensation of pins and needles in their extremities. Although it may feel as if your circulation is being cut off, this isn't the case. The tingling, believed to be caused by fluid accumulation pressing on nerve endings, is nothing to worry about. Changing your position may help. If the tingling interferes in any way with your functioning, report it to your practitioner.

CLUMSINESS

"Lately I've been dropping everything I pick up. Why am I suddenly so clumsy?"

Like the extra inches on your belly, the extra thumbs on your hands are part and parcel of being pregnant. As with so many pregnancy side effects, this temporary clumsiness is caused by the loosening of joints and the retention of water, both of which can make your grasp on objects less firm and sure. Other factors may include a lack of concentration as a result of the scatterbrain syndrome (see page 180) or a lack of dexterity as a result of carpal tunnel syndrome (see page 241).

Besides making a conscious effort to pick up things more carefully, there isn't much you can do about pregnancy "dropsies"—so it might be a good idea to let someone else handle the crystal for the next few months.

BABY KICKING

"Some days the baby is kicking all the time; other days he seems very quiet. Is this normal?"

Fetuses are only human. Just like us, they have "up" days, when they feel like kicking up their heels (and elbows and knees), and "down" days, when they'd rather lie back and take it easy. Most often, their activity is related to what you've been doing. Like babies out of the womb, fetuses are lulled by rocking. So when you're on the go all day, your baby is likely to be pacified by the rhythm of your routine, and you're likely not to notice much kicking—partly because baby's slowed down, partly because you're so busy. As soon as you slow down or relax, he or she is bound to start acting up (a pattern babies, unfortunately, tend to continue even after they're born). That's why most expectant mothers feel fetal movement more often in bed at night or when they're resting during the day. Activity may also increase after you've had a meal or snack, perhaps in reaction to the surge of glucose (sugar) in your blood. You may also notice increased fetal activity when you're excited or nervous (about to give a presentation, for example), possibly because the baby is stimulated by your adrenaline response.

Babies are actually most active

between weeks 24 and 28, when they're small enough to move around their uterine home. But their movements are erratic and usually brief, so they aren't always felt by the busy mother-to-be, even though they are visible on ultrasound. Fetal activity usually becomes more organized and consistent, with more clearly defined periods of rest and activity, between 28 and 32 weeks.

Don't be tempted to compare baby movement notes with other pregnant women. Each fetus, like each newborn, has an individual pattern of activity and development. Some seem always active; others mostly quiet. The activity of some fetuses is so regular their moms could set their watches by it; in others there's no discernible activity pattern at all. As long as there is no radical slowdown or cessation of activity, all variations are normal.

Research suggests that from the 28th week on it may be a good idea for mothers to test for fetal movements twice a day—once in the morning, when activity tends to be sparser, and once in the more active evening hours. Your practitioner may recommend a test or you can use this one: check the clock and start counting. Count movements of any kind (kicks, flutters, swishes, rolls). Stop counting when you reach ten, and note the time. Often, you will feel ten movements within ten minutes or so. Sometimes it will take longer.

If you haven't counted ten movements by the end of an hour, have some milk or a snack; then lie down, relax, and continue counting. If two hours go by without ten movements, call your practitioner without delay. Though such an absence of activity doesn't necessarily mean there's a problem, it can occasionally indicate fetal distress. In such cases, quick action may be needed.

The closer you are to your due date, the more important regular checking of fetal movements becomes.

"Sometimes the baby pushes so hard it hurts."

As your baby matures in the uterus, he or she becomes stronger and stronger, and those once butterflylike fetal movements pack more and more punch. Don't be surprised if you get kicked in the ribs or poked in the abdomen or cervix with such force it hurts. When you seem to be under a particularly fierce attack, try changing your position. It may knock your little linebacker off balance and temporarily stem the assault.

"The baby seems to be kicking all over. Could I be carrying twins?"

At some point in her pregnancy, just about every woman begins to think that she's carrying either twins or a human octopus. For most, of course, neither is true. Until a fetus grows to the point that its movements are restricted by the confines of its uterine home (usually at about 34 weeks), it's able to perform numerous acrobatics. So, while it may sometimes feel as if you're being pummeled by a dozen fists, it's more likely to be two fists that really get around—along with tiny knees, elbows, and feet.

For information on twins and how they are diagnosed, see page 164.

LEG CRAMPS

"I have leg cramps at night that interfere with my sleep."

Between your racing mind and your bulging belly, you probably have enough trouble sleeping without having to suffer from leg cramps. Unfortunately, these painful spasms, which occur most often at night, are very common among pregnant women in the second and third trimesters. Fortunately, there are ways of both preventing and alleviating them.

A STRETCHING EXERCISE TO WARD OFF LEG CRAMPS

Stand facing a wall, about two feet away from it. Lean forward and press your hands against the wall while keeping your heels on the floor. If you feel the stretching in your calves, you are doing it right. Hold for ten seconds, relax for five seconds, and repeat two or three times.

Because fatigue and fluid accumulation in the legs are thought to be possible contributing factors, wearing support hose during the day and alternating periods of rest (with your feet up) with periods of physical activity may be helpful in eliminating or reducing the frequency of leg cramps. And be sure to get adequate fluids (at least eight glasses a day).

If you do get a cramp in your calf, straighten your leg and flex your ankle and toes slowly up toward your nose. This should soon lessen the pain. (Doing this several times with each leg before retiring at night may even help ward off the cramps.) Standing on a cold surface sometimes works, too. If either technique reduces the pain, massage or local heat can then be used for added relief. If neither reduces it, don't massage your calves or apply heat. Do contact your practitioner if the pain continues, as there is a slight possibility that a blood clot may have developed in a vein, making medical treatment necessary (see Venous Thrombosis, page 510).

RECTAL BLEEDING AND HEMORRHOIDS

"I'm concerned about the rectal bleeding I've been having."

Bleeding is always a frightening symptom, especially during pregnancy—and particularly in an area so close to your birth canal. But unlike vaginal bleeding, rectal bleeding is not a sign of a possible threat to your pregnancy. During pregnancy, it's frequently caused by external or, less often, internal hemorrhoids and/or anal fissures (cracks in the anus). Hemorrhoids, which are varicose veins of the rectum, afflict between 20 and 50 percent of all pregnant women. Just as the veins of the legs are more susceptible to varicosities at this time, so are the veins of the rectum. Hemorrhoids (also called piles because of the resemblance these swollen veins sometimes bear to a pile of grapes or marbles) can cause itching and pain as well as bleeding. Anal fissures are also fairly common in pregnancy. They can accompany hemorrhoids or appear independently and are generally extremely painful. Constipation often causes or compounds both problems.

Don't try to self-diagnose rectal bleeding; it should always be evaluated by a physician. But if it does turn out that you do have hemorrhoids and/or fissures, you'll have an important role in treating them. Good self-care can often eliminate the need for more invasive medical therapy.

Avoid constipation. It is *not* a necessary component of pregnancy. Preventing constipation from the start is frequently an excellent way to prevent hemorrhoids and fissures completely (see page 156).

Take pressure off. Sleep on your side, not your back; avoid long hours of standing or sitting; don't strain when having a bowel movement or linger on the toilet (keep reading material out of the bathroom so you aren't tempted to just sit and read). Sitting with your feet on a step stool may make evacuation easier.

Lie down several times a day—if possible, on your left side—to take the pressure off your rectal veins for a while. Watch TV, read, and do paperwork in this position, if possible, when you can.

Do Kegel exercises regularly. These simple exercises improve circulation to the area (see page 193).

Soothe the area. To reduce discomfort, take warm sitz baths twice a day (see page 549). You can also apply witch hazel pads or ice packs to the site. Try both the hot and cold approach and use whichever you find more soothing, or alternate.

Don't use medications without medical advice. Use topical medications, suppositories, laxatives, or stool softeners only if prescribed by a doctor who knows you're pregnant. Do not take mineral oil, which can carry important nutrients out of your body.

Keep scrupulously clean. Wash the perineal area (from vagina to rectum) with warm water after bowel movements, always wiping from front to back. Use only white toilet paper (a cushiony two-ply is more soothing), and avoid aggressive wiping.

With good care, you can keep hemorrhoids from becoming chronic. They may be aggravated by delivery, especially if the pushing phase is long, but usually disappear postpartum if preventive measures are continued.

ITCHY ABDOMEN

"My belly itches constantly. It's driving me crazy."

Join the club. Pregnant bellies are itchy bellies, and they can become progressively itchier as the months pass and the skin is stretched taut across the abdomen. The result is dryness, causing very pronounced itching in some women. Try not to scratch, which will only make you itchier and could cause irritation. Lubricating lotion may ease the itch, but probably won't cure it. An anti-itching lotion (such as calamine or Aveeno) may provide more relief. If you itch *all over,* however, check with your practitioner.

PROTRUDING NAVEL

"My belly button used to be a perfect 'innie.' Now it's sticking all the way out. Will it stay that way even after I deliver?"

Protruding navels may not be preferred by the bikini set, but they're a sure thing when you're expecting. As the swelling uterus pushes forward, even the deepest "innie" is sure to pop like a timer on a turkey (except, on most women, the navel "pops" well before baby's "ready," often by the sixth month). Postpartum, your navel is likely to revert back in—though after all that stretching, it probably will be wider and a little less taut than it was before pregnancy. If this is your second pregnancy, your belly button may pop out sooner than it did in your first pregnancy.

COMPLEMENTARY AND ALTERNATIVE MEDICINE (CAM)

The days when alternative medicine was about as welcome in traditional medical practice as old wives' tales (and regarded with about as much credibility) are over. Today, these seemingly disparate branches of healing are no longer considered incompatible; in fact, more and more practitioners in both consider them complementary. Which is why Complementary and Alternative Medicine (CAM) is more and more likely to find a place—in some form—in your life and the life of your family.

The practitioners who practice complementary medicine take a broad view of health and well-being, examining and integrating the nutritional, emotional, and spiritual influences, as well as the physical ones. CAM also emphasizes the body's ability to heal itself—with a little help from some natural friends, including herbs, physical manipulation, the spirit, and the mind.

Since pregnancy is not an illness, but rather a "normal" part of life, it would seem that CAM might make a natural addition to traditional obstetrical care. And for an increasing number of women and their health care providers, it has. A variety of CAM practices are currently being used in pregnancy, labor, and delivery, with varying degrees of success, including the following:

◆ Acupuncture and acupressure, which can be used to relieve a number of pregnancy symptoms, including morning sickness and back pain, and which may provide pain relief in labor; also, electropuncture, which employs electrostimulation using acupuncture needles, and may help induce labor at term.

◆ Biofeedback, a method that helps patients learn how to control their biological responses to physical pain or emotional stress, and can be used safely to relieve a variety of pregnancy symptoms, including headache and other pains, insomnia, and possibly morning sickness. Biofeedback can also be used to lower blood pressure and combat depression, anxiety, and stress.

◆ Chiropractic medicine, which uses physical manipulation to help pregnant women battle back pain and sciatica.

◆ Massage, in the right hands (see page 214), can help relieve some of pregnancy's discomforts, including heartburn, headaches, backache, and sciatica, while preparing muscles for childbirth. It can also be used during labor and delivery to relax muscles between contractions and reduce the pain of back labor.

◆ Reflexology, a therapy in which pressure is applied to specific areas of the feet, hands, and ears to relieve a variety of aches and pains, has also been used to stimulate labor and reduce the pain of contractions. Since applying pressure to certain areas on or near the feet and on the hands can trigger contractions, it's very important that the reflexologist you visit be well trained and aware of your pregnancy, and that he or she avoids these areas before term.

◆ Hydrotherapy, or the therapeutic use of warm water (usually in a Jacuzzi tub), is used in many hospitals and birthing centers to help relax a laboring woman and reduce her discomfort. (Jets should be directed away from the vagina, however, to avoid forcing water inside.) Some women choose to give birth under water; see page 15.

◆ Aromatherapy, in which scented oils are used to heal body, mind, and spirit, is utilized by some practitioners during pregnancy; however, most experts advise caution, since some aromas (in this concentrated form) may be hazardous to pregnant women. (See page 213 for more.)

◆ Meditation, visualization, and relaxation techniques, all of which can help a woman safely through a variety of physical and emotional stresses during pregnancy, from the miseries of morning sickness to the pain of labor and delivery.

◆ Hypnosis, which can be useful in turning a breech birth (in conjunction with the more traditional external cephalic maneuver); in holding off premature labor; and in providing pain management during labor and delivery.

◆ Moxibustion, which combines acupuncture with heat (in the form of smoldering mugwort, an herb) to help turn a breech baby.

◆ Herbal remedies, which are "botanicals" that have been used since humankind first began looking for relief for ailments, and are today used by some practitioners to relieve pregnancy symptoms. Most experts, however, do not recommend herbal remedies for pregnant women, since adequate studies on safety have not yet been done. (See below.)

Clearly, CAM is making an impact in obstetrics. Even the most traditional ob-gyns are realizing that it's a force to be reckoned with, and one to begin incorporating into ob-business as usual. But in making CAM a part of your pregnancy, it's wise to proceed with prudence and with these caveats in mind:

◆ Complementary medications and herbal preparations are *not tested or approved* by the FDA. Because they haven't been thoroughly tested—as FDA-approved drugs are—their safety hasn't been clinically established. Which is not to say that there aren't complementary medications or herbal preparations that are safe to use in preg-

nancy, just that there is no official system in place to determine those that are and those that aren't. Until more is known, it makes sense to avoid taking any homeopathic or herbal medication or dietary supplement or aromatherapy treatment unless it has been specifically prescribed by a traditional practitioner who is knowledgeable in complementary medicines and who knows that you're pregnant. (This is also true once the baby is born, if you are breastfeeding.)

◆ Complementary procedures that are usually benign—or even beneficial—may not be safe during pregnancy. From therapeutic massage to chiropractic maneuvers, there are special precautions that must be observed when a patient is pregnant.

◆ Complementary and alternative medicine can still be strong medicine. Depending on how it's used, this potency can be therapeutic, or it can be hazardous. Keep in mind that "natural" is not synonymous with "safe" any more than "chemical" is synonymous with "danger." Have your practitioner help you navigate through the potential pitfalls and steer you toward CAM practices that can help—not hurt—when you're expecting.

For more information, contact: *Acupressure:* American Oriental Bodywork Therapy Association, (856) 782-1616, www. healthy.net/aobta; *Acupuncture:* National Acupuncture and Oriental Medicine Alliance, (253) 851-6896, www. acuall.org; *Biofeedback:* Association for Applied Psychophysiology and Biofeedback, (303) 422-8436, www.aapb.org; *Hypnotherapy:* American Board of Hypnotherapy, (800) 872-9996, www.hypnosis.com/abh/abh. html; *Reflexology*: Reflexology Association of America, (702) 871-9522, www. reflexology-usa.org.

Clogged Milk Duct

"I'm worried about a small, tender lump on the side of my breast. What could it be?"

Though you're still months away from nursing your baby, it sounds like your breasts are already gearing up. The result: a clogged milk duct. These red, tender-to-the-touch, hard lumps in the breast are very common even this early in pregnancy, and especially in second and subsequent pregnancies. Warm compresses (or letting warm water run on it in the shower) and gentle massage will probably clear the duct up in a few days, just as it will during lactation. Some experts suggest that avoiding underwire bras also helps— though do make sure you get ample support from the bra you do wear.

Keep in mind that monthly self-exams of your breasts shouldn't stop when you're pregnant. Though checking for lumps is trickier when you're expecting because of the changes your breasts are going through, it's still important to try. If you're uncertain about any lump, show it to your practitioner at your next visit.

Preeclampsia, or Toxemia

"Recently a friend of mine was hospitalized for toxemia. How can you tell if you have it?"

Fortunately toxemia, more commonly known as preeclampsia/eclampsia or pregnancy-induced hypertension (PIH), is uncommon. Even in its mildest form, it occurs in only 5 to 10 percent of pregnancies—and half of these cases are among women who came into pregnancy with chronic high blood pressure. Preeclampsia is more likely to occur in first pregnancies and beyond the 20th week of gestation. There may also be a genetic component; if your mother had

preeclampsia when she was pregnant with you, or your spouse's mother had preeclampsia when she was pregnant with him, you're slightly more likely to develop the condition. Diet may also play a role. Research has shown that women with preeclampsia are often found to be deficient in vitamins E and C (another reason to eat well when you're expecting). Finally, untreated gum disease can also play a role in preeclampsia.

In women who are receiving regular prenatal care, preeclampsia is diagnosed and treated early, preventing needless complications. Though routine office visits sometimes seem a waste of time in a healthy pregnancy, the earliest signs of preeclampsia can be picked up at such visits. In fact, researchers are hoping to develop a urine test (looking for low levels of a certain protein) that would predict who is at risk for preeclampsia.

Early symptoms of preeclampsia include sudden weight gain apparently unrelated to excess food intake, severe swelling of the hands and face, unexplained headaches, esophageal or stomach pain, or itching, and/or vision disturbances. If you experience any of these, call your practitioner. Otherwise, assuming you are getting regular medical care, there's no reason to worry about preeclampsia. See pages 186, 476, and 500 for more information on and tips for dealing with high blood pressure and preeclampsia.

Staying on the Job

"I was planning to work up until I deliver, but is that safe?"

Many women successfully mix business with baby-making right through the ninth month, without compromising the well-being of either occupation.

Still, some jobs are obviously safer and better suited to pregnant women than other jobs. And chances are the decision of whether or not you'll continue to work until delivery will have at least something to do with the kind of work you're involved in. If you have a desk job, you can probably plan to go straight from the office to the birthing room without any threat to you or your baby. A sedentary job that isn't particularly stressful may actually be less of a strain on you both than staying at home with a vacuum cleaner and mop, trying to tidy up the nest for your new arrival. And doing a small amount of walking—up to an hour or two daily, on the job or off—is not only harmless but may be beneficial (assuming you aren't carrying heavy loads as you go). Jobs that are strenuous, very stressful, and/or involve a great deal of standing, however, may be another matter—and are a matter of some controversy.

One study of pregnant doctors in arduous residency training programs found that although these women were on their feet sixty-five hours a week, they didn't seem to have any more pregnancy complications than women who worked many fewer and usually less stressful hours. Other studies, however, suggest that steady strenuous or stressful activity or long hours of standing after the 28th week—particularly if the expectant mother also has other children to care for at home—may increase the risk of certain complications, including premature labor, high blood pressure in the mother, and low birthweight in the baby.

Should women who stand on the job—salespeople, chefs, police officers, waitresses, doctors, nurses, and so on—work past the 28th week? Clearly, more study will need to be done before definitive answers to that question will be available. The American Medical Association recommends that women who work at jobs requiring more than four hours in a row a day on their feet should take a leave of absence (or switch to a desk job) by the 24th week, and that those who must stand for thirty minutes out of each hour should take a leave by the 32nd. But many practitioners feel this recommendation is too strict and impractical, and they permit women whose pregnancies are progressing normally and who feel fine to work longer. Standing on the job all the way to term, however, may not be a good idea, less because of the theoretical risk to the fetus than the real risk that such pregnancy discomforts as backache, varicose veins, and hemorrhoids will be aggravated.

It's probably a good idea to take early leave from a job that requires frequent shift changes (which can upset appetite and sleep routines, and worsen fatigue); one that seems to exacerbate any pregnancy problems, such as headache, backache, or fatigue; or one that increases the risk of falls or other accidental injuries. Some experts also recommend that a woman not stay past the 20th week at a job that requires pulling, pushing, climbing (stairs, poles, or ladders), or bending below the waist, if this kind of work is intensive; if it is moderate, then not past the 28th week. Lifting items that weigh 25 pounds or less, even repetitively, is usually not a problem, nor is lifting weights of up to 50 pounds intermittently (which should be reassuring to pregnant mothers of babies and preschoolers). But women in jobs requiring repetitive lifting of 50 pounds or more should probably take their leave by the 20th week and those who must repetitively lift 25 to 50 pounds by the 34th week. Those in jobs requiring only intermittent lifting of weights over 50 pounds should stop working by the 30th week.

Confused? Not sure which guidelines apply to you? Ask your practitioner for some help making the decision that's right for your situation. Keep in mind, too, that no matter how long you keep working, there are ways of reducing physical on-the-job stress during pregnancy. See page 112.

THE PAIN OF CHILDBIRTH

"I'm eager to become a mother, but not so eager to experience childbirth. Mostly, I worry about the pain."

Though almost every expectant mother eagerly awaits the birth of her child, fewer look forward to labor and delivery. Especially for those who've never experienced significant discomfort, the fear of this unknown is very real—and very normal.

There's no point in dreading the pain, but there's a lot to be said for being prepared for it. A woman who anticipates that labor will be incomparably exhilarating and instead ends up struggling through twenty-four hours of excruciating back labor may be suffering as much from disappointment as from pain. And because the pain is unexpected, she may have more trouble dealing with it.

In general, both women who fear pain the most and those who expect it the least have a harder time during labor and delivery than women who are realistic in their expectations and are prepared for any eventuality. If you prepare both your mind and your body, you should be able to reduce any anxiety you might be experiencing now, and at the same time help make your actual labor more comfortable.

Get educated. One reason earlier generations of women found labor so frightening was that they didn't understand what was happening to their bodies or why. Today, a good childbirth education class (see page 253) can reduce fear by increasing knowledge, preparing women and their coaches, stage by stage and phase by phase, for labor and delivery. If you can't take a class, read as much on the subject of labor and delivery as you can (try to touch on all the major schools of thought). What you don't know can hurt you more than it should.

Get moving. You wouldn't think of running a marathon without the proper physical training. Neither should you consider going into labor (which is a no less challenging feat) untrained. Work out faithfully with all the breathing and toning-up exercises your practitioner and/or childbirth educator recommends.

Put pain in perspective. There are at least two good things to be said about the pain of childbirth, no matter how intense. First, it has a definite time limit. Though it may be difficult to believe at the time, you will not be in labor forever. Average labor with a first child is between twelve and fourteen hours—and, for most women, only a few of those hours are likely to be *very* uncomfortable. (Though labor can sometimes run much longer, most doctors will not allow active labor to continue much beyond twenty-four hours, and will perform a cesarean at that point if adequate progress has not been made.) Second, unlike many other kinds of pain, it's a pain with a very definite *positive* purpose: contractions progressively thin and open your cervix, each contraction bringing you closer to the birth of your baby.

Don't feel guilty, however, if you lose sight of that purpose during very hard labor and care very little about anything but getting the whole thing over with. Most women feel that way at some point, and tolerance for pain *does not* reflect the depth of maternal love.

Don't plan on going it alone. Even if you don't feel very chatty—or even friendly—during labor, it will be comforting to know that your spouse (or a close friend or relative) is there to mop your brow, to feed you ice chips, to massage your back or neck, to coach you through contractions, or just be there for you to curse at. Your coach should attend childbirth classes with you. If that's not possible, he or she should at least read the section on labor and delivery beginning on page 337 and on the coach's role, starting on page 362, so that he or she will know what to expect.

With or without a coach, many women find that the support of a doula (see page 296) brings additional advantages.

Be ready to accept pain relief if it's needed. Asking for or accepting medication is not a sign of failure or of weakness. ("Mother" is not synonymous with "martyr.") In fact, sometimes pain relief is absolutely necessary to keep a laboring woman at her most effective. See page 276 for more on pain relief during labor and delivery.

And, hard as it is to believe as you try to breathe your way through those difficult contractions, it is true that most women put the pain of childbirth behind them pretty soon after the final push. (Or, at least, after they've shared their labor story two or three hundred times with friends and relatives.) Otherwise, there would be a lot of only-children out there.

LABOR AND DELIVERY

"I'm getting very anxious about labor and delivery. What if I forget everything I learn in childbirth education class?"

The advent of childbirth education probably did as much as any medical advancement in the past decades to improve the experience of women in labor. However, by creating a mystique of the perfect labor and delivery, it sometimes left parents-to-be feeling pressured to achieve that ideal. Couples prepared themselves for childbirth as if for a final exam. It's not surprising that many worried about failing, and thereby letting down not only themselves and each other but also their babies, their doctors or midwives, and especially their childbirth educators.

But fortunately most childbirth educators now present a more balanced and less dogmatic curriculum, one that acknowledges that there isn't just one way to experience childbirth. Most no longer portray labor and delivery as a test that a mother passes (she does her breathing exercises, has a vaginal delivery, and takes no medication) or fails (she is too panicked to remember her breathing exercises, accepts pain relief, and/or ends up with a cesarean). That's something you need to keep in mind, too. Even forgetting (because of pain and excitement) everything you're "supposed" to do won't change the outcome of the delivery or make you a failure.

Learn everything you can in your classes and from your reading, but don't lose sight of the fact that childbirth is a natural process, one that most women managed to stumble through successfully (if uncomfortably) for thousands of years before Mrs. Lamaze gave birth to her son, the doctor. And also remember that *natural* doesn't automatically mean "ideal" or "safe." In the days before modern medical technology, childbirth was a risky experience, one many mothers and many children did not survive. So take the "natural" route when you can, but be ready to accept help in the form of medical intervention when you need it, without feelings of guilt or failure. Remember, the most important goal of labor and delivery, and the only one that truly matters in the long run, is a healthy baby and a healthy mother.

"I'm afraid I'll do something embarrassing during labor."

The prospect of screaming, cursing loudly, or involuntarily emptying your bladder or bowel might seem embarrassing now. During labor, however, avoiding humiliation will be the farthest thing from your mind. Besides, nothing you can do or say during labor will shock or disgust your birth attendants, who've seen and heard it all before—and then some. So check your inhibitions when you check into the hospital or birthing center and feel free to do what comes naturally as well as what makes you most comfortable. If you are ordinarily a vocal, emotive person, don't try to hold in your moans or hold back your grunts and groans—or even your screams. On the other hand, if you're normally very soft-spoken or stoic and would prefer to whimper quietly into your pillow, don't feel obligated to outyell the woman in the next room.

"I have pretty definite ideas of what I'd like to happen during labor and delivery. I don't like the idea of losing control of the situation."

If you're a take-charge kind of person, the thought of handing control of your labor and delivery over to the medical staff can be a little unnerving. Of course you want them to take the best possible care of you and your baby. But you'd still like to maintain a modicum of control. And chances are you'll be able to, especially if you prepare thoroughly for labor and delivery by working hard now at your childbirth preparation exercises, becoming familiar with the birth process, and by developing a comfortable and productive rapport with your practitioner, if you haven't already. Setting up a birthing plan (see page 274), specifying what you would like to happen and not happen during a normal labor and delivery, also increases your control.

But with that said and done, it's important to understand that you won't necessarily be able to call *all* the shots during labor, no matter how well prepared you are and no matter what type of practitioner you are laboring with. The best-laid plans of obstetrical patients and their practitioners can give way to a variety of unforeseeable circumstances, and it makes sense to prepare for that possibility, too. For instance, you'd done your perineal massage faithfully (see page 330) in hopes of delivering without an episiotomy, but after three hours of pushing, your perineum refuses to budge. Or you'd planned to go through labor completely unmedicated, but an extremely long and trying active phase has sapped you of your strength. Learning when it's necessary to relinquish the reins—and be flexible—is in the best interest of you and your baby and is an important part of your childbirth education.

HOSPITAL TOURS

"I've always associated hospitals with sickness, and I'm pretty much terrified of them. How can I get more comfortable with the idea of giving birth in one?"

The labor and delivery floor is by far the happiest in the hospital. Still, if you don't know what to expect, you can arrive filled with trepidation. That's why the vast majority of hospitals and birthing centers encourage advance tours of maternity facilities by expectant couples. Inquire about such tours when you preregister. Some hospitals and birthing centers also have videotapes of the labor and delivery areas that you can borrow, and many have Web sites that offer virtual tours. You can also stop in for an informal peek during visiting hours; even if the actual labor and delivery area is off-limits then, you'll be able to view postpartum rooms and take a good look at the nursery. Besides making you feel more comfortable about the surroundings you'll be giving birth in, this will give you the opportunity to check out what newborns look like before you hold your own in your arms.

Chances are you'll be happily surprised by what you see when you pay your visit. Facilities vary from hospital to hospital and from birthing center to birthing center, but as competition for obstetrical patients increases, the range of amenities and services offered in many areas has become more and more impressive. Birthing rooms are becoming the rule, rather than the exception, in more and more hospitals (they've always been common at birthing centers staffed by midwives). See page 12 for more.

CLASSES FOR SECOND TIMERS

"This is my second pregnancy. Do I really need to take a childbirth education class again?"

Even seasoned pros stand to benefit from taking a childbirth education class. First of all, every labor and delivery is different, so what you experienced last time may not be what you can expect this time. Second, things change quickly in the delivery business, and they may have changed quite a bit, even if it's only been a couple of years since you were on a birthing bed. There

---

WHEN SOMETHING JUST DOESN'T FEEL RIGHT

Maybe it's a twinge of abdominal pain that feels too much like a cramp to ignore, a sudden change in your vaginal discharge, an aching in your lower back or in your pelvic floor—or maybe it's something so vague you can't even put your finger on it. Chances are nothing's wrong, but to play it safe, check pages 130 and 273 to see if a call to your practitioner is in order. If you can't find your symptoms on the list, it's probably a good idea to call anyway. Reporting odd symptoms could help identify early signs of premature labor or of other pregnancy complications, which could make a big difference in the outcome of your pregnancy. Remember, you know your body better than anyone.

---

may be different childbirth options available than there were last time; certain procedures that were routine may now be uncommon, certain procedures that were uncommon may now be routine. Taking another course may be especially important if you'll be using a different hospital or birthing center.

Chances are, however, that you won't have to sit in with the rookies. "Refresher" courses are available in most areas.

What It's Important to Know: CHILDBIRTH EDUCATION

In the middle of the last century, being prepared for childbirth meant that the baby's room was painted, the layette was ordered, and a suitcase packed with pretty nightgowns for the hospital stay was waiting at the door. It was the arrival of the child, not the childbirth experience, that was anticipated, planned for, and looked forward to. Women knew little of what to expect from labor and delivery; men knew even less. And since Mother was likely to be unconscious during the birth and Father was likely to be anxiously thumbing through magazines in the waiting room, their ignorance was of little consequence.

Now that general anesthesia is reserved mainly for emergency cesareans, waiting rooms are for nervous grandparents, and Mom and Dad can go through childbirth together, ignorance is neither wise nor acceptable. Preparing for childbirth has come to mean preparing for the labor and delivery experience as much as for the new baby. Expectant couples devour stacks of books and magazines, scour the Internet, and watch videos. They participate fully in their prenatal visits, seeking answers to all their questions, reassurance for all their worries. And, more often than not, they attend childbirth education classes.

Just what are these classes about, and why have they proliferated faster than six-month stretch marks? The original, pioneering classes were intended to explain a new approach to childbirth—without medication and without fear—and were commonly known as "natural childbirth" classes. Since then, there has been a shift in emphasis in many classes from natural childbirth (though it's still considered the ideal by many) to education and preparation for many of the possible eventualities of labor and delivery, so that whether the birth turns out to be medicated or unmedicated, vaginal or surgical, with an episiotomy or without one, parents will have an understanding of what is happening and will be able to participate as fully and as knowledgeably as possible.

The goals of most childbirth education classes today are:

♦ To impart accurate and balanced information about normal labor and delivery as well as about possible complications, common hospital procedures, and medical interventions, including various methods of pain relief. The goal: to reduce fears, improve ability to cope with pain, enhance decision-making skills, and thoroughly prepare the expectant couple for most labor and delivery scenarios.

♦ To teach specially designed techniques of relaxation, distraction, muscle control, and breathing—all of which can increase a couple's sense of being in control while contributing to the woman's endurance and a reduction in her perception of pain. These techniques will vary, depending on the type of class taken.

♦ To develop a productive working relationship between the mother and her coach, which, if maintained during labor and delivery, helps to provide a supportive environment that can, in turn, help the mother to minimize her anxieties and maximize her efforts during labor, as well as allow the coach to become an integral part of the experience.

BENEFITS OF TAKING A CHILDBIRTH CLASS

Just how much you as a couple will benefit from childbirth education depends on the course you take, on the instructor who teaches it, and on your own attitudes. In general, these classes work better for some than for others. Some couples thrive in group situations and find sharing feelings natural and helpful; others are uncomfortable in groups and find sharing difficult and uncomfortable. Many enjoy learning and practicing the relaxation and breathing techniques, while others feel that the repetition of such exercises is forced and intrusive, tension producing rather than tension alleviating. While many ultimately find these exercises effective in the control of pain during labor, an occasional couple may end up not using them at all. Just about every couple, however, stands to gain something from taking a *good* childbirth class—and certainly no couple has anything to lose by taking one. Some benefits include:

♦ The opportunity to spend time with other expectant couples: to share pregnancy experiences, compare progress, and swap tales of woes, worries, aches, and pains. It's also a chance to make friends with people-with-babies, for later enjoyment and sharing. Many classes hold "reunions" once everyone has delivered.

♦ Increased involvement of the father-to-be in the pregnancy, which is particularly important if he isn't able to attend prenatal visits. Classes will familiarize him with the process of labor and delivery so that he can be a more effective coach, and will allow him to meet other expectant fathers. Some courses include a special session for fathers only, which gives them the chance to express and find relief for the anxieties they may be reluctant to burden their partners with.

♦ A weekly chance to ask questions that come up between prenatal visits, or that you don't feel comfortable asking your practitioner.

♦ An opportunity to get hands-on instruction in breathing, relaxation, coaching techniques, and, sometimes, alternative approaches to pain relief and to get feedback from an expert as you learn. Mastering these coping strategies may help to decrease your perception of pain and, ideally, increase your ability to handle it during labor and delivery—which may translate into less need for medication.

♦ An opportunity to develop confidence in your ability to meet the strenuous demands of labor and delivery, through increased knowledge (which helps banish fear of the unknown). This sense of empowerment may enable you to feel more in control.

♦ The possibility of an improved, less stressful labor, thanks to all of the above. Couples who've had childbirth preparation generally rate their childbirth experiences as more satisfying overall than those who haven't.

♦ Possibly, a slightly shorter labor. Studies show that the average labor of women who have had childbirth education is somewhat shorter than that of women who haven't, probably because the training and preparation better enable them to work with, instead of against, contractions. (There is no guarantee of a short labor, only the possibility of a *shorter* one.)

CHOOSING A CHILDBIRTH CLASS

In some communities, where childbirth class options are limited, the choice is a relatively simple one. In others, the variety of offerings can be overwhelming and confusing. There are courses run by hospitals, by private instructors, by practitioners through their offices. There are "early bird" prenatal classes, taken in the first or second trimester, which cover such pregnancy topics as nutrition, exercise, fetal development, and sexuality; and there are down-to-the-wire six- to ten-week childbirth preparation classes, usually begun in the seventh or eighth month, which concentrate on labor, delivery, and post-partum mother and baby care.

If the pickings are slim, any childbirth class is probably better than none at all. If there is a selection of courses where you live, it may help to consider the following when making your decision:

Who sponsors the class? A class that is run by, is under the auspices of, or is recommended by your practitioner often works out best. Also useful could be a class provided by the hospital at which you'll be delivering. If the laboring and delivering philosophy of your childbirth education teacher varies greatly from that of the person or staff who will be assisting you during labor and delivery, you're bound to run into contradictions and conflicts. If differences of opinion do arise, make sure you address them with your practitioner well before your delivery date.

What's the size of the class? Small is best. Five or six couples to a class is ideal; more than ten or twelve may be too large. Not only can a teacher give more time and individual attention to couples in an intimate group—particularly important during the breathing and relaxation technique practice sessions—but the camaraderie in a small group tends to be stronger.

What is the curriculum like? Ask for a course outline and, if you can, sit in on a class. A good course will include a discussion of cesarean section (recognizing that 15 to 25 percent of students may end up having one) and of medication (recognizing, too, that some will need or want this). It will deal with the psychological and emotional as well as the technical aspects of childbirth.

What is the instructor's teaching style? Is it open-minded and flexible, or narrow-minded and dogmatic? Are the expectations set up for students realistic or unattainable? (If you're assured that taking the class will make labor short or free of interventions, for instance, beware.) Often there's no way to know for sure exactly what a teacher's philosophy of childbirth is until you take the class, but sitting in on one or talking to her before signing up can give you some idea of what you can expect.

What is the rate of drug-free labors among class "graduates"? This may be helpful information, but it can also be misleading. Does a low rate indicate that students were so well prepared in the various natural pain-reducing strategies that they rarely needed medication? Or were they so convinced that asking for medication was a sign of failure that they stoically withstood severe pain? Perhaps the best way to find the answer is to talk to some of the graduates.

How is the class taught? Are films of actual childbirths shown? Will you hear from mothers and fathers who've recently delivered? Is there discussion, or just lecture? Will there be ample opportunity for parents-to-be to ask questions? Is adequate time provided during class for practicing the various techniques that are taught?

CHILDBIRTH EDUCATION OPTIONS

Childbirth education classes in your area may be taught by nurses, nurse-midwives, or other certified professionals. Approaches may vary from class to class, even among those trained in the same programs. The most common classes include:

Lamaze. The Lamaze approach to childbirth education, probably the most widely used in the United States, was pioneered by Dr. Ferdinand Lamaze in the

1950s. Its foundation is the use of relaxation and breathing techniques by the laboring woman, along with the continuous support of a spouse (or other coach) and trained nurse to allow the laboring woman to experience a more natural childbirth. According to the Lamaze philosophy, birth is normal, natural, and healthy, and a woman's confidence and ability to give birth naturally can be either enhanced or diminished by the level of support she receives from her care provider as well as by the comfort of the birthing environment (which could be a birth center or home as well as a hospital). The goal of Lamaze training is active concentration based on relaxation and rhythmic breathing patterns. To help with concentration, women are encouraged to direct their attention to a focal point. Courses also cover comfortable labor and birthing positions; breathing, distraction, and massage techniques; communication skills; and other comfort measures, as well as information on the early postpartum period and breastfeeding. Though the Lamaze philosophy states that women have a right to give birth free from routine medical interventions, classes generally cover most common interventions (including pain relief) in order to prepare couples for any birthing scenario. A traditional Lamaze course consists of six 2- to 2½-hour sessions.

Bradley. This approach, where the husband-coached delivery originated, emphasizes excellent nutrition as the foundation of a healthy pregnancy and uses exercise to ease the discomforts of pregnancy and to prepare muscles for birth and breasts for nursing. In Bradley classes, women learn to mimic their nighttime sleeping position and breathing (which is deep and slow) for use during labor and to use relaxation techniques to make the first stage of labor more comfortable. The Bradley method employs deep abdominal breathing rather than panting; instead of using distraction and a focus of concentration outside the body to take the mind off discomfort, Bradley recommends that the laboring woman concentrate within and work with her body.

According to the Bradley technique, a woman's needs during labor are darkness, quiet, physical comfort aided by pillows, and closed eyes. Bradley teachers acknowledge that labor hurts, and they stress acceptance of pain. Medication is reserved for complications and cesareans (which are discussed so that parents can be prepared for any eventuality), and about 94 percent of Bradley graduates who have vaginal births go without it. The typical Bradley course runs twelve weeks, beginning in the sixth month, and most are taught by married couples. "Early bird" Bradley classes, which focus on matters prenatal, are available, as are classes that continue into the postpartum period, but neither is mandatory.

International Childbirth Education Association (ICEA) classes. These classes tend to be broader in scope, covering more of the many options available today to expectant parents in family-centered maternity care and newborn care. They also recognize the importance of individual freedom of choice, and so classes focus on a wide range of possibilities rather than on a single approach to childbirth. Teachers are certified through ICEA.

ALACE (Association of Labor Assistants and Childbirth Educators) programs. Founded by a midwife, ALACE champions a woman's right to a natural or unmedicated birth when at all possible and rejects routine interventions. Rather than try to teach expectant parents how to avoid labor and childbirth pain, classes

FOR INFORMATION ON PREGNANCY/ CHILDBIRTH CLASSES

Ask your practitioner about classes in your area, or call the hospital where you plan to deliver. If you are interested in pregnancy classes, ask at one of your early visits. The following organizations can also give you referrals to local classes.

Lamaze International: 2025 M Street, Suite 800, Washington, DC 20036-3309; (800) 368-4404; www.lamaze-childbirth.com.

International Childbirth Education Association: PO Box 20048, Minneapolis, MN 55420; (612) 854-8660; www.icea.org. (ICEA provides referrals from other groups as well.)

Bradley: American Academy of Husband-Coached Childbirth: PO Box 5224, Sherman Oaks, CA 91413-5224; (800) 4-A-BIRTH (422-4784); www.bradley birth.com.

ALACE: PO Box 382724, Cambridge, MA 02238; (617) 441-2500; www. ALACE.com.

Alexander Technique: American Society for the Alexander Technique: PO Box 60008, Florence, MA 01062; (800) 473-0620; www.alexandertech.com.

"At Home" Childbirth Education: The Childbirth Institute, (877) 31-BIRTH (312-4784); www.childbirthinstitute.com.

New Way Childbirth: (864) 244-4331; www.newwaychildbirth.com.

Association of Christian Childbirth Professionals: www.christianbirth.org.

The American Society of Clinical Hypnosis: 33 West Grand Avenue, Suite 402, Chicago, IL 60610; (312) 645-9810; www. asch.net.

Society for Clinical and Experimental Hypnosis, 3900 Vincennes Road, Suite 304, Indianapolis, IN 46268; sunsite.utk.edu/ ijceh/scehframe.htm.

provide coping tools to work *with* the discomfort.

Alexander technique. This approach, like that of ALACE instructors, views labor pain as normal, natural, and functional. The Alexander technique teaches women to cope with labor pain by learning to exercise conscious control over posture and movement and by reeducating the body to replace habitual patterns of tension with those of release.

Hypnobirthing. Classes, for individuals or groups, that teach how to use hypnosis to reduce discomfort and pain (and in some highly suggestible women to eliminate it entirely), achieve a deep state of relaxation, as well as improve mood and attitude during labor and childbirth, are becoming more available. Check with your practitioner or a national clinical hypnosis organization for names of certified hypnotherapists in your area. (For more on hypnobirthing, see page 281.)

Other childbirth classes. The range is wide. Childbirth Education Preparation (CEP) certifies nurses and practical nurses as childbirth educators who are trained to run classes that explain the many options, including Lamaze and Bradley, available to expectant parents during labor. In addition, there are Christian childbirth organizations that train childbirth educators, including the Association of Christian Childbirth Professionals, and there are childbirth education classes designed to prepare parents to deliver in a particular hospital, and classes sponsored by medical groups, health maintenance organizations (HMOs), or other health care provider groups. In some areas, prenatal classes, which cover all aspects of pregnancy as well as childbirth, are also offered, usually beginning in the first trimester.

Home study. If you are on bed rest, live in a remote area, or for some other reason cannot or do not want to attend a group class, there are other options. One is a complete Lamaze program on video available from Lamaze International. Another is the "At-Home" childbirth education program available from the Childbirth Institute (see box on the facing page). In addition to videos, this includes an illustrated manual, coaching cards for your coach, and an audiotape or CD that will allow you

to practice the relaxation and visualization skills you learned in class when you're in the car or the office or otherwise away from home (and will be usable during labor itself). Another option is the series of video and audiotapes put out by New Way Childbirth—which deals with prenatal "heart-to-heart" bonding as well as childbirth.

Weekend classes at resorts. These offer the same curriculum as typical classes, packed into a single weekend instead of spaced out over a series of weeks, and are a nice choice for those who can—and would like to—get away. In addition to promoting camaraderie among expectant parents (especially rewarding if you don't have other pregnant friends to talk to at home), these weekends can promote romance, too—a nice plus for twosomes who are about to become threesomes.

BACK TO SCHOOL

Of course, you've been studying up on childbirth techniques these days. But believe it or not, there's another class you should consider signing up for now: Infant CPR and First Aid. Sure, you don't actually have the baby yet—but there's no better time to learn how to keep that little bundle you're about to deliver safe and sound. First, because you won't have to line up a babysitter to attend class now. And second—and more importantly—because you'll be able to bring baby home secure in the knowledge that you have all the necesssary know-how at your fingertips in case of an emergency.

◆ ◆ ◆

CHAPTER 11

The Seventh Month

Approximately 28 to 31 Weeks

Welcome to your third—and final!—trimester. In this last stretch of pregnancy, you may continue to feel terrific. Or, if you're like many women, your aches and pains are starting to multiply; as the load you're carrying grows, so can the strain on your back, legs, and especially your psyche. Beginning this trimester also means you're just a few months away from labor and delivery, an event you should begin planning for, preparing for, and getting educated about. Time to sign up for those classes, if you haven't already.

What You Can Expect at This Month's Checkup

There are a couple of new items on the agenda at this month's checkup, along with the old standards. As you enter your last trimester, you can expect your practitioner to check the following, though there may be variations depending upon your particular needs and upon your practitioner's style of practice:[1]

- Weight and blood pressure

- Urine, for sugar and protein

- Fetal heartbeat

- Height of fundus (top of uterus)

- Size and position of fetus, by external palpation (feeling from the outside)

- Feet and hands for edema (swelling), and legs for protruding varicose veins

- Symptoms you have been experiencing, especially unusual ones

- Questions and problems you want to discuss—have a list ready

- Glucose screening test

- Blood test for anemia

1. See Appendix, page 545, for an explanation of the procedures and tests performed during office visits.

A LOOK INSIDE

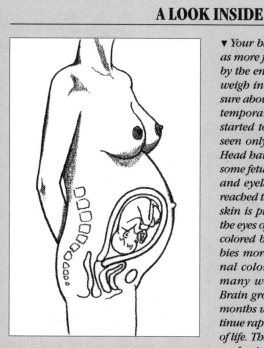

▲ *At the beginning of this month, your uterus is approximately 11 inches from the top of your pubic bone. By the end of the month, your baby's home has grown another inch in height and can be felt around 4½ inches above your belly button. You may feel that there is no more room for your womb to grow (it seems to have already filled up your abdomen), but you still have 8 to 10 more weeks of expansion ahead of you!*

▼ *Your baby is gaining weight rapidly, as more fat is deposited under the skin; by the end of this month he or she will weigh in at about 3 pounds and measure about 16 inches long. Lanugo (that temporary fuzz on baby's body) has started to disappear, and can now be seen only on the back and shoulders. Head hair is starting to grow (more in some fetuses than others) and eyebrows and eyelashes are present; nails have reached the tops of fingers and toes. The skin is pink and smooth. The irises in the eyes of light-skinned babies are now colored blue, and in dark-skinned babies more likely brown, though the final color won't be discernible until many weeks or months after birth. Brain growth in this and the next two months will be dramatic, and will continue rapidly through the first two years of life. The lungs, though still immature, are beginning to function; a baby born now has a very good chance of survival.*

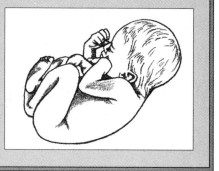

What You May Be Feeling

Y ou may experience all of these symptoms at one time or another, or only a few of them. Some may have continued from last month, others may be new. Still others may hardly be noticed because you've become so used to them. You may also have other, less common, symptoms.

PHYSICALLY

- Stronger and more frequent fetal activity
- Increasingly heavy whitish vaginal discharge (leukorrhea)
- Achiness in the lower abdomen or along the sides
- Constipation
- Heartburn, indigestion, flatulence, bloating
- Occasional headaches, faintness, or dizziness
- Nasal congestion and occasional nosebleeds; ear stuffiness
- Pink toothbrush from bleeding gums
- Leg cramps
- Backache
- Mild swelling of ankles and feet, and occasionally of hands and face
- Varicose veins of the legs
- Hemorrhoids (varicose veins of the rectum)
- Itchy abdomen
- Protruding navel
- Shortness of breath
- Difficulty sleeping
- Scattered Braxton Hicks contractions, usually painless (the uterus hardens for a minute, then returns to normal)
- Clumsiness (which increases the risk of falling)
- Enlarged breasts
- Colostrum, either leaking or expressed from nipples (though this premilk substance may not appear until after delivery)

EMOTIONALLY

- Increasing excitement
- Increasing apprehension about motherhood, baby's health, and labor and delivery
- Continued absentmindedness
- Increased dreaming and fantasizing about the baby
- Increased boredom and weariness with the pregnancy, or a sense of contentment and well-being, particularly if you're feeling great physically

What You May Be Concerned About

INCREASING FATIGUE

"I've heard women are supposed to feel terrific in the last trimester. I feel tired all the time."

"Supposed to" is a phrase that ought to be stricken from a pregnant woman's vocabulary. There's no one way you're supposed to feel at any time in pregnancy. Though some women feel less tired in the third trimester than in the first and second, many continue feeling fatigued or feel even more fatigued. Actually, there are probably more reasons

to feel tired than terrific in the last trimester. First of all, you're carrying around a lot more weight than you were earlier. Second, because of your increased bulk, you may be having trouble sleeping. You may also be losing sleep because your mind is overloaded with baby concerns, to-do lists, and fantasies. And if you have responsibilities other than carrying and nuturing and preparing for the new baby—such as taking care of other children, a job, or both—the fatigue factors multiply exponentially.

Fatigue is a normal part of this stage

of pregnancy, but that doesn't mean you should ignore it or resign yourself to being continuously exhausted. As always, fatigue is a signal from your body that you should slow down. Take the hint. Make rest and relaxation a priority as much as you can and cut back on any nonessential activities. You'll need every bit of strength you can save up for labor, delivery, and, more important, what follows.

Extreme fatigue that doesn't ease up when you get more rest should be reported to your doctor. Anemia (see page 187), which can trigger such fatigue, sometimes strikes at the beginning of the third trimester, which is why most practitioners repeat a routine blood test for it in the seventh month.

EDEMA (SWELLING) OF THE ANKLES AND FEET

"My ankles and feet seem to be swollen, especially when the weather is warm and at the end of the day. Is this a bad sign?"

Puffy ankles and tight shoes are what most pregnant women will be wearing in any season, and though these don't make for particularly attractive or comfortable fashion accessories, they are usually completely normal. While any degree of edema (swelling due to accumulation of fluids in the tissues) was once considered a potential danger sign in pregnancy, doctors now recognize that mild swelling of the ankles and feet is related to the normal and necessary increase in body fluids in pregnancy. In fact, 75 percent of women develop such edema at some point in their pregnancies.[2] It's especially common late in the day, in warm weather, or after standing

or sitting for a period of time. Most women find that much of the swelling disappears overnight or after several hours spent lying down.

Generally, this type of edema means nothing but a little discomfort. To ease it, avoid extended periods of standing; elevate your legs, if possible, when you're sitting; lie down for brief periods when you can, preferably on your left side; wear comfortable shoes or slippers; avoid elastic-top socks or stockings. Regular, practitioner-approved exercise breaks—such as periodic brisk five-minute walks up and down your office hallway—may help, too.

Wearing support panty hose can also bring relief—along with (often unwelcome) added warmth. Several types are available for pregnancy wear, including full panty hose (with roomy tummy space) and knee- or thigh-highs (which will at least be cooler to wear). When shopping, select the size based on your prepregnancy weight. Put the support hose on before you get up in the morning, while the swelling is down. In hot weather, powdering your legs and feet with a little cornstarch before you put the hose on may help to minimize sweating.

Help your system to flush out waste products by drinking at least eight to ten 8-ounce glasses of liquid a day. Paradoxically, drinking even greater amounts of liquids—up to a gallon a day—can help avoid excess water retention. It's no longer believed that salt restriction is wise during a normal pregnancy (though salt may be restricted for some women with high blood pressure), but *excessive* salt intake isn't any smarter and could increase fluid retention.

If your hands and/or face become puffy, or if edema persists for more than twenty-four hours at a time, you should notify your doctor. Such swelling may be insignificant, or—if accompanied by rapid weight gain, a rise in blood

---

2. One in 4 pregnant women never notice ankle swelling—and this can be completely normal, too.

pressure, and protein in the urine—it could signal the beginning of preeclampsia (pregnancy-induced hypertension; see page 500).

OVERHEATING

"I feel so warm most of the time, and I sweat a lot. Is this normal?"

With your basal metabolic rate (the rate at which your body expends energy at total rest) up about 20 percent during pregnancy, the heat's on. Not only are you likely to feel too warm in warm weather, you may feel overheated even in the winter, when everyone else is shivering. You will also probably perspire more, especially at night. This is a mixed blessing. While it helps to cool you off and rids your body of waste products, it is admittedly unpleasant.

For tips on how to keep your cool, see page 207.

FETAL HICCUPS

"I sometimes feel regular little spasms in my abdomen. Is this kicking, or a twitch, or what?"

Believe it or not, your baby's probably got hiccups, a phenomenon not uncommon among fetuses during the last

---

DON'T FORGET TO COUNT THOSE KICKS

Now that you're past the 28th week of pregnancy, you should make sure you feel baby movements every day. If you're too busy to notice fetal movement during the day, make sure you do the kick count test in the morning and evening (see page 243) and report any change in fetal movement to your practitioner.

---

half of pregnancy. Some get hiccups several times a day, every day. Others never get them at all. The same pattern may continue after birth.

But before you start holding a paper bag over your belly, you should know that hiccups don't cause the same discomfort in babies (in or out of the uterus) as they do in adults, even when they last twenty minutes or more. So just relax and enjoy this little entertainment from within.

SKIN ERUPTIONS

"As if it's not bad enough that I have stretch marks, now I seem to have some kind of itchy pimples breaking out in them."

Cheer up. You have less than three months left until delivery, when you'll be able to bid a grateful good-bye to most of the unpleasant side effects of pregnancy—among them, these new eruptions. Until then, it may help to know that although they may be uncomfortable, the lesions aren't dangerous to you or your baby. Known medically (and unpronounceably) as pruritic urticarial papules and plaques of pregnancy (try saying that fast three times), or PUPPP,[3] the condition generally disappears after delivery and doesn't recur in subsequent pregnancies. Though PUPPP most often develops in abdominal stretch marks, it sometimes also appears on the thighs, buttocks, or arms of the expectant mother. Show your rash to your practitioner, who may prescribe topical medication, an antihistamine, or a shot to ease any discomfort.

There are a variety of other skin conditions and rashes that can develop

---

3. PUPPP is now medically known as PEP (polymorphic eruption of pregnancy), but most doctors still refer to the condition as PUPPP.

during pregnancy. Though they should always be shown to your practitioner, they are rarely serious. Some will need to be treated; others will run a mild course and disappear after delivery.

ACCIDENTS

"I missed the curb today when I was out walking and fell belly first on the pavement. Could the fall have hurt the baby?"

A woman in the last trimester of pregnancy isn't exactly the most graceful creature on earth. A poor sense of balance (because her center of gravity keeps shifting forward) and looser, less stable joints contribute to her awkwardness and make her prone to minor falls—particularly belly flops. Also contributing to clumsiness are your tendency to tire easily, your predisposition to preoccupation and daydreaming, and the difficulty you may be having seeing past your belly to your feet—all of which makes those curbs easy to miss.

But while a curbside spill may leave you with multiple scrapes and bruises (particularly on your ego), it's extremely rare for a fetus to suffer the consequences of its mother's clumsiness. Your baby is protected by one of the world's most sophisticated shock absorption systems, comprised of amniotic fluid, tough membranes, the elastic, muscular uterus, and the sturdy abdominal cavity, which is girded with muscles and bones. For it to be penetrated, and for your baby to be hurt, you'd have to sustain very serious injuries—the kind that would very likely land you in the hospital.

Even though there's probably no harm done, you should let your practitioner know if you have a fall. You may be asked to come in so that your baby's heartbeat can be checked—mostly to set everybody's mind at ease.

On the extremely rare occasion when an accident does affect a pregnancy, it's most likely to involve separation (abruption) of the placenta. If you notice vaginal bleeding, leakage of amniotic fluid, abdominal tenderness, or uterine contractions, or if your baby seems unusually inactive, seek medical attention immediately. Have someone take you to the emergency room if you can't reach your practitioner.

LOWER BACK AND LEG PAIN (SCIATICA)

"I've been having pain on the right side of my back, running right down my hip and leg. What's that about?"

This sounds like another of the occupational hazards of expectant motherhood. The pressure of the enlarging uterus, which has been responsible for so many other discomforts, can also affect the sciatic nerve, causing lower back, buttock, and leg pain. Rest, and a heating pad applied locally, may help, as can performing standing Pelvic Tilts (page 194). Swimming can also relieve pressure on the nerve.

The pain of sciatica may pass as your baby's position changes, or it may linger until you've delivered. In severe cases, a few days of bed rest or special exercises may be recommended. Complementary and alternative treatments, such as chiropractic medicine, acupuncture, and therapeutic massage, may also be beneficial (see page 246).

ORGASM AND THE BABY

"After I have an orgasm, my baby usually stops kicking for about half an hour. Is sex harmful to him or her at this stage of pregnancy?"

Babies are individuals, even in the womb, and their responses to their parents' lovemaking vary. Some, perhaps like your baby, are rocked to sleep by the rhythmic motion of coitus and the uterine contractions that follow orgasm. Others, stimulated by the activity, may become more lively. Both responses are normal; neither indicates that the fetus is aware of what's going on or that he or she has been harmed in any way.

In fact, unless your practitioner has prescribed otherwise, you can continue enjoying lovemaking—and orgasms—until delivery. And you might as well while you can. Let's face it—it may be a while before it's as convenient to make love with your baby in the house again.

GLUCOSE SCREENING TEST

"My practitioner says I need to take a glucose screening test to check for gestational diabetes. Why would I need it—and what does the test involve?"

Don't feel too picked on. Almost all practitioners screen for gestational diabetes in almost all patients at about 28 weeks.[4] So chances are the test your practitioner ordered is just routine.

And it's simple, too, especially if you have a sweet tooth. You'll be asked to drink a very sweet glucose drink, which usually tastes like flat orange soda, one hour before having some blood drawn; you don't have to be fasting when you do this. Most women chugalug the stuff with no problem and no side effects; a few, especially those who don't have a taste for sweet liquids, feel a little nauseous afterwards. Researchers (perhaps

---

4. Those at higher risk for gestational diabetes, including older or obese mothers or those with a family history of diabetes, are screened earlier in their pregnancies and more often.

ANOTHER REASON TO EAT YOUR VEGETABLES

Want to raise a child who eats his or her vegetables? Make sure you eat yours now. Research shows that by the third trimester, fetuses can taste the flavors that make their way from their mothers' meals into amniotic fluid. And a recent study has suggested that what Mom eats while pregnant (and while breastfeeding, since breast milk picks up flavors the same way) influences a baby's future tastes. In the study, infants whose mothers had drunk carrot juice when they were pregnant or lactating lapped up cereal mixed with carrot juice more eagerly than infants of mothers who'd stayed away from carrots. Interesting science—and something to chew on next time the broccoli comes your way.

---

empathetic ones who've drunk the glucose drink themselves and vowed to find a tastier way) are now studying whether women can eat the glucose equivalent in jelly beans instead. So far, patients in the study have reported fewer side effects after the jelly bean challenge (though perhaps more toothaches).

If the blood work comes back with elevated numbers, which *suggests* the possibility that a woman might not be producing enough insulin to process the extra glucose in her system, the next level of test—the glucose tolerance test—is ordered. This fasting, three-hour test, which involves a higher-concentration glucose drink, is used to diagnose gestational diabetes. Symptoms that may also point to such a diagnosis include excessive hunger and thirst; frequent urination (even in the second trimester); recurrent vaginal infections; and an increase in blood pressure.

Gestational diabetes occurs in about 4 to 7 percent of expectant mothers, which gives it the dubious distinction of being the most common pregnancy complication. It's also, fortunately, one of the most easily managed. When blood sugar is closely controlled through diet, exercise, and, if necessary, medication, women with gestational diabetes can have perfectly normal pregnancies and healthy babies. In most (97 to 98 percent), the blood sugar abnormalities will disappear after delivery. Some of these women, however (and this is much more common in women who are obese), may be at higher risk of developing diabetes later in life. To reduce that risk, if you have gestational diabetes, take the following preventive measures postpartum: have regular medical checkups, maintain ideal weight, cultivate (or keep) good diet and exercise habits, and be familiar with the symptoms of the disease so any can be reported promptly to your physician. See page 499 for more on the condition and its management.

RESTLESS LEG SYNDROME

"As tired as I am at night, I can't seem to settle down because my legs feel so restless. I've tried all the tips for leg cramps, but they don't work. What else can I do?"

With so many other things coming between you and a good night's sleep in your last trimester, it hardly seems fair that your legs are, too. But for the up to 15 percent of pregnant women who experience—yes, it's got a name— restless leg syndrome (RLS), that's exactly what happens. The name captures it all—that restless, creeping, crawling, tingling feeling inside the foot and/or leg that keeps the rest of your body from settling down. It's most common at night, but it can also strike in the late after-noon—or pretty much any time you're lying or sitting down.

Experts aren't certain what causes RLS in some pregnant women, and they're even less sure of how to treat it. None of the tricks of the leg cramp trade—including rubbing or flexing—seem to bring relief. Medications are out, too, since those that are currently used to treat RLS aren't safe for use during pregnancy.

It's possible that diet, stress, and other environmental factors may contribute to the problem, so it may help to keep track of what you eat, what you do, and how you feel each day so that you can see what lifestyle habits, if any, bring on symptoms. Some women, for instance, find that eating carbohydrates late in the day can worsen RLS. It's also possible that iron-deficiency anemia may cause RLS, so it's worth asking your practitioner about testing to rule that out—as well as asking him or her for any other suggested treatments. And, of course, it couldn't hurt to try the sleep tips on page 183. Unfortunately, however, some women continue to find relief—and sleep—elusive. If you are one of them, RLS is something you may just have to put up with until delivery.

DREAMS AND FANTASIES

"I've been having so many vivid dreams—day and night — about the baby that I'm beginning to think I'm losing my mind."

Though the many dreams—night dreams and daydreams—you're dreaming now may make you feel as though you're losing your sanity, they're actually helping to keep you sane. Dreams and fantasies, both the horrifying and the heartwarming, are healthy and normal, and can help you to sort out worries and fears about motherhood in a nonthreatening way. Expectant dads may also have strange dreams and fantasies as they attempt to work out their conscious and subconscious anxieties about impending fatherhood.

The following are the most commonly reported dream and fantasy themes during pregnancy, and each expresses one or more of the deep-seated feelings and concerns that might otherwise be suppressed. Some probably sound familiar.

◆ *Oops! dreams.* Dreaming about losing or misplacing things (from your car keys to your baby); forgetting to feed the baby; missing a doctor's appointment; going out to shop and leaving baby home alone; being unprepared for the baby when it arrives can express the fear that you won't make an adequate mother.

◆ *Ouch! dreams.* Being attacked or hurt—by intruders, burglars, animals; falling down the stairs after a push or a slip—may represent a sense of vulnerability.

◆ *Help! dreams.* Dreams of being enclosed or unable to escape—trapped in a tunnel, a car, a small room; drowning in a pool, a lake of snowy slush, a car wash—can signify the fear of being tied down and deprived of freedom by the expected new family member.

◆ *Oh no! dreams.* Dreams about going off your pregnancy diet—gaining too much weight or gaining a lot of weight overnight; overeating; eating or drinking the wrong things or not eating the right things—are common among those trying to stick to a dietary regimen.

◆ *Ugh! dreams.* Dreaming about losing appeal—becoming unattractive or repulsive to your spouse or about your spouse finding someone else—

expresses the common fear that pregnancy will destroy your looks forever and drive away your partner.

◆ *Sexual dreams.* Dreams about sexual encounters—either positive or negative, pleasure- or guilt-provoking—may reflect the sexual confusion and ambivalence often experienced during pregnancy.

◆ *Memory dreams.* Dreaming of death and resurrection—lost parents or other relatives reappearing—may be the subconscious mind's way of linking old and new generations.

◆ *Life with baby dreams.* Dreaming about getting ready for the baby; loving and playing with the baby in a dream is practice parenting, bonding you with your baby prior to birth.

◆ *Imagining baby dreams.* Dreaming about what your baby will be like can represent a wide variety of concerns. Dreams about the baby being deformed, sick, or too large or too small express anxiety about its health. Fantasies about the infant having unusual skills (like talking or walking at birth) may indicate concern about the baby's intelligence and ambition for his or her future. Premonitions that the baby will be a boy or a girl could mean your heart's set on one or the other. So could dreams about the baby's hair or eye color or resemblance to one parent or the other. Nightmares of the baby being born fully grown could signify your fear of having to handle a tiny infant.

◆ *Labor dreams.* Dreaming about labor pain—or lack of it—or about not being able to push the baby out may reflect your fear of labor.

Though dreams and fantasies can be more anxiety-provoking in pregnancy than they are at other times, they can also be more useful. If you listen to what your parenthood fantasies are telling you about your feelings and deal with them now, you can make that transition into real-life parenthood more easily.

APPROACHING RESPONSIBILITY

"I'm beginning to worry that I won't be able to manage my job, my house, my marriage—and the baby, too."

Many a new mother has tried to be "superwoman"—handling a full workload at work; keeping the house in order, the refrigerator stocked, and food on the table; being a doting (read: sexy) partner and an exemplary mother; and leaping the occasional building at a single bound—but few have succeeded without sacrificing health and sanity, sometimes even their marriage.

How well you manage will depend on the decisions you make and the attitudes you develop, now and after your child arrives. It will help if you reconcile yourself to the idea that you can't do it all—and do it all well. It's a matter of deciding what your priorities are and arranging them in order of importance (no fair making them all number one). If baby, spouse, and job are top priorities, perhaps keeping the house clean will have to take a (messy) backseat for now. If full-time motherhood appeals to you and you can afford to stay home for a while, maybe you can put your career on hold temporarily. Or you might consider working part-time, as a compromise. Or switch to working from home, if possible.

It's also a matter of letting go of unrealistic expectations. Nobody's perfect, though initially you may have trouble accepting that reality. As much as you'll want to do everything right, you're certain to find that goal unattainable. Despite your best efforts, beds may go unmade and laundry unfolded, take-out may take over your dinner table, and getting "sexy" may mean finally getting around to washing your hair. Set your standards too high—even if you were able to meet them in your preparenting days—and you'll set yourself up for disappointment.

However you decide to rearrange

TO WORK OR NOT TO WORK?

If *that* is the question, don't be in a hurry to find the answer just yet. Though you definitely should start giving the matter some thought—talking it over with your spouse, consulting with friends who've gone back to work after having a baby and those who've opted not to, even making lists of pros and cons and financial considerations to ponder—you might be wise to put off the final decision until you've spent some time in your new job as a mother. For some women, just holding that newborn in their arms turns their previous thinking about returning to the workplace upside-down. For others, a completely different epiphany comes a few weeks into their maternity leave, as they begin to realize that full-time mothering isn't for them. So take your time, and make the decision that works for you. Remember, there is no *right* decision—each mother must follow her heart (pocketbook allowing). And remember, also, even your final decision isn't really final. Should you experience a change of heart months or even years into motherhood, you can *always* change your mind.

your life, it will be easier if you don't have to go it alone. Beside most successful moms is a dad who not only shares equally in household chores, but also is a full partner in parenting, in every department from diapering to bathing to cuddling. And what's good for you is even better for him: no matter how long his day at the office, there's no more fulfilling way to pass after-work hours than caring for and spending time with your child. If Dad's not available as much as you'd like (or isn't in the picture at all), then you are going to need to consider other sources of assistance: the baby's grandparents or other relatives, child care or household workers, baby-sitting co-ops, or day care centers.

PREMATURE LABOR

"Is there anything I can do to make sure that my baby won't be born early?"

It's far more likely your baby will be arriving late than early. In the United States, very few deliveries are premature or preterm—that is, before the 37th week of pregnancy. And most of these occur in women who are known to be at high risk for premature delivery.[5]

Still, as good as your chances of carrying to term already are, there's almost always room for improvement. The following risk factors, believed to be related to premature labor, are all controllable; eliminate any that apply to you, and you'll help give your baby the best chances of contentedly staying put in your uterus until term (between 38 and 42 weeks).

Smoking. Quit before conception or as early as possible in pregnancy. (But keep

in mind that quitting at any time in pregnancy is better than not quitting at all.)

Alcohol use. Avoid drinking beer, wine, and liquor.

Drug abuse. Don't take any medications—including over-the-counter or herbal preparations—without the approval of a physician who knows you are pregnant; don't take *any* nonmedicinal, "recreational," or illegal drugs at all.

Inadequate weight gain. If your prepregnant weight was normal, gain a minimum of 25 pounds; if you were *significantly* underweight before conceiving, you may need to gain closer to 35 pounds. Severely overweight women, with excellent nutrition and their practitioner's permission, may safely be able to gain less.

Inadequate nutrition. Follow a well-balanced diet throughout pregnancy. Be sure that your prenatal vitamin supplement contains zinc; some recent studies have linked zinc deficiency with preterm labor.

Gum infection. Take proper care of your teeth and gums and see a dentist at least once during your pregnancy to avoid gum disease.

Lots of standing, or heavy physical labor. If your job alone or your job plus housework requires you to stand for many hours each day, it may be advisable to cut back on the time you spend on your feet. Heavy physical labor and lifting may also need to be curtailed (see page 248).

Sexual intercourse (only for some women). Though most expectant mothers can continue to make love until delivery, those who are at *high risk* for premature delivery may be advised to abstain from intercourse and/or orgasm during the final two or three

5. The rate of premature deliveries is lower for white women (fewer than 6 in 100) and higher for black women (nearly 13 in 100), only partly for socioeconomic reasons.

months of pregnancy because, in these women, orgasm and/or the prostaglandins in sperm might trigger uterine contractions.

Other risk factors are not always possible to eliminate, but their effects can sometimes be modified.

Infection. Certain infections (rubella; some sexually transmitted diseases; and urinary tract, cervical, vaginal, and amniotic fluid infections) can put a mother-to-be at high risk for preterm labor. When the infection is one that could prove harmful to the fetus, early labor seems to be the body's way of attempting to rescue the baby from a dangerous environment. Antibiotics can often not only cure the infection, they can reassure the body that everything is okay and that "rescue" is not needed.

In the case of amniotic fluid infection, the body's immune response apparently triggers production of prostaglandins, which can initiate labor, as well as of substances that can damage the fetal membranes, leading to their premature rupture. If membranes do rupture prematurely, some practitioners routinely prescribe antibiotics for the mother as a precaution (whether or not an infection is apparent), though it's still unclear if that's helpful in preventing problems.

It's virtually impossible to prevent every infection, but there are many ways to minimize your chances of getting sick. Most preventive measures are common sense: stay away from people who are ill and make sure you get adequate rest and exercise, optimum nutrition, and regular prenatal care. Others, such as drinking plenty of water and urinating when you feel the urge to prevent bladder infection, may seem a little less obvious. Testing for and treating vaginal infections may also ward off preterm labor. And some doctors recommend using a condom during the last months of pregnancy to reduce the risk of infection that can trigger labor.

Hormonal imbalance. Just as it can trigger late miscarriage, an imbalance of hormones can trigger premature delivery. Treatment can prevent this.

Incompetent cervix. This condition, in which a weak cervix opens early (from the pressure of the growing fetus), often isn't diagnosed until after a woman has experienced late miscarriage or premature labor at least once. When the condition is diagnosed, the cervix will possibly be stitched closed at about the 14th week (see page 35 for more information).

Premature cervical effacement and dilation. In some women, for reasons unknown and apparently unrelated to an incompetent cervix, the cervix begins to thin out and open up early. Recent research suggests that at least some of this early effacement and dilation may be related to a shorter-than-normal cervix. Routine ultrasound examination of the cervix in the middle of pregnancy to uncover this condition in women who are at high risk is a common and probably useful procedure.

Uterine irritability. Research suggests that in some women the uterus is particularly irritable, and that this irritability makes it susceptible to untimely contractions. Some experts believe that if these women could be identified and monitored in the third trimester, it's possible that their premature labor could be prevented by full or partial bed rest and/or the use of medication to quiet the contractions.

Placenta previa (a low-lying placenta located near or over the cervix; see page 505). This condition, which can also activate premature labor, may be discovered in an ultrasound exam, or may not be suspected until bleeding is noted in mid- or late pregnancy. Once placenta previa is diagnosed, complete bed rest may head off a baby's early arrival.

Chronic maternal illness. Chronic conditions, such as high blood pressure, heart, liver, or kidney disease, or diabetes, put a mother at high risk for preterm delivery, but good medical and self-care (see Chapter 19), sometimes including bed rest, can often prevent it.

Extreme emotional stress. Sometimes the cause of stress can be eliminated or minimized (by quitting or cutting back at a high-pressure job or getting counseling for a shaky marriage, for example); sometimes it can't be eliminated (as when you lose your job or there's been a serious illness or death in the family). Still, all kinds of stress can be reduced with relaxation techniques, good nutrition, a balance of exercise and rest, and by talking the problem out, with your spouse or friends, your practitioner, a therapist, or in a support group run by a professional counselor (also see page 125).

Under age seventeen. Optimal nutrition and prenatal care can reduce the risk of early delivery by helping to compensate for the fact that the mother, like her fetus, is still growing.

Over age thirty-five. Optimal nutrition, good prenatal care, reduction of stress, and prenatal screening for genetic and obstetrical problems specific to women over thirty-five all reduce risk.

Low educational or socioeconomic level. Again, good nutrition and early access to and participation in culturally sensitive prenatal care, as well as the elimination of as many risk factors as possible, can decrease the risk.

Structural abnormalities of the uterus or large fibroids. These abnormalities may be due to the hormone DES being given to the expectant mother's mother during pregnancy,[6] to uterine surgery, to a birth defect affecting the shape or capacity of the uterus, or to other causes. Once the problem has been diagnosed, prepregnancy surgical repair can frequently prevent future preterm births.

Multiple gestations. Women carrying more than one fetus deliver an average of three weeks early (though it has been suggested that full term for twins may be 37 weeks, which might mean that three weeks early isn't early at all). Meticulous prenatal care, optimal nutrition, and the elimination of other risk factors, along with more time spent lying down and resting, and restrictions on activity as needed in the last trimester may prevent a too early birth.

Fetal abnormality. In some instances, prenatal diagnosis may pick up a defect that can be treated while the fetus is still in the uterus; sometimes correcting the problem can allow the pregnancy to continue to term.

History of premature deliveries. A diagnosed cause can be corrected; top-notch prenatal care, reduction of other risk factors, and limitations on activities may help to prevent a repeat. Though your having been born early is not a major risk factor for your child arriving ahead of schedule, your having been very small at birth may affect your own child's weight.

An unknown reason. Rarely, no identifiable risk factor is present. A perfectly healthy woman with a perfectly normal pregnancy who is taking perfectly good care of herself suddenly goes into labor early, for no apparent reason. Perhaps

---

6. If you are uncertain as to whether or not your mother received DES (diethylstilbestrol), and you were born before 1971, when the drug was prescribed for women with threatened miscarriage, ask your parents about the possibility.

someday a cause—and treatment—will be identified for all or some of such premature births, but for now they are labeled "cause unknown."

Research indicates that the use of home uterine monitoring for women at high risk of preterm labor doesn't improve the odds of carrying to term. Other research has found that weekly injections of a drug derived from the hormone progesterone does prevent early delivery in those at high risk. Education about the symptoms of preterm labor may also be helpful.

If, despite best efforts, preterm labor does begin, the delivery can often be held off until the baby is more mature. Even a brief delay can be very beneficial; each additional day the baby remains in the uterus until term improves its chances not just of survival but also of good health. So, though the chances of your baby arriving early are small—and are even smaller if you're not at high risk—it's still a good idea to familiarize yourself with the signs of premature labor and to alert your practitioner if you have the slightest suspicion that labor is beginning. Don't worry about bothering your practitioner; if you experience any of the following, call immediately, no matter what the day or hour:

♦ Menstrual-like cramps, with or without diarrhea, nausea, or indigestion

♦ Lower back pain or pressure, or a change in the nature of lower backache

♦ An achiness or feeling of pressure in the pelvic floor, the thighs, or the groin

♦ A change in your vaginal discharge, particularly if it is watery or tinged or streaked pinkish or brownish with blood

♦ Rupture of membranes (a trickle or gush of fluid from your vagina)

You can have some or all these symptoms and not be in labor, but only your practitioner can tell you for sure. If he or she suspects you're in labor, you will probably be examined promptly. For information about how premature labor is treated, see page 509.

And if you do end up among the small minority of women who deliver early, there's still good news. Thanks to modern medical care, your chances of bringing a healthy, normal baby home from the hospital will be excellent (though that trip home with the baby may have to be delayed days, weeks, or even months to increase those chances).

DON'T HOLD IT IN

Making a habit of not urinating when you feel the need increases the risk that your inflamed bladder may irritate the uterus and set off contractions, so don't hold it in. When you gotta go, go . . . promptly.

A LOW-BIRTHWEIGHT BABY

"I've been reading a lot about the high incidence of low-birthweight babies. Is there anything I can do to be sure I won't have one?"

Since most cases of low birthweight are preventable, you can do a lot—and, inasmuch as you're reading this book, chances are you already are. Nationally, 8 of every 100 newborns are categorized as low birthweight (under 5 pounds 8 ounces, or 2,500 grams), and slightly more than 1 in 100 babies as very low birth-weight (3 pounds 5 ounces, or 1,500 grams, or less). But that rate is much lower among informed women who are conscientious about both medical care and self-care (and are lucky enough to be able to afford the first and informed enough to do a good job on the second). Most of the common causes of low birthweight—use of tobacco, alcohol, or drugs (particularly cocaine) by the mother, poor nutrition, *excessive* anxiety,[7] and inadequate prenatal care, for example—are completely preventable. Many others, such as chronic maternal illnesses, can be controlled by a good working partnership between the mother and her practitioner. A major cause—premature labor—can also often be prevented (see page 270).

Of course, sometimes a baby is small at birth for reasons that no one can control: the mother's own low weight when she was born, for example, or an inadequate placenta, or a genetic disorder. A very short interval (less than nine months) between pregnancies may also be a factor. But even in these cases, excellent diet and prenatal care can often compensate. And when a baby does turn out to be small, the top-notch medical care currently available gives even the very smallest an increasingly good chance of surviving and growing up healthy.

If you think you have reason to worry about the possibility of having a low-birthweight baby, you should share your concern with your practitioner. An exam and/or an ultrasound will probably be able to reassure you that your fetus is growing at a normal pace. If it does turn out that your baby is on the small side, then steps can be taken to uncover the cause of the slow growth and, if possible, correct it (see page 502).

---

7. It appears that extremely excessive stress and worry can restrict blood flow (and thus nutrition) to the uterus.

A BIRTHING PLAN

"A friend who recently delivered said she worked out a birthing plan with her doctor before delivery. Should I?"

Birthing plans are becoming increasingly common as practitioners recognize that more and more women and their partners would like to be involved in making as many childbirth decisions as they possibly can. Some practitioners routinely ask expectant parents to fill out a birthing plan; most others are willing to discuss such a plan if a patient requests it. The typical plan combines the parents' wishes and preferences with what the practitioner and hospital or birthing center find acceptable—and what is feasible from a practical point of view. It's not a contract but a written understanding between practitioner and/or hospital or birthing center and patient, with the goal of bringing childbirth as close as possible to the patient's ideal while heading off unrealistic expectations, minimizing disappointment, and avoiding major conflict or miscommunication during labor and delivery.

A birthing plan may deal with a wide variety of topics; the precise content of each will depend on the parents, practitioner, and hospital or birthing center involved, as well as on the particular situation. Some of the issues that you may want to express your preferences about include the following (refer to the appropriate pages before making your decision):

◆ The locale of your labor and delivery—birthing room or LDRP (labor, delivery, recovery, postpartum room, for instance; see page 14)

◆ How far into your labor you would like to remain at home and at what point you would prefer to go to the hospital or birthing center

◆ Eating and/or drinking during active labor (page 346)

◆ Being out of bed (walking about or sitting up) during labor

◆ Wearing contact lenses during labor and delivery (usually not permitted if general anesthesia is required)

◆ Personalizing the atmosphere with music, lighting, items from home

◆ The use of a still camera or video camera

◆ The use of a mirror so you can see the birth

◆ The use of an IV (intravenous fluid administration; page 347)

◆ The use of pain medication and the type of pain medication (page 276)

◆ External fetal monitoring (continuous or intermittent); internal fetal monitoring (page 347)

◆ The use of oxytocin to induce or augment contractions (page 339)

◆ Delivery positions (page 357)

◆ Episiotomy; the use of steps to reduce the need for an episiotomy (page 352)

◆ Forceps or vacuum extractor use (page 354)

◆ Cesarean section (page 298)

◆ The presence of significant others (besides your spouse) during labor and/or at delivery

◆ The presence of older children at delivery or immediately after

◆ Suctioning of the newborn; suctioning by the father

◆ Holding the baby immediately after birth; breastfeeding immediately

◆ Postponing cutting the cord, weighing the baby, and/or administering eye drops until after you and your baby greet each other

◆ Having the father cut the cord

◆ Cord blood banking (see page 333)

You may also want to include some postpartum items on your birthing plan, such as:[8]

◆ Your presence at the weighing of the baby, the pediatric exam, and baby's first bath

◆ Baby feeding in the hospital (whether it will be controlled by the nursery's schedule or your baby's hunger; whether breastfeeding will be supported; whether supplementary bottles can be avoided)

◆ Management of breast engorgement if you're not breastfeeding (page 391)

◆ Circumcision (see *What to Expect the First Year*)

◆ Rooming in (see page 393)

◆ Other children visiting with you and/or with the new baby (see *What to Expect the First Year*)

◆ Postpartum medication or treatments for you or your baby

◆ The length of the hospital stay, barring complications (see page 394)

Of course, the most important feature of a good birthing plan is flexibility. Though chances are excellent that your plan can be carried out the way you draw it up, there are no guarantees. Since there is no way to predict in advance precisely how labor and delivery will progress (or

---

8. For more information on these postpartum issues, see *What to Expect the First Year.*

A BACKUP PLAN

Hopefully, once you've passed your approved birthing plan on to your practitioner, it will become part of your chart and find its way to your delivery. But just in case it doesn't make it in time, it's a very good idea to print up several copies of the plan to bring along to the hospital or birthing center, just so there's no confusion about your wishes. Your coach or doula can make sure that each new shift (with any luck, you won't have to labor through too many of these) is given a copy for reference. How it's passed along is important; thrusting it in the incoming nurse's face is probably not the best way to go. Instead, offer it in a pleasant, nonthreatening way, as in: "Would you like to see a copy of the birthing plan we drew up with the doctor?" Some expectant parents have found that placing the birthing plan in a small basket of goodies makes it even more welcome. Such a gift is also much appreciated by hardworking hospital personnel.

not progress), a birthing plan you design before the process begins may not end up being in the best interests of you and your baby, and may have to be changed at the last minute. It may also change because you have a change of mind (you were dead set against having an epidural, but once you find yourself in the thick of the contractions, you become dead set on having one). No matter how much of your birthing plan actually materializes, try to keep in mind that the priorities in any birth should be the health and safety of mother and child—and that all other considerations must be secondary.

What It's Important to Know: ABOUT CHILDBIRTH MEDICATION

On January 19, 1847, Scottish physician James Young Simpson splashed a half teaspoon of chloroform on a handkerchief and held it over the nose of a laboring woman. Less than half an hour later, she became the first woman to deliver while under anesthesia. There was only one complication: when the woman—whose first baby had been born after three days of painful labor—awoke, Dr. Simpson was unable to convince her that she'd actually given birth.

This revolution in obstetrical practice was welcomed by women but fought by both the clergy and some members of the medical profession, who believed that pain in childbirth (woman's punishment for Eve's indiscretions in Eden) was a burden that women were born to carry. Relief of the pain would be immoral.

But opponents didn't stand a chance of halting the revolution. Once word got around that childbirth didn't have to hurt, obstetrical patients wouldn't take "no pain relief" for an answer. It was no longer a question of whether anesthesia had a place in obstetrics, but of what kind of anesthesia would fill that place best.

The search for the perfect pain reliever—a drug that would eliminate pain without harming mother or child—was on. Enormous progress was made (and is still being made); analgesics and anesthetics became safer and more effective every year.

And then, during the 1950s and 1960s, the love affair between childbirth medication and obstetrical patients began to get shaky. Women wanted to be awake for their deliveries and to experience every sensation, even the painful ones. And they wanted their babies to arrive alert, not drugged from the effects of anesthesia.

Through the 1970s and into the 1980s, determined women waged war against recalcitrant physicians, the battle cry being "natural childbirth for all." Today enlightened practitioners and patients alike recognize that wanting relief from pain is natural, and that pain medication can therefore play a role in natural childbirth. When it comes to childbirth medication, mom (the one experiencing the pain) knows best—and should, when possible, be able to decide whether or not (or when) she wants pain relief.

Besides a mom's request for relief, there are other reasons why childbirth medication might be recommended:

♦ Labor is long and complicated, because the stress resulting from pain can lead to chemical imbalances that can interfere with contractions, compromise blood flow to the fetus, and exhaust the mother, reducing her ability to push effectively.

♦ The pain is more than the mother can tolerate, is interfering with her ability to push, or is so agitating that it is hindering the progress of labor.

♦ Forceps or vacuum extraction (to ease the baby out once its head is visible at the vaginal outlet; see page 354) is required.

♦ It's necessary to slow down a precipitous (too rapid) labor (see page 344).

A major concern of careful medicating in obstetrics is not only the safety of the direct recipient (the mother), but also that of the indirect recipient and innocent bystander (the baby). Occasionally, a baby whose mother has been given medication during delivery may be born drowsy, sluggish, unresponsive, and, far less often, with breathing and sucking difficulties and an irregular heartbeat. Studies show, however, that when drugs have been properly used, these adverse effects may be avoided entirely. When there is an effect, it typically disappears soon after birth. Even if a baby is so drugged, because excess medication or anesthesia has been used (which happens rarely), that he doesn't breathe spontaneously at birth, quick resuscitation (a simple procedure) will prevent long-term problems. Another concern in administering pain relief is how it will affect the progress of labor; medication given at the wrong time could slow or even stop progress.

Prudent use of any type of medication always requires a careful weighing of risk against benefit. In the case of obstetrical drugs used during labor and delivery, risks and benefits must be examined for both mother and baby, making the equation a more complicated one. In some instances, the risks of medications clearly outweigh the benefits they offer—such as when the fetus, because of prematurity or other factors, doesn't appear strong enough to cope with the combined stress of labor and drugs.

Most experts agree that when childbirth medication is used, benefits can be increased and risks reduced by:

♦ Selecting a drug that has minimal side effects and presents the least risk to mother and baby while still providing the desired pain relief; giving it in the smallest dose that will be effective; and administering it at the optimum time in the course of labor.

Exposure of the fetus to a general anesthetic, which may be used in emergency cesarean deliveries, is usually minimized by extracting the baby within minutes of administering the drug to the mother, before it has a chance to cross the placenta in significant amounts.

◆ Having an anesthesiologist or anesthetist administer anesthesia. (You have the right to insist on this if you are having general or regional—such as epidural, spinal—anesthesia.)

KINDS OF PAIN RELIEF MOST COMMONLY USED

A variety of anesthetics (substances that produce loss of sensation), analgesics (pain relievers), and ataraxics (tranquilizers) may be given during labor and delivery. Which drug, if any, will be administered will depend on the stage of labor, the patient's preference (except in an emergency), her past health history, and her present condition and that of her baby, as well as on the obstetrician's and/or anesthesiologist's preference and expertise. How effective the drug is in relieving pain will depend upon the woman (different drugs affect different people differently), the dosage, and other factors. Very rarely, a drug won't produce the desired effect, and will give little or no relief. Obstetrical pain relief is most commonly accomplished with the use of an epidural block or Demerol, but there are many other options that are available, some traditional, some from the growing area of complementary and alternative medicine (CAM):

The epidural block. The epidural, a regional nerve block, utilized for both vaginal and cesarean deliveries, is the most popular anesthetic for the relief of labor pain. More women ask for epidurals by name than for any other method of pain relief, with over 50 percent of women delivering at hospitals receiving one. The major reasons for the epidural's current surge in popularity are its relative safety (less drug is needed to achieve the desired effect), its ease of administration, and its patient-friendly results (local pain relief in the lower part of the body that allows you to be awake during the birth and alert enough to greet your baby immediately after it).

Before the epidural is administered, an IV of fluids is started (this is done to prevent the problem of low blood pressure, a side effect some women have with the epidural). In some hospitals (policies vary), a catheter (tube) is inserted into the bladder just before or just after administration of the epidural and stays in place to drain urine while the epidural is in effect (since the medication may suppress the urge to urinate). In other hospitals, the bladder is just drained intermittently, as deemed necessary by hospital personnel, with a catheter.

To administer the epidural, the woman's lower and mid-back are wiped with an antiseptic solution and a small area of the back is numbed with a local anesthetic. A larger needle is placed through the numbed area into the epidural space of the spine, usually while the mother lies on her left side, sits up and leans over a table to steady herself, or leans over her spouse, coach, or nurse. Some women will feel a little pressure as the needle is inserted. Others might feel a little tingling or a momentary shooting pain as the needle finds the correct spot. The needle is removed, leaving a fine catheter tube in place. The tube is taped to the woman's back so she can move from side to side. Three to five minutes following the initial dose, the nerves of the uterus begin to numb. After ten minutes, the woman begins to feel the full effect. The medication numbs the nerves in the entire lower part of the body and reduces pain significantly. Many women find they can push very effectively with an epidural. But if pushing turns out to be ineffective, the epidural can be stopped to allow a woman to have full control over the process. The medication can then be easily restarted after delivery to numb the repair of a tear or an episiotomy, if one is performed.

Blood pressure is checked frequently when an epidural is being administered. The potential for a sudden drop in blood pressure is the reason why an epidural is generally not used when there is a bleeding complication (such as placenta previa or abruptio placenta), severe preeclampsia or eclampsia, or fetal distress. In addition to the intravenous fluids, medication is sometimes given to counteract this side effect. Having the mother lie on her left side, so that her uterus leans to the left, may also help. Because an epidural is sometimes associated with slowing of the fetal heartbeat, continuous fetal monitoring is usually required.

Some other potential side effects of an epidural, though very infrequent, include shivering, numbness on one side of the body only (as opposed to complete pain relief), and postdelivery headaches. Epidurals also might not offer complete pain control for women experiencing back labor (when the fetus is in a posterior position, with its head pressing against the mother's back).

In the past, it has been suggested that the use of epidurals might slow or stop the progress of labor, increasing the need for cesarean, forceps, and vacuum deliveries. But recent studies have shown that isn't the case—epidurals apparently don't make a surgical delivery more likely. Overall, labor with an epidural may be somewhat longer, since the medication may cause contractions to become slightly sluggish. However, oxytocin may be administered to rev things up again *if* that becomes necessary.

While some practitioners recommend that an epidural be delayed until a woman is dilated to 4 centimeters to lower the risk of a cesarean, research shows that an early epidural not only doesn't up the chances for a c-section but also shortens the duration of labor. According to ACOG, a request for pain relief shouldn't be denied at any time during labor.

Another good option is the "walking epidural." The walking epidural uses a lower dose and a different mix of drugs than the traditional epidural, and though it diminishes pain, it does not diminish sensation or motor function, which means that the laboring woman can sense contractions, as well as get up and walk around if she wishes. Unfortunately, walking epidurals require the skill of a highly trained anesthesiologist and are not widely available at this time.

Other regional nerve blocks. *A pudendal block,* occasionally used to relieve early second-stage pain, is usually reserved for the vaginal delivery itself. Administered through a needle inserted into the vaginal area (while the mother lies on her back), it reduces pain in the region, but not uterine discomfort. It is useful when forceps or vacuum extraction is used, and its effect can last through episiotomy (if needed) and repair. It is frequently used in combination with Demerol or a tranquilizer to provide pain relief with relative safety—even when an anesthesiologist is not available.

A *spinal block* (for cesarean) and *low spinal,* or *saddle block* (for forceps-assisted or vacuum extraction vaginal delivery) is generally administered in a single dose just prior to delivery. The mother sits up or lies on her side while an anesthetic is injected into the fluid surrounding the spinal cord. There may be some nausea and vomiting while the drug is in effect, about 1 to 1½ hours. As with an epidural, there is a risk of a drop in blood pressure. Elevating the mother's legs, having her lie on her left side, administering intravenous fluids and, if necessary, medication may prevent or counteract this complication. After delivery, spinal-block patients, unlike those who've received an epidural, are usually required to remain flat on their backs for about eight hours, and a few may experience postspinal headache, which can be treated. As with epidurals, spinals are not usually used when there is placenta previa, abruptio placenta, pre-eclampsia or eclampsia, or fetal distress.

Analgesics. Meperidine hydrochloride, a powerful pain reliever commonly known under the trade name Demerol, is one of the most frequently used obstetrical analgesics. It is most effectively administered intravenously (injected slowly into an IV apparatus, so that its effects can be gauged) or intramuscularly (one shot, usually in the buttocks, though the medication may be repeated every two to four hours as needed). Demerol does not usually interfere with the contractions or their work, though with larger doses the contractions may become less frequent or weaker. It may actually help normalize contractions in a uterus that is functioning erratically. Like other analgesics, Demerol is not generally administered until labor is well established and false labor has been ruled out, but no later than two to three hours before delivery is expected. A woman's reaction to the drug and the degree of pain relief achieved varies widely. Some women find it relaxes them and makes them better able to cope with contractions. Others very much dislike the drowsy feeling it imparts, find it doesn't relieve pain, and find they are actually less able to cope. Side effects may include, depending on a woman's sensitivity, nausea, vomiting,

depression, and a drop in blood pressure. The effect Demerol will have on the newborn depends on the total dose and how close to delivery it has been administered. If it has been given too close to delivery, the baby may be sleepy and unable to suck; less frequently, respiration may be depressed and supplemental oxygen may be required. The baby's heart rate may also be affected, and this may be noted with external fetal heart monitoring. Any effects on the newborn are generally short-term and, if necessary, can be treated. Demerol may also be given postpartum to relieve the pain of an episiotomy repair, removal of the placenta, or a cesarean.

Other medications for relief of pain in labor and delivery. The following are used less frequently than the methods listed above.

Tranquilizers. These drugs (such as Phenergan and Vistaril) are used to calm and relax an extremely anxious woman so that she can participate more fully in childbirth. Tranquilizers can also enhance the effectiveness of analgesics, such as Demerol. Like analgesics, tranquilizers are usually administered once labor is well established, and considerably before delivery. But they are occasionally used in early labor if a mother's anxiety is impeding the progress of her labor. Women's reactions to the effects of tranquilizers vary. Some welcome the gentle drowsiness; others find it interferes with their control. Dosage definitely makes a difference. A small dose may serve to relieve anxiety without impairing alertness. A larger dose may cause slurring of speech and dozing between contraction peaks, making it difficult to use prepared childbirth techniques. Though the risks to a fetus or newborn from tranquilizers are minimal, it's a good idea for you and your coach to try nondrug relaxation techniques (such as meditation, massage, hypnosis) before asking for or accepting such medication.

General anesthesia. Once the most popular pain relief for delivery, general anesthesia, which puts the patient to sleep very rapidly, is used today almost exclusively for emergency surgical births, when there is no time for a regional anesthetic to be administered. It may also occasionally be used for delivering the head in a vaginal breech.

Inhalants (such as those used for analgesic effect) are used to induce general anesthesia—often in conjunction with injected agents. This is done by an anesthesiologist in an operating/delivery room. The mother is awake during the preparations and unconscious for however long it takes to complete the delivery (usually a matter of minutes). When she comes to, she may be groggy, disoriented, and restless. She may also have a cough and sore throat (due to the endotracheal tube; see below), experience nausea and vomiting, and find her bowels and bladder sluggish. A temporary drop in blood pressure is another possible side effect.

The major problem with general anesthesia is that as the mother is sedated, so is the fetus. Sedation of the fetus can be minimized, however, by administering the anesthesia as close to the actual birth as possible. That way the baby can be delivered before the anesthetic has reached him or her in amounts large enough to have an effect. Administering oxygen to the mother and tilting her to the side (usually the left side) can also help get oxygen to the fetus, minimizing the drug's effect.

Though women in labor were once routinely told not to eat and to limit liquids when in active labor because of the risk of vomiting and aspiration of vomited material if they ended up with general anesthesia, many hospitals and birthing centers no longer require such fasting. That's because aspiration is extremely rare—a risk of perhaps 7 in 10 million. And some suspect that fasting may not be good for a laboring woman and her baby. If you do have general anesthesia, an endotracheal tube will be inserted through your mouth into your throat to prevent even this slight possibility of aspiration. You may be given oral antacids just prior to the procedure to neutralize the acids in your stomach in case you do aspirate.

Complementary and alternative medicine (CAM) for pain relief. There are more and more options available to those seeking a nonmedical route to labor and delivery pain relief. These are aimed at reducing the perception of pain without the use of drugs. They are particularly good choices for women who would prefer not to use drugs during labor and childbirth or who are in drug or alcohol recovery and should not use mood-altering analgesics or tranquilizers:

Hypnosis. Despite the somewhat disreputable image it has developed on the nightclub circuit, hypnosis, in qualified hands, provides a legitimate, medically acceptable—and often highly successful—route to pain relief. There's really nothing mysterious about clinical hypnosis. It doesn't put you in a trance or put you under the control of another person. You are not asleep or dazed—you're simply able to relax and focus on your own inner processes. It's much like the state you are in when absorbed in a good TV movie, so absorbed you don't hear your spouse when he asks a question. Such natural hypnotic states happen all the time.

The type of hypnosis used during childbirth employs suggestions and the power of the mind to control labor and delivery discomfort. With successful hypnosis, a very high level of suggestibility is achieved, which (depending on an individual's degree of susceptibility and the type of hypnosis used) can do anything from simply making the patient more relaxed and comfortable to completely eliminating awareness of pain. It's believed that about 15 percent of the population is highly suggestible to hypnosis, 25 percent are highly resistant, and the rest fall somewhere in between; a very small percentage can even go through an unmedicated cesarean section without feeling pain. Those who are good candidates for hypnosis are generally those who enjoy a certain amount of solitude, who have a long attention span, and who have a vivid imagination.

Training for the use of hypnosis for childbirth pain relief should take place under a professional certified in the method. Avoid anyone without medically approved credentials, since hypnosis can be misused. You may be trained in auto- or self-hypnosis, or you may depend on the practitioner to make the suggestions during labor. Training should begin weeks or months in advance of your due date. If it begins in the first trimester, it can even be used to minimize such pregnancy symptoms as morning sickness. For resources on hypnosis, see page 247.

TENS (Transcutaneous Electrical Nerve Stimulation). TENS uses electrodes to stimulate nerve pathways to the uterus and cervix. It's theorized that this stimulation jams other sensory inputs along those pathways, such as pain. The intensity of stimulation is controlled by the patient, allowing her to increase it during a contraction and reduce it between contractions. While there is no scientific evidence that TENS is effective in reducing labor pains, it does seem to work for some women. Some hospitals are making TENS available, and it may be worthwhile checking to see if yours is one of them.

Acupuncture. Long popular in China and becoming more and more popular in the United States, acupuncture probably works according to the same principles as TENS, but the stimulation is supplied by needles inserted and manip-

ulated through the skin. Some studies have found that acupuncture can reduce the need for other forms of pain relief during labor and delivery.

Physical therapy. Massage, heat, pressure, counterpressure, or reflexology administered by a health professional or a loving spouse or friend (who has been advised of what is safe and what is not during labor) often lessens the perception of pain. These techniques may be taught in some childbirth classes.

Hydrotherapy can also be very effective in minimizing pain, which is why many hospitals and birthing centers have Jacuzzi tubs available for laboring women to use.

Alteration of risk factors for increased pain perception. A number of factors, emotional and physical, can affect how a woman perceives the pain of childbirth. Altering them can often increase comfort during labor (see page 360).

Distraction. Anything—watching TV, listening to music, meditating, practicing breathing exercises—that takes your mind off the pain can decrease your perception of it. So can focusing on an object (an ultrasound picture of your baby, a soothing landscape, a photo of a favorite place) or doing visualization exercises (for example, picturing your baby being pushed gently by contractions, preparing to exit the uterus, excited and happy).

MAKING THE DECISION

Women have more options in childbirth today than ever before. And with the exception of certain emergency situations, the decision of whether or not to have medication during labor and delivery will be largely yours. To try to make the best possible decision for you and your baby, you should:

◆ Discuss the topic of pain relief and anesthesia with your practitioner long before labor begins. Your practitioner's expertise and experience make him or her an invaluable partner—though not usually the deciding vote—in the decision-making process. Well before your first contraction, find out what kinds of drugs or procedures he or she uses most often, what side effects may be experienced, when he or she considers medication absolutely necessary, and when the option is yours.

◆ Recognize that, although childbirth is a natural experience that many women can go through without medication, it is not supposed to be a trial by ordeal or a test of bravery, strength, or endurance. The pain of childbirth has been described as the most intense in the human experience. Medical technology has given women the option of relief. Not only is such relief acceptable, it is sometimes preferable.

◆ Keep in mind that childbirth medication (or any medication) entails both benefits and risks, and it should be used only when the benefits outweigh the risks. Become familiar with CAM approaches and consider using them first, if possible, or use them in conjunction with medication (which generally means you will need less medication).

◆ Don't make up and close your mind in advance. Though it's fine to theorize what might be best for you under certain circumstances, it's impossible to predict what kind of labor and delivery you'll have, how you will respond to the contractions, and whether or not you'll want, need, or have to have medication. Even if you are so concerned about pain that you are sure you will need an epidural, it's worth trying some CAM approaches first—your labor may turn out to be more manageable than you'd thought.

If during labor you feel you need medication, discuss it with your coach and the nurse or doctor. But don't insist on it immediately. Try holding out fifteen minutes or so and putting that time to the best possible use, concentrating extra hard on your relaxation or breathing techniques and taking in all the comfort your coach can give you. You may find that with a little more support you can handle the pain, or that the progress you make in those fifteen minutes gives you the will to go on without help. If after waiting you find that you need the relief as much or even more, feel guilt-free to ask for it. If your physician decides that you need medication immediately, however, for your sake or your baby's, waiting may not be advisable.

Most important of all, remember that your well-being and that of your baby, not some preconceived, idealized childbirth scenario, are your number one priority (as they have been all through pregnancy). All decisions should be made with that priority in mind.

Remember, too, that no matter how difficult your labor and delivery, once you hold that little bundle of joy in your arms, the memory of the misery will quickly fade.

◆ ◆ ◆

CHAPTER 12

The Eighth Month

Approximately 32 to 35 Weeks

In this next-to-last month, you may still be relishing every pregnant moment, or you may be increasingly weary of carting around a watermelon-size belly everywhere you go (not to mention sleeping with it). Either way, you're sure to be preoccupied with, and excited about, the much-anticipated event: your baby's birth. Of course, you and your partner are likely experiencing a little trepidation along with your excitement, especially if this is your first foray into parenthood. Talking those very normal feelings through, preferably with friends or family members who've preceded you into parenthood, will help you realize that everyone feels that way the first time around.

What You Can Expect at This Month's Checkups

After the 32nd week, your practitioner may ask you to come in every two weeks so your progress and your baby's can be more closely watched. You can expect the following to be checked, depending upon your particular needs and upon your practitioner's style of practice:[1]

- Weight and blood pressure
- Urine, for sugar and protein
- Fetal heartbeat
- Height of fundus (top of uterus)
- Size (you may get a rough weight estimate) and position of fetus, by palpation (feeling from the outside)
- Feet and hands for edema (swelling), and legs for varicose veins
- Group B strep test
- Symptoms you have been experiencing, especially unusual ones
- Questions and problems you want to discuss—have a list ready

1. See Appendix, page 545, for an explanation of the procedures and tests performed during office visits.

A LOOK INSIDE

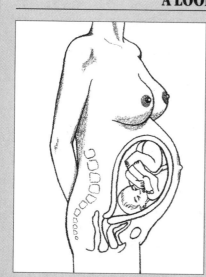

An interesting bit of pregnancy trivia: measurement in centimeters from the top of your pubic bone to the top of your uterus roughly correlates with the number of weeks you're up to; so, at 34 weeks, your uterus measures close to 34 centimeters from the pubic bone.

▶ *The fetus, at about 18 to 20 inches and 5 to 6 pounds (and gaining at a rate of ½ ounce a day), is looking plump and less wrinkly now as fat deposits fill out its adorable form; creases have formed around the wrists and neck, and the dimples you'll soon be kissing have started to appear on elbows and knees. With the uterine home increasingly cramped, baby has little room for gymnastics; you'll feel less vigorous kicking and more twisting and wiggling. Just like a newborn, the fetus will have regular periods of REM (or active sleep), deep sleep, active wakefulness, and quiet wakefulness. Brain growth continues at a fantastic clip. The lungs are approaching maturity, and a baby born now has an excellent chance of being completely healthy.*

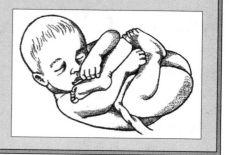

What You May Be Feeling

You may experience all of these symptoms at one time or another, or only a few of them. Some may have continued from last month, others may be new or hardly noticeable. You may also have other, less common, symptoms.

PHYSICALLY

- Strong, regular fetal activity
- Increasingly heavy whitish vaginal discharge (leukorrhea)
- Increased constipation
- Heartburn, indigestion, flatulence, bloating
- Occasional headaches, faintness, or dizziness
- Nasal congestion and occasional nosebleeds; ear stuffiness
- Bleeding gums
- Leg cramps
- Backache

- Pelvic pressure and/or achiness
- Mild swelling of ankles and feet, and occasionally of hands and face
- Varicose veins of legs
- Hemorrhoids
- Itchy abdomen
- Protruding navel
- Increasing shortness of breath as uterus crowds the lungs, which eases when the baby drops
- Difficulty sleeping
- Increasing "practice" (Braxton Hicks) contractions
- Increasing clumsiness

- Enlarged breasts
- Colostrum, either leaking or expressed, from nipples (though this premilk substance may not appear until after delivery)

EMOTIONALLY

- Increasing eagerness for the pregnancy to be over
- Apprehension about the baby's health, about labor and delivery
- Increasing absentmindedness
- Excitement—along with a little anxiety—at the realization that it won't be long now

What You May Be Concerned About

SHORTNESS OF BREATH

"Sometimes I have trouble breathing. Could this mean that my baby isn't getting enough oxygen?"

Shortness of breath doesn't mean you are short of oxygen, or that the baby is. Changes in the respiratory system during pregnancy actually allow women to take in *more* oxygen and to use it more efficiently. Still, most women experience varying degrees of difficulty breathing (some describe it as feeling a conscious need to breathe more deeply), particularly in the last trimester, when the expanding uterus presses against the diaphragm, crowding the lungs. Relief usually arrives when "lightening" occurs and the fetus settles down into the pelvis (in first pregnancies this generally occurs two to three weeks before delivery; see page 321). In the meantime, you may find it easier to breathe if you sit straight up instead of slumped over (which will

be easier on your back, too), sleep in a semi-propped-up position (with two or three pillows), and avoid overexertion.

Women who carry "low" throughout their pregnancies may never experience such exaggerated shortness of breath, and that's normal, too.

Shortness of breath that is severe, however, and is accompanied by rapid breathing, blueness of lips and fingertips, chest pain, and/or rapid pulse *isn't* normal and requires an immediate call to the doctor or trip to the emergency room.

BRAXTON HICKS CONTRACTIONS

"Every once in a while my uterus seems to bunch up and harden. What's going on?"

Practice, practice, practice. You are probably experiencing Braxton Hicks contractions, which usually begin to rehearse the pregnant uterus for labor sometime after the 20th week of pregnancy. These contractions are typically (though not always) felt earlier and are more intense in women who have had a previous pregnancy. In effect, your uterus is flexing its muscles, warming up in preparation for the real contractions, which will normally push your baby out at term. At first, you'll feel these practice contractions as a painless (but possibly uncomfortable) tightening of your uterus, beginning at the top and gradually spreading downward before relaxing. They usually last about fifteen to thirty seconds, but may last as long as two minutes or more.

As pregnancy draws to a close in the ninth month, Braxton Hicks contractions may become more frequent, intense, and sometimes even painful. Though they're not efficient enough to deliver your baby, Braxton Hicks contractions may get the prebirth processes of effacement and early dilation of the cervix started, thereby giving you a leg up on labor before it even begins.

To relieve any discomfort you may feel during these contractions, try changing your position—lying down and relaxing if you've been on your feet, or getting up and walking around if you've been sitting. You can also use this labor rehearsal to practice your breathing exercises and the various other childbirth techniques you've learned, which can make it easier to deal with the real contractions when they do arrive.

Though Braxton Hicks contractions are not true labor, they may be difficult for you to distinguish from the real thing (see About Prelabor, False Labor, Real Labor, page 334). They may also be difficult to differentiate from the kind of preterm uterine activity that precedes premature labor. So be sure to describe the contractions to your practitioner at your next visit. Report them immediately if they are very frequent (more than four per hour) and/or are accompanied by pain (back, abdominal, or pelvic) or by any kind of unusual vaginal discharge, or if you are at high risk for premature labor (see page 270).

NOT-SO-FUNNY RIB TICKLING

"It feels as though my son has his feet jammed up into my rib cage—and it really hurts."

In the later months, when fetuses run out of stretching room in their cramped quarters, the resourceful little creatures often do seem to find a snug niche for their feet between their mother's ribs, and that's one kind of rib tickling that *doesn't* tickle. Changing your own position may convince your baby to change his. A few Dromedary Droops (page 198) may dislodge him. Or try relocating him with this exercise: take a deep breath while you raise one arm over your head, then exhale while you drop your arm; repeat a few times with each arm.

If none of these tactics works, hang in there. When your little pain-in-the-ribs engages, or drops into your pelvis, which usually happens two or three weeks before delivery in first pregnancies (though not until labor begins in subsequent ones), he probably won't be able to reach his toes quite so high up.

STRESS INCONTINENCE

"I watched a funny movie last night and I seemed to be leaking urine every time I laughed. Is something wrong?"

In the last trimester, some women start to leak a little urine, usually only when they laugh (or cough, or sneeze, or are involved in strenuous activity). This is called stress incontinence, and is the result of the mounting pressure of the growing uterus on the bladder. Do make sure the leakage is urine, however, by giving it a sniff test; if it does not smell like urine, report it to your practitioner immediately, since there's a slight chance the leak is amniotic fluid. If you're certain it's urine you're leaking, mention the problem to your practitioner at the next visit.

In the meantime, these tips can help prevent or control stress incontinence to some degree:

◆ Avoid foods and beverages that could be bladder irritants, including coffee, other caffeinated beverages, citrus fruits and juices, tomatoes, spicy foods, carbonated drinks (including those that are sugar free), and alcohol in all forms.

◆ Do your Kegel exercises (see page 193) faithfully. These are useful for overcoming incontinence and are also helpful for firming up pelvic muscles for delivery and postpartum recovery. Since it may take weeks before you see an improvement, don't give up if you don't see results immediately. Just keep at it.

◆ Do Kegels or cross your legs when you feel a cough or sneeze coming on, or when you're about to do some heavy lifting.

◆ Take steps to avoid urinary tract infections (see page 453).

◆ Take steps to avoid constipation (see page 156), since impacted stool can put pressure on the bladder. Also, straining hard during bowel movements can weaken pelvic floor muscles.

◆ Keep your weight gain moderate. Excessive weight will only increase the pressure on your bladder.

Some women experience urge incontinence, the sudden, overwhelming need to urinate. If urge incontinence is plaguing you, try to alleviate the condition by training your bladder. Urinate more frequently—about every thirty minutes to an hour—so that you go before you feel that uncontrollable need. After a week, try to gradually extend the time between bathroom visits.

Remember to continue drinking at least eight glasses of fluids a day—even if you experience stress incontinence. Limiting your fluid intake will not help your bladder muscles keep the urine from leaking, and it may lead to urinary tract infections and/or dehydration.

BATHING

"My mother says I shouldn't take a bath this late in pregnancy. My doctor says it's okay. Who's right?"

This is one case where Mother, though well-intentioned, doesn't know best. It's likely that she is basing her warning on what her mother told her when she was pregnant with you. During grandma's time, you see, it was believed that dirty bathwater could travel up the vagina to the cervix late in pregnancy and cause an amniotic fluid infection.

But the tide has changed, putting pregnant women back in the bathwater. Today, it's believed that water does not enter the vagina unless it is forced, say from douching or jumping into a pool. Even if bathwater does enter the vagina, clinical studies have shown that the cervical mucous plug that seals the entrance to the uterus effectively protects the membranes that surround the fetus, the amniotic fluid, and the fetus itself from invading infectious organisms. Therefore, most practitioners permit tub baths in normal pregnancies. More and more allow—even encourage—baths in labor

LIFE-SAVING TESTS FOR NEWBORNS

Most babies are born healthy and stay that way. But a very small percentage of infants are born apparently healthy and then suddenly sicken. There are currently tests available for thirty neonatal (newborn) diseases, many of which are life-threatening if they aren't diagnosed and treated early on. There is an effort under way to push states to test for more of these illnesses, including PKU, congenital hypothyroidism, congenital adrenal hyperplasia, biotinidase deficiency, maple syrup urine disease, galactosemia, homocystinuria, and sickle-cell anemia.

In the meantime, if your state doesn't offer at least the core group of these tests, you can request that a private lab arrange testing. The lab will use blood that's collected in the hospital during your baby's routine heel-stick (when drops of blood are drawn from baby's heel after a quick stick with a needle).

In the very unlikely event your baby tests positive for any of the disorders, your baby's pediatrician and a genetic specialist can verify the results and begin treatment; early diagnosis and intervention can make a tremendous difference in the prognosis. Contact Baylor University Medical Center: 800-4BAYLOR (422-9567); www.baylor health.com/healthservices/metabolic/ (click on "Newborn Screening"); Mayo Medical Laboratories: www.mayoclinic. org/laboratorygenetics-rst/newborn screening.html; or Pediatrix Screening: 954-384-0175; www.pediatrixscreening.com.

(for hydrotherapy), and some will even deliver the baby underwater (see page 15). Just about everyone will okay showers right up to delivery.

Baths and showers, however, aren't totally risk free, particularly in the last trimester, when ungainliness can lead to slips and falls. To avoid such mishaps, bathe with care; be sure your tub or shower has a nonslip surface or use a slip-resistant mat; and have someone nearby, if possible, to help you in and out of the tub.

DRIVING

"I can barely fit behind the wheel. Should I still be driving?"

You can stay in the driver's seat as long as you fit there; moving the seat back and tilting the wheel up will help. Assuming you've got the room—and as long as you're not experiencing any dizzy spells or other symptoms that might interfere with the safe operation of your vehicle—driving short distances is fine up until delivery day.

Car trips lasting more than an hour, however, are probably too exhausting late in pregnancy, no matter who's driving. If you must take a longer trip, however, and have your practitioner's okay, be sure to shift around in your seat frequently and to stop every hour or two to get up and walk around. Doing Neck Relaxers and stretches (see pages 195, 201, and 202) may also keep you more comfortable.

Don't, however, try to drive yourself to the hospital while in labor. And don't forget the most important road rule: on any car trip, whether you are driver or passenger (and even if you're a passenger being driven to the hospital or birthing center in labor), fasten your seat belt.

GROUP B STREP

"My practitioner is going to test me for Group B strep infection. What does this mean?"

It means that your practitioner is playing it safe—and when it comes to Group B strep, safe is a very good way to play it.

Group B strep is a bacterium that can be found in the vaginas of healthy women. In carriers, it causes no harm. But in a newborn baby, who can pick it up while passing through the vagina during childbirth, Group B strep can cause very serious infection.

Since there are no symptoms in the Group B strep carrier, there's no way to tell whether an expectant mother has it unless she is tested. That's why many doctors now routinely test women between 35 and 37 weeks. (Testing done before 35 weeks isn't accurate in predicting who will be carrying GBS at the time of delivery.) If the test isn't offered, you can request it. Some doctors don't routinely test; instead they just treat women who arrive at the hospital in labor with certain risk factors (premature labor, membranes that have ruptured prematurely, or fever). Most doctors won't bother testing women who have previously delivered a baby with GBS; they'll proceed straight to treatment.

The GBS test is performed like a Pap smear, using a vaginal and rectal swab; women who test positive will be given IV antibiotics during labor. If GBS is detected in the urine, oral antibiotics will also be given in the last few weeks of pregnancy.

YOUR WEIGHT GAIN AND THE BABY'S SIZE

"I've gained so much weight that I'm afraid the baby will be very big and difficult to deliver."

Just because you've gained a lot of weight doesn't necessarily mean your baby has. There are many other variables, including genetics, your own birthweight (if you were born large, your baby is more likely to be, too), your prepregnancy weight (heavier women tend to have heavier babies), and the quality of the diet you've gained the weight on. Depending on those variables, a 35- to

40-pound weight gain can yield a 6- or 7-pound baby or a 25-pound weight gain can net an 8-pounder. On average, however, the more substantial the weight gain, the bigger the baby.

By palpating your abdomen and measuring the height of your fundus (the top of the uterus), your practitioner will be able to give you some idea of your baby's size, though such "guesstimates" can be off by a pound or more. An ultrasound may more accurately gauge size, but it may be off the mark, too.

Even if your baby is large, that doesn't automatically portend a difficult delivery. Though a 6- or 7-pound baby often makes its way out faster than an 8- or 9-pounder, most women are able to deliver a large baby vaginally and without complications. The determining factor, as in any delivery, is whether the baby's head (its largest part) can fit through the mother's pelvis.

Even if there is some suspicion of a mismatch between the fetal head and the mother's pelvis (cephalopelvic disproportion), the practitioner will allow the mother to go into labor naturally. This trial of labor is carefully monitored, and if baby's head descends and the cervix dilates at a normal rate, then the labor will be permitted to continue. If labor doesn't progress, it may, when appropriate, get a boost with the administration of oxytocin. If progress still isn't being made, a cesarean will usually be performed.

YOUR SIZE AND YOUR DELIVERY

"I'm five feet tall and very petite. I'm afraid I'll have trouble delivering a baby."

Fortunately, when it comes to giving birth, it's what's inside, not what's outside, that counts. The size and shape of your pelvis in relation to the size of your baby's head is what determines how difficult your labor will be. And you can't always judge a pelvis by its cover. A short, slight woman can have a roomier pelvis than a tall, stocky woman. Your practitioner can make an educated guess about its size, usually using rough measurements taken at your first prenatal exam. If there's some concern that your baby's head is too large to fit through your pelvis while you're in labor, ultrasound may be used to evaluate that possibility.

Of course, in general, the overall size of the pelvis, as of all bony structures, is smaller in people of smaller stature. For example, Asian women usually have smaller pelvises than women of Nordic descent. Luckily nature, in its wisdom, rarely presents an Asian woman with a Nordic-size baby—even when the father is a six-foot fullback. Instead, newborns are usually fairly well matched to the size of their mothers.

CARRYING BABY, EIGHTH MONTH

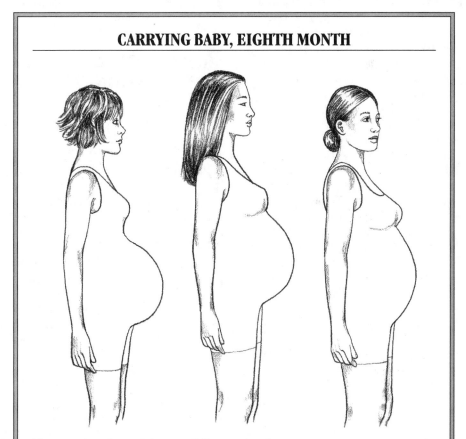

These are just three of the very different ways that a woman may carry near the end of her eighth month. The variations are even greater than earlier in pregnancy. Depending on the size and position of your baby, as well as your own size and weight gain, you may be carrying higher, lower, bigger, smaller, wider, or more compactly.

HOW YOU'RE CARRYING

"Everyone says I seem to be carrying small and low for the eighth month. Could it be that my baby isn't growing properly?"

It would be a good idea to make earplugs and blinders a part of every pregnant woman's maternity wardrobe. Wearing them for nine months would enable her to avoid the worry generated by the misguided commentary and advice of relatives, friends, and even strangers, and prevent invidious comparisons of her belly to those of other pregnant women who are larger, smaller, lower, or higher.

Just as no two prepregnant figures are proportioned in precisely the same way, no two pregnant silhouettes are identical. How you carry, both in size and shape, depends on a wide range of factors, including your prepregnancy profile (whether you started out tall or short, thin or not-so-thin, petite or voluptuous), how much weight you've gained, and what kind of diet you've gained it on. How you look on the outside is seldom an indication of the size of that precious cargo you're carrying on the inside. A petite woman carrying low and small may give birth to a larger infant than a bigger-boned woman carrying high and wide.

The only accurate assessments of your baby's progress and well-being are likely to come from your practitioner. When you're not in his or her office, keep your earplugs in and your blinders on, and you'll have a lot less to worry about.

"Everyone says I'm having a boy, because I'm all belly and no hips. I know that's probably an old wives' tale, but is there any truth to it at all?"

Predictions about the baby's sex—by old wives or others—have about a 50 percent chance of coming true. (Actually, a little better than that if a boy is predicted, since 105 boys are born for every 100 girls.) Good odds if you're placing a bet in Las Vegas; not necessarily good odds if you're basing your nursery paint selection on it.

That goes for "boy if you're carrying up front, girl if you're carrying wide," "girls make your nose grow, boys don't," and every other prediction not made from the pages of a baby's genetics report or from an ultrasound.

PRESENTATION AND POSITION OF THE BABY

"How can I tell if my baby is lying the right way for delivery?"

Playing "name that bump" (trying to figure out which are shoulders, elbows, bottom) may be better evening entertainment than TV, but it's not the most accurate way of determining your baby's position. Your practitioner can probably get a better idea than you, by palpating your abdomen with the flat of his or her trained hands for recognizable baby parts. The baby's back, for instance, is usually a smooth, convex contour opposite a bunch of little irregularities, which are the "small parts"—hands, feet, elbows. In the eighth month, the head has usually settled near your pelvis; it is round, firm, and when pushed down bounces back without the rest of the body moving. The baby's bottom is a less regular shape, and softer, than the head. The location of the baby's heartbeat is another clue to its position; if the presentation is headfirst, the heartbeat will usually be heard in the lower half of your abdomen; it will be loudest if the baby's back is toward your front. If there's any doubt about the position, ultrasound may be used for verification.

"My sister had a breech baby. Does that mean I might, too?"

There doesn't seem to be any genetic connection to a breech presentation. Though the causes of such a presentation are not fully understood, there are some factors that are known to increase the possibility that your baby will try to arrive bottom or feet first.

Breeches are more common when:

◆ The fetus is smaller than average or premature and not cradled snugly in the uterus

◆ There is more than one fetus

◆ The uterus is unusually shaped or contains fibroids, or is relatively relaxed because of having been stretched during previous pregnancies

◆ There is too much or too little amniotic fluid

◆ The placenta partly or fully covers the cervical opening (see Placenta Previa, page 505)

The vast majority of babies eventually settle into a head-down (vertex) presentation. Some of those who don't make this move on their own can be coaxed into position (see below). If your baby does turn out to be one of the 3 to 4 percent still in breech position at term, you should discuss the delivery possibilities with your practitioner—preferably *before* you go into labor.

"If my baby is breech, can anything be done to turn it?"

It's never too early to *prepare* yourself for the possibility of a breech birth, but it's definitely too early now to *resign*

yourself to one. Most babies settle into a head-down position between the 32nd and 36th weeks, but a few keep their parents and doctors guessing until only a few days before delivery.

The most frequently used and medically conventional approach to turning a fetus to a head-down position is external cephalic version (ECV), in which a physician attempts, with ultrasound guidance, to gently shift the fetus by applying his or her hands to the mother's abdomen. The condition of the fetus must be monitored continuously to be sure that the umbilical cord isn't accidentally compressed or the placenta disturbed. The procedure is best performed in the hospital before labor begins or very early in labor, when the uterus is still relatively relaxed. The more relaxed the uterus is, in fact, the more likely ECV is to be successful (which is why ECV works better in second and subsequent pregnancies than in first). Researchers are looking into the possibility that giving an epidural to women undergoing ECV may also increase the chances that the procedure will successfully turn their babies. Once turned, most fetuses stay head down, but a few do revert to breech before delivery.

When successful (as it is more than half the time), ECV can reduce the likelihood that a cesarean delivery will be necessary. For this reason ECV has become popular, with a majority of physicians using it at least occasionally. Some, however, still hesitate to use it because of the possibility of complications. Certainly, only a physician who has been trained to do ECV—and is prepared to do an emergency c-section if a problem arises—should attempt it.

Some nurse-midwives recommend doing exercises designed to encourage a breech baby to turn during the last eight weeks of pregnancy. Such exercises include Pelvic Tilts (page 194) or getting into the knee-chest position for twenty minutes, three times a day: kneel on your knees, keeping them slightly apart, and bend way over so your breasts touch the floor and your belly almost does. There's no medical proof that these exercises work, but there's also none to suggest that they do any harm. Some complementary and alternative medicine practitioners suggest moxibustion, a form of acupuncture plus heat, to help turn a breech baby.

"My doctor says the baby is in a breech position. How will this affect my labor and delivery?"

What is the best way to deliver a baby who ends up in a breech presentation come delivery day? At this point, the jury is still out, and no one can say definitively whether a vaginal delivery is better than a surgical one or vice-versa, though the most recent study seemed to give cesareans the edge. The vaginal route is believed to be perfectly safe in about one-third to one-half of breech births, but *only* if the doctor is experienced in the proper procedure for such deliveries (ask your practitioner if he or she performs vaginal breech deliveries and what his or her success rate is). Some studies of vaginal breech deliveries show that the potential added risk is not always from the delivery itself, but from the reason for the breech: for example, the baby is premature or undersize, there are multiple fetuses, or there is some other congenital problem.

Some physicians routinely perform

HOW DOES YOUR BABY LIE?

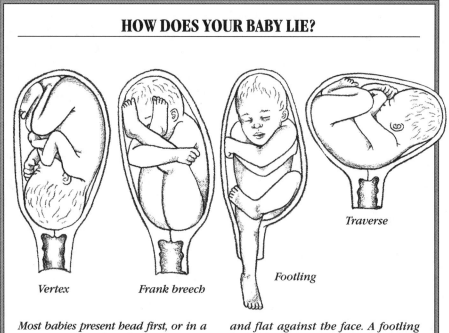

Vertex   *Frank breech*   *Footling*   *Traverse*

Most babies present head first, or in a vertex position. Breech presentations can come in many forms. A frank breech is when the baby is buttocks first, with his or her legs facing straight up and flat against the face. A footling breech is when one or both of the baby's legs are pointing down. A traverse position is when the baby is lying sideways in the uterus.

cesarean sections for breech presentation, believing, as the latest studies show, that this is the safest for the baby. Others are persuaded by their own experience that, under most circumstances, the way a breech baby is delivered doesn't affect the outcome. They will permit a trial of labor (in which labor that begins spontaneously is allowed to continue as long as it progresses normally) in breech deliveries, under the following conditions, some of which may be determined by ultrasound viewing:

◆ The baby is a frank breech (the legs are folded flat up against the face).

◆ The baby appears to be small enough (usually under 8½ pounds) for easy passage, but not so small (under 5½ pounds) that a vaginal delivery would be risky. Usually, breech babies under 36 weeks are delivered by cesarean.

◆ There is no evidence of placenta previa, prolapsed umbilical cord, or fetal distress that can't be easily remedied.

◆ The mother is ready and able to work hard during delivery, has no obstetrical or medical problem that could complicate a vaginal delivery, appears to have an adequate-size pelvis, and has no history of previous difficult or traumatic deliveries. Some physicians add the requirement that the mother be under thirty-five.

◆ The presenting part is engaged (has descended into the pelvis) as labor begins.

◆ The fetal head is not hyperextended (with the chin tipped back and pointed upward), but rather the chin is tucked down toward the chest.

◆ Everything (and everyone) is in readiness for an emergency surgical delivery should one suddenly become necessary.

When a vaginal delivery is to be attempted, labor is carefully monitored in a surgically equipped delivery suite. If all goes well, and the cervix is widening and the baby moving steadily down, labor is allowed to continue. If the cervix dilates too slowly or if other problems arise, the doctor and surgical team will perform a cesarean section in a matter of minutes. Continuous electronic fetal monitoring is absolutely essential to be sure the baby is doing well. Sometimes an epidural is administered to prevent the mother from bearing down too hard before she is fully dilated (which might lead to the cord being compressed between the baby and the pelvis). Occasionally, general anesthesia is administered to the mother when the baby is halfway delivered, to allow the baby to be delivered more quickly. Forceps may be used to keep the head properly flexed, and to help deliver it without pulling too much on the body or neck. A wide episiotomy is often routinely made to facilitate the entire process.

If the requirements for a trial of labor are not met or if, for any other reason, it is decided that a vaginal birth would be risky, a cesarean will be scheduled. Sometimes, however, labor begins before the assigned date and labor progresses so quickly that the baby's buttocks slip into the pelvis before surgery is begun. In that case, most doctors will attempt a vaginal delivery rather than a rushed and difficult cesarean.

The bottom line if your baby remains bottom down: you'll need to be flexible in your labor and delivery plans and prepared for any eventuality. Though the chances are good that you will be able to have a normal vaginal delivery, depending on various conditions,

BEST MEDICINE FOR LABOR?

Think three's a crowd? For many couples, not when it comes to labor and delivery. More and more are opting to share their birth experience with a doula, a woman trained as a labor companion. And for good reason. Recent studies show women who are supported by doulas are much less likely to require cesarean or forceps deliveries, induction, and pain relief. Births attended by doulas may also be shorter, with a lower rate of complications.

What exactly can a doula do for you? That depends on the doula you choose, at what point in your pregnancy you hire her, as well as on your preferences. Some doulas will become involved well before that first contraction strikes, helping with the design of a birthing plan, offering recommendations, and easing prelabor jitters. Many, on request, will come to the house to help a couple through early labor. Once at the hospital or birthing center, the doula takes on a variety of roles, again depending on the couple's needs

and wishes. Typically, her primary role is to offer continuous emotional and physical support and soothing and encouraging words during labor, as well as help with relaxation techniques and breathing exercises, advice on labor positions, massage, hand holding, pillow plumping, and bed adjusting. A doula can also serve as a mediator and an advocate, ready to speak for the laboring couple as needed, to translate medical terms and explain procedures, and to generally run interference with hospital personnel. She can offer information, too, and insight, which can be invaluable to first-time parents. She won't take the place of a coach (and a good doula won't make him feel like she's taking his place, either) or of the nurse on duty; instead, she will augment their support and services (especially important if the nurse assigned to you has several other patients in labor at the same time or if labor is long and nurses come and go as shifts change). She will also likely be the only person (besides the coach) who will

---

you may indeed end up having a cesarean. And, in fact, this is an eventuality that every pregnant woman should be prepared for anyway (see page 298).

TWIN LABOR AND DELIVERY

"I'm expecting twins. How will my labor and delivery be different from that of other women?"

There may not be any differences, other than the fact that you'll reap twice the reward for your efforts. Many twin deliveries turn out to be normal, vaginal, and uncomplicated.[2] Another

perk: twins tend to be quicker to deliver than single babies. Though active labor and the pushing phase are usually longer, the first phase is typically shorter, which means less total time from the first contraction to last push.

However, it's not surprising that there is more potential for complications during the delivery of twins, and that more precautions are routinely taken. Though most twins can be delivered vaginally (sometimes with the use of forceps to avoid putting the babies, who are often smaller than average, through excessive trauma), it is usually recommended that an anesthesiologist be on hand in case a cesarean becomes necessary. A pediatrician or a neonatologist usually stands by, too, ready to deal with any immediate problems in the newborns. Both fetuses may be monitored during labor, one ex-

---

2. With each increase in the number of fetuses, however, the likelihood of a surgical delivery increases.

stay by the laboring woman's side throughout labor and delivery—a friendly and familiar face from start to finish. And many doulas don't stop there. They can also offer support and advice postpartum on everything from breastfeeding to baby care.

Though an expectant father may fear that hiring a doula will relegate him to third wheel status, this isn't the case. A good doula is also there to help the coach relax so he can help his partner relax. She'll be there to answer questions he might not feel comfortable broaching with a doctor or nurse. She'll be there to provide an extra set of hands (most fathers only have one set) when the mother-to-be needs her legs and back massaged at the same time, or when she needs both a refill on ice chips and help breathing through a contraction. She'll be an obliging and cooperative member of their labor team—ready to pitch in, but not to push him aside and take over.

How do you locate a doula? Many birthing centers and hospitals keep lists of doulas, and so do some practitioners. Ask friends who've recently used a doula for recommendations, or check on-line for local doulas. Once you've tracked down a candidate, arrange a consultation before you hire her to make sure both of you are comfortable with her. Ask her about her experience, her training, what she will do and what she won't do, what her philosophies are about childbirth (if you're planning on asking for an epidural, for instance, you won't want to hire a doula who discourages the use of pain relief), whether she will be on call at all times and who covers for her if she isn't, whether she provides pregnancy and/or postpartum services, and what her fees are. For more information or to locate a doula in your area, contact Doulas of North America: (206) 324-5440; www.dona.com.

An alternative to a doula, which could also be beneficial, is a female friend or relative who has gone through pregnancy and delivery herself and with whom you feel totally comfortable. The plus there: her services will be free. The drawback: she probably won't be quite as knowledgeable.

ternally and the other internally, with a scalp electrode (see page 347).

With twins, as you will soon find out, you can always expect the unexpected. And these surprises can start at delivery. Because there is more than one baby, and possibly more than one set of circumstances, there may be more than one type of delivery. For instance (assuming the twins are dwelling in separate sacs), the first infant's amniotic sac may rupture spontaneously, but the other twin's may have to be ruptured artificially. Or the first baby might arrive easily via the vaginal route, but the second, lying crosswise and unturnable, might have to be delivered with a cesarean.

In most vaginal deliveries, the second twin comes along within twenty minutes of its sibling—though occasionally the wait is much longer. If number two is a slowpoke, the physician may administer oxytocin or use forceps to speed up delivery, or may perform a cesarean. If the second baby is in a breech position, the physician might have to reach into the uterus and turn it headfirst. Once both twins are born, the placenta or placentas usually separate, and can be delivered quickly. But sometimes placental delivery is slow and requires some help from the physician.

"I'm carrying twins and I've been hearing a lot about twins arriving prematurely. Is this true?"

Yes, twins do tend to arrive earlier than singletons. After all, as cozy as it can be for your little ones in the uterus, it can also get pretty crowded as they grow. Though there's nothing you can do about your babies' cramped conditions, there's plenty you—and your doctor—can do to try to delay that early arrival (see pages 167 and 270). Keep in mind, however, that since the ideal term for twins may be 37 weeks, delivering three weeks early is probably not early at all for twins.

TRIPLET DELIVERY

Does carrying triplets mean I absolutely will have a cesarean?

Three may be a crowd, but that crowd can exit vaginally under certain conditions. Cesarean is most often used for triplet delivery, but some recent studies indicate that a vaginal delivery can be an option if triplet A (the one nearest the "exit") is in a head-down presentation, fetal monitoring is possible, and there are no other obstetrical contraindications (such as preeclampsia in the mother or fetal distress in one or more of the babies). In some cases, the first baby or the first and second may be delivered vaginally, and the final one may require a cesarean. Of course, more important than having all three of your babies exit vaginally is having all four of you leaving the delivery room in good condition. Any route to that outcome should be considered a successful one.

CESAREAN SECTION

"My doctor just told me I might have to have a cesarean. Are cesareans more dangerous than vaginal births?"

Though popular lore has it that the cesarean section got its name because Julius Caesar came into the world via his mother's abdomen, that's virtually impossible. In those days, delivering a baby surgically was apparently invariably fatal for the mother. So though Julius might have survived such an operation, his mother wouldn't have—and it is known that Mrs. Caesar lived for many years after his birth.

Today, however, cesareans are nearly as safe as vaginal deliveries for the mother, and in difficult deliveries or when there's fetal distress, they are often the safest delivery mode for the baby. Even though it is technically considered major surgery, a cesarean carries relatively minor risks—closer to those of a tonsillectomy than of a gallbladder operation, for instance—that can generally be treated easily.

Cesareans aren't inherently dangerous for the baby, either. In fact, when a surgical delivery is truly *necessary,* the baby is at least as safe, and often safer,

HOSPITALS AND CESAREAN RATES

Cesarean rates vary from hospital to hospital. Though major medical centers often have very high rates because they do a lot of high-risk deliveries, when these high-risk births are adjusted for, these hospitals, equipped with staff obstetricians and neonatal intensive care units, generally have relatively low rates of cesarean deliveries. And, in fact, a fully staffed hospital can take a wait-and-see attitude. Some small community hospitals have higher rates because they don't have around-the-clock staff able to perform emergency cesareans at any hour. So if there's any suspicion that a vaginal delivery might not succeed or that an emergency might arise, the anesthesiologist and others needed for a surgical delivery may be called in to perform a cesarean before it is certain that it is needed. Discuss with your practitioner the cesarean rate at the hospital you've chosen, and ask whether there are any special procedures in place to discourage unnecessary cesarean deliveries.

MAKING THE CESAREAN BIRTH A FAMILY AFFAIR

Family-centered cesarean birth is becoming more commonplace across the country, with the vast majority of practitioners and hospitals relaxing the old "wait in the waiting room" rules for cesarean deliveries. During a nonemergency cesarean, most now make it possible for the mother to be awake, the father to be in attendance, and the new family to get to know each other in the period just after birth, just as they would after an uncomplicated vaginal delivery. Studies show that this "normalizing" of surgical delivery helps couples feel better about the experience, reduces the possibility of postpartum depression and low self-esteem in the mother, and allows the bonding process to begin sooner.

arriving that way rather than through the vaginal route. Every year thousands of babies who might not have survived the journey through the birth canal (or might have survived impaired) are lifted from an incision in their mothers' abdomens sound and unscathed.

In most ways, babies delivered via cesarean don't differ from those delivered vaginally, though cesarean babies do have the edge in initial appearance. Because they don't have to accommodate to the narrow confines of the pelvis, they usually have nicely rounded, not pointy, heads. Apgar scores, which rate an infant's condition one and five minutes after birth, are comparable in babies born vaginally and those born by cesarean. Cesarean-born babies do have the slight disadvantage of not having some of the excess mucus squeezed out of their respiratory tracts in the birthing process, but this mucus can be easily suctioned after delivery. Though minor lacerations do occasionally occur during a surgical delivery, especially when the baby is in a breech position or the membranes are already ruptured, only very, very rarely is any serious damage sustained by a baby during cesarean delivery—much more rarely than during vaginal deliveries.

Occasionally a mother who has had a cesarean will harbor feelings that can temporarily interfere with the establishment of bonding: she may feel resentment toward the baby who deprived her of the birth experience she had been looking forward to and brought such insult to her body.[3] She may feel jealousy toward mothers who've delivered "naturally." She may even feel guilty for what she perceives as "failing" at the job of birthing. Or she may incorrectly assume that the cesarean-born infant is unusually fragile (few are) and become overprotective. All of these feelings can be harmful, and can prevent a new mother from enjoying and bonding with her new baby early on. If they occur, it is important to confront and resolve them, seeking professional help if necessary.

But often you can avoid such negative attitudes right from the start—even before labor begins. First, by recognizing that the method by which a baby is delivered in no way reflects on either you or your child. Second, by making sure that if a surgical delivery becomes necessary, it interferes with parent-baby bonding as little as possible. Long before you go into labor, let your doctor know that if you have a cesarean you would like to be able to hold or even nurse the baby on

---

3. Women who deliver vaginally may also resent their babies, almost always temporarily, because of the pain of delivery.

the operating table or, if that's not possible, in the recovery room. Detail your wishes in your birthing plan, too, if you have one (see page 274). If you wait until delivery day to state your case, you may not have the strength or opportunity to make it. Planning ahead for this possibility also gives you the chance to question contrary hospital rules, such as those requiring every cesarean-delivered newborn, even healthy ones, to spend some time in the neonatal intensive care unit. If you present a strong argument in a rational, calm way, you may be able to effect a change in, or an exception to, such rules.

If, good intentions notwithstanding, you turn out to be too tired to participate in any serious mother-baby bonding right after delivery (and many women are, whether they've had abdominal or vaginal deliveries), or if your baby needs to be observed or cared for in the neonatal intensive care unit for a while, don't worry. There is no evidence that bonding must begin immediately after birth (see page 392).

"I've always wanted a completely natural birth experience, but I'm worried I'll end up needing a cesarean."

If cesareans are so safe, and sometimes lifesaving, why do most pregnant women dread the prospect of having one? Partly because major surgery, even when it's routine and very low-risk, is still scary. But mostly because, though most expectant mothers spend months preparing for natural childbirth, many don't prepare at all for the very real possibility that they'll have a surgical delivery instead. They devour childbirth primers but bypass the chapters on cesarean section. They ask dozens of questions about natural delivery in childbirth class but hesitate to ask one about surgical birth. They look forward to holding their spouse's hand as they pant and push their baby into the world—not to lying passively, and possibly unconscious, as sterile instruments extract the baby. When suddenly faced with a cesarean, they feel deprived of control over the birth of their baby and of the birth experience they'd planned for. Occasionally, feelings of frustration, disappointment, anger, and guilt are ushered in along with the medical technology, marring the delivery and the postpartum period.

But that's not how it has to be. Several steps taken now can make the prospect of a cesarean less ominous. Even if you have no reason to believe that you might end up needing a cesarean, learning all you can about cesarean sections before delivery—from your practitioner, in your childbirth class (which should include cesareans in its curriculum), and through reading—will help to prepare you and to ease your fears. If you do have some reason to believe a cesarean section might be necessary, do even more homework; if you can find one, take a full preparatory class in cesareans.

Becoming educated about cesarean sections has another benefit, too. It will allow you, assuming an emergency situation doesn't exist, to have an informed dialogue with your practitioner should he or she recommend a surgical delivery, either before labor begins or while it's in progress.

Whether you're preparing for a scheduled cesarean or just for the possibility of one, there are also a number of issues you might want to talk over in advance of labor with your doctor or the physician your nurse-midwife is affiliated with. Don't be put off by assurances that you aren't likely to need a cesarean; explain that you want to be prepared, just in case. Let the doctor know that you would like to be part of the decision-making team (if time allows) should a cesarean seem necessary.

Of course, most pregnant women would not select a cesarean as their delivery of choice, and almost 4 out of 5 will end up delivering vaginally. But for those who don't, there's no reason for disappointment or feelings of guilt or failure. Any delivery (vaginal or abdominal, medicated or unmedicated) that yields a healthy mother and baby is an unqualified success.

"Why are cesarean rates so high these days?"

Does it seem like everybody (and their sister . . . and their neighbor) is having a c-section these days? That's because cesarean rates in the U.S. are at an all time high. Over 27 percent of women can expect to have a surgical delivery now, and if the past few years are any indication of future trends, you can expect those numbers to continue climbing. This upswing has reversed a downward trend that brought the c-section rate down to a low of 20 percent in the mid 1990s, as many practitioners (and hospitals) pushed hard to limit the number of cesareans performed, with expectant moms urging them on.

Many factors contribute to these soaring cesarean rates, which many would argue are much too high.

Changes in obstetrical practice. First of all, cesarean delivery has become an extremely quick and safe option—and in most instances mothers can be awake and alert during their baby's surgical birth. Second, the fetal monitor, and a variety of other tests, can more accurately (though not infallibly) indicate when a fetus is in trouble and needs to be delivered in a hurry. Third, with more expectant mothers exceeding the recommended weight gain of 25 to 35 pounds, more large babies, who may be more difficult to deliver vaginally, are arriving. Then there is the trend toward noninterventionist obstetrics. Though letting nature set its own pace, rather than hurrying it by rupturing membranes, using oxytocin, or employing forceps, often allows for a more natural birth, it can also result in stalled labors, which can lead to cesareans. In addition, there are the increasing ranks of older women and others with chronic medical problems who are now able to have successful pregnancies but are more likely to require cesarean deliveries. Finally, a major factor in the burgeoning cesarean rate is the repeat cesarean. Though VBAC (vaginal birth after cesarean) is still considered a viable option, fewer doctors and hospitals are allowing women to try one and more are scheduling surgeries over a trial of labor, for a variety of reasons (see page 27).

Physician preparation and attitude. Though there had been an overall effort in the medical community to reduce the numbers of unnecessary cesareans, the system is obviously still far from perfect. For instance, a physician inadequately trained to read the fetal monitor may decide to do a cesarean the instant a negative reading is picked up on the monitor (without double-checking to be sure the baby, and not the fetal monitor, is in trouble). Or a malpractice-shy physician may perform a cesarean to cover him- or herself when a vaginal delivery shows even the slightest potential for problems. (More lawsuits against obstetricians are instituted for *not* performing a cesarean—and consequently getting a bad result—than for performing one.)

Maternal attitude. Since cesareans are so safe, and can prevent the pain of labor and possible injury during vaginal delivery (small though the risk is), some women (particularly those who've had one before) prefer them to vaginal deliveries and actually request them.

Safety of mother and/or baby. Most doctors perform cesareans not for convenience, or for money, or for fear of malpractice, but because they believe, as some studies show, that in certain circumstances a surgical delivery is the best way to protect either the mother or the baby.

In spite of the many legitimate reasons for cesareans, there is general agreement in the medical community that a significant number of unnecessary cesareans are presently being performed. In an effort to shift the cesarean trend back toward the downswing, many experts and women's groups, as well as some insurers, medical groups, and other individuals are encouraging that women and their practitioners:

◆ Ask for a second opinion, when feasible, before a c-section is performed

◆ Push hard for the hospital and doctor to allow a VBAC (see page 27) assuming the conditions are right

◆ Have greater patience with a slow labor and/or a long pushing phase, especially in women who received epidurals, assuming mother and baby are doing well, before resorting to surgery

◆ Better train physicians in interpretation of fetal monitor readings, so that surgery won't be performed unnecessarily

◆ Use a variety of more reliable techniques (such as fetal scalp stimulation, scalp electrodes, biophysical profile, or acoustical stimulation; see page 324) to confirm any fetal distress suggested by readings on a fetal monitor

◆ Consult (either in person or by faxing results) with other experts when fetal monitor results are ambiguous and the condition of the fetus is questionable

◆ Institute a peer review system, wherein all first-time cesareans are carefully studied afterwards on a case-by-case basis and doctors found to be doing unnecessary cesareans face disciplinary action

◆ Have a doula (see page 296) or one-on-one nursing care on hand during labor. This probably reduces the risk of a surgical delivery by helping a laboring woman to become more fully relaxed, thus enabling her to work more efficiently with her contractions

◆ Better train medical residents in VBAC, external cephalic version (ECV, to turn breech babies), the vaginal delivery of breech babies, and the use of forceps or vacuum extraction

"Do you generally know in advance that you are going to have a cesarean, or is it usually last minute?"

M ost women won't know whether or not they will have a cesarean until they are well into labor. Occasionally, however, a cesarean may be scheduled before labor begins, if the indications are clear. The most common of these include:

◆ A previous cesarean (see page 26), if the reason for it still exists and can't be surmounted (maternal disease or an abnormally shaped pelvis, for example)

◆ A previous cesarean with a classical vertical uterine incision, which could rupture during delivery, rather than a low horizontal one. The type of incision made in the uterus has no relationship to the type of incision made in the abdomen—so if you don't know for sure, it may be necessary to contact the doctor who performed the original surgery or to check your old medical records to learn the kind of incision that was made.

♦ Induction of labor in a woman who has previously had a cesarean (see page 27)

♦ A fetal illness or abnormality that makes labor and vaginal delivery unacceptably risky or traumatic (not all fetal illnesses do)

♦ Maternal diabetes, in cases where preterm delivery is deemed necessary and it is found that the cervix is not ripe enough for the induction of labor

♦ Other maternal illness (including heart disease and respiratory disorders), if the physician determines a vaginal delivery would be risky

♦ HIV infection in the mother (page 39), which can be passed on to the fetus during vaginal birth

♦ An *active* herpes infection (page 36), especially a primary one, if there is evidence of cervical or genital lesions, and if active external lesions cannot be covered and isolated from the field of vaginal delivery

♦ Placenta previa (when the placenta partially or completely blocks the cervical opening; see page 505), since labor can cause such a placenta to detach prematurely, which could result in hemorrhage

♦ Abruptio placenta (page 516), when there is an extensive separation of the placenta from the uterine wall and the fetus is in danger if not delivered immediately

♦ Probable cephalopelvic disproportion (when a fetus's head is believed too large to pass through its mother's

pelvis; see page 369), suggested either by the size of the baby on ultrasound examination and the size of the pelvis as seen on X ray or CT scan or MRI pelvimetry, or by a previous difficult delivery. Though either the ultrasound on the baby or the pelvimetry test alone doesn't adequately predict a problem, the two tests combined (known as the "fetal pelvic index") do. Other indications that point to the possibility, but not the certainty, of a cesarean:

♦ Maternal hypertension (page 476) or kidney disease, if it appears the mother may be unable to tolerate the stress of labor

♦ Unusual fetal presentation, such as a feet-first (footling) breech or a transverse (crosswise, with the shoulder first) presentation, which can make a vaginal delivery difficult or impossible (see page 292)

♦ Maternal obesity or diabetes

Cesareans may also be scheduled before labor begins when prompt delivery is necessary and either there is no time to induce labor or it is believed that mother and/or baby will be unable to tolerate its stresses. Any of the following might necessitate such a delivery:

♦ Preeclampsia or eclampsia (page 500) that doesn't respond to treatment

♦ A postmature fetus (two or more weeks overdue; see page 324) when the uterine environment has begun to deteriorate

♦ Fetal or maternal distress, due to any cause

In most cases, however, it isn't until active labor that the possible need for a

CESAREAN QUESTIONS TO DISCUSS
WITH YOUR DOCTOR

◆ When labor isn't progressing, will it be possible, assuming it isn't an emergency situation, to try other alternatives before a cesarean is resorted to—for example, oxytocin to stimulate contractions, or squatting to make pushing more effective?

◆ If the fetal monitor suggests the baby may be in trouble, will other tests be used to verify the monitor readings before a cesarean is decided upon? Will it be possible, time permitting, to get a second opinion?

◆ If the reason for the proposed cesarean is a breech presentation, will trying to turn the baby in the uterus (using external cephalic version or another technique; page 293) be tried first?

◆ What kinds of anesthesia might be used? A general anesthesia, which puts you to sleep, is occasionally necessary when time is of the essence, but epidural or spinal anesthesia is usually safer and will allow you to remain awake during a nonemergency abdominal delivery. (See About Childbirth Medication, page 276.)

◆ Will a low transverse incision in the uterus be used whenever possible, so that a vaginal delivery can be attempted next time around? You may also want to know, for cosmetic reasons, if the abdominal incision (which is unrelated to that in the uterus) will be a low, or "bikini," one.

◆ Can your coach be present if you are awake? If you are asleep?

◆ Can your nurse-midwife (if you have one) or doula be with you, too?

◆ Will you and your spouse be able to hold the baby immediately after birth (if you are awake and all is well), and will you be able to nurse in the recovery room? If you're asleep, will your spouse be able to hold the baby?

◆ If the baby doesn't need special care, can he or she room in with you?

◆ After an uncomplicated cesarean birth, how much recovery time will you need both in and out of the hospital? What physical discomforts and limitations can you expect to experience?

cesarean becomes apparent. Then the most likely reasons include:

◆ Failure of labor to progress (the cervix hasn't dilated quickly enough) after 16 to 18 hours (some practitioners will wait longer), or a prolonged pushing stage, especially when the baby and/or mother are not doing well. In most cases, physicians will try to give sluggish contractions a boost with oxytocin before resorting to a cesarean.

◆ Fetal distress signaled by the fetal monitor or other tests of fetal well-being (see page 347)

◆ A prolapsed umbilical cord (page 521), which if compressed could cut off oxygen to the fetus, causing fetal distress

◆ A ruptured uterus, which could be fatal to the fetus if immediate surgical delivery isn't performed

◆ Previously undiagnosed case of placenta previa or abruptio placenta, particularly if there is a risk of excessive bleeding

If your practitioner says that a cesarean section will be necessary in your case, ask for a detailed explanation of the reasons. Ask, too, if any alternatives are open to you. Depending on the set of circumstances, a trial of labor is often possible. If you come away from your consultation uncomfortable about the reason given for the cesarean, you should ask for, and get, another opinion. Different doctors sometimes follow different protocols when it comes to planned surgical deliveries.

YOUR SAFETY DURING CHILDBIRTH

"I know medical science has taken most of the risk out of giving birth, but I'm still afraid of dying during delivery, which my grandmother did when my mom was born."

There was a time when mothers routinely risked their lives to have children; they still do in many parts of the world. In the United States today, however, the risk to a mother's life in labor and delivery is minuscule, particularly among healthy women who receive regular prenatal care.

In short, even if your pregnancy falls into the highest-risk category—and certainly if it doesn't—you're worrying without reason. Labor and delivery have never been safer for mothers and babies.

BANKING YOUR OWN BLOOD

"I'm worried about the possibility of needing a transfusion during delivery and receiving contaminated blood. Can I store my own blood beforehand?"

First of all, there is very little likelihood you will need a blood transfusion. A woman typically doesn't lose enough blood during a vaginal or cesarean birth to cause a problem, since in pregnancy blood volume is up 40 to 50 percent anyway. Second, the risk of contracting HIV or hepatitis C (the diseases most commonly transmitted through the blood) from a transfusion in the United States today is very low since all donated blood is screened by some very accurate tests. Third, because facilities for autologous (self) blood donations are expensive and priority is given to those about to undergo major high-risk surgery, women who are about to deliver may not even be accepted for such a donation.

If, however, you have reason to believe that you may be at high risk for blood loss during delivery, you can speak to your doctor about the possibility of making an autologous blood donation—but be aware that donating the blood late in pregnancy could pose a problem because it could excessively lower your blood volume or lead to anemia. Or you can plan to have a relative or friend with compatible blood make a directed donation (one to a specific person, namely you) prior to delivery. Keep in mind, however, that not every hospital is equipped for or willing to oblige with directed donations, and that the risk of contracting HIV or hepatitis C from a blood transfusion isn't any lower when the donation is from a friend or family member than when it's from the general blood supply. If the blood hasn't gone through a screening process, the risk may be higher.

To reduce the risk of excessive blood loss during delivery, take precautions during the last trimester by avoiding consumption of any substance that can increase bleeding (most of which are not recommended for use in pregnancy anyway). These include aspirin and any over-the-counter or prescribed medication containing aspirin (read labels carefully or check with your practitioner); ibuprofen (and products containing it); vitamin E (beyond that in your prenatal supplement); ginkgo biloba (an herbal preparation); and medications (such as cough syrups) containing alcohol.

If your opposition to receiving blood transfusions from others is based on religious beliefs or other intractable reasons, then discuss the issue with your practitioner now—don't wait until you are ready to go into labor. Some hospitals and some physicians use techniques that make "bloodless" surgery safer.

TRAVEL SAFETY

"I may have to make an important business trip this month. Is it safe for me to travel this late in pregnancy, or should I cancel?"

B efore you schedule your trip, schedule a call or visit to your practitioner. Different practitioners have differing points of view on the matter of travel in the last trimester. Whether yours will encourage you or discourage you from hitting the road—or the rails or the skies—at this point in your pregnancy will probably depend on that point of view, as well as on several other factors. First and most important is the kind of pregnancy you've been having; you're more likely to get the green light if it has been uncomplicated. How far along you are (most practitioners advise against flying after the 36th week) and whether you are at any increased risk at all for premature labor will also weigh into the recommendation. Second, and also very important, is how you've been feeling. Pregnancy symptoms that multiply as the months pass also tend to

multiply as the miles pass; traveling can lead to increased backache and fatigue, aggravated varicose veins and hemorrhoids, and added emotional and physical stress. Other considerations include how far and for how long you will be traveling (and how long you will actually be in transit), how demanding the trip will be physically and emotionally, as well as how necessary the trip is (optional trips or trips that can be easily postponed until well after delivery may not be worth making now). If you're traveling by air, you'll also need to factor in the restrictions—if any—of the airline you choose. Some will not let you travel in the ninth month without a letter from your practitioner affirming that you are not in imminent danger of going into labor while in flight; others are more lenient.

If your practitioner gives you the go-ahead, there are still plenty of other arrangements you'll need to make besides the travel ones. See page 223 for tips to ensure happy (and safer, and more comfortable) trails for the pregnant you. Getting plenty of rest will be especially important. But most critical this late in the game will be making sure you have the name, phone number, and address of a recommended obstetrician or nurse-midwife (and the hospital or birthing center he or she delivers at) at your destination—one, of course, whose services will be covered by your insurance plan should you end up requiring them.[4] If you're traveling a long distance, you may also want to consider the possibility of bringing along your spouse; on the remote chance that if you do end up going into labor at your destination, at least you won't have to deliver without him.

---

4. If your insurer will not cover such emergency care, it would be prudent to get medical travel insurance.

RELATIONSHIP WITH YOUR SPOUSE

"The baby isn't even born yet, and already my relationship with my husband seems to be changing. We're both so wrapped up in the upcoming birth and the baby, instead of in each other, the way we used to be."

All spousal relationships, to differing degrees, undergo some alterations in dynamics and a reshuffling of priorities after baby makes three, but studies show that the shock of this upheaval is usually less stressful if the couple begins the process during pregnancy. So, though the change you're noticing in your relationship may not seem like a change for the better, it's one you're better off experiencing now, rather than after your baby is born. Couples who overly romanticize the notion of a cozy threesome, and who don't anticipate at least some disruption of romance, often find the reality of life with a demanding newborn harder to deal with.

But while it's very normal—and healthy—to be wrapped up in the pregnancy and your expected extra-special delivery, you shouldn't let this new facet of your life *completely* block out the others, especially the most important one: your relationship. Now is the time to learn to combine the care and feeding of your baby with the care and feeding of your marriage. Regularly reinforce romance. At least once a week, do something together—see a movie, have dinner out, visit some galleries—that has nothing to do with childbirth or babies. While you're layette shopping, stop in the men's department and buy a little something special (and unexpected) for your husband. When you leave the practitioner's office after your next visit, pull out a pair of tickets for a show your spouse is eager to see or a sports event you know he'd love to attend. At dinner spend at least some time asking about his day, talking about yours, discussing the day's headlines—all without indulging in baby talk even once. Bring massage oil to bed now and then, and rub each other the right way; even if you're not in the mood for sex, this kind of touching can keep you close. None of this flame fanning will make the upcoming wonderful event any less special, but it will remind you both that there's more to life than Lamaze and layettes.

Keeping this in mind now will make it easier to keep the love light burning later, when you're taking turns walking the floor at 2 A.M. And that love light is, after all, what will make the cozy nest you're busily preparing for your baby a bright, happy, and secure one. (Tips to fan the flame postpartum can be found in *What to Expect the First Year*.)

MAKING LOVE NOW

"I'm confused. I hear a lot of conflicting information about sexual intercourse in the last weeks of pregnancy."

The problem is that existing medical evidence on the subject is confusing and conflicting. It is widely believed that neither intercourse nor orgasm alone precipitates labor unless conditions are ripe (though many impatient-to-deliver couples have enjoyed trying to prove otherwise). For that reason, most physicians and midwives allow patients with normal pregnancies to make love, assuming they're still interested, right up until delivery day. And most couples apparently can do so without any problems arising, so to speak.

Even though a recent study discounted the long-held theory that sex late in pregnancy can increase the risk of premature delivery for those at *high risk,* some practitioners still prescribe last-trimester abstinence for such women, just to be on the safe side. Another safety measure that has been suggested—and some practitioners recommend this to all couples, regardless of risk—is the use of condoms in the last eight weeks of pregnancy. It appears that condoms can effectively prevent possible infection during intercourse, as well as keep the irritant prostaglandins in semen from triggering premature contractions.

Ease your confusion by checking with your practitioner to see what the latest medical consensus is. If you get a green light, then by all means make love—if you want to and feel comfortable about it. If the light is red (and it probably will be if you are at high risk for premature delivery, have placenta previa or abruptio, are experiencing unexplained bleeding, or if your membranes have ruptured), then foster intimacy in other ways. Try a romantic rendezvous at a candlelit restaurant or walking hand-in-hand under the stars. Or an evening at home, cuddling under an afghan in front of the TV, or soaping each other in the shower. Or use massage as the medium. And while that kind of sublimation may not quite satisfy, try to remember that you have a whole lifetime of lovemaking ahead (though the pickings may continue to be slim in that department at least until baby's sleeping through the night).

What It's Important to Know:
ABOUT BREASTFEEDING

Before the twentieth century, nearly every baby was fed at the breast; there was no other choice. But in the early 1900s, women began to demand rights they'd never had—to vote, to work, to smoke cigarettes, to let down or bob their hair, to peel off confining undergarments, and to set their sights outside the kitchen and the nursery. Breastfeeding was old-fashioned, it was restricting, and it represented all that women sought freedom from. It was considered not only a form of slavery, but the feeding style of the poor, who couldn't afford to buy the ingredients to prepare formula. To the modern middle-class woman, bottle-feeding was the best thing since store-bought sliced bread.

Ironically, it was the revitalized women's movement of the 1960s and '70s that brought breastfeeding back into vogue. Women wanted not only freedom but control—control of their lives and control of their bodies. They knew that control was gained through knowledge, and knowledge told them that breastfeeding was best for their babies and, on the whole, for themselves. Today breastfeeding rates are rising higher still, particularly among those who are familiar with its many benefits.

WHY BREAST IS BEST

There is no question that under normal circumstances, breastfeeding is best for your baby. It provides the perfect food and the perfect food delivery system. The known benefits of human breast milk are many:

It's custom made. Tailored to the needs of human infants, breast milk contains at least 100 ingredients that are not found in cow's milk and that cannot be precisely duplicated in commercial formulas. Breast milk is individualized for each infant; raw materials are selected from the mother's bloodstream as needed, altering the milk's composition from day to day, feeding to feeding, as the baby grows and changes. The nutrients are matched to an infant's needs and its ability to handle them. For example, breast milk contains one-third the mineral salts of high-sodium cow's milk, making it easier for a baby's kidneys to handle. It also contains less phosphorus than cow's milk; the higher phosphorus content of cow's milk is linked to a decreased calcium level in the formula-fed infant's blood.

It goes down easily. The proportion of protein in mother's milk is lower (1.5 percent) than in cow's milk (3.5 percent), making it more digestible. The protein itself is mostly lactalbumin, which is more nutritious and digestible than the major protein component of cow's milk, caseinogen. The amount of fat in the two milks is similar, but the fat in mother's milk is more easily broken down and used by the baby. Infants also have an easier time absorbing the important micronutrients in breast milk than in cow's milk (in which the nutrients are designed to be absorbed by the young calf).

It's safe. You can be sure that the milk served up directly from your breast isn't improperly prepared, contaminated, or spoiled.[5]

It's a tummy soother. Nursed babies are almost never constipated, because of the easier digestibility of breast milk. They

also rarely have diarrhea, since breast milk seems both to destroy some diarrhea-causing organisms and to encourage the growth of beneficial flora in the digestive tract, which further discourage digestive upset. On a purely esthetic note, the bowel movements of a breastfed baby are sweeter-smelling (at least until solids are introduced) and less apt to cause diaper rash.

It's a fat flattener. Not only is breastfeeding less likely to cause overweight infants, but having been nursed as a baby appears to be related to lower rates of obesity later in life. It may also be linked to lower cholesterol readings in adulthood.

It's a brain booster. Breastfeeding appears to slightly increase a child's IQ at least through age fifteen. This may not only be related to the brain-building fatty acids (DHA) it contains, but to the closeness and mother-baby interaction that is built into breastfeeding (which fosters intellectual development).

It keeps allergies on hold. Virtually no baby is allergic to breast milk (though some can have allergic reactions to a certain food or foods in their mothers' diets, including cow's milk). On the other hand, beta-lactoglobulin, a substance contained in cow's milk, can trigger an allergic response, with a variety of possible symptoms ranging from mild to severe. Soy milk formulas, which are often substituted when an infant is allergic to cow's milk, stray even further in composition from what nature intended, and can also cause an allergic reaction. Studies also show that breastfed infants are less likely to get childhood asthma than those babies fed formula.

It's an infection preventer. Not only are breastfed babies less subject to diarrhea, but also to lower respiratory

---

5. As long as you don't have any disease that contraindicates breastfeeding.

infection, urinary tract infections, ear infections, and septicemia (an infection of the blood)[6] in the first year of life. Protection is partially provided by the transfer of immune factors in breast milk and in the premilk substance, colostrum. Breastfeeding also appears to somewhat lower the risk for childhood leukemia. And it improves the immune response to immunizations for most diseases (such as tetanus, diphtheria, and polio).

It builds stronger mouths. Because nursing at the breast requires more effort than sucking on a bottle, breastfeeding encourages optimum development of jaws, teeth, and palate. Also, recent studies show that babies who are breastfed are less likely to get cavities later on in childhood than those who are not.

There are benefits from breastfeeding for you, the mother, as well:

Convenience. Breastfeeding requires no advance planning or packing, no equipment; it is always available (at the park, on an airplane, in the middle of the night), at just the right temperature. Thanks to the fact that nursing in public has become more accepted and more common, you and your baby, with a little discretion and a big napkin, can dine at the same restaurant table. When you and baby aren't together (if you work outside the home, for instance), milk may be expressed in advance and stored in the freezer for bottle feedings as needed.

Economy. There are no bottles, nipples, or formula to buy; there are no half-emptied bottles or opened cans of formula

to waste. There is also a saving in terms of health care costs. Whether you pay them yourself, or your health care insurer does, treating the additional illnesses that may be more likely to strike the average formula-fed baby can cost plenty.

Speedy recovery. Breastfeeding helps speed the shrinking of the uterus back to its prepregnant size and decreases the flow of lochia (the postpartum vaginal discharge), which means less blood loss. It also enforces rest periods for the new mother—particularly important, as you will discover, during the first six postpartum weeks.

Speedy return to prepregnancy shape. Nursing can help burn off the fat accumulated during pregnancy. If you are careful to consume only enough calories to keep your milk supply and energy up (see page 404), and make certain that all those calories come from nutritious foods, you can fill all of your infant's nutritional needs while recovering your own figure.

Period postponement. Breastfeeding suppresses ovulation and menstruation, at least to some degree. Though it shouldn't be relied on for birth control, it may postpone resumption of your periods for several months at least, as long as you are breastfeeding exclusively.

Bone building. Nursing can improve mineralization in your bones after weaning and reduces the risk of hip fracture after menopause, assuming you're taking in enough calcium to fill your needs and milk-making requirements.

Cancer risk reduction. Feeding your baby via the breast can reduce your risk of some cancers down the road. Women who breastfeed have a lower risk of developing uterine cancer and premenopausal breast cancer.

---

6. There are a number of studies that suggest that a very wide range of diseases may be lower in breastfed children, including bacterial meningitis, botulism, necrotizing enterocolitis, SIDS, diabetes, Crohn's disease, ulcerative colitis, lymphoma, and other chronic digestive diseases.

The biggest and best bonus. Breast-feeding brings you and your baby together, skin to skin, eye to eye, *at least* six to eight times a day. The emotional gratification, the intimacy, the sharing of love and pleasure, can not only be very fulfilling and make for a strong mother-child relationship, but it may also enhance your baby's brain development. (A note to mothers of twins: all the advantages of breastfeeding are doubled for you. See page 408 for tips that can make breastfeeding easier.)

For more information on breast-feeding, contact your local La Leche League or call (800) La-Leche (525-3243). Or reach them on the Web at www.laleche.org.

WHY SOME PREFER THE BOTTLE

There are women today who choose not to nurse. And though the advantages of bottle-feeding seem to be dwarfed by those of breastfeeding, they can be real and convincing for some women.

More shared responsibility. Bottle-feeding allows the father to share the feeding responsibilities and its bonding benefits more easily. (Although the father of a breastfed baby can derive the same benefits, assuming his baby will take a bottle at all, by feeding a bottle of expressed mother's milk and getting involved in other baby-care activities, such as bathing and rocking.)

More freedom. Bottle-feeding doesn't tie the mother down to her baby. She's able to work outside the home without worrying about pumping and storing milk, travel a few days without the baby, even sleep through the night—because someone else can feed her baby. (Of course, these options are also open to

---

THE BREAST: SEXUAL OR PRACTICAL?

Or can it be both? If you think about it, having two or even more roles in life is not unusual—even roles that are very different, that require different skills and different attitudes (lover and mother, for example). You can look at the different roles of the breast—one sexual and one practical—in the same way: each is important, neither is mutually exclusive. In deciding whether or not to breastfeed, keep this in mind.

---

breastfeeding moms who express milk or supplement with formula.)

Potentially, more romance. Bottle-feeding doesn't interfere with a couple's sex life (except when baby wakes up for a feeding at the wrong time). Breast-feeding, on the other hand, can. First, because lactation hormones can keep the vagina relatively dry (though vaginal lubricants can remedy the problem); and second, because leaky breasts during lovemaking are a turnoff to some couples. For bottle-feeding couples, the breasts can play their strictly sensual role rather than their utilitarian one.

Fewer dietary constraints. Bottle-feeding doesn't dictate your diet or cramp your eating style. You can eat all the spicy foods and cabbage you want (though many babies don't object to these tastes in breast milk, and some actually relish them), you don't have to limit your intake of milk products if your baby can't handle them, you can have a daily glass of wine or a cocktail, and you don't have to worry about as many nutritional requirements.

Less embarrassment for the modest. If you're uncomfortable about the intimate contact with your infant that breastfeeding requires and about the possibility of nursing in public, breast-feeding may be hard to imagine. These hangups, though, are often quickly hung up; many women who opt to try breast-feeding soon find it becomes second nature, even in the most public places.

Less stress. Some women feel they are too impatient or tense by nature to breastfeed. If they give it a try, however, some find (once breastfeeding is well established) that nursing is actually very relaxing and surprisingly easy.

MAKING THE CHOICE TO BREASTFEED

For more and more women today, the choice is clear. Some know they will opt for breast over bottle long before they even decide to become pregnant. Others, who never gave it much thought before pregnancy, choose breastfeeding once they've read up on its many bene-fits. Some women teeter on the brink of indecision right through pregnancy and even delivery. A few women, convinced that nursing isn't for them, still can't shake the nagging feeling that they ought to do it anyway.

For all undecided women, here's a suggestion: try it—you may like it. You can always quit if you don't, but at least you will have eased those nagging doubts. Best of all, you and your baby will have reaped some of the most im-portant benefits of breastfeeding, if only for a brief time.

But do be sure to give breastfeed-ing a fair trial. The first few weeks can be challenging, even for the most ardent breastfeeders, and are always a learning process on both sides of the breast. A full month, or even six weeks, of nursing is generally needed to establish a

SMOKING AND BREASTFEEDING?

Nicotine does pass into the breast milk, so if you smoke and want to breastfeed, the best thing you can do for you and your baby is to quit smoking. If you can't quit (it's tough, but it can be done; see page 61), then you should still opt for breastfeeding, since it pro-tects your baby to some extent from some of the dangers of secondhand smoke. But you can further reduce the risk of your smoking to your baby by:

◆ Cutting back and smoking fewer cigarettes

◆ Smoking lower-nicotine brands

◆ Feeding your baby at least ninety-five minutes after your last ciga-rette, so that there will be little or no nicotine in your breast milk when your baby latches on

◆ Not smoking when you nurse; better still, never smoking in your child's presence. (Smoking around your baby can greatly increase the risk of respiratory problems and SIDS.)

successful feeding relationship and to give a mother time to decide whether she's comfortable with it or not.

MIXING BREAST AND BOTTLE

Some women who choose to breast-feed find—for one reason or an-other—that they can't or don't want to do it exclusively. Maybe exclusive breast-feeding doesn't turn out to be practical in the context of their lifestyle (too many business trips away from home, or a job that otherwise makes pumping a logistical nightmare). Maybe it proves to be too difficult (they suffer from multiple breast infections or from a chronic shortage of milk). Fortunately, neither breastfeeding nor bottle-feeding is an all-or-nothing proposition—and for some women, combining the two is a compromise that works. If you choose to do the combo, keep in mind that you'll need to wait until breastfeeding is well established (at least two to three weeks, but preferably five or six) before introducing formula. For more information on combining breast and bottle, see *What to Expect the First Year.*

WHEN YOU CAN'T OR SHOULDN'T BREASTFEED

Unfortunately, the option of breastfeeding isn't open to every new mother. Some women can't or shouldn't nurse their newborns. The reasons may be emotional or physical, due to the mother's health or the baby's, temporary (in which case breastfeeding can sometimes begin later on) or long-term. The most common maternal factors that *may* prevent or interfere with breastfeeding include:

◆ Serious debilitating illness (such as cardiac or kidney impairment, or severe anemia) or extreme underweight—though some women manage to overcome the obstacles and breastfeed their babies.

◆ Serious infection, such as active untreated tuberculosis (after two weeks of treatment, breastfeeding should be okay); in the meantime, breasts can be pumped (and milk discarded) so a supply will be established once breastfeeding begins.

◆ Chronic conditions that require medications that pass into the breast milk and might be harmful to the baby, such as antithyroid, anticancer, or antihypertensive drugs or mood-altering drugs, such as lithium, tranquilizers, or sedatives. If you take any kind of medication, check with your physician before beginning breastfeeding. In some cases, a change of medication or spacing of doses may make breastfeeding possible.[7]

◆ Exposure to certain toxic chemicals in the workplace; check with OSHA (see page 77) for specific information.

◆ AIDS, or HIV infection, which can be transmitted via body fluids, including breast milk.

◆ Drug abuse—including the use of tranquilizers, cocaine, heroin, methadone, marijuana, or the abuse of alcohol (an occasional drink is okay).[8]

◆ A deep-seated aversion to the idea of breastfeeding. (But again, some women who feel this way change their minds once they hold their babies to the breast. Talking to other women who also felt uncomfortable before deciding to give breastfeeding a try may help, too.)

Some conditions in the newborn may make breastfeeding difficult, but not

---

7. A temporary need for medication, such as penicillin, even at the time you begin nursing, does not eliminate the chances of your breastfeeding. Women who need antibiotics during labor or due to a breast infection (mastitis) can continue to breastfeed while on the medication.

8. But be aware that when a mother has had alcohol, her baby gets less milk and generally sleeps less well. To minimize these problems, avoid breastfeeding for at least two hours after having an alcoholic drink.

A LITTLE SUPPORT GOES A LONG WAY

It only takes two to breastfeed, but it often takes three to make it happen. A recent study showed that when fathers are supportive of breastfeeding, moms are likely to try that approach 96 percent of the time; when they are ambivalent, only about 26 percent give it a try. Fathers: *take note!*

(with the right medical support) impossible. They include:

♦ Disorders such as lactose intolerance or phenylketonuria (PKU), in which neither human *nor* cow's milk can be digested. In the case of PKU, babies can be breastfed if they also receive supplemental phenylalanine-free formula; with lactose intolerance (which is extremely rare at birth), mother's milk can be treated with lactase to make it digestible.

♦ Cleft lip and/or cleft palate, and other mouth deformities that interfere with sucking. Though the success of breastfeeding depends somewhat on the type of defect, with special help, nursing is usually possible.

Very rarely, there are no contraindications to breastfeeding, but it just doesn't work—no matter how hard mother and baby work at it. The milk supply isn't adequate, perhaps because of insufficient glandular tissue in the breast.

If you end up not being able to nurse your baby—even if you very much wanted to—there's no reason to add guilt or feelings of inadequacy to your disappointment. In fact, it's important that you don't, to avoid letting those feelings interfere with the very important process of getting to know and love your baby (a process that by no means must include breastfeeding). Instead, put those feelings aside, pick up the bottle (and your baby), and read on.

BOTTLE-FEEDING WITH LOVE

Though breastfeeding is a good experience for both mother and child, there is no reason why bottle-feeding can't be, too. Millions of happy, healthy babies have been raised on the bottle. When you can't, or don't wish to, breastfeed, the danger lies not in the bottle, but in the possibility that you might communicate any frustration or guilt you feel to your baby. Know that, with but a little extra effort, love can be passed from mother to child through the bottle as well as through the breast. Make every feeding a time to cuddle your baby, just as you would if you were nursing (don't prop the bottle and let your baby feed alone in a crib or infant seat). And when it's practical, make skin-to-skin contact by opening your shirt and letting the baby rest against your bare breast while suckling on the bottle.

♦ ♦ ♦

The Ninth Month

Approximately 36 to 40 Weeks

Finally. The month you've been waiting for and working toward (and possibly, worrying about just a little bit) since that pregnancy test came back positive is here at last. Chances are you're at once very ready (To hold that baby! To see my toes again! To sleep on my stomach!) and not ready at all. Yet despite the inevitable flurry of activity (more practitioner appointments, a layette to shop for, projects to finish at work, paint colors to pick for baby's room), you may find that the ninth month seems like the longest month of all. Except, of course, if you don't deliver by your due date. In that case, alas, it's the tenth month that's the longest.

What You Can Expect at This Month's Checkups

You'll be spending more time than ever at your practitioner's office this month (stock up on some good waiting-room reading), with appointments scheduled weekly. These visits will be more interesting—the practitioner will estimate baby's size and may even venture a prediction about how close you are to delivery—with the excitement growing as you approach D day. In general, you can expect your practitioner to check the following, though there may be variations, depending upon your particular needs and upon your practitioner's style of practice:[1]

◆ Your weight (gain generally slows down or stops)

◆ Your blood pressure (it may be slightly higher than it was at midpregnancy)

◆ Your urine, for sugar and protein

◆ Your feet and hands for edema (swelling), and legs for varicose veins

---

1. See Appendix, page 545, for an explanation of the procedures and tests performed.

- Your cervix (the neck of your uterus), by internal examination, to see if effacement (thinning) and dilation (opening) have begun; if there's suspicion of infection, a culture may be done

- The height of the fundus

- The fetal heartbeat

- Fetal size (you may get a rough weight estimate), presentation (head or buttocks first), position (front or rear facing), and descent (is presenting part engaged) by palpation (feeling with the hands)[2]

- Questions and problems you want to discuss, particularly those related to labor and delivery—have a list ready. Include frequency and duration of Braxton Hicks contractions, if you've noted any, and other symptoms you have been experiencing, especially unusual ones.

You can also expect to receive a labor and delivery protocol (when to call if you think you are in labor, when to plan on heading to the hospital or birthing center) from your practitioner; if you don't, be sure to ask for these instructions.

What You May Be Feeling

You may experience all of these symptoms at one time or another, or only a few of them. Some may have continued from last month, others may be new. Still others may hardly be noticed because you are used to them and/or because they are eclipsed by new and more exciting signs indicating that labor may not be far off.

PHYSICALLY

- Changes in fetal activity (more squirming and less kicking, as the fetus has progressively less room to move around)

- Vaginal discharge (leukorrhea) becomes heavier and contains more mucus, which may be streaked red with blood or tinged brown or pink after intercourse or a pelvic exam or as your cervix begins to dilate

- Constipation

- Heartburn, indigestion, flatulence, bloating

- Occasional headaches, faintness, dizziness

- Nasal congestion and occasional nosebleeds; ear stuffiness

- Bleeding gums

- Leg cramps at night

- Increased backache and heaviness

- Buttock and pelvic discomfort and achiness

- Increased swelling of ankles and feet, and occasionally of hands and face

- Itchy abdomen, protruding navel

- Varicose veins of the legs

- Hemorrhoids

- Easier breathing after the baby drops

- More frequent urination after the baby drops, putting pressure on the bladder once again

- Increased difficulty sleeping

---

2. If these can't be determined by palpation, the practitioner may order an ultrasound.

- More frequent and more intense Braxton Hicks contractions (some may be painful)
- Increasing clumsiness and difficulty getting around
- Colostrum, either leaking or expressable from nipples (though this premilk substance may not appear until after delivery)
- Fatigue or extra energy (nesting syndrome), or alternating periods of each
- Increase in appetite, or loss of appetite

EMOTIONALLY

- More excitement, more anxiety, more apprehension, more absent-mindedness
- Relief that you're almost there
- Irritability and oversensitivity (especially with people who keep saying: "Are you *still* around?")
- Impatience and restlessness
- Dreaming and fantasizing about the baby

A LOOK INSIDE

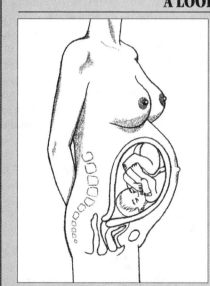

▲ *Your uterus is right under your ribs now—and your measurements aren't really changing that much from week to week anymore; the top of your uterus is around 38 to 40 centimeters from the top of your pubic bone. Your weight gain slows down or even stops as D day approaches. Your abdominal skin is stretched as far as you think it can go, and you're probably waddling more now than ever, possibly because the baby has dropped in anticipation of impending labor.*

▼ *Baby's gearing up to make a move. Halfway through this month, he or she will officially be considered "full term" and ready to be born. During the month, growth continues to be rapid, with about 2 inches and 2½ pounds being added; at birth, body fat will have increased to about 15 percent. At this point, your baby has pretty much run out of kicking space, but it's still important to keep track of those squirms and wiggles. Most babies have settled into a head-down birthing position in the ninth month; many babies of first-timers will "drop" into the mother's bony pelvis (which serves as the starting gate for labor and delivery) by about 38 weeks. In their last month of service, the umbilical cord has now grown to over 2 feet in length and the placenta weighs in at about a pound and a half.*

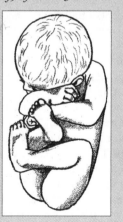

What You May Be Concerned About

CHANGES IN FETAL MOVEMENTS

"My baby used to kick so vigorously, and I can still feel him moving, but he seems less active now."

When you first heard from your baby, way back in the fourth or fifth month, there was ample room in the uterus for acrobatics, and lots of kicking and punching. Now that conditions are getting a little cramped, his gymnastics are curtailed. In this uterine straitjacket, there is room for little more than turning, twisting, and wiggling. And once the head is firmly engaged in the pelvis, baby will be even less mobile. It's not important what kind of fetal movement you feel at this stage, as long as you note activity every day. If, however, you feel *no* activity (see below) or a sudden spurt of very panicky activity, check with your practitioner.

"I've hardly felt the baby kick at all this afternoon. Should I be alarmed?"

It could be that your baby has settled down for a nap (fetuses, like newborns, have periodic interludes of deep sleep) or that you've been too busy or too active to notice any movements. For reassurance, check for activity in a more formal way, by performing the test on page 243. It's a good idea to repeat this test routinely a couple of times each day throughout the last trimester. Ten or more movements during each test period mean that your baby's activity level is normal. Fewer suggests that medical evaluation might be necessary to determine the cause of the inactivity—so contact your practitioner at once if that's the case. Though a baby who is relatively inactive in the womb can be perfectly healthy, inactivity at this point sometimes indicates fetal distress. Picking up this distress early and taking steps to intervene medically can often prevent serious consequences.

"I've read that fetal movements are supposed to slow down as delivery approaches. My baby seems more active than ever. Could that mean he's going to be hyperactive?"

Before birth is too soon to start worrying about hyperactivity. Studies show that fetuses who are very active in the womb are no more likely than quieter fetuses to be hyperactive in childhood, though they may well turn out to be very active children.

Research also contradicts the notion that the average fetus becomes lazy just before delivery. In late pregnancy, there is generally a gradual decline in the number of movements (from about 25 to 40 an hour at 30 weeks to 20 to 30 at term), probably related to tighter quarters, a decrease in amniotic fluid, and improved fetal coordination. But unless you're counting every single movement, you're not likely to notice a significant difference.

URINARY FREQUENCY—AGAIN

"During the last few days, it seems like I'm in the bathroom constantly. Is it normal to be urinating this frequently now?"

It sounds like you're being revisited by your old friend, urinary frequency. Though many women urinate frequently throughout pregnancy, this annoying symptom is most common and most pronounced when there is pressure on the bladder. This happens early in pregnancy, when the uterus is still low in the pelvic

CHOOSING A PEDIATRICIAN

Choosing a pediatrician (or a family practitioner) is one of the most important decisions you'll make as a parent—and actually, you shouldn't wait until you become a parent to make it. Sifting through your choices and making your selection now, before your baby starts crying at 3 A.M., will ensure that your transition to parenthood will be that much easier. It will also allow for an informed—not hasty—decision.

If you're not sure where to begin your search, ask your practitioner (if you've been content with him or her) or friends, neighbors, or co-workers who have young children for recommendations. Or contact the hospital or birthing center where you'll be delivering (you can call the labor and delivery floor or pediatrics, and ask a nurse on duty for some suggestions; no one gets a better look at doctors than nurses do). Of course, if you're on a health insurance plan that limits your choices, you'll have to glean from that list.

Once you've narrowed your choices down to two or three, call for consultations; most pediatricians or family practitioners will oblige. Bring a list of questions about issues that are important to you, such as office protocol (for instance, whether there are call-in hours for nervous new parents, or when you can expect calls to be returned), breastfeeding support, circumcision, the use of antibiotics, whether the doctor handles all well-baby visits or whether they are typically handled by nurse practitioners in the practice. Also important to know: Is the doctor board certified? Which hospital is the doctor affiliated with—and will he or she be able to care for the newborn in the hospital? For more questions to ask and issues to consider, see *What to Expect the First Year.*

cavity, and late, after the baby has engaged, settling back into the pelvis in preparation for childbirth. As long as frequency isn't accompanied by signs of infection (see page 453), it's completely normal.

Don't be tempted to cut back on fluids in an attempt to cut back on your trips to the bathroom—and, as always, go as soon as you feel the urge. But do be sure that you keep the nighttime route to the toilet illuminated by a night-light and free of stumbling blocks—shoes, books, area rugs, or other items that can trip you up—and that you make those nocturnal trips in bare feet, not in slippery slippers or socks.

NESTING INSTINCT

"I've heard about the nesting instinct. Is it for real?"

The need to nest can be as real and as powerful an instinct for some humans as it is for our feathered and four-legged friends. If you've ever witnessed the birth of puppies or kittens, you've probably noticed how restless the laboring mother becomes just before delivery—frantically running back and forth, furiously shredding papers in a corner, and finally, when she feels all is in order, settling into the spot where she will give birth. Many expectant mothers do experience the uncontrollable urge to ready their "nests," too, just prior to childbirth. For some it's subtle—all of a sudden, it becomes vitally important to clean out the refrigerator and make sure there's a six-month supply of toilet paper in the house. For others, this unusual burst of manic energy plays itself out in behavior that is dramatic, sometimes irrational, and often humorous (at least, to those observing it)—cleaning every crevice of the nursery with a toothbrush, rearranging the contents of the kitchen cabinets alphabetically, ironing everything that isn't tied down or being worn, or folding and refolding baby's clothes for hours on end.

Though it isn't a reliable predictor of when labor will begin, nesting usually intensifies as the big moment approaches—perhaps as a response to increased adrenaline circulating in the expectant mother's system. Keep in mind, however, that not all women experience the nesting instinct—and that those who don't are just as successful in both childbirth and child rearing as those who do. The urge to slump in front of the television during the last few weeks of pregnancy is as common as the urge to clean out closets, and just as understandable.

If a nesting urge does strike, make sure it's tempered by common sense and caution. Suppress that overwhelming urge to paint the baby's nursery yourself; let someone else climb the ladder with the bucket and roller while you oversee from afar. Don't let overzealous home cleaning exhaust you, either—you'll need energy reserves for both labor and a new baby. Most important of all, keep the limitations of your species in mind. Although you may share this nesting instinct with members of the animal kingdom, you are still only human, and you can't expect to get everything done before that little bundle of joy arrives at your nest.

BLEEDING OR SPOTTING

"Right after my husband and I made love this morning, I began to bleed. Does this mean that labor is beginning—or is the baby in some kind of danger?"

Any new symptom—particularly bleeding and spotting—in the ninth month immediately raises two anxiety-provoking questions: "Is it time?" and

"Is something wrong?" The answers to these questions in your case depend on the type of bleeding you're experiencing and the circumstances that surround it.

Pinkish-stained or red-streaked mucus appearing soon after intercourse or a vaginal examination, or brownish-tinged mucus or brownish spotting appearing within forty-eight hours after the same, is usually just a result of the sensitive cervix being bruised or manipulated. This is normal and not a danger sign, although it should be reported to your practitioner, who may advise that you abstain from intercourse until after delivery.

Bright red bleeding or persistent spotting could be originating at the placenta and requires immediate medical evaluation. Call your practitioner at once. If he or she can't be reached, have someone take you to the hospital.

Pinkish- or brownish-tinged or bloody mucus *accompanied* by contractions or other signs of oncoming labor (see About Prelabor, False Labor, Real Labor, page 334), whether it follows intercourse or not, could be signaling the start of labor. Put in a call to your practitioner.

MEMBRANES RUPTURING IN PUBLIC

"I'm really worried that my water will break in public."

You're not alone. The idea of the "bag of waters," or membranes, breaking on a bus, in a crowded department store, or in the workplace is as mortifying to most pregnant women as that of losing bladder control in public. In fact, pregnancy lore has it that one woman became so obsessed with her worry that she began carrying a jar of pickles in her handbag, ready to be dropped at the first telltale trickle of amniotic fluid. ("Oops, sorry those pickles are making such a mess!")

But before you start rummaging through your cupboards for the garlic dills, there are two things you should know. First, the rupture of membranes before labor begins is uncommon—occurring in less than 15 percent of pregnancies. And once they do break, the flow of amniotic fluid is unlikely to be heavy except when you are lying down (something you aren't likely to do in public). When you are walking or sitting, the fetal head tends to block the opening of the uterus like a cork in a wine bottle.

And second, should your membranes rupture and the amniotic fluid gush suddenly, you can be sure that those around you will not point, shake disapproving heads, or—worse—chuckle. Instead they will (as you would if you were a bystander) either offer you assistance or discreetly ignore you. Keep in mind, after all, that no one is likely to overlook the fact that you're pregnant and therefore to mistake amniotic fluid for anything else.

Also keep in mind that some women whose membranes rupture prior to labor never experience a gushing of amniotic fluid when their membranes rupture—partly because of the cork effect, partly because there are no contractions to force the fluid out. All they notice is a trickle, either constant or intermittent.

Wearing a panty liner or maxi pad (or even, if you're really worried, an incontinence diaper) in the last weeks may give you a sense of security, as well as keep you fresh as your vaginal discharge (leukorrhea) increases. You also might want to place heavy towels, a plastic sheet, or hospital "chucks" under your bedsheets in the last few weeks, just in case your water breaks in the middle of the night. Many a mattress has been ruined by amniotic fluid.

LIGHTENING AND ENGAGEMENT

"If I'm past my 38th week and haven't dropped, does it mean I'm going to be late?"

"Dropping," also called "lightening," occurs when the fetus descends into the pelvic cavity. Lightening is a sign that the presenting part, usually the head, is engaged in the upper portion of the bony pelvis. In first pregnancies, this lightening generally takes place two to four weeks before delivery. In women who have had children previously, it rarely occurs until they go into labor. But as with almost every aspect of pregnancy, exceptions to the rule are the rule. A first-time mother can drop four weeks before her due date and deliver two weeks "late," or she can go into labor without having dropped at all.

Often, lightening is quite apparent. You might note that your belly seems to be lower and tilted farther forward. The happy consequences: as the upward pressure of the uterus on the diaphragm is relieved, taking a deep breath becomes easier, and with the stomach less crowded, eating a full meal becomes more comfortable. Of course, these welcome changes are offset by the discomforts caused by pressure on the bladder, the pelvic joints, and the perineal area: increased frequency of urination, difficult mobility, a sensation of increased perineal pressure, and sometimes pain. Sharp little shocks or twinges may be felt when the fetal head presses on the pelvic floor. Some women sense a rolling in the pelvis when the baby's head turns. And often, because her center of gravity has shifted again, a pregnant woman feels more off-balance once lightening has occurred.

It is possible, however, for lightening to occur without your realizing it. If, for instance, you were carrying low to begin

BE PREPARED

These days it almost goes without saying that becoming educated about childbirth is one of the best ways to prepare for this momentous experience. So by all means make sure you and your coach are as educated as you can be: read the next chapter, along with any other materials on labor and delivery you can get your hands on; watch videos; take a childbirth class together. But don't let your preparedness stop there. Be as prepared for matters practical and esthetic, and plan, too, for your entertainment. Consider, for example: Are you interested in having the event videotaped (preferably by a third party, so that your coach will not have to be di-verted from his primary role), or will a few photos suffice? Will music soothe your soul when your soul needs it most, or will you prefer some peace and quiet? What will distract you best between contractions—playing a game of cards, checking e-mail on your laptop, watching reruns of your favorite sitcoms on TV? (Of course, also be prepared for the possibility that once those contractions begin, you may have little patience for distractions.) Don't forget to include the materials you'll need for the activities you've planned (including film for that camera!) in the suitcase you'll be bringing to the hospital or birthing center (see page 328).

with, your pregnant silhouette might not alter noticeably. Or if you never experienced difficulty breathing or getting a full meal down or if you always urinate frequently, you might not notice any obvious difference.

Your practitioner will rely on two basic indicators to determine whether or not your baby's head is engaged: First, on internal examination, the presenting part is felt in the pelvis; second, on palpating the head externally, it is found to be fixed in position, no longer "floating" free.

How far the presenting part has progressed through the pelvis is measured in "stations," each a centimeter long. A fully engaged baby is said to be at "zero (or 0) station"—that is, the fetal head has descended to the level of the prominent bony landmarks on either side of the midpelvis. A baby who has just begun to descend may be at −4 or −5 station. Once delivery begins, the head continues on through the pelvis past 0 to +1, +2, and so on, until it begins to "crown" at the external vaginal opening at +5. Though a woman who goes into labor at 0 station probably has less pushing ahead than the woman at −3, this isn't invariably true, since station isn't the only factor affecting the progression of labor.

Though the engagement of the fetal head strongly suggests that the baby can get through the pelvis without difficulty, it's no guarantee; conversely, a fetus that is still floating going into labor is not necessarily going to have trouble. And in fact, the majority of fetuses that haven't yet engaged when labor begins come through the pelvis smoothly. This is particularly true in women who have already delivered one or more babies previously.

WHEN YOU WILL DELIVER

"I just had an internal exam and the doctor said I'll probably be going into labor very soon. Can she really tell exactly how close I am?"

Your practitioner can make a prediction about when you'll give birth, but it's still just an educated guess. There are clues that labor is getting closer, which a practitioner looks for beginning in the ninth month, both by palpating the abdomen and doing an internal exam. Has lightening or engagement taken place? What level, or station, has the baby's presenting part descended to? Have effacement (thinning of the cervix) and dilation (opening of the cervix) begun? Has the cervix begun to soften and move to the front of the vagina (another indicator that labor is getting closer) or is it still firm and positioned to the back?

But "soon" can mean anywhere from an hour to three weeks or more. Ask the woman whose euphoria at being told by her practitioner, "You'll be in labor by this evening" turns to depression as weeks more of pregnancy pass with nary a contraction. Or the woman who drags home from the doctor's office resigned to another long month of pregnancy after being told that "labor is weeks away," only to give birth the following morning. The fact is that engagement, effacement, and dilation can occur gradually, over a period of weeks or even a month or more

in some women and overnight in others. So these signs can't be used to accurately pinpoint the start of labor.

If it's important to have a more accurate idea when you will deliver (for example, if you are past your due date), a more formal evaluation of readiness for delivery may be done. One evaluation combines the Bishop score, which includes the degree of cervical dilation and effacement (each graded 0–3), the station the presenting part has reached (0–3), and cervical texture and position (each graded 0–2) with the measurement of cervical length. When the Bishop is 6 or more and the cervical length 26 mm or less, the chances are good that spontaneous labor will start within seven days. Or your doctor may check for a substance called "fetal fibronectin" (FFN) in your cervical-vaginal secretions (though the FFN test, which is very expensive and not all that reliable, is usually reserved for women who are at risk for preterm labor). Presence of FFN usually indicates an imminent delivery. But, again, no guarantees.

DO-IT-YOURSELF LABOR INDUCTION?

Some things, it appears, are best left to nature, or at least to qualified medical personnel. Many do-it-yourself techniques for inducing labor have been suggested, but most are either ineffective, have drawbacks, or both. For instance, nipple stimulation appeared to work in one study. In the study, women who from 39 weeks on stimulated their nipples for three hours or more daily were much less likely to carry past their due dates (and, with twenty-one or more hours a week spent on nipple stimulation, were also probably much less likely to have time for a life). However, since nipple stimulation can not only induce labor but produce very strong contractions (much as oxytocin can), it's

not a technique that should be carried out without medical supervision—even if you can find the hours in your day for it. In other words, don't try this at home.

Other techniques for bringing on labor that you may have heard about are unproven in the success department; they include: sexual intercourse (it may or may not work, but at least you can have fun trying); walking a lot (as long as activity hasn't been restricted by your practitioner); raspberry leaf tea (do not use this before your due date, as it may trigger early contractions); a single dose of castor oil (again, check with your practitioner; many women say it just produces bowel cramps, not contractions).

HOW IS BABY DOING?

Doctors are daily discovering new ways of checking up on babies while they're still in the uterus. These tests may be performed at 41 or 42 weeks when the baby is presumed overdue, or earlier in pregnancy (anytime after the 26th week of pregnancy) when there is some concern about the condition of the fetus. Testing may be repeated periodically when the problem that prompted the testing in the first place persists. Some tests may also be performed during labor, as needed.

The most common prenatal tests of the condition of the fetus are:

At-home fetal movement assessment. A mother's record of fetal movements (see page 243), though not foolproof, can provide some indication of how her baby is doing, and can be used to screen for possible problems. Ten movements in a two-hour period or less is usually reassuring. If the mother doesn't note adequate activity, other tests are then performed.

The nonstress test (NST). The mother is hooked up to the fetal monitor just as she would be if she were in labor, and the response of the fetal heart to fetal movements is observed. If, during the nonstress test, the heart rate doesn't react to movement or the baby doesn't move at all, or if other signs of a problem are noted, the results are considered nonreassuring (which doesn't mean the fetus is in distress, only that its condition needs further evaluation). A weakness of the NST (and of electronic fetal monitoring) is that the accuracy of the test depends on the skill of the person interpreting it. (Note: If the expectant mother has smoked recently, the results may be distorted.)

Fetal acoustical stimulation (FAS), or vibroacoustic stimulation (VAS). This nonstress test, in which a sound-and-vibration-producing instrument is placed on the mother's abdomen to determine the fetus's response to sound or vibrations, has been found to be more accurate than traditional nonstress tests and is useful in evaluating the results of other tests.

The contraction stress test (CST), or oxytocin challenge test (OCT). If a nonstress test is ambiguous, your practitioner may order a stress test. This test, done at a hospital, tests how the baby responds to the "stress" of uterine contractions to get some idea of

---

So feel free to pack your bags, but don't keep the motor running in the car. Like every pregnant woman who proceeded you into the birthing room, you will still have to play the waiting game, knowing for certain only that your day, or night, will come—sometime.

THE OVERDUE BABY

"I'm a week overdue. Is it possible that I might never go into labor on my own?"

The magic date is circled in red on the calendar; every day of the 40 weeks that precede it is crossed off with great anticipation. Then, at long last, the big day arrives—and, as in about half of all pregnancies, the baby doesn't. Anticipation dissolves into discouragement. The baby carriage and crib sit empty for yet another day. And then a week. And then, in 10 percent of pregnancies, most often those of first-time mothers, two weeks. Will this pregnancy never end?

Though women who have reached the 42nd week might find it hard to believe, no pregnancy on record ever went on forever—even before the advent of labor induction. (It's true an occasional pregnancy progresses to the 44th week or even slightly beyond, but today a large majority are induced before they go past the 42nd.)

Studies show that about 70 percent

how the baby will handle full-blown labor. In this somewhat more complex and time-consuming test (it may take up to three hours), the mother is hooked up to a fetal monitor. If contractions are not occurring on their own, they are given a push via the intravenous administration of oxytocin, or by stimulation of the mother's nipples (with hot towels and, if necessary, manually by the mother). How the fetus responds to contractions indicates its probable condition and that of the placenta. This rough simulation of the conditions of labor can, if the results are unequivocal, allow a prediction to be made about whether or not the fetus can safely remain in the uterus and whether it can meet the strenuous demands of true labor. (This test is not suitable for women in preterm labor or those at high risk for preterm labor; those with premature rupture of the membranes; those who have had uterine surgery or a classic incision made during a cesarean delivery; and those who have been diagnosed with placenta previa.)

A biophysical profile (BPP). A BPP generally evaluates, through the use of ultrasound, four aspects of life in the uterus: fetal breathing, fetal movement, fetal tone, and amniotic fluid volume. When all these are normal, the baby is probably doing fine. If any of these are abnormal or unclear, an assessment of the fetal heart rate by a nonstress test will be given to provide a more accurate picture of the baby's condition.

The "modified" biophysical profile. The modified biophysical profile combines the NST with an evaluation of the quantity of amniotic fluid. A low level of amniotic fluid may indicate that the fetus is not producing enough urine and that the placenta may not be functioning well. If the fetus reacts appropriately to the nonstress test and levels of amniotic fluid are adequate, it's likely that all is well.

Umbilical artery Doppler velocimetry. This noninvasive ultrasound test looks at the flow of blood through the umbilical artery. A weak, absent, or reverse flow indicates the fetus is not getting adequate nourishment and is probably not growing well.

Other tests of fetal well-being. These include regular ultrasound exams to document fetal growth; amniotic fluid sampling (through amniocentesis); fetal electrocardiography or other tests (to assess the fetal heart); and fetal scalp stimulation (which tests how a fetus reacts to pressure on, or pinching of, the scalp).

of apparent postterm pregnancies aren't postterm at all. They are only believed to be late because of a miscalculation of the time of conception, usually thanks to irregular ovulation or a woman's uncertainty about the exact date of her last menstrual period. And in fact, when early ultrasound examination is used to confirm the due date, diagnoses of postterm pregnancy drop dramatically from the long-held estimate of 10 percent to about 2 percent.

When a pregnant woman appears to be postterm (technically 42 weeks or more, though some doctors will take action sooner), the practitioner, in evaluating the situation, considers two major factors. One, is the estimated due date accurate? It's reasonably certain that it is if it has consistently correlated with various benchmarks of a pregnancy's progress, including the size of the uterus, the height of the fundus (the top of the uterus), the timing of the first fetal movements felt by the mother, and the first fetal heartbeats detected by the practitioner. Early pregnancy ultrasound or blood tests for hCG levels may also be looked at to help confirm the correct gestational age.

The second factor usually considered is whether the fetus is continuing to thrive. Many babies continue to grow and thrive well into the tenth month (although this growth can be a problem if the baby becomes too large during this time to pass easily through the mother's pelvis). Occasionally, however, the once ideal environment in the uterus begins to deteriorate when a baby is postterm. The aging placenta fails to supply adequate nutrition and oxygen, and production of amniotic fluid drops off, dangerously reducing levels of fluid in the uterus. Under these conditions, it becomes difficult for the fetus to continue doing well.

Babies born after spending time in such an inhospitable environment are called postmature. They are thin for their length, with skin that is dry, cracked, peeling, loose, and wrinkled, having lost the protective cheesy vernix coating common in term newborns. Being "older" than other new arrivals, they have longer nails and more abundant hair, and are generally open-eyed and alert. Those with longer stays in a deteriorating uterus may have a temporary greenish staining of the skin and umbilical cord, from having passed their first bowel movement (meconium) in utero. Those who have been in the postterm uterus the longest may have yellow staining.

Because they are usually larger than 40-week babies, with wider head circumferences, and because they may be somewhat compromised by insufficient oxygen and nutrition or by possibly having inhaled meconium, postmature babies are at increased risk of having a difficult labor and are more likely to be delivered by cesarean. They may also need some special care in the neonatal intensive care nursery for a short time after birth. Still, the vast majority of those born at 42 weeks after uncomplicated pregnancies are at no greater risk of permanent problems than babies born at 40 weeks.

To avoid any added risk to the fetus, many practitioners will choose to induce labor (see page 339) when it has been determined with certainty that a pregnancy is past 41 weeks and the cervix is

found to be ripe (soft and ready to dilate). Delivery by induction or cesarean will also be initiated, whether the cervix is ripe or not, if complications such as hypertension or diabetes threaten the mother, or if meconium staining, suspected inadequate fetal growth, or other problems threaten the fetus. If the cervix is not ripe, the practitioner may choose to try to ripen it by administering a drug, such as prostaglandin E-2 gel.

Or he or she may choose to wait it out a little longer, performing one or more tests (see box, page 324) to see if the fetus is still doing okay in the uterus, and repeating these tests once or twice a week until labor begins.

Some practitioners will wait until 42 weeks or even a bit longer before deciding to circumvent Mother Nature—assuming the fetus continues to pass its tests and the mother is doing well. If at any point test results show that the placenta is no longer doing its job or that the level of amniotic fluid has become inadequate, or if there are any other signs that either mother or baby is in trouble, the practitioner will take action and, depending upon the situation, induce labor or perform a cesarean section. Fortunately for anxious expectant mothers, few pregnancies are allowed to go more than a matter of days beyond 42 confirmed weeks.

There are measures that are sometimes recommended to reduce the likelihood that a baby will deliver postterm, but both have drawbacks. One—daily nipple stimulation—can be handled by the mother at home (see box, page 323), but is risky because it could trigger overly strong contractions. The other—stripping of the fetal membranes—calls for the manual separating of the chorionic membranes surrounding the fetus from the lower section of the uterus and must be performed by the practitioner. Many physicians believe stripping the

SOME REASSURANCE ABOUT AN UNREASSURING TEST RESULT

Remarkable strides have been made in the field of fetal testing. Today, doctors have at their fingertips numerous procedures that can help determine how a baby is doing in utero. Still, as quickly evolving a science as it is, it is not yet a perfect one. And in many cases it proves far from perfect. While false negatives (a result that indicates everything is okay when it actually isn't) are fairly rare on these tests, false positives (a result that indicates a problem when there isn't one) are very common. In other words, while a good test result is almost a certain sign that a baby is doing well, a poor test result is not automatically a sign that a baby is having problems. Poor test results on any of the available tests *should be* followed up by one or more other tests in order to see whether fetal distress is actually present.

Because false positives are so common—and because a misdiagnosis of fetal distress can lead to unnecessary intervention (such as the surgical delivery of a baby who could have safely withstood a normal vaginal one)—the medical community has taken to labeling poor test results, previously automatically tagged as "fetal distress," as *"unreassuring."* An unreassuring test result doesn't rule out fetal distress, but it definitely doesn't diagnose it, either. Which means that "unreassuring" really isn't as unreassuring as it sounds.

membranes is not advisable because of the risks of rupturing them or causing infection. But recent studies indicate this procedure, which induces labor by triggering certain body chemicals, including prostaglandins, is safe and effective *if* the cervix is dilated. It's not uncommon to experience contractions or spotting following the procedure.

PLANNED INDUCTION OF LABOR

"A lot of my friends are having labor induced instead of waiting for it to start naturally. Is this becoming more common?"

Childbirth trends seem to be as difficult to keep up with—or predict—as fashion trends these days, and that's certainly true when it comes to labor induction. For many years, a large percentage of doctors routinely induced labor so that births would come at a convenient time, making the induction rate high. Then, as the natural childbirth movement began to take hold in the obstetrical community, routine induction, like so many interventions, fell out of favor. The FDA withdrew approval for the use of oxytocin (the drug most often used for inducing labor) for inductions that were elective (performed for reasons other than medical necessity, such as convenience). Patients and, eventually, most doctors came to recognize the benefits of letting nature take its course, and the number of inductions dropped dramatically.

But recently, inductions have been on the rise again. Though the reasons for this retro trend aren't all clear, there are a couple of likely explanations. Changes in obstetrical practice are definitely playing a role; more doctors are choosing to induce pregnancies that go beyond 42 weeks. But it does appear that convenience is once again a factor, and not only the physician's convenience. More and more women seem anxious to schedule

WHAT TO TAKE TO THE HOSPITAL OR BIRTHING CENTER

Though you could show up with just your belly and your insurance card, traveling *that* light to the hospital or birthing center probably isn't the best idea. Pack your bags early (so you won't be turning the house upside-down for your favorite CD when the contractions are coming five minutes apart) with as many (or as few) of the following as you'd like:

For the Labor or Birthing Room

◆ This book; the *What to Expect Pregnancy Organizer,* which has ample room for labor-and-delivery note keeping. A pen and pad may also be useful for jotting down questions and answers on procedures and on your condition and your baby's; instructions for when you go home; and the names of staff members who have taken care of you.

◆ Several copies of your birthing plan (see page 274) so that attendants will know your preferences.

◆ A watch or clock with a second hand for timing contractions.

◆ A radio or a CD or cassette player, along with some of your favorite tunes, if music soothes and relaxes you.

◆ A camera, tape recorder, and/or video equipment, if you don't trust your memory to capture the moment (and if the hospital or birthing center rules allow media coverage of births—most do).

◆ Entertainment. Cards, a laptop, a puzzle, a handheld video game player, or whatever diversions you think will keep you from focusing too much on your labor.

◆ Favorite lotions, oils, or anything else you'd like to be massaged with.

◆ A tennis ball or plastic rolling pin, for firm countermassage should lower backache be a problem.

◆ A pillow of your own to make you more comfortable during and after labor.

◆ Sugarless lollipops or candies to keep your mouth moist (though sugared candies are sometimes recommended, they will only make you thirstier).

◆ A toothbrush, toothpaste, and mouthwash (you may find yourself desperate for a freshen-up after eight hours or so).

◆ Heavy socks, should your feet become cold.

◆ Comfortable slippers with nonskid bottoms, in case you feel like doing some walking during labor and so you can do some strolling in the halls later, between baby feedings.

◆ A hairbrush, if you find having your hair brushed comforting or you just want to avoid postpartum tangles.

◆ A "scrunchie," clip, or hairband, if your

their babies' births into their busy lives—between projects at work, for instance, or at a time of day when they can be sure of having a baby-sitter available for an older child. Women in group practices may prefer to schedule delivery when their favored practitioner is on call.

Though these scheduling concerns are often compelling, the benefit of addressing them probably does not outweigh the risk, however small, associated with induction. In fact, the American College of Obstetricians and Gynecologists, bucking this trend, has issued guidelines recommending that, whenever possible, induction not be performed until at least 39 weeks, and then only when benefits outweigh risks.

hair is long, to keep it out of your face and tangle free.

♦ A couple of sandwiches or other snacks for your coach, so he won't have to leave your side in search of sustenance.

♦ A change of clothes for your coach, for comfort's sake, and if he plans to sleep over in the hospital.

♦ A bottle of champagne or bubbly cider labeled with your name, for celebrating (your coach can ask the nurse to put it in the fridge), though depending on the hour you deliver, you may be more in the mood for orange juice.

For Postpartum

♦ A robe and/or nightgowns, if you'd rather wear your own than the hospital's. Make sure it opens in the front for easier breast-feeding. Be forewarned, however, that though pretty nightgowns can boost your spirits, they may get bled on and stained.

♦ Toiletries, including shampoo, tooth-brush, mouthwash, toothpaste, lotion (your skin may be dry from a loss of flu-ids), body wash or a bar of your favorite soap in a carrying case, deodorant, hair-brush, hand mirror, makeup, and any other essentials of beauty and hygiene.

♦ Your favorite brand of maxi pads, though pads will also be provided by the hospital. Don't use tampons.

♦ A couple of changes of underwear and a nursing bra.

♦ All the entertainment listed above, plus

books (including a baby naming book if that decision's still up in the air).

♦ A supply of snacks: raisins, nuts, whole-wheat crackers, cereal bars, and other healthy treats to keep you regular in spite of a hospital diet and to keep you from starving when hunger strikes between meals or while you're breastfeeding in the middle of the night.

♦ List of phone numbers of family and friends to call with the good news; a phone card or calling card number or cell phone (though some hospitals don't allow them).

♦ Music to relax you while breastfeeding.

♦ A going-home outfit for you, keeping in mind that you'll still be sporting a siz-able abdomen. (You'll probably look like you're at least five months pregnant; plan accordingly.)

♦ A going-home outfit for baby—a ki-mono or stretch suit, T-shirt, booties, a receiving blanket, and a heavy bunting or blanket if it's cold; diapers will probably be provided by the hospital, but take along an extra, just in case.

♦ Infant car seat. Most hospitals will not let you leave with the baby unless he or she is safely strapped into an approved rear-facing infant car seat. (Besides, it's the law.)

♦ A camera and film (or a disposable cam-era) for all those photo ops.

♦ A baby book to record those special firsts in.

♦ A copy of *What to Expect the First Year*.

PLAN-AHEAD PAIN RELIEF

"At my hospital, you can sign up ahead for an epidural. Everybody's doing it, and I'm tempted, too, just so I won't have to go through all that pain. Is there any reason not to?"

Wait long enough, and just about everything comes back into style. Stiletto heels. Short skirts. Narrow ties. And, as you've noticed, childbirth pain relief. While women a generation ago fought hard for the right to give birth without drugs, many women today are rallying for the right to give birth without pain, or at least without a lot of pain,

MASSAGE YOUR WAY TO AN EASIER LABOR

Impatiently waiting for labor to start? Don't just sit there—massage your perineum! Perineal massage, long recommended by midwives, may help to stretch your perineum in preparation for childbirth, minimize "stinging" when baby's head crowns, and may even help you avoid an episiotomy or tears. And it's simple to do. Start by washing your hands thoroughly with soap and water (or if your spouse will be performing the massage for you, make sure his hands are clean). Well-trimmed nails are also a good idea. Then lubricate your thumbs (or his thumbs or index fingers) with K-Y jelly and insert them just inside your vagina. Press downward (towards the rectum) and slide your thumbs across the bottom and then up the sides of the perineum (or have your spouse do so). Repeat daily during the last weeks of pregnancy. *Note:* a little discomfort or a burning sensation is normal when you do this, but stop if you feel sharp pain. Also note that perineal massage certainly isn't something you have to do (if you don't feel comfortable with the concept, it seems too weird, or you just don't have the time); though anecdotal evidence has long supported its effectiveness, clinical research has not yet backed it up. As always, different strokes work for different folks.

without pain relief, while often seemingly the ideal for both mother and baby, isn't always in their best interest (as when pain becomes so intense or has gone on so long that it actually interferes with the progress of labor). But, despite their recent surge in popularity, routine sign-up-in-advance epidurals aren't always in mother's and baby's best interest, either. It's simply impossible to predict whether you'll need pain relief before the pain has actually begun. And while epidurals are safer and more effective than ever before, they, like every childbirth intervention, carry some degree of inherent risk that must be weighed against the potential benefit.

In other words, while it's wise to prepare for the possibility that you'll need an epidural, and to learn all you need to know about them, deciding in advance to sign up for one probably isn't. For much more on pain relief during labor and delivery, see page 276.

FEAR OF ANOTHER LONG LABOR

"I had a forty-eight-hour labor my first time around, and finally delivered after four and a half hours of pushing. Though we both came out of it okay, I dread going through that torture again."

Anyone brave enough to go back into the ring after such a challenging first round deserves a break. And chances are good that you'll get one. Of course, though the odds of an easier childbirth are significantly improved the second time around, there are no sure bets in labor and delivery rooms. Your baby's position or other factors may alter these odds. Short of a crystal ball, there's no way to predict precisely what will happen this time around.

much as their great-grandmothers did when childbirth medication first came into style.

But the problem with styles is that they don't always take into account the best interest of the consumer (as many who've worn those stiletto heels and lived to regret it can attest). Giving birth

But second and subsequent labors and deliveries are usually easier and shorter than first ones—often dramatically so. Less resistance will be met from your now roomier birth canal and your laxer muscles, and though the process won't be effortless (it rarely is), it probably will seem like less of an ordeal. The most marked difference may be in the amount of pushing you have to do; second babies often pop out in a matter of minutes rather than hours.

ADVANCE PLANNING

How far along in labor should you be before calling your practitioner? Should you call if your water breaks? How can you make contact if the contractions start outside of regular office hours? Should you call first and then head for the hospital or birthing center? Or the other way around? Are there any other specifics of labor and delivery logistics your practitioner wants you to keep in mind? Discuss all of these issues with your practitioner at your next appointment and write down the answers as you get them; otherwise you're sure to forget the instructions when the labor pains start coming.

Also be sure you know the best route to your place of delivery, roughly how long it will take to get there at various times of the day, and what kind of transportation is available if you don't have someone to drive you. (Don't plan on driving yourself.) And if there are other children at home, or an elderly relative, or a pet, be sure you've made plans for their care in advance.

Keep a copy of all the above information in your handbag and in the suitcase you've packed, as well as on your refrigerator door or bedside table.

BREASTFEEDING

"My breasts are very small and my nipples are flat. Will I be able to breastfeed?"

As far as hungry babies are concerned, satisfaction comes in all kinds of packages. Breasts don't have to be centerfold-shaped or -sized, and they can come equipped with almost any kind of nipple—small and flat, large and pointy, even inverted. All combinations of breast sizes and nipple shapes have the capacity to produce and dispense milk. The quantity and quality is not in the least dependent on outward appearance. So don't let fallacies and old wives' tales about what kinds of breasts can and cannot satisfy a baby discourage you from breastfeeding.

And don't listen to anyone (old wives or otherwise) who tells you that your nipples need to be prepped for nursing with breast shells, hand manipulation, or a manual breast pump. Not only are these preparatory techniques often less effective than *no treatment*, but they can do more harm than good. The shells, besides being embarrassingly conspicuous, can cause sweating and rashes. Hand manipulation and pumping can stimulate contractions and, occasionally, even trigger breast infection.

Some experts do recommend not soaping your nipples and areola—just rinsing with water—during the last months of pregnancy. Soap tends to dry the nipples and may make early breastfeeding a little more difficult. If your breasts are dry or itchy, a mild cream or lotion may feel soothing, but avoid getting it on the nipple or areola. If your nipples are dry, try applying a lanolin-based cream such as Lansinoh.

If, once you deliver, you find your baby has trouble latching on to your flat nipples, pumping briefly with an electric pump before feedings for a few days may help to draw the nipples out. In some cases, it may be necessary to continue this pumping (with an electric or hand pump) for a longer period. And remember, the baby shouldn't suckle just on the nipple, but on the areola that surrounds it, so be sure the latch-on includes the dark area around the nipple.

"My mother says she had milk leaking from her breasts in the ninth month; I don't. Does this mean I won't have any milk?"

The thin, yellowish discharge that some pregnant women can express, or may notice leaking from their breasts, is not milk. It is a *premilk* called colostrum. Richer in protein and lower in fat and milk sugar than the breast milk that arrives three or four days after delivery, it contains antibodies that may be important in protecting the baby against disease.

Many women, however, don't have any noticeable colostrum until *after* delivery. (Even then, they may not be aware of it until baby starts to feed.) This in no way predicts a lack of milk or difficulty in nursing.

BREAST SURGERY AND NURSING

"I had a breast reduction done several years ago. Will I be able to breastfeed my baby?"

Many women who have had breast reductions are able to breastfeed, though most don't produce enough milk to nurse exclusively. Whether you will be able to breastfeed your baby—and how much you'll need to supplement your milk supply with formula—will depend at least in part on how extensive

the reduction was, where the incision was made, and how the procedure was performed. Check with your surgeon. If care was taken to preserve milk ducts and nerve pathways, chances are good that you'll be able to produce at least some milk.

Even if your surgeon isn't particularly reassuring, there's no harm in giving breastfeeding a try. Increase your chances of success by reading up on breastfeeding and working with a lactation consultant who is familiar with the challenges of nursing after a breast reduction. Closely monitoring your baby's intake (by keeping an eye on growth and the number of dirty and wet diapers) will be especially important. If you don't end up making enough milk, using a nursing supplementation system (which allows you to breastfeed and supplement with formula at the same time) can encourage milk production while ensuring that your baby gets enough to eat. Remember, any amount of breastfeeding— even if it doesn't turn out to be baby's only or even primary source of nutrition—is beneficial.

"I have breast implants. My doctor says that they shouldn't interfere with breastfeeding, but I'm still worried that I won't be able to nurse."

Breast augmentation is far less likely to interfere with breastfeeding than a breast reduction. But while many women with implants are able to nurse exclusively, a significant minority may not produce enough milk. To make sure your supply meets your baby's demand, you'll need to keep close tabs on his or her growth and the number of dirty and wet diapers accumulated daily. And don't worry about the type of implants you have. Studies have shown that silicone from breast implants does not get into breast milk.

CONSIDERING CORD BLOOD BANKING

Though it is still experimental, some parents are deciding to have blood from their newborn's umbilical cord and placenta harvested and stored in case the stem cells should be needed at a future time for the treatment of a serious disease in the child or another family member.

Cord blood harvesting, a painless procedure that takes less than five minutes and is done after the cord has been clamped and cut, is completely safe for mother and child (as long as the cord is not clamped and cut prematurely), but storage is quite expensive and the benefits for low-risk families are not at all clear.

For these reasons, ACOG doesn't recommend cord blood banking, and the American Academy of Pediatrics (AAP) doesn't recommend private cord blood storage unless a family member has a medical condition that might be helped by a stem cell transplant now or in the near future. These conditions include leukemia, lymphoma, and neuroblastoma; sickle-cell anemia, aplastic anemia, and thalassemia illness; Gaucher's disease and Hurler's syndrome; Wiskott-Aldrich syndrome, and severe hemoglobinopathy. The AAP does, however, support parents donating the cord blood to a bank for general use by the public. This costs the donor nothing and could save a life.

If you are interested in storing or donating cord blood, contact the International Cord Blood Foundation at (650) 635-1456; www.cordblooddonor.org; the Cord Blood Registry at (888) 267-3256; www. cordblood.com; the National Marrow Donor Program at www.marrow.org; or www.parentsguidecordblood.com

MOTHERING

"Now that the baby's arrival is so close, I'm beginning to worry about how I'm going to take care of it. I've never even held a newborn before."

Most women are not born mothers (any more than men are born fathers), instinctively knowing how to soothe a crying baby, change a diaper, or give a bath. Motherhood—parenthood, for that matter—is a learned art, one that requires practice to make perfect (or rather *near*-perfect, since there's no such thing as a *perfect* parent). For centuries, that practice commonly took place at an early age, when female children learned to care for younger siblings or other infants in the family, much as they learned to bake bread and mend socks.

Today, a high percentage of fully grown women have never kneaded bread dough, taken a needle to a worn sock, or held—let alone taken care of—an infant. Their training for motherhood comes on the job, with a little help from books, magazines, the Internet, and, if they're lucky enough to find one locally, a baby care class. Which means that for the first week or two (and often much longer) the new mom feels out of her element as the baby does more crying than sleeping, the diapers leak, and many a tear is shed over the "no-tears" shampoo.

Slowly but surely, however, the new mom begins to feel like an old pro. Her trepidation turns to assurance. The baby she was afraid to hold (won't it break?) is now cradled casually in her left arm while her right pays bills or pushes the vacuum cleaner. Dispensing vitamin drops, giving baths, and slipping squirming arms and legs into sleepers have ceased to be dreaded ordeals. Like all the daily tasks of parenting an infant, these have become second nature. She's a mother, and—difficult though it may be to imagine—you will be one, too.

Though nothing can make those first days with a first baby a cinch, starting the learning process before delivery can make them seem a little less overwhelming. Any of the following can help moms- (and dads-) to-be ease into their new roles: visiting a newborn nursery and viewing the most recent arrivals; holding, diapering, and soothing a friend's or family member's infant; reading up on a baby's first year;[3] and watching a video or taking a class in baby care.

What It's Important to Know:
ABOUT PRELABOR, FALSE LABOR, REAL LABOR

It always seems so simple on TV. Somewhere around 3 A.M., the pregnant woman sits up in bed, puts a knowing hand on her belly, and reaches over to rouse her sleeping husband with a calm, almost serene, "It's time, honey."

But how, you wonder, does this woman know it's time? How does she recognize labor with such cool, clinical confidence when she's never *been* in labor before? What makes her so sure she's not going to get to the hospital, be examined by the resident, found to be nowhere near her time, and be sent home, amid snickers from the night shift, just as pregnant as when she arrived? The script, of course.

On our side of the screen (with no script in hand), we're more likely to awaken at 3 A.M. with complete uncertainty. Are these really labor pains, or just more Braxton Hicks? Should I turn on the light and start timing? Should I bother to wake my spouse? Do I drag my practitioner out of bed at 1 A.M. to report what might really be false labor? If I do and it isn't time, will I turn out to be the pregnant woman who cried "labor" once too often, and will anybody take me seriously when it's for real? Or will I be the only woman in my childbirth class not to recognize labor? Will I leave for the hospital too late, maybe giving birth in the back of a taxicab (film at 11!). The questions multiply faster than the contractions.

The fact is that most women, worry though they might, *don't* end up misjudging the onset of their labor. The vast majority, thanks to instinct, luck, or no-doubt-about-it killer contractions, show up at the hospital neither too early nor too late, but at just about the right time. Still, there's no reason to leave your deliberations up to chance. Becoming familiar in advance with the signs of prelabor, false labor, and real labor will help to allay the concerns and clear up the confusion when those contractions (or are they?) begin.

No one knows exactly what triggers labor (and more women are concerned with "when" than "why") but it's believed that a combination of fetal, placental, and maternal factors are involved. This very intricate process begins with the fetus, whose brain sets off a relay of chemical messages (which probably translate into something like, "Mom, let me out of here!") that kick off a chain reaction of hormones in the mother. These hormonal changes in turn pave the way for the work of prostaglandins and oxytocin, substances that trigger contractions when all labor systems are "go."

---

3. *What to Expect the First Year* should be helpful.

PRELABOR SYMPTOMS

The physical changes of prelabor can precede real labor by a full month or more—or by only an hour or so. Prelabor is characterized by the beginning of cervical effacement and dilation, which your practitioner can confirm on examination, as well as by a wide variety of related signs that you may notice yourself:

Lightening and engagement. Usually somewhere between two and four weeks before the onset of labor in first-time mothers, the fetus begins to descend into the pelvis (see page 321). This milestone is rarely reached in second or later births until labor is about to commence.

Sensations of increasing pressure in the pelvis and rectum. Crampiness (similar to menstrual cramps) and groin pain are particularly common in second and later pregnancies. Persistent low backache may also be present.

Loss of weight or cessation of weight gain. Weight gain might slow down in the ninth month; as labor approaches, some women even lose a bit of weight, up to two or three pounds.

A change in energy levels. Some ninth-monthers find that they are increasingly fatigued. Others experience energy spurts. An uncontrollable urge to scrub floors and clean out closets has been related to the "nesting instinct," in which the female of the species prepares the nest for the impending arrival (see page 319).

A change in vaginal discharge. You may find that your discharge increases and thickens.

Pink, or bloody, show. As the cervix effaces and dilates, capillaries frequently rupture, tinting the mucus pink or streaking it with blood. This "show" usually means labor will start within twenty-four hours—but it could be as much as several days away.

Loss of the mucous plug. As the cervix begins to thin and open, the "cork" of mucus that seals the opening of the uterus becomes dislodged. This gelatinous chunk of mucus can be passed through the vagina a week or two before the first real contractions, or just as labor begins.

Intensification of Braxton Hicks contractions. These practice contractions (see page 286) may become more frequent and stronger, even painful.

Diarrhea. Some women experience loose bowel movements just prior to the onset of labor.

FALSE LABOR SYMPTOMS

Real labor probably has *not* begun if:

♦ Contractions are not at all regular and don't increase in frequency or severity.

♦ Contractions subside if you walk around or change your position.

♦ Show, if any, is brownish.[4] (This kind of discharge is often the result of an internal exam or intercourse within the past forty-eight hours.)

♦ Fetal movements intensify briefly with contractions. (Let your practitioner know immediately if activity becomes frantic.)

---

4. Bright red blood requires immediate consultation with your practitioner.

REAL LABOR SYMPTOMS

When contractions of prelabor are replaced by stronger, more painful, and more frequent ones, the question arises: "Is this the real thing or false labor?" It is probably real if:

◆ The contractions intensify, rather than ease up, with activity and aren't relieved by a change in position.

◆ Contractions become progressively more frequent and painful, and generally (but not always) more regular. However, not every contraction will necessarily be more painful or longer (they usually last about thirty to seventy seconds) than the previous one, but the intensity does build up as real labor progresses. Nor does frequency always increase in regular, perfectly even intervals—but it does increase.

◆ Contractions may feel like gastrointestinal upset and be accompanied by diarrhea. Early labor contractions can also feel like heavy menstrual cramps. Pain may be just in the lower abdomen or in the lower back and abdomen, and it may also radiate to the legs (particularly the upper thighs). Location, however, is not as reliable an indication, because false labor contractions may also be felt in these places.

◆ Show is present and pinkish or blood-streaked.

◆ Membranes rupture, though in 15 percent of labors, the waters break—in a gush or a trickle—before labor begins, and in many others, membranes do not rupture spontaneously and are ruptured artificially by the practitioner.

WHEN TO CALL THE PRACTITIONER

When in doubt, call. Even if you've checked and rechecked the above lists, you may still be unsure whether you're really in labor. If you *are* unsure, call your practitioner, unless you'd like an unplanned home birth. He or she will probably be able to tell from the sound of your voice, as you talk through a contraction, whether it's the real thing. (But only if you don't try to cover up the pain in the name of stoicism or good manners.) Fear of embarrassment if it turns out to be a false alarm shouldn't prevent your calling your practitioner. Nobody's going to laugh at you. You wouldn't be the first patient to misjudge her labor signs, and you certainly won't be the last.

Call anytime, night or day, if all signs indicate that you're ready to go to the hospital. Don't let an overdeveloped sense of guilt or politeness keep you from waking your practitioner up in the middle of the night. People who deliver babies for a living don't expect to work only 9 to 5.

Your practitioner has probably specified that you should call when your contractions have reached a particular frequency—say five, eight, or ten minutes apart. Call when at least some are that frequent. Don't wait for perfectly even intervals; they may never come. Don't assume that if you're not sure it's real labor, it isn't. Err on the side of caution and call.

Your practitioner has probably also instructed you to call as soon as possible if your membranes rupture but labor has not begun. If your due date is still several weeks away, if there is a cord prolapse (see page 521), or the amniotic fluid is stained greenish brown, call *immediately*. If you can't reach your practitioner, then head for the hospital.

◆ ◆ ◆

CHAPTER 14

Labor and Delivery

I t takes nine months to grow a baby, and only a matter of hours (though they may seem like *very long* hours) to bring one into the world. Yet it's those hours that seem to occupy the minds of expectant women (and their partners) most. More questions and concerns revolve around the process of labor and delivery than around any other aspect of pregnancy. When will labor start? More important, when will it end? Will I be able to tolerate the pain? Will I need an epidural? A fetal monitor? An episiotomy? What if I don't make any progress? What if I progress so quickly that I don't make it to the hospital?

You'll find answers to your questions and reassurance for your concerns in this chapter. These answers, teamed with a lot of support from your partner and your birth attendants (doctors, midwives, nurses, doulas), and the knowledge that labor and delivery have never been safer and more manageable than they are today, should help prepare you for most anything that labor and delivery might bring your way. *And* help you to keep in mind that what's really important is the end result: that new baby of yours.

What You May Be Concerned About

MUCOUS PLUG AND BLOODY SHOW

"I think I lost my mucous plug. Should I call my practitioner?"

D on't send out for the champagne just yet. The mucous plug—the clear, globby, gelatinous blob-like barrier that has "corked" your cervix throughout your pregnancy—occasionally becomes dislodged as dilation and effacement begin.

Though the passage of the plug (which not every woman experiences, and which has no bearing on the eventual progress of labor) is a sign that your body's preparing for the big day, it's not a reliable signal that the big day has arrived—or even that it's imminent. At this point, labor could be one, two, or even three weeks away, with your cervix continuing to open gradually over that time. In other words, there's no need to call your practitioner or frantically pack your bags.

"I have a pink mucous discharge. Does it mean labor's about to start?"

Passage of "bloody show," a mucous discharge tinged pink or brown with blood, is usually a sign that your cervix is effacing and/or dilating and that the process that leads to delivery is well under way. But it's a process with an erratic timetable that will keep you in suspense until the first true contractions. Based on averages, chances are good that you'll feel those contractions within twenty-four to forty-eight hours. But, because everyone's timetable is different, labor might also be less than an hour away, with dilation occurring rapidly. Or a few days away, with it taking its sweet time. So the suspense continues.

If your discharge should suddenly become bright red, especially if it seems to amount to more than an ounce (about 2 tablespoons), contact your practitioner immediately. Actual bleeding could indicate premature separation of the placenta (see page 516) or placenta previa (see page 505), both of which require prompt medical attention.

RUPTURE OF MEMBRANES

"I woke up in the middle of the night with a wet bed. Did I lose control of my bladder, or did my water break?"

A sniff of your sheets will probably clue you in. If the wet spot smells sort of sweet (not like urine, which has the harsher odor of ammonia), it's likely to be amniotic fluid. Another clue that the membranes surrounding your baby and containing the amniotic fluid he or she's been living in for nine months have probably ruptured: you continue leaking the pale, straw-colored fluid (which won't run dry because it continues to be produced until delivery, replacing itself every

three hours). You are more likely to notice the leaking while you are lying down; it usually stops, or at least slows, when you stand up or sit down, since the baby's head acts as a cork, blocking the flow temporarily. The leakage is heavier—whether you're sitting or standing—if the break in the membranes is down near the cervix than if it is higher up.

Your practitioner has probably given you instructions on what to do and when to call if your water breaks. Follow those instructions, as well as the precautions listed below. As always, if you're not sure what to do, err on the side of caution and call your practitioner.

"My water just broke, but I haven't had any contractions. When is labor going to start, and what should I do in the meantime?"

Most women whose membranes rupture before labor begins can expect to feel that first contraction within twelve hours of that first trickle; most others can expect to feel it within twenty-four hours. So it's likely that labor is on the way—and soon.

About 1 in 10, however, find that labor takes a little longer to get going. Because, as time passes, the risk of infection to baby and/or mother through the ruptured amniotic sac increases, most physicians will induce labor (see facing page) within twenty-four hours of a rupture if a woman is at or near her due date, though a few will induce as early as six hours after. Many women who have experienced a rupture actually welcome a sooner-than-later induction, preferring it to twenty-four hours of wet waiting.

The first thing you should do if you experience a trickle or flow of fluid from your vagina (besides grab a towel and a box of maxi pads) is call your doctor or nurse-midwife (unless he or she has instructed otherwise). In the meantime, keep the vaginal area as clean as possible to avoid infection. Don't have sexual relations (not that there's much chance you'd want to right now); use a pad (not a tampon) to absorb the flow; don't try to do your own internal exam; and, as always, wipe from front to back when you use the toilet.

Rarely, when the membranes rupture prematurely and the presenting part is not yet engaged in the pelvis (most likely when the baby is breech or preterm), the umbilical cord becomes "prolapsed"—it is swept into the opening of the uterus (the cervix), or even down into the vagina, with the gush of amniotic fluid. If you can see a loop of umbilical cord at your vaginal opening, or think you feel something inside your vagina, get immediate medical attention (see page 521).

DARKENED AMNIOTIC FLUID (MECONIUM STAINING)

"My membranes ruptured, and the fluid isn't clear—it's greenish-brown. What does this mean?"

Your amniotic fluid is probably stained with meconium, a greenish-brown substance that comes from your baby's digestive tract. Ordinarily, meconium is passed after birth as the baby's first stool. But sometimes—particularly when the fetus has been under stress in the womb, and very often when it is past its due date—the meconium is passed prior to birth into the amniotic fluid.

Meconium staining alone is not a sure sign of fetal distress, but because it suggests the possibility there might be a problem, notify your practitioner immediately. The meconium could also indicate that *you* are at increased risk of

infection around the time of delivery and should be watched more carefully.

INADEQUATE AMNIOTIC FLUID

"My doctor said that my amniotic fluid is low and that she needs to supplement it. Should I be concerned?"

Usually Mother Nature keeps the uterus well stocked with a self-replenishing supply of amniotic fluid. Fortunately, even when levels do run low during labor, medical science can step in and supplement that natural source with a saline (salt) solution pumped directly into the amniotic sac through a catheter into the uterus. This procedure, called amnioinfusion, may also be used when there is moderate or very thick meconium staining of the amniotic fluid.

Because it improves uterine conditions, amnioinfusion can significantly reduce the possibility that a surgical delivery will become necessary due to fetal distress or another complication.

LABOR INDUCTION

"My doctor wants to induce labor. I'm upset because I had wanted a natural delivery."

There are a variety of medical situations in which it is probably wise—or even necessary—to deliver a baby before nature appears ready, willing, and able to do so. In some cases, a cesarean section is the best way to accomplish this. In other cases, when there's no immediate risk to baby (due to distress, for instance), both baby and mother are deemed able to tolerate labor, and the practitioner has reason to believe that a vaginal delivery is possible, induction is usually the first choice. For example:

♦ When a fetus isn't thriving—because of inadequate nourishment, postmaturity (being in the uterus ten days to two weeks beyond the estimated due date), low levels of amniotic fluid, or any other reason—and is mature enough to do well outside the uterus

♦ When tests suggest that the placenta is no longer functioning optimally and the uterus is no longer a healthy home for the fetus

♦ When the membranes rupture in a term pregnancy and labor doesn't begin within twenty-four hours thereafter (though some practitioners will induce much sooner)

♦ When the amniotic fluid is infected

♦ When a pregnancy has gone two or more weeks past a due date that is considered accurate

♦ When the mother has diabetes and the placenta is deteriorating prematurely, or when it's feared her baby will be very large—and thus difficult to deliver—if carried to full term

♦ When the mother has preeclampsia (toxemia) that cannot be controlled with bed rest and medication, and delivery is necessary for her sake and/or her baby's

♦ When the mother has a chronic or acute illness, such as high blood pressure or kidney disease, that threatens her well-being or that of her baby if the pregnancy continues

♦ When the fetus is afflicted with severe Rh disease that necessitates early delivery

In addition, an induction may be scheduled for the woman who might not make it to the hospital or birthing center on time once labor has started, either because she lives a long distance away or because she's had a previous very short labor.

The first and most important step in ensuring a successful induction is ripening the cervix—making it soft and ready for labor. Ripening the cervix is usually accomplished by administering a hormonal substance such as prostaglandin E-2 in the form of a vaginal gel (or a vaginal suppository in tablet form).[1] In this painless procedure, using a syringe, the gel is placed in the vagina close to the cervix. After a few hours of letting the gel do its work, the woman is checked to see if her cervix is getting softer and beginning the process of effacement and dilation. If it isn't, a second dose of the prostaglandin gel is administered. Most women respond well to the gel, and in many cases, the gel is enough to get contractions and labor started.[2] If the cervix is sufficiently ripened but contractions have not begun, the induction process continues.

The next step some practitioners take is to artificially rupture the membranes (the "bag of waters," also known as the amniotic sac) that surround the fetus (see page 351). Other practitioners may strip the membranes, a process that involves separating the membranes from the cervix. While stripping the membranes is not intended to break the bag, it sometimes does. It may also be painful for some women.

More often, medications like oxytocin (Pitocin) are used to induce labor

---

1. Some practitioners use mechanical agents to ripen the cervix, such as a catheter with an inflatable balloon, graduated dilators, or even an herb (laminaria japonicum) that, when inserted into the cervix, gradually opens the cervix as it absorbs fluid around it.

2. Outpatient cervical ripening (where the woman uses cervical ripening agents at home) is being studied now and might be done more often in the future.

once the cervix is ripe (if contractions haven't yet begun). Oxytocin is a hormone produced naturally by the maternal pituitary gland throughout pregnancy. As pregnancy progresses, the uterus becomes more and more sensitive to the hormone. When the cervix is ripe, oxytocin is capable of initiating (or augmenting; see box, page 342) a labor that closely mimics one that occurs naturally. New studies show that giving oxytocin at the same time as prostaglandins (so that induction and cervical ripening go hand in hand) shortens the overall length of labor, though most physicians still wait until the cervix is ripe before administering the oxytocin.(The drug misoprostol, given through the vagina, appears to be as or more effective as prostaglandin gel and oxytocin. Studies show that giving misoprostol decreases the amount of oxytocin needed and shortens labor.)

Oxytocin is generally administered through an intravenous drip (IV), a safe and easy way to precisely control the rate at which the medication enters the mother's body. Usually the induction begins slowly, with very little oxytocin being given, and the reactions of the uterus and the fetus carefully monitored. (A doctor or nurse must be in attendance at all times during induction.) The rate of infusion is increased gradually until effective contractions are established. Should the woman's uterus prove extremely sensitive to the drug and be overstimulated into either too long or too powerful contractions, this method allows the infusion rate to be reduced or discontinued entirely. Contractions usually begin about thirty minutes after oxytocin has been started. They're generally more regular and more frequent than those of a naturally occurring labor, right from the start. If, after six to eight hours of oxytocin administration, labor hasn't begun or progressed, the procedure will probably be terminated in favor of an alternative approach, usually a cesarean section. If contractions become well established and continue on their own, the oxytocin is also discontinued.

It is often possible to predict ahead of time whether or not induction will be successful using the Bishop score. Research also suggests that women at term who test positive for cervical fetal fibronectin (FFN) are more likely to have a successful induction. (For more on the Bishop score and FFN, see page 323.)

Induction of labor is inappropriate when immediate delivery is necessary, when there is any doubt that the fetus can fit through the mother's pelvis, or when VBAC is being tried (see page 27). The procedure also is avoided when the placenta is near or covering the opening of the uterus (placenta previa), there is a prolapsed cord, the fetus is lying sideways, there is a genital herpes infection, and, generally, in women who have had six or more previous births or who have a vertical uterine scar from a past cesarean section, since they are at greater risk for uterine rupture from very strong contractions. Some physicians will also not attempt induction when a woman is carrying multiple fetuses or when a baby is in the breech position. The American College of Obstetricians and Gynecologists recommends that when labor is induced, the physician be ready and available to perform an emergency cesarean, if one is needed.

Some women find the sudden onset of hard labor that sometimes occurs with induction unpleasant; some even feel cheated by the artificially shortened duration of their laboring experience. Others are relieved by such a down-to-business birth. With their coach at their side, they go through their induced labor otherwise naturally, using all the breathing exercises and other coping mechanisms learned in childbirth classes—

GIVING MOTHER NATURE A BOOST

Sometimes a woman goes into labor on her own, but for one reason or another, her contractions are either not effectively dilating the cervix or are too sluggish for labor to progress as it should. Often the physician will administer oxytocin to stimulate stronger and more effective contractions that will get the labor back on track.

recognizing that labor, no matter how it's triggered, is labor. Giving some thought in advance to the possibility of induced labor may help you to cope with it more effectively.

CALLING YOUR PRACTITIONER DURING LABOR

"I just started getting contractions and they're coming every three or four minutes. I feel silly calling my practitioner, who said we should spend the first several hours of labor at home."

Better silly than sorry. Most first-time mothers-to-be (whose labors often begin slowly, with a gradual buildup of contractions) can safely count on spending the first several hours at home. But if your contractions start off strong—lasting at least forty-five seconds and coming more frequently than every five minutes—your first several hours of labor may very well be your last, especially if you're not a first-timer. Chances are that much of the first stage of labor has passed painlessly, and that your cervix has dilated significantly during that time. This would mean that not calling your

practitioner, chancing a dramatic dash to the hospital or birthing center at the last minute or not getting there in time, would be considerably sillier than picking up the phone now.

Before you do, however, it is best to have timed contractions for about forty-five minutes to an hour (unless, of course, your contractions started off so close together that waiting this long would be asking for trouble). Be clear and specific about their frequency, duration, and strength when you report them. Since your practitioner is used to judging the phase of labor in part by the sound of a woman's voice as she talks through a contraction, don't try to downplay your discomfort or put on a brave front or maintain a calm tone of voice when you describe your situation. Let the contractions speak for themselves, unchecked by any sense of decorum.

If you feel you're ready but your practitioner doesn't seem to think so, don't take "wait" for an answer. Ask if you can go to the hospital or to your practitioner's office and have your progress checked. (See When to Call the Doctor in the About Prelabor, False Labor, Real Labor section, page 334.) You can take your suitcase along "just in case," but be ready to turn around and go home if you've only just begun to dilate.

IRREGULAR CONTRACTIONS

"In childbirth class we were told not to go to the hospital until the contractions were regular and five minutes apart. Mine are less than five minutes apart, but they aren't at all regular. I don't know what to do."

Just as no two women have exactly the same pregnancies, no two women have exactly the same labors. The labor often described in books, in childbirth education classes, and by practitioners is what is typical—and close to what many women can expect. But far from every labor is true-to-textbook, with contractions regularly spaced and predictably progressive.

If you are having strong, long (forty to sixty seconds), frequent (mostly five minutes apart or less) contractions, even if they vary considerably in length and time elapsed between them, do not wait for them to become "regular" before calling your practitioner or heading for the hospital, no matter what you've heard or read. It's possible that your contractions are about as regular as they are going to get, and that you are well into the active phase of your labor. Waste no time in calling your practitioner and getting to the hospital; she who hesitates in a case like this could end up with an unscheduled home birth.

BACK LABOR

"The pain in my back since my labor began is so bad that I don't see how I'll be able to make it through delivery."

What you're probably experiencing is known in the birthing business as "back labor." Technically, back labor occurs when the fetus is in a posterior position, with the back of its head pressing against the mother's sacrum—the rear boundary of the pelvis. It's possible, however, to experience back labor when the baby is not in this position, or to continue to experience it after the baby has turned from a head-to-the-back to head-to-the-front position[3]—possibly because the area has already become a focus of tension.

When you're having this kind of

pain—which often doesn't let up between contractions and can become excruciating during them—the cause is not a crucial consideration. How to relieve it, even slightly, is. There are several measures that may help; all are at least worth trying:

Taking the pressure off your back. Try changing your position. Walk around (though this may not be humanly possible once contractions are coming fast and furiously), crouch or squat, get down on all fours, do whatever is most comfortable and least painful for you. If you feel you can't move and would prefer to be lying down, lie on your left side, with your back well rounded—in a sort of fetal position.

Heat or cold, applied by your coach or attendant. Use a hot-water bottle wrapped in a towel, warm compresses, a heating pad, or ice packs or cold compresses—whichever soothes best. Or alternate heat and cold, if you find that most helpful.

Counterpressure. Have your coach experiment with different ways of applying pressure to the area of greatest pain, or to adjacent areas, to find one or more that seem to help. He can try his knuckles, or the heel of one hand reinforced by pressure from the other hand on top of it, using direct pressure or a firm circular motion. Pressure can be applied while you are sitting or while you are lying on your side. The relief you may get from really intense counterpressure will be well worth any black-and-blue marks you find the morning after.

Acupressure. This treatment, which has its roots in ancient Chinese medicine, is probably the oldest form of pain relief. For back labor, it involves applying strong finger pressure just below the center of the ball of the foot.

Massage. Aggressive massage to the area

---

3. This change occurs in most deliveries. When it doesn't, the doctor may be able to rotate the fetus or, failing this, try a forceps delivery (see page 354).

may spell relief either in place of counterpressure or alternated with it. A rolling pin or a tennis ball can be used for especially firm massage (although you will probably be pretty sore afterward). Oil or powder can be applied periodically to reduce possible irritation.

Other alternative pain relievers. If you've had some experience with meditation, visualization, self-hypnosis, or reflexology for pain, try these. They often work. Acupuncture can also help relieve pain, but you will have had to plan ahead to take advantage of this option.

Medicinal pain relief. If nothing helps and the pain continues to be excruciating, talk to your practitioner about the possible forms of pain relief available at your stage of labor.

HAVING A SHORT LABOR

"Can a short labor be harmful to the baby?"

Short labor isn't always as short as it seems. Often the expectant mother has been having painless contractions for hours, days, even weeks, contractions that have been dilating her cervix gradually. By the time she finally feels one, she is well into the transition stage of labor (see the Stages and Phases of Childbirth, beginning on page 357). This slow-buildup, quick-resolution labor places no extra strain on the fetus.

Occasionally the cervix dilates very rapidly, accomplishing in a matter of minutes what most cervixes (particularly those of first-time mothers) take hours to do. But even with this abrupt, or precipitous, kind of labor (one that takes three hours or less from start to finish), there is rarely any threat to the baby. There is no evidence to support the notion that an infant must go through some

minimum amount of labor in order to arrive in good condition.

Once in a great while, however, an extremely rapid labor does deprive the fetus of oxygen or other needed gases, or results in tearing or other damage to the mother's cervix, vagina, or perineum. So, if your labor seems to start with a bang—with contractions strong and close together—get to the hospital or birthing center quickly. Medication may be helpful in slowing contractions a bit and easing the pressure on your baby and on your own body.

NOT GETTING TO THE HOSPITAL IN TIME

"I'm afraid that I won't get to the hospital in time."

Fortunately, most of those sudden deliveries you've heard about take place in the movies and on television. In real life, deliveries, especially those of first-time mothers, rarely occur without ample warning. But once in a great while, a woman who has had no labor pains, or just erratic ones, suddenly feels an overwhelming urge to bear down; often she mistakes it for a need to go to the bathroom.

As remote as the possibility is that this will happen to you, it's a good idea for both you and your coach to become familiar with the basics of an emergency delivery (see boxes on facing page and page 348). Once that's done, relax—with the knowledge that a sudden and quick delivery is an extremely remote possibility.

ENEMAS

"I've heard that enemas early in labor aren't really necessary, and that they interfere with natural birth."

At one time, enemas were administered routinely in early labor as part of the hospital admissions procedure. The theory was that emptying the bowels *before* delivery would allow for less cramped conditions in the birth canal (caused by a full bowel pressing against it), and would speed baby's trip down it. It was also believed that the enema (by stimulating a bowel movement before delivery) might spare the laboring woman the "embarrassment" of eliminating on the delivery table and might also lessen her inhibitions about pushing as well as prevent contamination of the sterile birthing setup by the feces.

Today, thankfully, enemas are no longer routine, and for good reason. First of all, it is now recognized that it's not likely a full rectum will compress the birth canal if a woman has had a bowel movement in the past twenty-four hours—and, in fact, many labors begin with loose, frequent bowel movements that effectively clear out the colon. Second, the use of disposable sterile gauze pads during delivery to whisk away any fecal matter that does make its way out virtually eliminates the threat of contamination. Finally, though an enema may reduce the likelihood that feces will be pushed out on the birthing bed, it doesn't eliminate it entirely. Which is nothing to be embarrassed about any-

EMERGENCY DELIVERY IF YOU'RE ALONE

1. Try to remain calm. You *can* do this.

2. Call 911 (or your local emergency number) for the emergency medical service. Ask them to call your practitioner.

3. Find a neighbor or someone else to help, if possible.

4. Start panting to keep yourself from pushing.

5. Wash your hands and the vaginal area, if you can.

6. Spread some clean towels, newspapers, or sheets on a bed, sofa, or the floor, and lie down to await help.

7. If despite your panting the baby starts to arrive before help does, gently ease it out by pushing each time you feel the urge.

8. As the top of the baby's head begins to appear, pant or blow (do not push), and apply very gentle counterpressure to your perineum to keep the head from popping out suddenly. Let the head emerge gradually—never pull it out. If there is a loop of umbilical cord around the baby's neck, hook a finger under it and gently work it over the baby's head.

9. Next take the head gently in two hands and press it very slightly downward (*do not* pull), pushing at the same time, to deliver the front shoulder. As the upper arm appears, lift the head carefully, feeling for the rear shoulder to deliver. Once the shoulders are free, the rest of the baby should slip out easily.

10. Place the baby on your abdomen, or if the cord is long enough (don't tug at it), at your breast. Quickly wrap the baby in blankets, towels, or anything else that is available (preferably something clean; something recently ironed is relatively sterile).

11. Don't try to pull the placenta out. But if it emerges on its own before emergency assistance arrives, wrap it in towels or newspaper, and keep it elevated above the level of the baby, if possible. There is no need to try to cut the cord.

12. Keep yourself and your baby warm and comfortable until help arrives.

way, since it's a normal part of childbirth. After all, to paraphrase the popular proverb: bowel movements happen . . . during delivery.

SHAVING THE PUBIC AREA

"Is it still considered necessary to have your pubic hair shaved before labor? I don't like the idea."

How you wear your pubic hair at delivery is entirely up to you nowadays, since shaving of the pubic area has pretty much been abandoned in U.S. hospitals. It was once believed that pubic hair harbored bacteria that could infect the baby as it passed through the vaginal outlet and that shaving was the only way to effectively eliminate that risk. But since the entire area surrounding the vagina is swabbed with an antiseptic solution prior to delivery, infection isn't a likely problem anyway. And, in fact, some studies have shown a higher rate of infection among women who are shaved prior to delivery than among those who aren't, probably because the small—sometimes microscopic—nicks that even very careful shaving can produce may serve as excellent breeding grounds for bacteria. From the woman's point of view, the humiliation of being shaved and the postpartum burning and itching as the hair grows back are additional reasons this procedure of the past is best left there. (Of course, if you typically shave or wax your pubic hair and you prefer it that way, there's no reason why you can't continue to do so in pregnancy—just be extra wary of cuts and irritation.)

Some doctors still feel that shaving facilitates performing and repairing an episiotomy, by providing a clearer area in which to work. But most find clipping the hair with scissors or pushing it back as they work gives them an adequate view.

On the slight chance that your doctor is one of the few still ordering patients shaved, ask in advance. If you object, don't wait until you arrive at the hospital to make your feelings known. Include your preferences in your birthing plan.

EATING AND DRINKING DURING LABOR

"I've heard conflicting stories about whether it's permissible to eat and drink during labor."

That's not surprising, since there are conflicting views. At one time, eating and drinking once labor began were strictly prohibited for fear that food in the digestive tract might be breathed in (aspirated) should emergency general anesthesia be necessary. Some doctors and hospitals still take that position. (They usually permit only ice chips to help hydrate the laboring woman, supplemented as needed by intravenous fluids.) More, however, do allow liquids and light solids during a low-risk labor, reasoning that a woman in labor needs both fluids and calories to stay strong and do her best work.

The number of studies on the subject is few, but the one study that looked at the aspiration risk (which only exists if general anesthesia is used, and it rarely is) found it to be extremely low: 7 in 10 million births. And there have been no studies showing a benefit from fasting during labor; fasting can, in fact, increase stress levels and cause dehydration. Some studies have also shown that women who are allowed to eat and drink during labor have shorter labors by an average of ninety minutes, are less likely to need oxytocin to speed up labor, require fewer pain medications, and have babies with higher Apgar scores than women who don't eat. Though you may have little or no appetite, an occasional light snack—

fruit Popsicles, gels, or juices, cooked fruit, dry toast, or clear broth are ideal choices—may well help keep your energy up at a time you need it most. So do discuss this issue with your practitioner and include it in your birthing plan.

ROUTINE IVS

"When we had our tour of the hospital, I saw a woman being wheeled from the delivery room with an IV attached. Is that necessary with a normal labor and delivery?"

Thanks to TV hospital dramas and war movies, we readily associate IVs (intravenous setups) with wounded GIs, rapidly fading heroines with fatal illnesses, and heroes soundly thrashed by jealous lovers. But it's hard to associate an IV with normal childbirth.

Yet in some hospitals, it is routine to administer an IV containing a simple solution of nutrients and fluid to a woman in labor. This is done partly to be certain that the woman does not become dehydrated from lack of fluids or weak from lack of food during labor (if eating and drinking aren't allowed; see the previous question), partly to provide ready access for medication should the need arise (it can be injected right into the IV bottle or line, instead of into the patient). In these instances, the IV is precautionary, intended to prevent a problem from developing.

Many doctors and midwives, on the other hand, prefer to wait until there is a clear need for an IV—for instance, because the labor has been lengthy and the mother-to-be is running out of energy, or if an epidural is on the agenda. Check your practitioner's policy in advance, and if you strongly object to having a routine IV, say so. It may be possible to hold off until the need, if any, arises.

If it's your practitioner's policy to give IVs routinely and there's no room for discussion, or if you end up needing one, don't despair. The IV is only slightly uncomfortable as the needle is inserted and thereafter should barely be noticed. When it's hung on a movable stand, you can take it with you to the bathroom or on a stroll down the corridors. (If at any point the IV site becomes sore or painful, inform your practitioner or nurse immediately.)

Though you can't always make the decision about whether or not you should have an IV, you do have a right to know what the IV is infusing into your veins. Ask the nurse or doctor who inserts it. Or have your labor partner read the label on the bottle. Occasionally medication may be ordered without your being consulted. If this happens, ask to speak to your practitioner as soon as possible. Better still, have your coach or doula do the talking for you.

FETAL MONITORING

"I've heard that fetal monitoring can lead to unnecessary cesareans and also makes labor more uncomfortable. Will I have to have it?"

For someone who's spent the first nine months of his or her life floating peacefully in a warm and comforting amniotic bath, the trip through the narrow confines of the maternal pelvis will be no joyride. Your baby will be squeezed, compressed, pushed, and molded with every contraction.

It is because there is an element of risk in this stressful journey that fetal monitors—which assess how a fetus is doing during labor by gauging the response of its heartbeat to the contractions of the uterus—first came into common use. For a while, some hospitals continuously electronically monitored all labor and delivery patients. Most others monitored at least half of the patients,

EMERGENCY DELIVERY: TIPS FOR THE COACH

At Home or in the Office

1. Try to remain calm, while at the same time comforting and reassuring the mother. Remember, even if you don't know the first thing about delivering a baby, a mother's body and her baby can do most of the job on their own.

2. Call 911 (or your local emergency number) for the emergency medical service; ask them to call the practitioner.

3. Have the mother start panting, to keep from pushing.

4. If there's time, wash the vaginal area and your hands with detergent or soap and water (use an antibacterial product, if you have one handy).

5. If there's no time to get to a bed or table, place newspapers or clean towels or folded clothing under the mother's buttocks. Protect delivery surfaces, if possible, with a plastic tablecloth, shower curtain, newspapers, towels, or similar material. A dishpan or basin can be placed under the mother's vagina to catch the amniotic fluid and blood.

6. If there is time, place the mother on the bed (or desk or table) so that her buttocks are slightly hanging off, her hands under her thighs to keep them elevated. If available, a couple of chairs can support her feet. A few pillows or cushions under her shoulders and head will help to raise her to a semi-sitting position, which can aid delivery. If you are awaiting emergency help and the baby's head hasn't appeared, however, having the mother lie flat may slow delivery until help arrives. Protect delivery surfaces, if possible, as described in number 5.

7. As the top of the baby's head begins to appear, instruct the mother to pant or blow (not push), and apply very gentle counter-pressure to her perineum to keep the head from popping out suddenly. Let the head emerge gradually—never pull it out. If there is a loop of umbilical cord around the baby's neck, hook a finger under it and gently work it over the baby's head.

8. Next take the head gently in two hands and press it very slightly downward (*do not* pull), asking the mother to push at the same time, to deliver the front shoulder. As the upper arm appears, lift the head carefully, watching for the rear shoulder to deliver. Once the shoulders are free, the rest of the baby should slip out easily.

---

particularly those in high-risk categories, who had meconium-stained amniotic fluid, who were receiving oxytocin, who had an epidural, or who were having a difficult labor.

A review of the research, however, now suggests that in low-risk labors and deliveries, these high-tech instruments are no better at spotting problems than the Doppler (see page 163). As long as the Doppler is used to check the baby's heartbeat at regular intervals (every fifteen to thirty minutes during labor and every five minutes during delivery), it can be just as effective in assessing fetal condition. (In some hospitals, however, cutbacks in nursing staff may mean that fetal heart checks are not done frequently enough. If you are not hooked up to a fetal monitor, your coach or doula should make sure that your baby's heartbeat is checked at the recommended intervals.)

Because routine continuous electronic fetal monitoring is believed to have led to an increase in unnecessary cesareans in some hospitals (when results are misread or readings are not confirmed with other tests), and is viewed by some as

9. Place the baby on the mother's abdomen, or if the cord is long enough (don't tug at it), at her breast. Quickly wrap the baby in blankets, towels, or anything else that is available (preferably something clean; something recently ironed is relatively sterile).

10. Don't try to pull the placenta out. But if it emerges on its own before emergency assistance arrives, wrap it in towels or newspaper, and keep it elevated above the level of the baby, if possible. There is no need to try to cut the cord.

11. Keep both mother and baby warm and comfortable until help arrives.

En Route to the Hospital

If you're in your own car and delivery is imminent, pull over. If you have a cell phone with you, call for help. If not, turn on your hazard warning lights or turning signal. If someone stops to help, ask him or her to get to a phone and call 911 or the local emergency medical service. If you're in a cab, ask the driver to radio for help.

If possible, you should help the mother into the back of the car. Place a coat, jacket, or blanket under her. Then, if help has not arrived, proceed as for a home delivery. As soon as the baby is born, continue to the nearest hospital in a hurry.

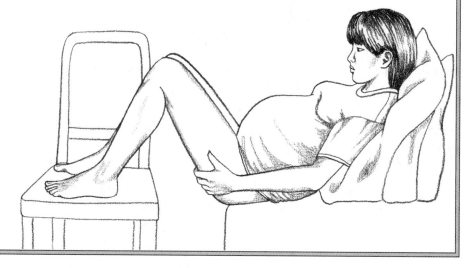

just another technological intrusion into the birthing process (replacing a one-on-one nurse with an impersonal machine), the practice seems to be slowly falling out of favor in the obstetrical community. Though some doctors and hospitals continue to monitor routinely, the American College of Obstetricians and Gynecologists states that in low-risk pregnancies, intermittent fetal heart checks are an acceptable alternative to continuous electronic fetal monitoring.

So if yours is a low-risk delivery, there's a good chance you won't have continuous electronic fetal monitoring or that you'll never even encounter a fetal monitor during your birth experience. If, however, you or your baby are at high risk (or if you've been induced or have an epidural), it's almost certain that you'll meet up with one at some point in your labor or delivery. Either way, it's a good idea to become familiar with the types of monitoring and how they work.

External monitoring. In this type of monitoring, used most frequently, two devices are strapped to the abdomen. One, an ultrasound transducer, picks up the fetal heartbeat. The other, a pressure-sensitive gauge, measures the intensity and duration of uterine contractions. Both are connected to a monitor, which displays or prints out the readings. External fetal monitoring doesn't confine a laboring woman to bed, hooked up to a machine like Frankenstein's monster, for hours on end. In most cases, monitoring is required only intermittently, which means the mother-to-be can have freedom of movement between readings. Some hospitals are equipped with portable monitors that can be hooked up to the patient's clothing, allowing her to walk around while data on her baby's well-being is sent back to her bedside or a nursing station.

During the second (pushing) stage of labor, when contractions may come so fast and furiously that it's hard to know when to push and when to hold back, the monitor can be used to accurately signal the beginning and end of each contraction. Or the use of the monitor may be all but abandoned during this stage, so as not to interfere with the mother's concentration. In this case, the fetal heart rate is checked periodically with a Doppler.

Internal monitoring. When more accurate results are required—such as when there is reason to suspect fetal distress—an internal monitor may be used. In this type of monitoring, an electrode that transmits a reading of the fetal heartbeat is attached to the baby's scalp. Since the electrode must be passed through the cervix, internal monitoring is possible only once dilation has reached at least 1 or 2 centimeters and the membranes have ruptured. Contractions can be measured either with the pressure gauge strapped to the mother's abdomen or with a fluid-filled catheter (tube) inserted

into the uterus. Because an internal monitor can't be periodically disconnected and reconnected, it limits mobility somewhat—but changes in the mother's position are still possible.

Sometimes internal monitoring employs telemetry, a technology that reads and transmits vital signs via radio waves. This technique, pioneered in the space program, allows the laboring woman to be monitored without being confined by equipment. She is totally mobile—able to strike any position she finds comfortable, to go to the bathroom, or even to take a stroll.

Like any invasive medical procedure (one that enters or intrudes upon the body), internal fetal monitoring entails some risks. There is a slight risk of infection, and in some instances the baby later develops a rash, or occasionally an abscess, on the site where the electrode was placed, and, very rarely, may even be left with a permanent bald spot. Because of the risks, however small—and because it's possible that the insertion of the electrode causes momentary pain or discomfort to the baby—internal fetal monitoring is best used only when its benefits are significant.

With both internal and external types of monitoring, a printout that indicates that the fetus is doing well is virtually always accurate. On the other hand, readings that point to trouble are much less accurate. So, if the monitor signals trouble, it's most likely a false alarm.

False alarms—which can actually come in the form of a loud (and potentially scary-sounding) beep if the monitor has been preset to alert personnel when a variation in heart rate occurs—are common. Sometimes, the false alarm comes because the monitor isn't working right; sometimes because it's misread; sometimes because contractions have suddenly picked up intensity and frequency. Even when the monitors do detect an actual problem, it's often one that's easily rectified. For example, frequently an abnormal heart rate reading is simply a result of the mother's position putting pressure on a major blood vessel or her baby's cord, interfering with blood flow. In that case, having her change her position (to her left side) brings the readings back to the normal range quickly. If administration of oxytocin is causing the variation, reducing the dosage or terminating the infusion completely will generally clear it up. Another easy fix that often does the trick: giving oxygen to the mother.

An experienced and knowledgeable obstetrician will take many factors into account before concluding that a baby is actually in trouble. If the abnormal readings continue, several possible next steps can be taken. If the fetus seems in imminent danger, the physician may opt for an immediate cesarean delivery. If there's time, further evaluation will be undertaken. First, some speedy testing will be done to verify the monitoring results: the amniotic fluid will be checked for meconium; pH levels in a fetal blood sample, taken from the scalp, will be assessed; and/or the response of the fetal heart to sound stimulation, or to pressure on or pinching of the fetal scalp, will be evaluated. Since direct access to the fetus is necessary in order for some of these tests to be performed, the membranes will be ruptured artificially at this point, if they haven't already ruptured spontaneously or been ruptured earlier. In addition, the mother's medical and obstetrical history may be reviewed to determine if the fetal heart rate abnormalities might be related to maternal infection or chronic disease or to medication the mother is taking, rather than to actual fetal distress. In some cases, the monitor printout may be faxed to a consulting expert for a second opinion. If fetal distress is confirmed, then an immediate cesarean is usually called for. In some situations, the physician may first administer drugs to try to improve the condition of the fetus while it's still in the uterus. When successful, this approach allots everyone additional time to prepare for a cesarean delivery,[4] enhances the chances of delivering an alert baby, and in some cases may even allow a vaginal delivery to continue.

A new device recently approved by the FDA can provide doctors a more reliable picture of conditions in the uterus. The OxiFirst fetal monitor is a thin probe placed through the cervix and next to the baby's cheek that measures the baby's blood oxygen levels. It is useful in cases where the fetal heart monitor is difficult to interpret and when additional information can help decide if labor should continue or if a cesarean is needed. The equipment is new, however, and the majority of hospitals don't use it yet.

ARTIFICIAL RUPTURE OF MEMBRANES

"I'm afraid that if my water doesn't break on its own, the doctor will have to rupture the membranes artificially. Won't that hurt?"

Most women don't feel a thing when their membranes are artificially ruptured, particularly if they're already in labor (there are far more significant pains to cope with then). A few do experience a little discomfort, but that's more likely from the introduction into the vagina of the amniohook (the instrument used to perform the procedure) than from the rupture itself. Chances are, all you'll really notice is a gush of water,

4. Among other benefits, this extra time may allow for an epidural, rather than the general anesthesia usually necessary in emergency surgeries.

followed soon (at least that's the hope) by harder and faster contractions that will get your baby moving. (Artificial rupture of the membranes is also performed to allow for other procedures, such as internal fetal monitoring and forceps delivery, when necessary.)

Many practitioners wait until the cervix has dilated to 5 centimeters before rupturing membranes that haven't broken spontaneously, though some will take amniohook in hand by 3 or 4 centimeters if labor is progressing too slowly. If there's no compelling reason to rupture them (labor's moving along just fine), you and your practitioner may decide to hold off until even later on. Occasionally, membranes stay stubbornly intact throughout delivery (the baby is born with the bag of waters still surrounding him or her, and the doctor or midwife must then rupture the membranes upon delivery to allow the baby to take its first breath)—and that's fine, too.

THE SIGHT OF BLOOD

"The sight of blood makes me feel faint. What if I pass out while I'm watching my delivery?"

The sight of blood makes many people feel weak in the knees. But, remarkably, even the most squeamish women—and most of their mates—manage to get through their own deliveries without smelling salts.

First of all, there isn't all that much blood—not much more than you see when you're menstruating (a little more with an episiotomy or a tear). Second, you're not really a spectator at your delivery; you'll be a very active participant, putting every ounce of your concentration and energy into pushing your baby those last few inches. Caught up in the excitement and anticipation (and, let's face it, the pain and fatigue), you are un-

likely to notice, much less be unsettled by, any bleeding. If you ask friends who are new mothers, few will be able to tell you just how much blood, if any, there was at their deliveries.

If you feel strongly that you don't want to see any blood, simply avert your eyes from the mirror (if one has been provided for you) if and when an episiotomy is performed, and at the moment of birth. Instead, just look down past your belly for a good view of your baby as it emerges. From this vantage point, virtually no blood will be visible. (Some fathers, too, worry about how they'll handle viewing the birth. If your spouse is anxious about this aspect of delivery, have him take a look at page 442.)

AN EPISIOTOMY

"Will having an episiotomy make delivery easier for me and safer for my baby?"

At one time, there was little question that the answer was yes. In fact, since the middle of the last century, this minor surgical procedure (during which an incision is made in the perineum to enlarge the vaginal opening just before the emergence of the baby's head) was considered fairly routine by many physicians. But obstetrics is an evolving science, and opinion on this procedure (and many others) has evolved with it. The American College of Obstetricians and Gynecologists currently recommends that an episiotomy should *not* be performed routinely.

The reason for the turnaround is simple: apparently, the long-perceived benefits of the procedure actually do not exist. Historically, the episiotomy, which originated in Ireland in 1742 to help facilitate difficult births, was thought to prevent many complications in the mother, including tearing of the perineum and urinary and fecal incontinence. In the newborn, it was believed that episiotomies reduced the risk of birth trauma (from the fetal head pushing long and hard against the perineum) that could lead to cerebral palsy and other neurological damage. But recent studies have found infants fare as well without an episiotomy, and experience no more trauma to the head after a prolonged second stage of labor. And mothers, too, seem to do as well, if not better, without it. Average *total* labor seems no longer. And the mothers often experience less blood loss, less infection, less fecal and urinary incontinence, and less perineal pain after delivery. Nor are they at higher risk of postpartum complications than women with episiotomies.

But while routine episiotomies are no longer recommended, there is still a place for them in certain obstetrical scenarios. Episiotomies may be indicated when a baby is large and needs a roomier exit route, when forceps or vacuum delivery need to be performed, or for the relief of shoulder dystocia (in which a shoulder gets stuck in the birth canal during delivery).

There are two basic types of episiotomies: the median and the mediolateral. The median incision is made directly back toward the rectum. In spite of its advantages (it provides more exit space per inch of incision, heals well and is easier to repair, causes less blood loss, and results in less postpartum discomfort or infection), it is less frequently used in the United States because it has a greater risk of tearing completely through to the rectum. To avoid this tearing, most physicians prefer the mediolateral incision, which slants away from the rectum, especially in first births.

To reduce the possibility that you'll need an episiotomy and to ease delivery without one, it's a good idea to do Kegel exercises (see page 193) and perineal massage (see page 330) for six to eight weeks before your due date. During labor, the following can also help: warm compresses to lessen perineal discomfort; perineal massage; a standing or squatting position, exhaling or grunting while pushing to facilitate stretching of the perineum; and avoiding regional anesthesia, which makes the perineal muscles flaccid. During the pushing phase, one of the attendants will probably use perineal support—applying gentle counterpressure to the perineum so the baby's head doesn't push out too quickly and cause an unnecessary tear.

If you haven't already, discuss the episiotomy issue with your practitioner. It's likely he or she will agree that the procedure should not be performed routinely. Document your feelings about episiotomies in your birthing plan (see page 274) so that all hospital personnel will be aware of them. But keep in mind that, occasionally, episiotomies do turn out to be necessary, and the final decision should be made not before you go into labor, but in the delivery or birthing room, with your well-being and the safe delivery of your baby the prime considerations.

BEING STRETCHED BY CHILDBIRTH

"I'm concerned about my vagina stretching and tearing. Will I ever be the same again?"

The vagina is a remarkably elastic organ, whose accordion-like folds open for childbirth. It is normally so narrow that inserting a tampon may be difficult, yet it can expand to allow the passage of a 7- or 8-pound baby. Over a period of weeks following delivery, it returns to close to its original size.

The perineum, the area between the vagina and the rectum, is also elastic, but less so than the vagina. Massage during the months prior to delivery may help increase its elasticity and reduce stretching. Likewise, exercising the pelvic muscles during this period may enhance their elasticity, strengthen them, and hasten their return to normal tone.

Many couples report that sex after delivery is even more satisfying than it was before, thanks to the increased muscular awareness and control the woman has developed as a result of prepared childbirth training. In other words, you may not be the same after childbirth—you may be even better!

Most women find that the slight increase in roominess they experience postpartum is imperceptible and does not interfere with sexual enjoyment. For those who were unusually small before conception, it can be a real plus, as intercourse may become more pleasurable. Very occasionally, however, in a woman who was "just right" before, childbirth does stretch the vagina enough to reduce sexual enjoyment. Often, the vaginal muscles tighten up again with the passage of time. Faithfully doing Kegels after delivery, at frequent intervals during the day—while showering, washing the dishes, walking with the baby, driving the car, sitting at your desk—should help speed the process. If after six months the vagina still seems too slack, talk to your doctor about other possible treatments.

STIRRUPS DURING DELIVERY

"I really hate having my feet in stirrups. Do I have to during delivery?"

Few if any women who've had a pelvic exam have anything good to say about stirrups. Fortunately, most won't have to encounter them during delivery—for several reasons. First, birthing beds have, for the most part, taken the place of the stirrup-equipped delivery table. Second, a variety of birthing positions have replaced the standard woman-on-her-back, legs-up-and-spread attitude. Third, there is strong antistirrup sentiment among women who, like yourself, want as much control and dignity during childbirth as possible. Besides which, women today are much better prepared for childbirth than they were in generations past; the stirrups that once kept them from thrashing around in pain and fear of the unknown are now largely unnecessary.

Still, a few physicians continue to ask their patients to use the stirrups during delivery because they believe this allows room for maneuvering—particularly during a forceps, vacuum, or breech delivery. And some women still find stirrups help while they push by keeping their thighs open and back. As always, different strokes work for different laboring folk.

Discuss the issue of stirrups with your practitioner in advance. It's very likely that your wishes in this matter will prevail.

FORCEPS AND VACUUM EXTRACTION

"I've heard that a lot more doctors are doing forceps deliveries or using vacuum extraction. Is this safe?"

It was in 1598 that British surgeon Peter Chamberlen the Elder designed the first pair of forceps and used the tong-shaped instrument to grasp a baby's head and ease it out of the birth canal when a difficult delivery might otherwise cost both mother and infant their lives. Instead of writing himself up in the latest obstetrical journal, however, Dr. Chamberlen kept his discovery a secret, privy only to four generations of Chamberlen medical men and their patients, many of them royalty. Indeed, the use of forceps might have ended forever with the career

OUTLET FORCEPS AND VACUUM EXTRACTOR

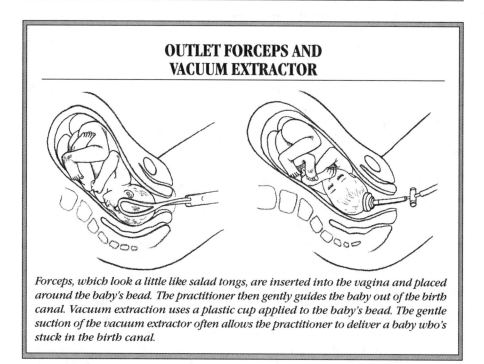

Forceps, which look a little like salad tongs, are inserted into the vagina and placed around the baby's head. The practitioner then gently guides the baby out of the birth canal. Vacuum extraction uses a plastic cup applied to the baby's head. The gentle suction of the vacuum extractor often allows the practitioner to deliver a baby who's stuck in the birth canal.

of the last Chamberlen doctor had a hidden box of instruments not been uncovered beneath a floorboard in the family's ancestral home in the mid-1800s.

For a while, near the end of the last century, there were those who believed the use of forceps should have died with those Chamberlen doctors. Concern that forceps might do more harm than good—and might even be responsible for serious injuries to both infants and mothers—gave these instruments more negative than positive press. But the latest studies have shown that forceps deliveries are no more or less likely to be associated with bad outcomes than other forms of delivery, and that they have a place in modern obstetrics.

Like any other childbirth intervention, forceps should be used only by a physician experienced in the procedure and only when valid indications exist. Most commonly, these include prolonged labor or prolonged second-stage labor (see page 368); maternal distress (the

mother is exhausted; can't push well; or has heart, muscular, neurological, or respiratory disease that prevents her from pushing); an abnormal fetal heart rate; vaginal bleeding from a suspected placental abruption; or cord prolapse.

Before a forceps delivery is attempted, it's necessary for the mother's cervix to be fully dilated and effaced, for her membranes to have ruptured, and for the fetal head to be engaged. In addition, all should be in readiness for a cesarean section should a trial of forceps fail. Once those conditions are met, the mother is given a local anesthetic to numb the perineal area. Then the curved tongs are cradled one at a time around the temples of the crowning head, and the baby is gently delivered.

The vacuum extractor, an alternative to forceps, has a plastic cup that is placed on the baby's head to gently pull him or her out of the birth canal. It is becoming much more popular in obstetrical practices, with its use probably outpacing that of forceps. Indications for vacuum extraction are similar to those for forceps delivery, and both the vacuum extractor and forceps have been found to be as safe for the baby as a cesarean is. The vacuum extractor shouldn't be used if the pregnancy is under 34 weeks, or if there is a breech or face presentation. If the procedure isn't working or if the cup keeps slipping off, the effort will be abandoned. As with forceps procedures, the physician performing a vacuum extraction should be well trained in its application and ready to do a cesarean if the procedure fails.

If during delivery your doctor suggests the need for forceps or vacuum extraction to speed things up, you might want to ask if you can rest for several contractions (time permitting) before trying again; such a break might give you the second wind you need to push your baby out effectively. You can also try changing your position: get up on all fours, or squat; the force of gravity might shift the baby's head.

Any questions you have about the possible use of forceps or vacuum extraction during your delivery should be discussed with your practitioner now, before you go into labor. He or she should be able to allay any concerns you might have.

APGAR SCORE

"I've heard some of my friends who just had babies discuss the Apgar score. What's an Apgar?"

It's your baby's first test. The Apgar was developed in 1952 by Dr. Virginia Apgar, a noted anesthesiologist, to enable medical personnel to quickly evaluate the condition of a newborn. At one minute after birth, a nurse or doctor checks the infant's Appearance (color), Pulse (heartbeat), Grimace (reflex), Activity (muscle tone), and Respiration. Hence the eponymous acronym AP-GAR. Babies who score above 6 are fine. Those who score between 4 and 6 often need resuscitation, which generally includes suctioning their airways and administering oxygen. Those who score un-

APGAR TABLE

SIGN	POINTS		
	0	1	2
Appearance (color)*	Pale or blue	Body pink, extremities blue	Pink all over
Pulse (heartbeat)	Not detectible	Below 100	Over 100
Grimace (reflex irritability)	No response to stimulation	Grimace	Lusty cry
Activity (muscle tone)	Flaccid (weak or no activity)	Some movement of extremities	A lot of activity
Respiration	None	Slow, irregular	Good (crying, breathing)

*In non-Caucasian children, the color of mucous membranes of the mouth, of the whites of the eyes, and of the lips, palms, hands, and soles of feet will be examined.

der 4 require more dramatic lifesaving techniques.

The Apgar test is administered once again at five minutes after birth. If the score is 7 or better at this point, the outlook for the infant is very good. If it's lower, it means the baby needs some careful watching, but is still very likely to turn out fine.

Other tests will also be performed on your newborn. For more information, see *What to Expect the First Year.*

LABOR POSITIONS

"I know you're not supposed to lie on your back during labor. But what position is best?"

The best labor position is the one that's best for you. And with the exception of lying flat on your back—which can not only slow down labor but also compress major blood vessels, possibly interfering with blood flow to the fetus—almost any position or combination of positions can end up working well. Particularly efficient are upright positions that employ the forces of gravity, speeding dilation and baby's descent; studies show that they can actually shorten labor. These include standing, sitting (in bed, on a exercise ball, in your coach's arms), squatting or half kneeling, half squatting (on the floor or on the bed), and straddling a chair. While the latest research shows that walking during labor probably does not speed up the process any more than standing (or another upright position), it also does no harm and may in fact reduce discomfort. Some women also find that kneeling on all fours (on a bed or on the floor) brings some measure of relief.

If you are more comfortable lying down in bed while laboring, lie on your left side to promote more efficient circulation, and do Pelvic Tilts periodically (see page 194).

What It's Important to Know:
THE STAGES AND PHASES OF CHILDBIRTH

Few pregnancies seem as though they could have been lifted right from the pages of an obstetrical text—with morning sickness that vanishes at the end of the first trimester, first fetal movements felt at precisely 20 weeks, and lightening that occurs exactly two weeks before the onset of labor. Likewise, few childbirth experiences mirror the textbook case—commencing with mild regular contractions that progress at a predictable pace to delivery. Yet just as it's helpful to have a general idea of what a typical woman can expect when she's expecting, it's helpful to know what an average childbirth is like—as long as you are prepared for the likelihood of variations that will make your experience yours alone.

Childbirth is divided (more loosely by nature, more formally by obstetrical science) into three stages. The *first stage* is labor, divided into three phases: early (or latent), active, and transitional, ending with the full dilation (opening) of the cervix; the *second stage* is delivery, culminating in the birth of the baby; and the *third stage* is delivery of the placenta, or afterbirth. The whole process averages about fourteen hours for first-time mothers, about eight hours for women

LABOR POSITIONS

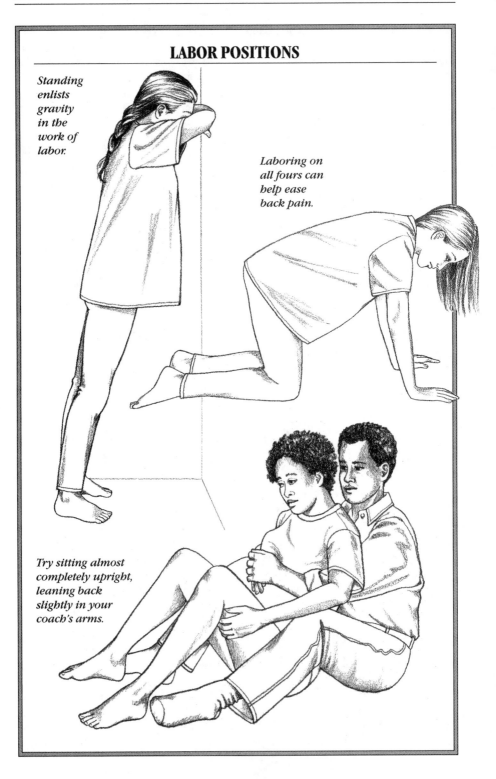

Standing enlists gravity in the work of labor.

Laboring on all fours can help ease back pain.

Try sitting almost completely upright, leaning back slightly in your coach's arms.

STAGES AND PHASES OF LABOR

STAGE ONE: Labor
  Phase 1: Latent or Early—thinning (effacement) of cervix and dilation to 3 centimeters
  Phase 2: Active—dilation of cervix to 7 centimeters
  Phase 3: Transitional—dilation of cervix to 10 centimeters (fully dilated)

STAGE TWO: Delivery of the baby

STAGE THREE: Delivery of the placenta

who have already had children—but the range is enormous, from a few hours to a few days.

Unless labor is cut short by the need for a cesarean, all women who carry to term go through all three phases of the first stage. Some, however, may not recognize that they are in labor until the second, or even the third, phase because their initial contractions are mild or painless. The third phase is complete once the cervix has dilated to a full 10 centimeters. For a very few women, all of dilation passes unnoticed; they don't realize they're in labor until they feel the urge to push that signals the second, or delivery, stage.

The timing and intensity of contractions can help pinpoint which phase of labor you are in at any particular time. Periodic internal exams, to check on the progress of dilation, will confirm the progress.

If labor doesn't seem to be progressing along the typical course, some doctors will augment Mother Nature's efforts by administering oxytocin, and if that fails, will preempt her entirely with a cesarean. Others may allow more time before taking such action, as long as both mother and baby are doing well.

THE FIRST STAGE OF CHILDBIRTH: LABOR

THE FIRST PHASE: EARLY, OR LATENT, LABOR

This is usually the longest and, fortunately, the least intense phase of labor. The dilation (opening) of the cervix to 3 centimeters and the accompanying effacement (thinning out) that characterize this phase can be reached over a period of days or weeks without noticeable or bothersome contractions, or over a period of two to six hours (and, less commonly, up to twenty-four hours) of unmistakable labor.

Contractions in this phase usually last thirty to forty-five seconds, though they can be shorter. They are mild to moderately strong, may be regular or irregular (ranging between five and twenty minutes apart), and become progressively closer together, but not necessarily in a consistent pattern. Some women don't notice them at all.

You will probably be told to go to the hospital at the end of this phase or the beginning of the next.

What you may feel or notice. The most common signs and symptoms in Phase One include: backache (either constant or with each contraction), menstrual-like cramps, indigestion, diarrhea, a sensation of warmth in the abdomen, and bloody show (a blood-tinged mu-

PAIN PERCEPTION
IN PERSPECTIVE

There's no question that labor contractions hurt. But there's no reason why they should hurt more than they have to. The amount of pain you perceive can actually be increased or decreased by a number of factors that are largely within your control, especially with a little planning and a lot of perspective.

Your perception of pain may be increased by:	It may be decreased by:
Being alone	Having the company and support of those you love, and/or of experienced medical personnel
Fatigue	Being well rested (try not to overdo things during the ninth month); trying to rest and relax between contractions
Hunger and thirst	Eating and drinking lightly during early labor; sucking ice chips, drinking fluid, and snacking throughout, if permitted
Thinking about and expecting pain	Turning your mind to other thoughts and distractions (though not during pushing); thinking of contractions in terms of how much they accomplish, rather than how much they hurt; and remembering that no matter how intense the discomfort, it won't last forever
Anxiety and stress; tensing up during contractions	Using relaxation, meditation, or visualization techniques between contractions; concentrating on your breathing and pushing efforts during them
Fear of the unknown	Learning as much as you can about labor and delivery in advance; taking childbirth one contraction at a time; and not worrying about what's to come
Self-pity	Thinking about how lucky you are and about the wonderful reward ahead
Feeling out of control and helpless	Having good childbirth preparation; knowing enough to feel some measure of control and confidence

cousy discharge). You may experience all of these, or just one or two. The amniotic membranes may rupture before the onset of contractions, but it is more likely that they will rupture (or be artificially ruptured) sometime during labor itself.

Emotionally, you may feel excitement, relief, anticipation, uncertainty, anxiety, fear; some women are relaxed and chatty, others tense and apprehensive.

WHAT YOU CAN DO

♦ Relax. Your practitioner has probably told you not to call until you are in more active labor. Or may have suggested that you call early on if labor begins during the day or if your membranes rupture. Definitely call immediately, however, if your membranes rupture and the amniotic fluid is murky or greenish, if you have any bright red vaginal bleeding, or if you feel no fetal activity (it may be hard to notice because you are distracted by contractions, so you might want to try the test on page 243). Although you may not feel like it, it's best if you, not your coach, make the call and talk to your practitioner. A lot can be lost in third-party translations.

♦ If it's the middle of the night, try to sleep. It's important to rest now, because you probably won't be able to later on in labor. And you needn't fear that you'll sleep through the next phase; the contractions will be too insistent. If sleep eludes you, don't just lie in bed timing contractions; that will only make labor seem longer. Instead, get up and do things around the house that will distract you. Clean out a closet; put sheets on the bassinet; finish packing your bag for the hospital; take a shower; make

your coach a sandwich to take along; play solitaire; visit a pregnancy chatroom to see if anyone else is in the same boat.

♦ If it's daytime, go about your usual routine, as long as it doesn't take you far from home. If you have nothing planned, find something to keep you occupied. Try some of the distractions suggested above, take a walk, watch TV, make and freeze a meal or two for easy postpartum dining. Put your coach on alert, but, if he's at work, it's not necessary for him to come running home—yet. If you're using a doula, now's a good time to give her a call, too.

♦ Make yourself comfortable. Take a warm bath (if your membranes have ruptured, check with your practitioner first) or a shower (but be careful not to slip); use a heating pad if your back is aching—but do not take aspirin or ibuprofen (acetaminophen is okay if your practitioner approves) and do not lie on your back.

♦ Eat a light snack if you're hungry (broth, toast with jam, a fruit Popsicle, or something else your practitioner has suggested). Don't eat heavily, and avoid hard-to-digest foods, such as meats, full-fat dairy products, and other fatty foods. Not only will digesting a heavy meal compete with the birthing process for body resources, but eating heavily may be against your practitioner's recommendations. You may also want to avoid anything acidic, such as orange juice.

♦ Time contractions (from the beginning of one to the beginning of the next) for half an hour, if they seem to be getting closer than ten minutes apart, and periodically even if they

ON TO THE HOSPITAL OR BIRTHING CENTER

Getting to the hospital or birthing center. Sometime near the end of the early phase or the beginning of the active phase (probably when your contractions are five minutes apart or less, sooner if you live far from the hospital or if this isn't your first baby), your practitioner will tell you to pick up your bag and get going. Getting to the hospital or birthing center will be easier if your coach is reachable anywhere, anytime by cell phone or beeper and can get to you quickly (*do not try to drive yourself to the hospital*);* you've planned your route in advance; are familiar with parking regulations (if parking is likely to be a problem, taking a cab may be more sensible); and know which entrance will get you to the obstetrical floor most quickly. En route, try stretching out on the rear seat with a pillow under your head, your seat belt fastened loosely beneath your belly, and, if you have chills, a blanket covering you.

Hospital or Birthing Center Admission. Procedures will vary, but you can probably expect something like the following:

♦ If you've preregistered (and it's best if you have), this process will be brief; if you're in active labor, your coach can take care of it.

♦ Once in the labor and delivery suite or birthing unit, your nurse for the shift will take you to a labor or birthing room. Sometimes, you may be brought first to a triage (assessment) room, where your cervix will be checked or your contractions monitored for some time to see if you're actively in labor or not. Depending on hospital regulations, your coach and other family members may be asked to wait outside while you are being admitted and "prepped." (Note to the coach: this is a good time to make a few priority phone calls, to get a snack if you haven't brought one, and to arrange for stowing luggage for the hospital stay and for chilling the celebratory champagne or sparkling cider. If you aren't called in to the labor or birthing room within twenty minutes or so, remind someone at

don't. But don't be a continuous clock watcher.

♦ Remember to urinate frequently, even if you're not feeling the urge to. A full bladder could inhibit the progress of labor.

♦ Use relaxation techniques (see page 127) if they help, but don't start your breathing exercises yet, or you will become bored and exhausted long before you really need them.

FOR THE COACH: WHAT YOU CAN DO

If you're around during this phase, here are some ways you can help. If a doula's also on site, she can share in any or all of these:

♦ Practice timing contractions. The interval between contractions is timed from the beginning of one to the beginning of the next. Time them periodically, and keep a record. When they are coming less than ten minutes apart, time them more frequently.

♦ Be a calming influence. During this early phase of labor, your most important function is to keep the expectant mother relaxed. And the best way to do this is to keep yourself relaxed, both inside and out. Your own anxiety can be transferred to her unwittingly, communicated not just through words but through touch. Doing relaxation exercises together or giving her a gentle, unhurried massage may

the nurses' station that you are waiting. Be prepared for the possibility that you will be asked to put on a sterile gown over your clothes.)

◆ Your nurse will take a brief history, asking, among other things, when the contractions started, how far apart they are, whether your membranes have ruptured, and, possibly, when and what you last ate.

◆ Your nurse will ask for your signature (or your spouse's) on routine consent forms.

◆ Your nurse will give you a hospital gown to change into and might request a urine sample. She will check your pulse, blood pressure, respiration, and temperature; look for leaking amniotic fluid, bleeding, or bloody show; listen to the fetal heartbeat with a Doppler or hook you up to a fetal monitor, if this is deemed necessary. She may also evaluate the position of the fetus and take a fetal blood sample.

◆ Depending on the policies of your prac-

titioner and hospital, and hopefully your preferences, an IV may be started.

◆ Your nurse, your practitioner, or a staff doctor will examine you internally to see how dilated and effaced your cervix is. If your membranes haven't ruptured spontaneously and you are at least 3 or 4 centimeters dilated (many practitioners prefer to wait until the cervix has dilated to 5 centimeters), your membranes may be artificially ruptured—unless you and your practitioner have decided to leave them intact until later in labor. The procedure is generally painless; all you will feel is a warm gush of fluid.

If you have any questions—about hospital policy, about your condition, about your practitioner's plans—that haven't been answered before, now is the time for you or your coach to ask them.

---

* If, for any reason, you can't reach your coach, you should have a backup driver or the number of a car service or taxi company to call. Your coach can then meet you at the hospital.

help. It's too soon, however, to have her begin using breathing exercises.

◆ Offer comfort, reassurance, and support. She'll need them all from now on.

◆ Keep your sense of humor, and help her keep hers; time flies, after all, when you're having fun. It'll be easier to Ïaugh now than when contractions are coming fast and hard.

◆ Try distraction. Suggest activities that will help keep both your minds off her labor: playing board games or cards, doing a puzzle, watching a silly sitcom or a mindless movie, studying name-your-baby books, taking short walks.

◆ Keep up your own strength so you'll be able to reinforce hers. You should

eat periodically, even if her eating is restricted. Prepare a sandwich to bring along to the hospital, if you'd prefer not to leave her side for the cafeteria—but avoid anything with an overpowering or lingering odor.

THE SECOND PHASE: ACTIVE LABOR

The second, or active, phase of labor is usually shorter than the first, lasting an average of two to three and a half hours (with, again, a wide range considered normal). The contractions are more concentrated now, accomplishing more in less time. As they become stronger, longer (forty to sixty seconds, with a distinct peak of about half that time), and more frequent (generally three to four minutes apart, though the pattern may not be regular), the cervix dilates to 7 centimeters. There is less time to rest between contractions.

You will probably be in the hospital or birthing center early in this phase—unless, as occasionally happens, dilation of the cervix occurs over a period of a week or two, in which case labor may not be apparent to you until the next phase (transition).

What you may feel or notice. The most common signs and symptoms in this phase include increasing discomfort with contractions (you may be unable to talk through them now), increasing backache, leg discomfort, fatigue, and increasing bloody show. You may experience all of these, or just one or two. Your membranes may rupture (or be ruptured) during this phase, if they haven't earlier.

Emotionally, you may feel restless and find it more difficult to relax; or your concentration may become more intense, and you may become completely absorbed in the work at hand. Your confidence may begin to waver, and you may feel as if labor is never going to end; or you may feel excited and encouraged that things are really starting to happen. Whatever your feelings, accept them and get ready to start getting "active."

WHAT YOU CAN DO

♦ Start your breathing exercises, if you plan to use them, as soon as contractions become too strong to talk through. (If you have never practiced any of these exercises, some simple breathing suggestions from the nurse or doula may help make you more comfortable.) If the exercises seem to make you uncomfortable or more

tense, however, don't feel that you have to use them. Women gave birth without them for centuries.

♦ If your practitioner permits it, drink clear beverages frequently to replace fluids and to keep your mouth moist. If you're hungry, and again if you have your practitioner's okay, have a light snack of a nonfat, nonfibrous food (fruit Popsicles, sorbet, Jell-O, or applesauce, for example). If your practitioner prohibits anything else by mouth, sucking on ice chips can serve to refresh. Some doctors and hospitals, however, still use IVs to keep laboring patients hydrated (see page 347).

♦ Make a concerted effort to relax between contractions. This will become increasingly difficult as they come more frequently, but it will also become increasingly important as your energy reserves are taxed. Use the relaxation techniques you (hopefully) learned in childbirth class, or those on page 127.

♦ Walk around, if possible, or at least change positions frequently, seeking those that provide the most comfort. (See page 357 for suggested labor positions.)

♦ Remember to urinate periodically; because of tremendous pelvic pressure, you may not notice the need to empty your bladder.

♦ If you feel you need some pain relief, don't be afraid to discuss it with your attendants. They may suggest waiting for fifteen minutes or half an hour before having it administered—at which point you may have made so much progress that you won't need it, or you may have found renewed strength and no longer want it.

FOR THE COACH: WHAT YOU CAN DO

If a doula is present, she can help out with many of these. Discuss ahead of time who will do what.

♦ Hand a copy of the birthing plan (see page 274) drawn up by your laboring partner to each nurse or other attendant at the birth, so they are aware of her preferences. If the shift changes, make sure the new attendants receive a copy.

♦ If possible, keep the door of the labor or birthing room closed, the lights low, and the room quiet to promote a restful atmosphere. Soft music, if permitted, may also help (unless she prefers to watch TV). Continue encouraging relaxation techniques between contractions. And stay as calm as possible yourself—possibly doing some breathing or meditation exercises, too.

♦ Keep track of the contractions. If your partner in labor is on a monitor, ask the practitioner or the nurse to show you how to read it. Later, when contractions are coming one on top of the other, you can announce each new contraction as it begins. (The monitor may detect the tensing of the uterus before a laboring woman can.) You can also encourage your partner by telling her when each peak is ending. This will give both of you some sense of control over the labor. If there is no monitor, learn to recognize the arrival and departure of contractions with your hand on her abdomen.

♦ Breathe with her through difficult contractions, if that helps her. Don't pressure her to do the breathing exercises if she is uncomfortable with them, they make her tense, or they annoy her.

♦ If she complains of any symptoms of hyperventilation (dizziness or lightheadedness, blurred vision, tingling and numbness of fingers and toes), have her exhale into a paper bag (the nurse will be able to supply one) or into cupped hands. She should then inhale the exhaled air. After repeating this several times, she should feel better. If she doesn't, inform a nurse or your practitioner at once.

♦ Offer constant verbal reassurance (if it doesn't make her more edgy); praise, but don't criticize, her efforts (think what you'd like her to say if your roles were reversed). Particularly if progress is slow, suggest that she take her labor one contraction at a time, and remind her that each pain brings her closer to seeing the baby. If she finds such comments irritating, however, skip them.

♦ Massage her abdomen or back, or use counterpressure or any other techniques you've learned, to make her more comfortable. (Back massage, while she sits up, may help to shorten labor.) Take your cues from her; let her tell you what kind of stroking or touching or massage helps. If she prefers not to be touched at all (some women find it annoying), then it might be best to comfort her verbally.

♦ Don't pretend the pain doesn't exist, even if she doesn't complain; she needs your support and understanding. But don't tell her you know how it feels (you don't, if you haven't gone through labor yourself).

♦ Remind her to relax between contractions.

♦ Remind her to try to urinate at least once an hour.

◆ If it's allowed, be sure she has an ample supply of ice chips to suck on or fluids to sip or light foods to snack on, and offer them to her periodically.

◆ Use a damp washcloth, wrung out in cold water, to help cool her body and face; refresh it often.

◆ If her feet are cold, offer to get out a pair of socks and put them on for her (reaching her feet isn't easy for her).

◆ Continue with distractions she finds helpful between contractions (card or video games, light conversation, music, TV, reading aloud), as well as encouragement and support.

◆ Suggest a change of position; take her for a walk down the corridors, if that's possible.

◆ Don't take it personally if she doesn't respond to—or even seems irritated by—your attempts to comfort her. Ease up, if that's what she seems to prefer. A woman's moods during labor are even more mercurial than during pregnancy—and for good reason. Stand by to offer support as she needs and wants it, and expect that what she needs and wants will change from moment to moment. Remember that your role is important, even if you sometimes feel superfluous or in the way.

◆ Serve as her go-between with medical personnel as much as possible. Intercept questions from them that you can answer, ask for explanations of procedures, equipment, use of medication, so you'll be able to tell her what's happening. For instance, now might be the time to find out if a mirror will be provided so that she can view the delivery. Be her advocate when necessary, but try to fight her battles quietly, perhaps outside the room, so that she won't be disturbed or upset.

◆ If she requests medication, communicate her request to the nurse or practitioner, but suggest a waiting period before it's administered. During that time, the practitioner will probably want to discuss the need for pain relief and do an internal exam to check on the progress of labor anyway. It's possible that an encouraging progress report or some time to think it over may give your labor partner renewed strength to continue unmedicated. Don't be disappointed, however, if she and the practitioner decide that medication is needed. Remember, labor isn't a test of pain endurance that she will fail if she asks for or accepts medication. Allowing severe pain to continue can actually slow or even stop labor.

WHAT HOSPITAL PERSONNEL MAY DO

◆ Provide a relaxed, comfortable, supportive environment and answers to your questions and concerns. (Don't hesitate to voice any you may have or ask your coach or doula to do so.)

◆ Continue monitoring the baby's condition with a Doppler or electronic fetal monitor, and through observation of the amniotic fluid (greenish-brown staining is a sign of possible fetal distress). The baby's position may also be checked by palpating the abdomen.

◆ Continue checking your blood pressure.

◆ Periodically evaluate the timing and strength of contractions and quantity and quality of bloody discharge. (The pads on the bed will be replaced as needed.) When there is a change in the pattern or intensity of contractions, or the show becomes more bloody, an internal exam will be done to check the progress of your labor.

◆ Possibly, stimulate labor if it is progressing very slowly, by the use of oxytocin or artificial rupture of the membranes, if they are still intact.

◆ Administer pain relief as needed and desired.

THE THIRD PHASE: ADVANCED ACTIVE OR TRANSITIONAL LABOR

Transition is the most demanding phase of labor. Suddenly the intensity of the contractions picks up. They become very strong, two to three minutes apart, and sixty to ninety seconds long—with very intense peaks that last for most of the contraction. Some women, particularly women who have given birth before, experience multiple peaks. You may feel as though the contractions never completely disappear, and that you can't completely relax between them. The final 3 centimeters of dilation, to a full 10 centimeters, will probably take place in a very short time: on average, fifteen minutes to an hour.

What you may feel or notice. In transition, you are likely to feel strong pressure in the lower back and/or perineum. Rectal pressure, with or without an urge to push or move your bowels, may cause you to grunt involuntarily. You may feel either very warm and sweaty or chilled and shaky, or alternate between the two. Your bloody vaginal show will increase as more capillaries in the cervix rupture; your legs may be crampy and cold and

may tremble uncontrollably. You may experience nausea and/or vomiting, and drowsiness may overcome you between contractions as oxygen is diverted from your brain to the site of the delivery. Some women also feel tightening in their throat or chest. Not surprisingly, at this point you may feel exhausted.

Emotionally, you may feel vulnerable and overwhelmed; as though you're reaching the end of your rope. In addition to frustration over not being able to push yet, you may feel discouraged, irritable, disoriented, restless, and have difficulty concentrating and relaxing (it may seem impossible to do either). You may also find excitement reaching a fever pitch in the midst of all the stress.

WHAT YOU CAN DO

◆ Hang in there. By the end of this phase, which is not far off, your cervix will be fully dilated, and it will be time to begin pushing your baby out.

◆ Instead of thinking about the work ahead, try to think about how far you've come.

◆ If you feel the urge to push, pant or blow instead, unless you've been instructed otherwise. Pushing against a cervix that isn't completely dilated can cause it to swell, which can delay delivery.

◆ If you don't want anybody to touch you unnecessarily, if your coach's once comforting hands now irritate you, don't hesitate to let him know.

◆ If you find them useful, use breathing techniques you have learned that are appropriate for this stage of labor (or ask the nurse or doula for guidance).

◆ Try to relax between contractions (as much as is humanly possible) with slow, rhythmic chest breathing.

IF YOU AREN'T MAKING PROGRESS

Progress in labor is measured by the dilation, or opening, of the cervix and the descent of the fetus through the pelvis. Good progress requires three main components: strong uterine contractions that effectively dilate the cervix; a baby that is in position for an easy exit; and a pelvis that is sufficiently roomy to permit the passage of the baby.

If one or more of these factors is not present, abnormal (or dysfunctional) labor, in which progress is slow or nonexistent, generally occurs. There are several types of abnormal labor:

Prolonged latent phase—when little or no dilation has occurred after twenty hours of labor in a first-time mother, or after fourteen hours in one who has delivered previously. Sometimes progress is slow because labor hasn't really begun and the contractions felt are those of false—not true—labor (see page 335). Sometimes the reason is overmedication before labor was well established. There is also the theory that the cause may sometimes be psychological: a woman panics when labor begins, triggering the release of chemicals in the nervous system that interfere with uterine contractions.

In general, the practitioner may suggest trying to stimulate a slow first phase of labor with activity (such as walking) or with just the opposite (sleep and rest, possibly aided by the use of relaxation techniques and, if you're too agitated to relax naturally, an alcoholic drink or the administration of a sedative). This will also help rule out false labor (the contractions of false labor usually subside with activity, a nap, or an alcoholic beverage). It is important to remember to urinate periodically throughout labor, as a full bladder can interfere with the baby's descent. Full bowels may do the same, so if you haven't moved your bowels in twenty-four hours, an enema may be helpful.

Once true latent-phase labor has been established, it may be speeded up with the administration of oxytocin, prostaglandin E-2, or another labor stimulator. If attempts to stimulate labor are unsuccessful, your practitioner may have to consider the possibility that there is a mismatch between the fetus's head and your pelvis (cephalopelvic disproportion, or CPD).

Most physicians will perform a cesarean after twenty-four or twenty-five hours (sometimes sooner) of labor if sufficient progress has not been made by that time; some will wait longer, as long as both mother and baby are doing well.

Primary dysfunction of active phase (phase 2)—when the second, or active, phase of la-

---

FOR THE COACH: WHAT YOU CAN DO

Again, the doula, if one is present, can share these tasks with you.

- Be specific and direct in your instructions to your partner in labor, without wasting words. She may find small talk annoying now. If she rejects your efforts to help and comfort her, don't take it personally. Give her the space she needs for as long as she needs it, but stand by in case she changes her mind or you're otherwise needed.

- Offer lots of encouragement and praise, unless she prefers you to keep quiet. At this moment, eye contact or touch may communicate more expressively than words.

- Touch her only if she finds it comforting. Abdominal massage may be offensive now, though counterpressure applied to the small of her back may provide some measure of relief for back pain.

bor progresses very slowly (less than 1 to 1.2 centimeters of dilation per hour in women having their first babies, and 1.5 centimeters per hour in those who've had previous deliveries). If any progress, even if it's slow, is being made, many practitioners will let the uterus set its own pace, on the theory that the woman will eventually deliver naturally, as two-thirds of those who experience primary dysfunction do. A laboring woman *may* be able to speed up the work of her uterus by walking or otherwise staying off her back, and keeping her bladder empty. Intravenous fluids may be administered during a lengthy labor to avoid dehydration (see page 347).

Secondary arrest of dilation—when, during active labor, there is no progress for two hours or more. In about half of these cases, it is estimated, disproportion exists between the fetal head and the pelvis (CPD), necessitating a cesarean delivery. In most other cases, the administration of oxytocin or another labor stimulator (such as rupturing the membranes) will reestablish labor, particularly when the cause of the labor slowdown is simply exhaustion. Again, it may be possible to contribute to the battle against sluggish labor by utilizing gravity (sitting upright, squatting, standing, or walking) and by keeping your bladder empty.

Abnormal descent of the fetus—when the baby moves down the birth canal at a rate of less than 1 centimeter per hour in women having their first babies, or 2 centimeters per hour in others. In most such cases delivery will be slow, but otherwise uneventful. Again, stimulation with a labor-inducing drug and/or rupturing of the membranes may be used—assuming there are no contraindications.

Prolonged second stage—one that lasts longer than two hours in a first-time mother who hasn't had an epidural, three hours in one who has (the cutoff may come sooner in second and subsequent deliveries). Many physicians routinely use forceps or vacuum extraction or perform a cesarean when a second stage goes beyond two hours; others allow the spontaneous vaginal delivery to continue much longer if steady progress is being made and both mother and fetus (whose conditions are being carefully monitored) are doing well. Rotation of the head (so that it faces back and will better fit through the pelvis) may also be attempted, either manually or with forceps. Gravity, again, can help; a semi-sitting or semi-squatting position may be most effective for delivery.

It's important to note that for a woman who has had an epidural, the expectations for the progress of labor are different. Everything—both first and second stage—will probably take longer.

- Breathe with her through every contraction if it seems to help her through them.

- Remind her to take it one contraction at a time. Again, she may need you to tell her when each begins and ends.

- Help her rest and relax between contractions, touching her abdomen lightly to show her when a contraction is over. Remind her to use slow, rhythmic breathing in between contractions, if she can.

- If her contractions seem to be getting closer and/or she feels the urge to push—and she hasn't been examined recently—inform the nurse or practitioner. She may be fully dilated.

- Offer her ice chips or a sip of water or juice frequently, if allowed, and mop her brow with a cool damp cloth often.

- Keep your eye on the prize. It's been a long haul for you both. But it won't be long before the pushing begins—and that anticipated moment arrives.

WHAT HOSPITAL PERSONNEL MAY DO

◆ Continue providing comfort and support.

◆ Continue monitoring your condition and that of the fetus.

◆ Continue noting duration and inten-sity of contractions, and the cervical progress you are making.

◆ Prepare for delivery, ultimately mov-ing you to a delivery room if you are not delivering in the same room where you've been laboring.

THE SECOND STAGE OF CHILDBIRTH: PUSHING AND DELIVERY

Up until this point, your active participation in the birth of your child has been negligible. Though you've undeniably taken the brunt of the abuse in the proceedings, your cervix and uterus (and baby) have done most of the work. But now that di-lation is complete, your help is needed to push the baby the remainder of the way through the birth canal and out. This generally takes between half an hour and an hour, but can sometimes be accom-plished in ten (or even fewer) short min-utes or in two, three, or even more very long hours.

The contractions of the second stage are usually more regular than the contractions of transition. They are still about sixty to ninety seconds in dura-tion, but sometimes farther apart (usu-ally about two to five minutes) and possibly less painful—though some-times they are more intense. There now should be a well-defined rest period be-tween them, although you may still have trouble recognizing the onset of each contraction.

What you may feel or notice. Common in the second stage is an overwhelming urge to push—although not every woman feels it. You may experience a burst of renewed energy (a second wind) or fatigue; tremendous rectal pressure; very visible contractions, the uterus rising noticeably with each; an increase in bloody show; a tingling, stretching, burning, or stinging sensa-tion at the vagina as the head crowns; and a slippery wet feeling as the baby emerges.

Emotionally, you may feel relieved that you can now start pushing (though some women feel embarrassed, inhib-ited, or scared); you may also feel exhil-arated and excited or, if the pushing stretches on for much more than an hour, frustrated or overwhelmed. In a pro-longed second stage, you may find your preoccupation is less with seeing the baby than with getting the ordeal over with; this is a natural, and temporary, re-action, which in no way reflects on your capacity for motherly love.

WHAT YOU CAN DO

◆ Get into a pushing position (which one will depend on hospital policy, your practitioner's predilection, the bed or chair you are in, and, hope-fully, what is most comfortable and effective for you). A semi-sitting or semi-squatting position is often the best because it enlists the aid of grav-ity in the birthing process and may afford you more pushing power.

A BABY IS BORN

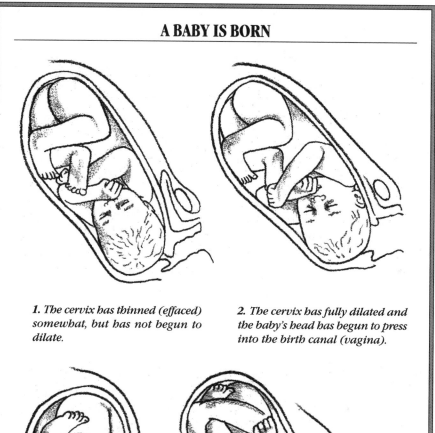

1. The cervix has thinned (effaced) somewhat, but has not begun to dilate.

2. The cervix has fully dilated and the baby's head has begun to press into the birth canal (vagina).

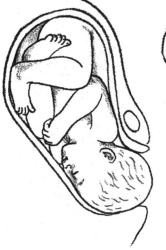

3. To allow the narrowest diameter of the baby's head to fit through the mother's pelvis, the baby usually turns sometime during labor. Here the slightly molded head has crowned.

4. The head, the baby's broadest part, is out. The rest of the delivery should proceed quickly and smoothly.

Sometimes, if the pushing isn't moving your baby down the birth canal, it may be helpful to change positions. If you've been semi-inclined, for example, you might want to get up on all fours or try squatting.

- Give it all you've got. The more efficiently you push, and the more energy you pack into the effort, the more quickly your baby will make the trip through the birth canal. But keep your efforts controlled, coordinating your rhythm closely with the instructions of your practitioner, nurse, or doula. Frantic, disorganized pushing wastes energy and accomplishes little. Avoid pushing with your upper body, which could result in chest pain after delivery. Instead, focus on a point below the navel and imagine you're pushing from there or that you are pushing out a bowel movement. Try not to involve your face in the process—straining with your face as you push could leave you with black-and-blue cheeks and bloodshot eyes.

- Don't let inhibition or embarrassment break the pushing rhythm. Since you're bearing down on the whole perineal area, anything that's in your rectum may be pushed out, too; trying to avoid this while you're pushing can impede your progress. A little involuntary evacuation (or passage of urine) is experienced by nearly everyone in delivery. No one else in the room will think twice about it, and neither should you. Sterile pads will whisk away any excretion immediately.

- Do what comes naturally. Push when you feel the urge, unless otherwise instructed. Take a few deep breaths while the contraction is building. As the contraction peaks, take another and hold it. Then push with all your might until you can no longer *comfortably* hold your breath, or try exhaling as you push. You may feel as many as five urges to bear down with each contraction. Follow each urge, rather than trying to hold your breath endlessly and push through an entire contraction (or while someone counts to ten); breath-holding for long periods of time can exhaust you and may deprive the fetus of oxygen. Taking several deep breaths as the contraction wanes will help restore your respiratory balance. If nothing seems to be coming naturally—and pushing doesn't for every woman—your practitioner, nurse, or doula will help direct your efforts, and redirect them if you lose your concentration.

- Relax your entire body, including your thighs and perineum, as you push. Tenseness works against your pushing efforts.

- Stop pushing when you're instructed to (as you may be, to keep the baby's head from being born too rapidly). Pant or blow instead.

- Rest between contractions, with the help of your coach and the attendants. If you are really exhausted, especially when the second stage drags on, your practitioner may suggest that you not push for several contractions so you can rebuild your strength.

- Don't become frustrated if you see the baby's head crown, and then disappear again. Birthing is a two-steps-forward, one-step-backward proposition.

- Remember to keep an eye on the mirror (if one is available) once there's something to look at. Seeing your baby's head crown (and reaching down and touching it) may give you the inspiration to push when the pushing gets tough. Besides, unless your coach is videotaping, there won't be any replays to watch.

FOR THE COACH: WHAT YOU CAN DO

Once again, these responsibilities can be shared with a doula.

- Continue giving comfort and support, but don't feel hurt if the object of your efforts doesn't seem to notice you're there. Her energies are necessarily focused elsewhere.

- Guide her pushing and breathing, using the cues that you have both become familiar with during childbirth preparation; or relay instructions from the nurse or practitioner.

- Don't feel intimidated by the finesse and expertise of the professional medical team around you. Your presence is important, too. And, in fact, your whispered "I love you" may be more valuable to her at this stage than anything they can offer.

- Help her to relax between the contractions—with soothing words, a cool cloth applied to forehead, neck, and shoulders, and, if feasible, back massage or counterpressure to help ease backache.

- If you are allowed to do so, continue to supply ice chips or fluids to moisten her parched mouth as needed.

- Support her back while she's pushing, if necessary; hold her hand, wipe her brow—or do whatever seems to help her. If she slips out of position, help her back into it.

- Periodically point out her progress.

As the baby begins to crown, remind her to keep an eye on the mirror so she can have visual confirmation of what she is accomplishing; when she's not looking, or if there's no mirror, give her inch-by-inch descriptions. Take her hand and touch the head together for renewed inspiration.

- If you're offered the opportunity to "catch" your baby as he or she emerges or, later, to cut the cord, don't be afraid. Both are relatively easy—and you'll get step-by-step directions and backup from the attendants. You should know, however, that the cord can't be snipped like a piece of string. It's tougher than you may think.

WHAT HOSPITAL PERSONNEL MAY DO

- Move you to the room in which you will deliver, if you aren't already there. If you're in a birthing bed, they'll simply remove the foot of the bed to prepare for delivery.

- Give you support and direction as the delivery progresses.

- Continue to check the condition of the fetus periodically, perhaps by attaching the fetal monitor briefly. In some cases, it may be attached throughout this stage to monitor contractions as well as the baby. Or it may not be used at all; a Doppler may be used instead to check your baby's heartbeat every five minutes.

- About the time the head crowns, prepare for the delivery—spreading sterile drapes and arranging instruments, donning surgical garments and gloves, sponging the perineal area with antiseptic. Midwives generally just don gloves and do no draping.

A FIRST LOOK AT BABY

Those who expect their babies to arrive as round and smooth as a Botticelli cherub may be in for a shock. Nine months of soaking in an amniotic bath and a dozen or so hours of compression in a contracting uterus and cramped birth canal take their toll on a newborn's appearance. Those babies who arrived via cesarean section have a temporary edge as far as appearance goes.

Fortunately, most of the less-lovely newborn characteristics that follow are temporary. One morning, a couple of months after you've brought your wrinkled, slightly scrawny, puffy-eyed bundle home from the hospital, you'll wake to find that a beautiful cherub has taken its place in the crib.

Oddly shaped head. At birth the infant's head is, proportionately, the largest part of the body, with a circumference as large as the chest. As the baby grows, the rest of the body will catch up. Often the head has molded to fit through the mother's pelvis, giving it an odd, possibly pointed "cone" shape; pressing against an inadequately dilated cervix can further distort the head by raising a lump. The lump will disappear in a day or two, the molding within two weeks—at which point your baby's head will begin to take on that cherubic roundness.

Newborn hair. The hair that covers the head at birth may have little resemblance to the hair the baby will have later. Some newborns are virtually bald, some have thick manes, but most have a light cap of soft hair. All will eventually lose their newborn hair (though this may not be apparent), which is gradually replaced by new growth, possibly of a different color and texture.

Vernix caseosa coating. The cheesy substance that coats the fetus in the uterus is believed to protect the skin from the long exposure to the amniotic fluid. Premature babies have quite a bit of this coating at birth; postmature babies have almost none, except in the folds of their skin and under their fingernails.

Swelling of the genitals. This is common in

- Perform an episiotomy just before the head is delivered, but *only* if necessary (see page 352). First a local anesthetic will be injected into the perineum to anesthetize it. This will be done at the height of a contraction, when the pressure of the baby's head naturally numbs the area; the incision will also be made at the height of a contraction and, if the perineum is anesthetized (or if you've had an epidural), will probably be painless.

- Elect to try vacuum extraction or forceps to ease the baby's head out, if necessary. Usually a regional anesthetic will be administered if an epidural or other block hasn't already been given, to ease the pain of a forceps delivery.

- Once the baby's head emerges, quickly suction the nose and mouth to remove excess mucus, then assist the shoulders and torso out.

- Clamp and cut the umbilical cord (or invite your coach to do so) shortly after the delivery, probably with the newborn lying across your abdomen. Some practitioners prefer to wait until the placenta is delivered or the cord has stopped pulsating before cutting the cord. You may also have a chance to cuddle with your baby at this point to help transition him or

both male and female newborns, and is particularly pronounced in boy babies delivered via cesarean. The breasts of newborns, male and female, may also be swollen (occasionally even engorged, secreting a white or pink substance nicknamed "witch's milk") due to stimulation by maternal hormones. The hormones may also stimulate a milky-white, even blood-tinged, vaginal secretion in girls. These effects are normal, and disappear in a week to ten days.

Lanugo. Fine downy hair, called lanugo, may cover the shoulders, back, forehead, and temples of full-term babies. This will usually be shed by the end of the first week. Such hair can be more abundant, and will last longer, in a premature baby and may be gone in a postmature one.

Puffy eyes. Swelling around the newborn's eyes, normal for someone who's been soaking in amniotic fluid for nine months and then squeezed through a narrow birth canal, may be exacerbated by the ointment that is used to protect the eyes from infection. It disappears within a few days. Caucasian babies' eyes are usually, but not always, a slate blue, no matter what color they will be later on. In darker-skinned babies, the eyes are usually brown at birth.

Birthmarks and skin lesions. A reddish blotch at the base of the skull, on the eyelid, or on the forehead, called a salmon patch, is very common, especially in Caucasian newborns. Mongolian spots—bluish-gray pigmentation of the deep skin layer that can appear on the back, buttocks, and sometimes the arms and thighs—are more common in Asians, southern Europeans, and blacks. These markings will eventually disappear, usually by the time a child is four years old. Hemangiomas, elevated strawberry-colored birthmarks, vary from tiny to about quarter-size or even larger. They will eventually fade to a mottled pearly gray, then disappear entirely. Coffee-with-cream colored (café au lait) spots can appear anywhere on the body; they are usually inconspicuous, and don't fade. A variety of rashes, tiny "pimples," and whiteheads may also mar the newborn complexion, due to maternal hormones, but all are temporary. You may also notice skin dryness and cracking, due to first-time exposure to air; these too will pass.

her into the world. In fact, studies show that infants who have skin to sking contact with their mothers immediately following delivery sleep longer and exhibit less stressful body movements hours later.

♦ Provide initial protective care for the newborn: evaluate his or her condition, and rate it on the Apgar scale at one minute and five minutes after birth (see page 356); give a brisk, stimulating, and drying rubdown; identify the baby by taking his or her footprints and your fingerprint for hospital records, and by attaching an identifying band to your wrist and/or ankle and that of your baby; administer nonirritating eye ointment to the newborn to prevent infection; weigh, then wrap the baby to prevent heat loss. (In some hospitals some of these procedures may be omitted; in others many will be attended to later, so you can have more time to bond with your newborn.)

♦ Present your now cleaned-up baby to you and your coach. Unless there is a problem, you should both be able to hold and cuddle your baby. You may, if you wish to, try breastfeeding (but don't worry if you and/or your baby don't catch on immediately— see Getting Started Breastfeeding, page 398).

THE THIRD STAGE OF CHILDBIRTH: DELIVERY OF THE PLACENTA, OR AFTERBIRTH

The worst is over, and the best has already come. All that remains is tying up the loose ends, so to speak. During this final stage of childbirth (which generally lasts anywhere from five minutes to half an hour or more), the placenta, which has been your baby's life support inside the womb, will be delivered. You will continue to have mild contractions of approximately one minute's duration, though you may not feel them. The squeezing of the uterus separates the placenta from the uterine wall and moves it down into the lower segment of the uterus or into the vagina so you can then push it out. Once the placenta is delivered, any necessary stitching up of an episiotomy or naturally occurring tears will be taken care of.

What you may feel or notice. Now that the work of labor and delivery is done, you may feel fatigue or, conversely, a burst of renewed energy. If you've been deprived of food and drink, you are likely to be very thirsty and, especially if labor has been long, hungry. Some women experience chills in this stage; all experience a bloody vaginal discharge (called lochia) comparable to a heavy menstrual period.

For many women, the immediate emotional reaction is a sense of relief. There may also be exhilaration and talkativeness; elation, tempered by a new sense of responsibility; impatience at having to push out the placenta or submit to the repair of the episiotomy or tear, though you may be too excited or tired to care. Some women feel a strong closeness to their spouses and an imme-

diate bond with their new baby; others feel somewhat detached (who is this stranger sniffing at my breast?), even resentful (how this creature has made me suffer!), particularly after a difficult delivery. This doesn't mean, incidentally, that you won't come to love your baby intensely. (See page 393.)

WHAT YOU CAN DO

- Help expel the placenta, if necessary, by pushing when directed.

- Be patient during repair of any episiotomy or tears.

- Nurse or hold the baby, once the cord is cut. In some hospitals, and under some circumstances, the baby may be kept in a heated bassinet for a while or be held by the coach while the placenta is being expelled.

- Take pride in your accomplishment, relax, and enjoy! And don't forget to thank your coach, who may be feeling overwhelmed, underappreciated, or left out.

FOR THE COACH: WHAT YOU CAN DO

If a doula is present, she can continue to help out, concentrating on the more practical aspects of postdelivery care while you spend some quality time together with the two stars of the show.

- Offer some well-earned words of praise to the new mom—and congratulate yourself, as well, for a job well done.

- Begin bonding with the baby with

some holding, cuddling, and whispered words or songs. Remember, this child has probably heard your voice a lot during his or her stay in the uterus and is familiar with its sounds. Hearing it will bring comfort.

◆ Don't forget to do some cuddling and bonding with the new mother, too.

◆ Ask for an ice pack to soothe her perineal area—if the nurse doesn't offer one.

◆ Ask for some juice for the new mom; she may be very thirsty. After she's been rehydrated, and if both of you are in the mood, break out the bubbly—champagne or sparkling cider, depending on your preference. (Limit the champagne for mom if she's dehydrated or if she's breastfeeding.)

◆ If you've brought along the necessary equipment, take baby's first still photos or capture your amazing newborn on video.

WHAT HOSPITAL PERSONNEL MAY DO

◆ Help deliver the placenta. The exact procedure will vary depending upon the practitioner and the situation. Some will pull the cord gently with one hand while pressing and kneading the uterus with the other; others will exert downward pressure on the top of the uterus, asking you to push at the appropriate time. Many physicians will use oxytocin, by injection or IV, after delivery (some will begin the IV earlier, when the forward shoulder delivers) to encourage uterine contractions, which will speed expulsion of the placenta, help shrink the uterus back to size, and minimize bleeding.

◆ Examine the placenta to be sure it is intact. If it isn't, the practitioner will inspect the uterus manually for placental fragments and remove any that remain.

◆ Cut the cord, if it wasn't cut earlier.

◆ Stitch an episiotomy or tear, if any. A local anesthetic (if none was previously given, or if it has worn off) will probably be injected to numb the area. You will feel a pinch.

◆ Check your vagina to remove clots or sponges used during episiotomy repair.

◆ Sponge-bathe the lower part of your body, help you into a clean gown, and help you put on a maxi pad (they may call it a "perineal pad"). You may be given an ice pack to minimize perineal swelling.

◆ When you and baby are finished getting acquainted (after about an hour), they will probably whisk baby off to the nursery (at least temporarily) and transfer you to a postpartum room (unless you have delivered in an LDRP—a labor, delivery, recovery, postpartum—room).

◆ Deliver the baby to the nursery for a bath, a more complete pediatric exam, and some routine protective procedures (including a heel stick and a hepatitis B shot). If you have rooming-in, the baby will be returned as soon as possible and tucked into a bassinet next to your bed.

CONGRATULATIONS—
YOU'VE MADE IT!
NOW RELAX AND ENJOY
YOUR NEW BABY.

Breech Delivery

As far as the mother and coach are concerned, labor and vaginal delivery of a breech baby don't differ much from that of a vertex (head-down) baby; tips for coping and comforting are virtually identical. The activities of the hospital staff will be different, however, and will vary further depending on the type of breech position and the delivery procedure that the practitioner elects to follow.

Up to the second stage, a vaginal breech labor progresses about the same as a head-down labor. But it is always considered a trial of labor, allowed to proceed only as long as it progresses normally. Because of the ever-present possibility that a cesarean may become necessary, you will probably be transferred to a delivery/operating room at the end of the first stage. Depending on your baby's exact breech position, your doctor will determine the safest and most effective way to proceed (see page 294). A common procedure in the vaginal breech delivery is to allow the baby to deliver naturally, until the legs and lower half of the torso are out. After a local anesthetic is administered, then the shoulders and head are delivered, with or without the aid of forceps.

A large episiotomy is usually necessary with a breech, but occasionally it can be avoided. The delivery position for a vaginal breech birth will vary, again depending on the situation and on your practitioner's experience. Some find they have more control if the woman is flat on her back, legs up in stirrups.

Once the baby is delivered, the proceedings continue as with a head-first birth.

Cesarean Section: SURGICAL DELIVERY

You won't be able to participate actively at a cesarean delivery the way you would at a vaginal one. In fact, your most important contribution to the comfort and success of your baby's cesarean birth can be made before you arrive at the hospital, possibly before you even know that you're having a cesarean. That contribution is preparation. Being prepared both intellectually and emotionally for a cesarean, in case it should become necessary, will help minimize any disappointment you may feel and make your surgical delivery experience a more positive one.

Thanks to regional anesthesia and the liberalization of hospital regulations, most women (and often their coaches) are able to be spectators at their cesarean deliveries. Because they aren't preoccupied with pushing or discomfort, they are often able to relax (at least to some degree) and enjoy the birth. This is what you can expect in a typical cesarean birth:

◆ Your abdomen may be shaved and will be washed down with an antiseptic solution. A catheter (a narrow tube) will be inserted into your bladder to keep it empty and out of the surgeon's way.

♦ In the operating room, sterile drapes will be arranged around your exposed abdomen. If you are to be awake for the delivery, a screen will be put up at about shoulder level so that you won't have to see the incision being made.

♦ An IV infusion will be started (if it isn't already in) to provide speedy access if additional medications or fluids are needed.

♦ Anesthesia will be administered: either an epidural or a spinal block (both of which numb the lower part of your body but don't knock you out) or, if time is of the essence, a general anesthetic (which does put you to sleep but is sometimes necessary in an emergency when it becomes critical to deliver the baby immediately).

♦ If your coach is going to attend the delivery, he will be suited up in sterile garb. He will sit near your head, so

IS THERE A PEDIATRICIAN IN THE ROOM?

Unless there is reason to believe there may be something wrong with the baby, it appears that there is no more need to have a pediatrician routinely on hand at a cesarean section than at a vaginal birth. Apgar scores appear to be about the same following both types of deliveries, and babies do equally well.

that he can give you emotional support and hold your hand; he will have the option of viewing the actual surgery. (Whether or not you know in advance that you are going to have a cesarean, it's a good idea to discuss with your doctor ahead of time the conditions under which your spouse will or will not be allowed to be with you during surgery. Usually, if general anesthesia is used, the coach will be asked to wait outside the operating room.)

♦ If yours is an emergency cesarean, things may move very quickly. Try to stay calm and focused in the face of all that activity and don't let it worry you—that's just the way things work in a hospital sometimes. Be prepared for the possibility that hospital policy, and concern for the safety of you and your baby, may dictate that your coach leave during the delivery, which takes only about five or ten minutes.

♦ Once the physician is certain that the anesthetic has taken effect, an incision (usually a horizontal bikini cut) is made in the lower abdomen, just above the pubic hairline. If you are awake, you may feel a sensation of being "unzipped," but no pain.

♦ A second incision (either vertical or horizontal)[5] is then made, this time in your uterus. The amniotic sac is opened, and, if it hasn't already ruptured, the fluid is suctioned out; you may hear a sort of gurgling or swooshing sound.

---

5. A transverse (horizontal) incision is usually preferred because it is in the lower, thinner part of the uterus and results in less bleeding. But in some instances, when the placenta is low in the uterus or your baby is in an unusual position, a vertical incision may be needed.

◆ The baby is then eased out, either manually or with forceps, usually while an assistant presses on the uterus. With an epidural (though not likely with a spinal block), you will probably feel some pulling and tugging sensations, as well as some pressure. If you're eager to see your baby's arrival, ask the doctor if the screen can be lowered slightly, which will allow you to see the actual birth, but not the more graphic details.

◆ Your baby's nose and mouth are then suctioned; you'll hear the first cry, and if the cord is long enough, you will be allowed a quick glimpse.

◆ The cord will be quickly clamped and cut, and while the baby is getting the same routine attention that a vaginally delivered infant receives, the doctor removes the placenta.

◆ Now the doctor will quickly do a routine check of your reproductive organs and stitch up the incisions that were made. The uterine incision will be repaired with absorbable stitches, which do not have to be removed. The abdominal incision may be closed with either stitches or surgical staples.

◆ An injection of oxytocin may be given intramuscularly or into your IV bottle, to help contract the uterus and thus control bleeding. IV antibiotics may be given to minimize the chances of infection.

◆ Depending upon your condition and the baby's, as well as hospital rules, you may or may not be able to hold the baby right there in the delivery room. If you can't, perhaps your spouse can. If the infant has to be whisked away to the ICU nursery, don't let it get you down. This is standard in many hospitals following a cesarean and doesn't necessarily indicate a problem with a baby's condition. And as far as bonding is concerned (no matter what you may hear), later can be just as good as sooner.

◆ ◆ ◆

Part 3

LAST BUT NOT LEAST

CHAPTER 15

Postpartum: The First Week

The moment you've waited for and labored for has finally arrived. That little bundle of joy is finally in your arms, instead of in your belly. You are officially a mother. But keep in mind that this transition from pregnancy to postpartum comes with more than just a baby. It comes, too, with a variety of symptoms (good-bye pregnancy aches and pains, hello postpartum ones)—and a variety of questions (Why am I sweating so much? Why do I still look six months pregnant? Whose breasts are these anyway?).

What You May Be Feeling

During the first week postpartum, depending on the type of delivery you had (easy or difficult, vaginal or cesarean) and other individual factors, you may experience all, or only some, of the following:

PHYSICALLY

◆ Bloody vaginal discharge similar to your period (lochia)

◆ Abdominal cramps (afterpains) as the uterus contracts

◆ Exhaustion

◆ Perineal discomfort, pain, numbness, if you had a vaginal delivery (especially if you had stitches; pain is worse with sneezing and coughing) or a cesarean following a lengthy labor

◆ Pain around the incision and, later, numbness in the area, if you had a cesarean (especially a first one)

◆ Discomfort sitting and walking if you had an episiotomy, a repair of a tear, or a cesarean

◆ Difficulty urinating for a day or two; difficulty and discomfort with

- bowel movements for the first few days; constipation

- General soreness, especially if pushing was difficult

- Bloodshot eyes; black-and-blue marks around eyes, on cheeks, elsewhere, from vigorous pushing

- Sweating, possibly profuse, particularly at night

- Breast discomfort and engorgement about the third or fourth day postpartum

- Sore or cracked nipples, if you are breastfeeding

EMOTIONALLY

- Elation, depression, or swings between the two

- Feelings of inadequacy and trepidation about mothering, especially if you're breastfeeding

- A feeling of being overwhelmed by the physical and emotional and practical challenges facing you

- Frustration, if you're still in the hospital and would like to leave (or if you've been discharged but the baby has to stay in the hospital for a few extra days)

What You May Be Concerned About

BLEEDING

"I'd been told to expect a bloody discharge after delivery, but when I got out of bed for the first time and saw the blood running down my legs, I was really frightened."

Grab a pile of pads, and relax. This discharge of leftover blood, mucus, and tissue from your uterus, known as lochia, is normally as heavy as (and sometimes even heavier than) a menstrual period for the first three to ten postpartum days. And though it'll probably seem more copious than it really is, it may total up to two cups before it begins to taper off. A sudden gush on getting out of bed in the first few days is common, and no cause for concern. And since blood and an occasional blood clot are the predominant ingredients of lochia during the immediate postpartum period, your discharge can be quite red for anywhere between five days to three weeks, gradually turning to a watery pink, then to brown, and finally to a yellowish white.

Maxi pads, not tampons, should be used to absorb the flow, which may continue on and off for just a couple of weeks or as long as six weeks. In some women, light bleeding continues for three months. The flow is different for every woman.

Breastfeeding and the intravenous administration of oxytocin (routinely ordered by some doctors following delivery) may reduce the flow of lochia by encouraging uterine contractions and helping to shrink the uterus back to normal size more quickly. The contraction of the uterus after delivery is important because it pinches off exposed blood vessels at the site where the placenta separated from the uterus, preventing excessive bleeding (which is *not*, by the way, what you're experiencing).

If you are in the hospital and you notice any of the signs of postpartum hemorrhage listed on page 525 (some of which may also indicate infection), notify a nurse. If any of these signs occur once you are home, call your practitioner without delay; if you can't reach him or her, go to the emergency room (in the hospital at which you delivered, if possible) immediately.

YOUR POSTPARTUM CONDITION

"I look and feel more like I've been in a boxing ring than in a birthing room. How come?"

You probably worked harder birthing your child than most boxers work in the ring. So it isn't surprising that, thanks to powerful contractions and strenuous pushing during delivery, you look and feel as though you've gone several rounds. Many women do, particularly following a labor that was long and/or difficult. Not uncommon postpartum are:

◆ Pelvic soreness as a result of stretching

◆ Soreness at the site of incisions (episiotomy or cesarean) or repair of a perineal tear. The pain is usually gone in seven to ten days, though in some cases it may continue for a month or more.

◆ Black and/or bloodshot eyes from pushing with the face more than the lower part of your body; dark glasses will do a cover-up job in public until the eyes return to normal, and cold compresses for ten minutes several times a day may hasten that return

◆ Bruises, ranging from tiny dots on the cheek to larger black-and-blue marks on the face or upper chest area—also usually due to vigorous "face" or "chest" pushing

◆ Achiness in the chest and/or difficulty taking a deep breath due to straining of the chest muscles during strenuous pushing (hot baths, showers, or a heating pad may reduce discomfort)

◆ Pain and tenderness in the area of the tailbone (coccyx) either because

of injury to the muscles of the pelvic floor or because the tailbone is actually fractured (heat and massage may help)

◆ General allover achiness (again, heat may help)

Though looking and feeling like you've taken a beating is normal postpartum, you should report without delay any of the above as well as any other unusual or uncomfortable symptoms you notice to the nurse or your practitioner.

AFTERPAINS

"I've been having cramplike pains in my abdomen, especially when I'm nursing."

Unfortunately, contractions don't end immediately upon delivery of your child, and neither does the discomfort they cause. What you are probably experiencing are afterpains, which are triggered by the contractions of the uterus as it shrinks (from about 2½ pounds to just a couple of ounces) and makes its normal descent back into the pelvis following the birth of your baby. You can keep track of the shrinking size of your uterus by pressing lightly under your navel. By the end of six weeks, you probably won't feel it at all.

The afterpains are more likely to be felt by, and be more intense in, women whose uterine muscles are lacking in tone because of previous births or excessive stretching (as with a multiple pregnancy). These pains can be more pronounced during nursing, when contraction-stimulating oxytocin is released. Acetaminophen or another mild analgesic may be prescribed if necessary, but the pain should subside naturally within four to seven days. If analgesics don't relieve the symptoms, or if they persist for more than a week, see your practitioner to rule out other postpartum problems, including infection.

PAIN IN THE PERINEAL AREA

"I didn't have an episiotomy, and I didn't tear. Why am I so sore down below?"

You can't expect some 7 pounds of baby to pass through the perineum unnoticed. Even if the perineum was left intact during the baby's arrival, the area has still been stretched, bruised, and generally traumatized; and discomfort, ranging from mild to not so mild, is the very normal result. You may even find that sitting down is uncomfortable for a few days.

It's also possible that in pushing your baby out, you developed hemorrhoids and, possibly, anal fissures, which can range from uncomfortable to seriously painful. See page 244 for tips on dealing with hemorrhoids.

"My episiotomy site is so sore, I'm afraid my stitches are infected. But how can I tell?"

The perineal soreness experienced by all vaginal deliverees (and, sometimes, by those who had a difficult labor before undergoing a cesarean) is likely to be compounded if the perineum was torn or surgically cut. Like any freshly repaired wound, the site of an episiotomy or laceration will take time to heal—usually seven to ten days. Pain alone during this time, unless it is very severe, is not an indication that an infection has developed.

Infection is possible, but very unlikely if good perineal care has been practiced. While you're in the hospital, a nurse will check the perineum at least

once daily to be certain that there is no inflammation or other indication of infection. She will also instruct you in postpartum perineal hygiene, which is important in preventing infection not only of the repair site but of the genital tract as well. For this reason, the same precautions apply for those who were neither torn nor had an episiotomy. Follow this ten-day plan for the care of the perineum:

- ◆ Use a fresh maxi pad at least every four to six hours. Secure it snugly so that it doesn't slide back and forth.

- ◆ Avoid dragging germs from the rectum toward the vagina while removing the pad.

- ◆ Pour or squirt warm water (or an antiseptic solution, if one was recommended by your practitioner or nurse) over the perineum *while* urinating to reduce burning and *after* both urinating and defecating to keep the area clean. Pat dry with gauze pads, or with the paper wipes that come with some hospital-provided sanitary pads, always from front to back.

- ◆ Keep your hands off the area until healing is complete.

Though discomfort is likely to be greater if you've had a repair (with itchiness around the stitches possibly accompanying soreness), the suggestions below are usually welcomed by all recently delivered mothers. To relieve pain in the perineal area:

Ice it. To reduce swelling, use chilled witch hazel pads, a surgical glove filled with crushed ice, or a maxi pad with a built-in cold pack, applied to the site every couple of hours during the first twenty-four hours following delivery.

Heat it. Warm sitz baths for twenty minutes three times a day, hot compresses on a similar schedule, or heat lamp exposure will ease discomfort.[1]

Numb it. Use local anesthetics in the form of sprays, creams, ointments, or pads recommended by your practitioner; mild pain relievers, such as acetaminophen, may be prescribed.

Keep off it. To decrease strain on the area, lie on your side, when possible, and avoid long periods of standing or sitting. Sitting on a pillow or inflated tube (usually marketed to hemorrhoid sufferers) may also help, as may tightening your buttocks before sitting.

Keep it loose. Tight clothing, especially underwear, can rub and irritate the wound, increasing pain.

Exercise it. Kegel exercises (see page 193), done as frequently as possible after delivery and right through the postpartum period, will stimulate circulation to the area, promoting healing and improving muscle tone. (Don't be alarmed if you can't feel yourself doing them; the area will be numb right after delivery. Feeling will return to the perineum gradually over the next few weeks.)

If the perineum becomes very red, very painful, and swollen, or if you detect an unpleasant odor coming from the area, you may have developed an infection. Call your practitioner immediately.

DIFFICULTY URINATING

"It's been several hours since I gave birth, and I haven't been able to urinate yet."

1. Use a heat lamp only under supervision in the hospital; to use at home, ask for instructions from your practitioner on how to avoid burns.

Urinating doesn't come easily for most women during the first twenty-four postpartum hours. Some women feel no urge at all; others feel the urge but are unable to satisfy it. Still others manage to urinate, but with accompanying pain and burning. There are a host of reasons why bladder function often becomes such an effort after delivery:

◆ The holding capacity of the bladder increases because it suddenly has more room to expand—thus the need for urination may be less frequent.

◆ The bladder may have been traumatized or bruised during delivery due to pressure created by the fetus, and become temporarily paralyzed. Even when it's full, it may not send the necessary signals of urgency.

◆ Drugs or anesthesia may decrease the sensitivity of the bladder or the alertness of the mother to its signals.

◆ Pain in the perineal area may cause reflex spasms in the urethra (the tube through which the urine exits), making urination difficult. Edema (swelling) of the perineum may also interfere with urination.

◆ The sensitivity of the site of an episiotomy or laceration repair can cause burning and/or pain with urination. Burning may be alleviated somewhat by standing astride the toilet while urinating so that the flow comes straight down, without touching sore spots. Squirting warm water on the area while you urinate (the nurse can provide you with a squirt bottle) can also decrease discomfort.

◆ Any number of psychological factors may inhibit urination—fear of pain on voiding, lack of privacy, embarrassment or discomfort over using a bedpan or needing assistance at the toilet.

As difficult as urination may be after delivery, it's essential that the bladder be emptied within six to eight hours, to avoid urinary tract infection, loss of muscle tone in the bladder from overdistension, and bleeding (because an overfull bladder can hinder the proper descent of the uterus). Therefore, the nurse will ask you frequently after delivery if you've urinated. She may request that you void for the first time postpartum into a container or bedpan, so that she can measure your output, and may palpate your bladder to make sure it's not distended.

If you haven't urinated within eight hours or so, your physician may order a catheter (a tube inserted into your urethra) to empty the bladder of urine. You may be able to avoid this with the following:

◆ Be sure you're taking plenty of fluids—what goes in is more likely to go out.

◆ Take a walk. Getting up from bed and going for a slow stroll as soon after delivery as you're allowed will help get your bladder (and your bowels) moving.

◆ If you're uncomfortable with an audience, have the nurse wait outside the bathroom while you urinate. She can come back in when you've finished, to give you a demonstration of perineal hygiene.

◆ If you're too weak to walk to the bathroom and must use a bedpan, ask for privacy; be sure the nurse has warmed the pan (if it's metal) and given you warm water to pour over the perineal area (which may stimulate the urge). It will also help to sit on the pan, instead of lying on it.

◆ Warm the perineal area in a sitz bath or chill it with ice packs, whichever seems to induce urgency for you.

◆ Turn the water on while you try. Running water in the sink really does encourage your own faucet to flow.

After twenty-four hours, the problem of too little generally becomes one of too much. Postpartum women begin urinating frequently and copiously as the excess body fluids of pregnancy are excreted. If urinating is still difficult, or if output is scant during the next few days, it's possible you have a urinary tract infection. The symptoms of a bladder infection include pain and/or burning with urination that continues even after the sensitivity of the episiotomy or laceration repair has lessened; frequency and urgency with little urine passed; and, sometimes, a low-grade fever. Symptoms of a kidney infection are more severe, and may include a fever of 101°F to 104°F and mid-back pain on one or both sides—usually in addition to the symptoms of a bladder infection. Your physician will want to begin antibiotic treatment specific to the infection-causing organism, if infection is confirmed. You can help speed recovery by drinking plenty of extra fluids, particularly cranberry juice.

"I can't seem to control my urine. It just leaks out."

The physical stress of childbirth can put a lot of things temporarily out of commission, including the bladder. Either it can't let go of the urine or it lets go of it too easily, as in your case. Such leakage (or urinary incontinence) occurs because of loss of muscle tone in the perineal area. Kegel exercises, which are recommended for everyone postpartum anyway, can help restore the tone and help you regain control over the flow of urine. See page 287 for more tips on dealing with incontinence; if it continues, consult your practitioner.

THAT FIRST BOWEL MOVEMENT

"I delivered two days ago and I haven't had a bowel movement yet. Although I've felt the urge, I've been too afraid that straining would open my stitches."

The passage of the first bowel movement after childbirth is a milestone every newly delivered woman is anxious to put behind her. And the longer it takes, the more anxious—and the more uncomfortable—she's likely to become.

Several physiological factors may interfere with the return of normal bowel function after delivery. For one thing, the abdominal muscles that assist in elimination have been stretched during childbirth, making them flaccid and sometimes temporarily ineffective. For another, the bowel itself may have been traumatized by delivery, leaving it sluggish. And, of course, it may have been emptied before or during delivery, and probably remained empty because you didn't eat much solid food during labor.

But perhaps the most potent inhibitors of postpartum bowel activity are psychological: the unfounded fear of splitting open the stitches; the concern over making hemorrhoids worse; the natural embarrassment over lack of privacy in the hospital; and the pressure to "perform," which often makes performance all the more elusive.

Although reregulating your system is rarely effortless, it isn't necessary to suffer helplessly. There are steps you can take to resolve the problem:

Don't worry. Nothing keeps you from moving your bowels more effectively than worrying about moving your bowels. Don't worry about opening the stitches—you won't. And don't worry if it takes a few days to get things moving; that's okay, too.

Request roughage. If you're still in the hospital, select whole grains and fresh fruits and vegetables from the menu. Supplement with bowel-stimulating food brought in from outside. Apples, raisins and other dried fruit, nuts, bran muffins, and small boxes of bran cereal will help. Chocolate—so often a gift to new moms—will only worsen constipation. If you're home, make sure you're eating regularly and well—and that you're getting your fill of fiber.

Keep the liquids coming. Not only must you compensate for fluids lost during labor and delivery, you must take in additional liquids—especially water and fruit juices (particularly apple and pear)—to help soften stool if you're constipated.

Get off your bottom. An inactive body encourages inactive bowels. You won't be running marathons the day after delivery, but you should be able to take short strolls through the corridors. Kegel exercises, which can be practiced in bed almost immediately after delivery, will help tone up not only the perineum but also the rectum. At home, take walks with baby; also see page 426 for postpartum exercise ideas.

Don't strain. Straining won't break open any stitches you have, but it can lead to hemorrhoids. If you do have hemorrhoids, you may find relief with sitz baths, topical anesthetics, suppositories, or hot or cold compresses.

Use stool softeners. Many hospitals send women home with both a stool softener and a laxative—so if all else fails, these may help.

The first few bowel movements may pass with great discomfort. But as stools soften and you become more regular, the discomfort will ease and eventually end.

"Since delivery, I've been embarrassed to find that I can't control my bowel movements. I also keep passing gas involuntarily."

Though they certainly can be embarrassing, postpartum fecal incontinence and gas are not uncommon. During labor and childbirth the muscles and nerves in the area are stretched and sometimes damaged, leaving them unable to go about business as usual. In most cases, the problem takes care of itself as the muscles and nerves get back to normal; you can speed that recovery by performing your Kegels faithfully. If the problem continues, talk to your doctor about possible treatment solutions. Sometimes biofeedback works (see page 246); sometimes surgery is necessary. Following surgery with Kegels improves the outcome still more.

EXCESSIVE PERSPIRATION

"I've been waking up at night soaked with perspiration. Is this normal?"

It's messy, but normal. New moms are sweaty moms; perspiration is one of the ways the body rids itself of pregnancy-accumulated fluids during the week following delivery. Often perspiration continues to be an uncomfortable problem for several weeks, because of the postpartum hormonal adjustments. Don't worry about it; but do make sure fluids that you do need are replaced—particularly if you're breastfeeding, but even if you're not—by taking extra liquids. An absorbent towel over your pillow may help make you more comfortable if you do most of your perspiring during the night.

As a precaution, it's a good idea to take your temperature, and to report it to your doctor if it's over 100°F.

ADEQUACY OF YOUR MILK SUPPLY

"It's been two days since I delivered, and nothing comes out of my breasts when I squeeze them, not even colostrum. I'm worried about my baby—is he going to starve?"

Not only is your baby not starving, he isn't even hungry yet. Babies aren't born with an appetite, or with immediate nutritional needs. And by the time your baby begins to hunger for a breastful of milk (on the third or fourth day postpartum), you will undoubtedly be able to oblige.

Which isn't to say that your breasts are empty now. Colostrum, which provides your baby with enough nourishment (for now) and with important antibodies his or her own body can't yet produce (and also helps to empty baby's digestive system of excess mucus and the bowels of meconium), is definitely present in the tiny amounts necessary. A teaspoon or so per feeding is all your baby needs at this point. But until the third or fourth postpartum day, when your breasts begin to swell and feel full (indicating the milk has come in), it's not that easy to express by hand. A day-old baby, eager to suckle, is better equipped to extract this premilk than you are.

ENGORGED BREASTS

"My milk finally came in, leaving my breasts three times their normal size—and so hard and painful that I can't bear to put on a bra. Is this what I have to look forward to until I wean my baby?"

If swollen, painfully tender, sometimes throbbing, granite-hard breasts were indeed what mothers had to look forward to for the duration of the breastfeeding experience, most babies would be weaned before they entered their

WHEN TO CALL YOUR PRACTITIONER

Few women feel their physical and emotional best after delivering a baby—that's just par for postpartum. Especially in the first six weeks after delivery, experiencing a variety of aches, pains, and other unpleasant symptoms is common, and rarely a sign of a problem. Fortunately, what isn't common is having a serious postchildbirth complication. Still, all recent deliverees should be aware of symptoms that might point to a postpartum complication, just in case. Call your practitioner immediately if you experience any of the following:

◆ Bleeding that saturates more than one pad an hour for more than a few hours. If you can't reach your doctor immediately, have someone take you to the emergency room, or call 911 or your local emergency medical service. En route or while waiting for emergency help to arrive, lie down and keep an ice pack (or a zip-locked plastic bag filled with ice cubes and a couple of paper towels to absorb the melting ice) on your lower abdomen (directly over your uterus, if you can locate it), if possible.

◆ Large amount of *bright* red bleeding any time after the first postpartum week. But don't worry about light menstrual-like bleeding for up to six weeks (in some women as much as twelve) or a flow that increases when you're more active or when you're nursing.

◆ Lochia that has a foul odor. It should smell like a normal menstrual flow.

◆ Numerous or large (lemon-size or larger) blood clots in the lochia. Occasional small clots in the first few days, however, are normal.

◆ A complete absence of lochia during the first two weeks postpartum.

◆ Pain or discomfort, with or without swelling, in the lower abdominal area beyond the first few days after delivery.

◆ Persistent pain in the perineal area, beyond the first few days.

◆ After the first twenty-four hours, a temperature of over 100°F for more than a day. But a brief temperature elevation up to 100.4°F right after delivery (due to dehydration) or a low-grade fever no higher than 101°F at the time your milk comes in is of no concern.

◆ Dizziness.

◆ Nausea and vomiting.

◆ Localized pain, swelling, redness, heat, and tenderness in a breast once engorgement has subsided, which could be signs of mastitis or breast infection. Begin home treatment (page 406) while waiting to reach the doctor.

◆ Localized swelling and/or redness, heat, and oozing at the site of a cesarean incision.

◆ Difficult urination; pain or burning when urinating; a frequent urge to urinate that yields little result; scanty and/or dark urine. Drink plenty of water while trying to reach the doctor.

◆ *Sharp* chest pain, which could indicate a blood clot in the lungs (not to be confused with chest achiness, which is the usual result of strenuous pushing). Call 911 or your local emergency medical service if you can't reach your doctor immediately.

◆ Localized pain, tenderness, and warmth in your calf or thigh, with or without redness, swelling, and pain when you flex your foot—which could be signs of a blood clot in a leg vein (page 510). Rest, with your leg elevated, while you try to reach your doctor.

◆ Depression that affects your ability to cope, or that doesn't subside after a few days (see page 414); feelings of anger toward your baby, particularly if those feelings are accompanied by violent urges.

second week of life. The engorgement (sometimes accompanied by a slight fever),[2] caused by the milk's arrival, can make nursing agonizing for the mother and, if the nipples are flattened by the swelling, frustrating for the baby. The condition may be aggravated when the first nursing session is postponed because either mother or baby isn't up to it.

Happily, the engorgement and its distressing effects, which sometimes extend to the armpits, gradually diminish once a well-coordinated milk supply-and-demand system is established—within a matter of days. Nipple soreness, too—which usually peaks at about the twentieth feeding—generally diminishes rapidly as the nipples toughen up from frequent nursing. Some women may also experience nipple cracking and bleeding. This, with proper care (see page 405), is also usually only temporary.

Until nursing becomes as gratifying and fulfilling as you had hoped it would be—and, believe it or not, painless—there are some steps you can take to reduce the discomfort and speed the establishment of a good milk supply (see Getting Started Breastfeeding, page 398).

ENGORGEMENT IF YOU'RE NOT BREASTFEEDING

"I'm not nursing. I understand that drying up the milk can be painful."

Whether you nurse or not, your breasts will probably become engorged (overfilled) with milk around the third or fourth postpartum day. This can be uncomfortable, even painful. However, it is blessedly temporary.

---

2. If the fever is over 101°F, let your practitioner know.

Some physicians used to rely on hormones or other drugs to suppress lactation. But the drugs have serious side effects and are not reliable (they sometimes fail to relieve engorgement, and if they do, it frequently returns when the medication is discontinued), so the FDA has recommended against their use. Since postpartum breast engorgement is a natural process, it is best to let nature resolve it, which it always does eventually.

Your breasts are designed to produce milk only as needed. If the milk isn't used, production ceases. Though sporadic leaking may continue for several days, or even weeks, severe engorgement shouldn't last more than twelve to twenty-four hours. During this time, ice packs, mild pain relievers, and a supportive bra may help. Avoid hot showers, which stimulate milk production.

FEVER

"I've just returned home from the hospital and I'm running a fever of about 101°F. Could it be related to childbirth?"

It was in 1847 that Dr. Ignaz Semmelweiss, a young Viennese physician, proposed that if birth attendants washed their hands before delivering babies, the risk of childbirth-related infection could be greatly reduced. So, thanks to Dr. Semmelweiss, the chances of a new mother developing a postpartum infection today are extremely slight. And thanks to Sir Alexander Fleming, the British scientist who developed the first infection-fighting antibiotics, the occasional case that does occur is easily cured.

The most severe cases of infection usually begin within twenty-four hours of delivery. A fever on the third or fourth day could possibly be a sign of postpartum infection—but it could also be caused by a nonpostpartum-related illness. A low-grade fever (of about 100°F) occasionally accompanies engorgement when your milk first comes in. It also occasionally accompanies the combination of excitement and exhaustion that's common in the early postpartum period. But as a precaution, report any fever that lasts more than four hours during the first three postpartum weeks to the doctor—even if it's accompanied by obvious cold or flu symptoms or vomiting—so that its cause can be determined and any necessary treatment started. See page 526 if postpartum infection is suspected or diagnosed.

BONDING

"My new son was premature and is going to be in a neonatal intensive care unit for at least two weeks. Will it be too late for good bonding when he gets out?"

Bonding, the process of attachment between a mother and her newborn child, for a while became a cause célèbre in childbirth circles. The term originated in the 1970s, when some studies began to show that the separation of an infant from its mother immediately after birth posed a threat both to their lifelong relationship and to the infant's future relationships with others. Many very positive changes in postchildbirth procedure have come about because of this work. Today, most hospitals and birthing centers encourage new mothers to hold their babies moments after birth, and to cuddle and nurse them for anywhere from ten minutes to an hour or more, instead of whisking the newborns off to the nursery the moment the cord is cut. They also encourage rooming-in, giving parents a chance to spend almost full-time with their newborn.

But as sometimes happens with the popularization of a good idea, the concept of bonding soon became misunderstood and abused, with some unfortunate results. Mothers who have an emergency surgical delivery or a complicated vaginal one and are unable to hold their babies immediately after birth may fear that their parent-child relationship will be tarnished. The same worry may plague parents whose babies must be in neonatal intensive care for several days or weeks, giving them few bonding opportunities. Some parents have become so frantic about the necessity for instant bonding that they demand it even at risk to their infants.

Of course, initial bonding in the delivery room is wonderful. This early meeting of mother and baby gives them a chance to make contact, skin to skin, eye to eye. It's the first step in the development of a lasting parent-child connection. But only the first step. And this step doesn't have to take place at the moment of birth. It can take place later in a hospital bed, or through the portholes of an incubator, or even weeks later at home. When your parents were born, they probably saw little of their mothers and even less of their fathers until they went home—often ten days after birth—and the vast majority of this generation grew up with strong, loving family ties. Mothers who have had the chance to bond at birth with one child and not with another usually report no difference in their feelings toward the children. And adoptive parents, who often don't meet their babies until hospital discharge (or even much later), foster bonds just as strong as a birth parent's. Some experts believe, in fact, that bonding, in most cases, doesn't really take place until somewhere in the second half of the baby's first year. Certainly it is a complex process that isn't accomplished—or forever compromised—in minutes or days.

The fact is that it's never too late to tie the bonds that bind. So, instead of wasting energy regretting the time you've lost, prepare to make the most of the lifetime of mothering you have ahead.

That doesn't mean you shouldn't try to touch, talk to, or possibly hold your baby even while he or she's in the NICU (neonatal intensive care unit). Most hospitals not only allow parent-child contact in such situations, they encourage it. Talk to the nurse in charge of the NICU and see how you best can get close to your newborn during this trying time. For more on the care of premature babies, see *What to Expect the First Year.*

"I've been told that bonding brings mother and child closer together, but every time I hold my baby, she seems like a stranger to me."

Love at first sight is a concept that flourishes in romantic books and movies but rarely materializes in real life. The kind of love that lasts a lifetime usually requires time, nurturing, and plenty of patience to develop and deepen. And that's as true for the love between a newborn and its parents as it is between a man and a woman.

Physical closeness between mother and child immediately after birth does not guarantee instant emotional closeness. Feelings of affection don't flow as quickly and surely as lochia; those first few postpartum seconds aren't automatically bathed in the glow of maternal love. In fact, the first sensation a woman experiences after birth is far more likely to be relief than love—relief that the baby is normal and, especially if her labor was difficult, that the ordeal is over. It's not at all unusual to see that squalling and unsociable infant as a stranger— with very little connection to the cozy, idealized little fetus you carried for nine months—and to feel little more than ambivalent toward him or her. One study found that it took an average of over two

weeks (and often as long as nine weeks) for mothers to begin having strong positive feelings toward their newborns.

Just how you react to your newborn at your first meeting and later may depend on a variety of factors: the length and intensity of your labor; whether you received tranquilizers and/or anesthetics during labor; your previous experience (or lack of it) with infants; your feelings about having a child; your relationship with your spouse; extraneous worries that may preoccupy you; your general health; and, probably most important of all, your personality. *Your* reaction is normal for *you.*

And as long as you feel an increasing sense of comfort and attachment as the days go by, you can relax. Some of the best relationships get off to slow starts. Give yourself and your baby a chance to get to know and appreciate each other, and let the love grow naturally and unhurriedly.

If you don't feel a growing closeness after a few weeks, or if you feel anger or antipathy toward your baby, discuss these feelings with your pediatrician. It's important to get help working them out early on.

ROOMING-IN

"In childbirth class, having the baby room in with me sounded like heaven. Since I gave birth, it's been more like hell. I can't get the baby to stop crying — yet what kind of mother would I be if I asked the nurse to take her?"

You would be a very human mother. You've just completed the more-than-Herculean task (in fact, Hercules couldn't have done it) of giving birth and are about to embark on an even greater challenge: child rearing. Needing a bit of rest in between is nothing to feel guilty about.

Full-time rooming-in is a wonderful option in family-centered maternity care—but you are not a failure or a bad mother if you don't enjoy, or feel too tired for, rooming-in right now. Of course, some women handle it with ease. They may have had easy deliveries that left them feeling exhilarated instead of exhausted. Or they may have had experience caring for newborns, either their own or other people's. For these women, an inconsolable infant at 3 A.M. may not be a joy, but it's not a nightmare, either. However, for a woman who's been without sleep for forty-eight hours, whose body has been left limp from an enervating labor, and who's never been closer to a baby than a diaper ad, such predawn bouts can leave her wondering tearfully: "Why did I ever decide to become a mother?"

Playing the martyr can raise motherly resentments against the baby, feelings the baby will be likely to sense. So, don't be pushed into having the baby room-in if you don't think you want it; and if you've committed yourself to trying it, don't feel you can't change your mind. Partial rooming-in (during the day but not at night) may be a good solution for you. Or you might prefer to get a good night's sleep the first night and start rooming-in on the second. (Do make sure, however, that if you're breastfeeding, your baby is brought in for all feedings, not given a supplementary bottle.)

Be flexible. Be more concerned with the quality of the time you spend with your baby in the hospital than the quantity. Round-the-clock rooming-in will begin soon enough at home. And if you are sensitive to your needs now, by then you should be a bit more emotionally and physically ready to deal with it. But again, you will need some extra support. Ideally, your spouse should pick up the baby for the middle-of-the-night feedings, do any necessary diaper changing, bring her to you, and then deliver her back to her crib. If you don't have a partner, then you should try to get other

HOSPITAL STAYS

How long you and your baby stay in the hospital will depend on the kind of delivery you had, your condition, and your baby's. By federal law, you have the right to expect your insurer to pay for forty-eight hours following a normal vaginal delivery, ninety-six hours following a cesarean. If both you and your baby are in fine shape and you are eager to go home early—because of other children or just because you feel you'd be more comfortable at home—you may be able to arrange with your practitioner for an early discharge. In that case, plan on having a home nurse visit (your insurance plan may pay for it) or taking your newborn for an office visit to the doctor within a few days, just to be sure no problems have cropped up. The baby's weight and general condition will be assessed (including a check for jaundice). There should also be an evaluation of how feeding is going—keeping and bringing along a feeding diary will help.

If you do stay the full forty-eight or ninety-six hours, take advantage of the opportunity to rest as much as possible. You'll need it when you get home.

help—paid or volunteer—to stay with you for at least a few nights, while you recover from childbirth.

RECOVERY FROM A CESAREAN SECTION

"What will my recuperation from a cesarean be like?"

Recovery from a cesarean section is similar to recovery from any abdominal surgery—with a delightful difference: instead of losing an old gallbladder or appendix, you gain a brand-new baby.

Of course there's another difference, slightly less delightful. In addition to recovering from surgery, you'll also be recovering from childbirth. Except for a neatly intact perineum, you'll experience all the same postpartum discomforts over the next weeks (lucky you!) that you would have had if you'd delivered vaginally—afterpains, lochia, perineal discomfort (if you went through a lengthy labor before the surgery), breast engorgement, fatigue, hormonal changes, hair loss, excessive perspiration, and, possibly, the baby blues.

As for your surgical recovery, you can expect the following in the recovery room:

Anesthesia aftereffects. Until your anesthesia wears off, you will be observed carefully in the recovery room. You may be very shaky and sensitive to temperature changes. If you've had a general anesthetic, your memory of this time may be fuzzy or totally absent. Since everyone responds differently to drugs—and each drug is different—whether you are clearheaded and alert in a few hours or not for a day or two will depend upon the medications you were given and your reaction to them. If you feel disoriented, or have hallucinations or bad dreams, your coach or an understanding nurse can help you get back to reality when you waken.

It will take longer for epidural or spinal anesthesia to wear off—which they usually do from the toes up. You will be encouraged to wiggle your toes and move your feet as soon as you can. If you've had a spinal block, you will have to stay flat on your back for about eight to twelve hours. You may be allowed to have both your spouse and your baby visit with you in the recovery room.

Pain around your incision. Once the anesthesia wears off, your wound, like any wound, is going to hurt—though just how much depends on many factors, including your personal pain threshold and how many cesareans you've had. (The first is usually the most uncomfortable.) You will probably be given pain relief medication as needed, which may make you feel woozy or drugged. It will also allow you to get some needed sleep. You needn't be concerned if you're nursing; the medication won't pass into your colostrum, and by the time your milk comes in, you probably won't need any heavy painkillers. If the pain continues for weeks, as it sometimes does, you can safely rely on over-the-counter pain relief. Ask your practitioner for a recommendation. To encourage healing, also try to avoid heavy lifting and even driving for the first few weeks after the surgery.

Possibly, nausea, with or without vomiting. This isn't always a problem, but if it is, you may be given an antiemetic preparation to prevent vomiting. (If you vomit easily, you might want to talk to your doctor about prescribing such a medication and/or Relief Bands—a drug-free device worn on the wrist that blocks postoperative nausea in many patients—before nausea appears.)

Breathing and coughing exercises. These help rid your system of any leftover general anesthetic, and help to expand your lungs and keep them clear to prevent pneumonia. Such necessary lung calisthenics may be very uncomfortable if you do them correctly. You may be able to minimize this discomfort by "splinting" your incision with a pillow.

Exhaustion. You're likely to feel somewhat weak after surgery, partly due to loss of blood, partly due to the anesthetic. If you went through some hours of labor before the surgery, you are almost certain to feel even more worn out.

Regular evaluations of your condition. A nurse will periodically check your vital signs (temperature, blood pressure, pulse, respiration), your urinary output and vaginal flow, the dressing on your incision, and the firmness and level of your uterus (as it shrinks in size and makes its way back into the pelvis). She will also check your IV and urinary catheter.

Once you have been moved to your room, you can expect:

Continuing evaluation of your condition. Your vital signs, your urinary output and vaginal flow, your dressing, and your uterus, as well as your IV and catheter (as long as they remain in place) will be checked regularly.

Removal of the catheter. Removal will probably take place shortly after surgery. Urination may be difficult, so try the tips on page 387. If they don't work, the catheter may be reinserted until you can urinate by yourself.

Afterpains. These start about twelve to twenty-four hours after delivery. See page 384 for more about these postpartum contractions.

A *slow* return to a normal diet. While it used to be routine (and still is in some hospitals and with some physicians) to keep women on IV fluids for the first twenty-four hours after a cesarean and limited to clear liquids for a day or two after that, resuming solids much sooner may be a better bet. Research has shown that women who started back on solids earlier (gradually, but beginning as early as four to eight hours post-op) have that first bowel movement earlier, and are generally ready to be released from the hospital twenty-four hours sooner than those kept on fluids only. Procedures may vary from hospital to hospital and from physician to physician; your condition after the surgery may also play a part in deciding when to pull the plug on the IV and when to pull out the silverware. Keep in mind, too, that reintroduction of solids will come in stages. You'll start with fluids by mouth,

moving on next to something soft and easily tolerated (like Jell-O), and on (slowly) from there. But your diet will have to stay on the bland and easily digested side for at least a few days; don't even think about having someone smuggle in a Big Mac yet. Once you're back on solids, don't forget to push the fluids, too—especially if you're breastfeeding.

Referred shoulder pain. Irritation of the diaphragm following surgery can cause a few hours of sharp shoulder pain. An analgesic may help.

Possible constipation. Since the anesthesia and the surgery may slow your bowels down, it may be a few days until you pass any stool, and that's normal. You may also experience some painful gassiness because of the constipation. A stool softener or mild laxative may be prescribed to help move things along. Try some of the tips given on page 388. Chewing gum stimulates digestive reflexes and gets your system back to normal, so grab a stick of gum, too. If you haven't had a movement by the fifth day, a suppository may do the trick.

Abdominal discomfort. As your digestive tract (temporarily put out of commission by surgery) begins to function again, trapped gas can cause considerable pain, especially when it presses against your incision line. The discomfort may be worse when you laugh, cough, or sneeze. Ask the nurse or doctor to suggest some possible remedies. Narcotics are not usually recommended because they can prolong the problem, which ordinarily lasts just a day or two. You may get a small enema or a suppository to help release the gas. Or you may be advised to walk up and down the corridor. Lying on your left side or on your back, your knees drawn up, taking deep breaths while holding your incision may help. If the pain remains severe, a tube may be inserted in your rectum to allow the gas to escape.

Encouragement to exercise. Before you are out of bed, you will be encouraged to wiggle your toes, flex your feet to stretch your calf muscles, push against the end of the bed with your feet, and turn from side to side. You can also try these: (1) Lie flat on your back, bend one knee (with that foot flat on the bed), and then extend the other leg while tightening your abdomen slightly. Slide the bent leg slowly back down; repeat with the other leg. (2) Lie on your back, knees bent, feet flat on the bed, and raise your head for about thirty seconds. (3) On your back, knees bent and feet flat on the bed, tighten your abdomen, and reach with one arm across your body to the other side of the bed, at about waist level. Then switch to the other side.

These exercises are intended to improve circulation, especially in your legs, and prevent the development of blood clots. (But be prepared for some of them to be quite painful, at least for the first twenty-four hours or so.)

To get up between eight and twenty-four hours after surgery. With the help of the nurse, you'll sit up first, supported by the raised head of the bed. Then, using your hands for support, you'll slide your legs over the side of the bed and dangle them for a few minutes. Then, slowly, you'll be helped to step down on the floor, your hands still on the bed. If you feel dizzy (which is normal), sit right back down. Steady yourself for a few more minutes before taking a couple of steps and then take them slowly; the first few may be extremely painful. Stand as straight as you can, even if the temptation is great to hunch over to ease the discomfort. Though you may need help the first few times you get up, this difficulty in getting around is temporary. In fact, you may soon find yourself more mobile than the vaginal deliveree next door—and you will probably have the edge in sitting.

To wear elastic stockings. These improve circulation and are also intended to prevent blood clots in the legs.

To spend time with your baby. You can't lift the baby yet, but you can cuddle and feed. (If you're nursing, place the baby on a pillow over your incision or lie on your side while nursing.) Depending on how you feel, and on hospital regulations, you may be able to have modified rooming-in. Some hospitals even allow full rooming-in; having your spouse bunking with you, too, will be a big help.

To take sponge baths. Until your stitches are removed (or absorbed), you probably won't be allowed a real bath or shower.

Removal of stitches. If your stitches or clips aren't self-absorbing, they will be removed about four or five days after delivery. The procedure isn't very painful, although you may find it uncomfortable. When the dressing is off, look at the incision with the nurse or doctor; ask how soon you can expect the area to heal, which changes will be normal, and which might require medical attention.

In most cases, you can expect to go home about four days postpartum. But you will continue to need help both with baby care and self-care. Try to have someone with you at all times during the first couple of weeks.

BACKACHE

"My sister said she had a bad back-ache after delivery because she had an epidural. I have a backache, too, but I didn't have an epidural."

It was once believed that only women who had had epidurals suffered from postpartum backaches. But studies show that backache is just as common among women who labor and deliver without an epidural. Your aches are probably related to those sagging abdominal muscles (you must have noticed they're not what they once were), which are too weak right now to support your back properly. Postpar-

tum exercises (see Getting Back into Shape, page 426) will help build up those muscles and get your back back into shape. In the meantime, avoid heavy lifting (except for your baby).

What It's Important to Know: GETTING STARTED BREASTFEEDING

Ever since Eve put Cain to suckle for the first time, breastfeeding has been coming naturally to mothers and their newborns. Right?

Well, not always—at least not immediately. Though nursing does come naturally, it comes naturally a little later for some mothers and babies than for others. Sometimes there are physical factors that foil those first few attempts; at other times it's just a simple lack of experience on the part of both participants. But whatever might be keeping your baby and your breasts apart, it won't be long before they're in perfect synch—as long as you don't give up first. Some of the most mutually satisfying breast-baby relationships begin with several days—or even weeks—of fumbling, of bungled efforts, and of tears on both sides.

Knowing just what to expect and how to deal with setbacks can help ease the mutual adjustment. Taking a prenatal class in breastfeeding will be useful, as will the following:

◆ Start as soon as possible after birth. Right in the delivery room is best, when feasible. (See Breastfeeding Basics, page 400.) But sometimes mother's not in any condition to nurse, and sometimes baby isn't— neither of which means they won't be able to start successfully later. (And even if you and the baby feel well, this first nursing experience

won't necessarily go smoothly. You both have a lot to learn.)

◆ Enlist the support of your practitioner in advance to be sure that you will be allowed to nurse in the birthing or delivery room if all goes normally. Also, arrange for full or partial rooming-in, or for a demand-feeding schedule (a nurse brings the baby to you when he or she is hungry).

◆ Get some professional help, if you can. Hopefully, a lactation specialist will join you during at least a couple of your first baby feedings to provide hands-on instruction, helpful hints, and perhaps literature. If this service isn't offered to you, ask if a lactation consultant or a nurse who is knowledgeable about breastfeeding can observe your technique, and redirect you if you and your baby are not on target. If you leave the hospital before getting such help, your technique should be evaluated by someone with breastfeeding expertise—either the baby's doctor, a home nurse, or an outside lactation consultant[3]—within a few days. You can also find empathy and advice by calling your local La Leche League chapter.

---

3. For a lactation consultant near you, contact the International Lactation Consultant Association (ILCA), 1500 Sunday Drive, Suite 102, Raleigh, NC 27607; (919) 787-5181; www.ILCA.org.

- Limit visitors to allow more nursing opportunities. If the baby is rooming in full-time, this may mean limiting visiting privileges to just your spouse—which is probably for the best anyway, since it allows the three of you to get to know each other while maintaining the relaxed atmosphere needed for learning-to-nurse sessions.

- Be patient if your baby is still recovering from delivery. If you received anesthesia or had prolonged, difficult labor, you can expect your baby to be drowsy and sluggish at the breast for a few days. Not to worry—he or she will soon pick up the pace. There's no danger baby will starve in the meantime, since newborns have little need for nourishment during the first days of life. What they do need, though, is nurturing. Cuddling at the breast is just as important as suckling.

- Make sure your baby's appetite and sucking instinct aren't sabotaged between feedings. It's routine in some hospital nurseries to quiet a crying baby between mother's feedings with a bottle of sugar water. This can have a twofold detrimental effect. First, it satisfies the baby's still-delicate appetite for hours. Later, if your baby is brought to you too full to nurse, your breasts aren't stimulated to produce milk, and a vicious cycle—one that interferes with the establishment of a good demand-and-supply system—begins. Second, because the rubber nipple requires less effort, the baby's sucking reflex may become lazy. Faced with the greater challenge of tackling the breast, he or she may just give up. Formula feedings can also interfere with nursing. So issue strict orders—through your baby's doctor—that, as recommended by the American Academy of Pediatrics, supplementary feedings not be given to your baby in the nursery unless medically necessary. You may even want to put a sign in the baby's bassinet that reads: "Breastfeeding only—no bottles please."

- Nurse on demand. Get in at least eight to twelve feedings a day—even if the demand isn't yet up to that level. Not only will this keep your baby happy, it will increase your milk supply to meet the demand as it grows. Imposing a four-hour feeding schedule, on the other hand, can worsen breast engorgement early on and result in an undernourished child later.

- Nurse for as long as baby wants. It used to be recommended that keeping initial feeding short (five minutes on each breast) would prevent sore nipples by toughening them up gradually. Sore nipples, however, result from improper positioning of the baby on the breast and have little to do with the length of the feeding. Most newborns require ten to forty-five minutes to complete a feeding. As long as your positioning is correct, there is no need to restrict your nursing time. Ideally, at least one breast should be emptied at each feeding—this is more important than being sure that baby feeds from both breasts.[4] So don't pull the plug just because your baby has fed for fifteen minutes on breast number one—wait until he or she seems ready to quit. Then offer the second breast, but don't force it. Remember to start the next feeding on the breast that baby nursed from last and didn't empty completely.

---

4. If the breast isn't emptied, the baby doesn't get the hind milk, which contains more calories to support weight gain than the milk that comes in earlier.

BREASTFEEDING BASICS

1. Pick a quiet location. Until you and your baby have breastfeeding down pat, set yourselves up in an area that has few distractions and a low noise level.

2. Have a drink—of milk, juice, or water—at hand to replenish fluids. Avoid hot drinks (which could scald you or your baby, should they spill); if you don't want a cold drink, opt instead for something lukewarm. Add a healthy snack, if it's been a while since your last meal.

3. As you become more comfortable with breastfeeding, you can keep a book or magazine handy to occupy you during long feeding sessions. (But don't forget to put your reading matter down periodically so you can interact with your nursing infant.) Turning on the TV, however, can be too distracting, especially in the early weeks. So can talking on the phone; turn down the ringer and let voice mail pick up messages—or have someone else answer.

4. Get into a position that's comfortable for you and your baby. If you're sitting up, a pillow across your lap can help raise your baby to a comfortable height. Make sure, too, that your arms are propped up on a pillow or chair arms; trying to hold 6 to 8 pounds without support can lead to arm cramps and pain. And elevate your legs, if you can.

5. Position your baby on her side, facing your nipple. Make sure baby's whole body is facing you—tummy to tummy—with ear, shoulder, and hip in a straight line. You don't want your baby's head turned to the side; rather, it should be straight in line with her body. (Imagine how difficult it would be for you to drink and swallow while turning your head to the side. It's the same for your baby.) Proper positioning is essential to prevent nipple soreness and breastfeeding difficulties.

6. Lactation specialists recommend two nursing positions during the first few weeks. The first is called the *crossover hold*: Hold your baby's head with the opposite hand (if nursing on the right breast, hold your baby with your left hand). Your hand should rest between your baby's shoulder blades, your thumb behind one ear, your other fingers behind the other ear. Using your right hand, cup your right breast, placing your thumb above your nipple and areola (the dark area) at the spot where your baby's nose will touch your breast. Your index finger should be at the spot where your baby's chin will touch the breast. *Lightly* compress your breast so that your nipple points slightly toward your baby's nose. You are now ready to have the baby latch on (see step 7).

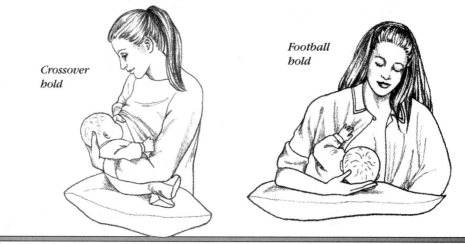

Crossover hold

Football hold

The second position is called the *football hold*:* Position your baby at your side in a semi-sitting position facing you, with his or her legs under your arm (your right arm if you're nursing on the right breast). Support your baby's head with your right hand and cup your breast as you would for the crossover hold.

As soon as you're comfortable with nursing, you can add the *cradle hold,* in which your baby's head rests in the crook of your arm and the *side-lying position,* in which you and your baby lie on your sides, tummy to tummy. This position is a good choice when you're nursing in the middle of the night.

7. Gently tickle your baby's lips with your nipple until his or her mouth is opened very wide—like a yawn. Some lactation specialists suggest directing your nipple toward your baby's nose and then down to the upper lip to get your baby to open his or her mouth very wide. This prevents the lower lip from getting tucked in during nursing. If your baby turns away, gently stroke his or her cheek on the side nearest you. The rooting reflex will make baby turn his or her head toward your breast.

8. Once the baby's mouth is opened wide, move your baby closer. Do not move your

---

*The football hold, also called the clutch hold, is especially useful if you've had a cesarean and want to avoid placing your baby against your abdomen; or your breasts are large; or your baby is small or premature; or if you are nursing twins.

breast toward the baby. Many latching-on problems occur because mom is hunched over baby, trying to shove breast into mouth. Instead, keep your back straight and bring your baby to your breast.

9. Don't stuff the nipple in an unwilling mouth; let your baby take the initiative. It might take a couple of attempts before your baby opens his or her mouth wide enough to latch on properly.

10. Be sure the baby latches on to both the nipple and the areola that surrounds it. Sucking on just the nipple won't compress the milk glands and can cause soreness and cracking. Also be sure that it's the nipple that your baby is busily milking. Some infants are so eager to suck that they will latch on to any part of the breast (even if no milk is forthcoming), causing a painful bruise.

11. If your breast is blocking your baby's nose, *lightly* depress the breast with your finger. Elevating your baby slightly may also help provide a little breathing room. But as you maneuver, be sure not to loosen his or her grip on the areola.

12. Check for swallowing. Milk is flowing if there is a strong, steady, rhythmic motion visible in your baby's cheek.

13. If your baby has finished suckling but is still holding on to your breast, pulling it out abruptly can cause injury to the nipple. Instead, break the suction first by depressing your breast or by putting your finger into the corner of the baby's mouth to admit some air.

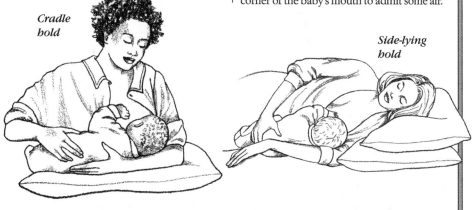

Cradle hold

Side-lying hold

- Don't let sleeping babies lie if it means that they'll sleep through a feeding. Some babies, especially in the first few days of life, may not wake often enough for nourishment. If it's been three hours since your newborn last fed, then it's time for a wake-up call. Here's one way to accomplish this. First, unwrap your baby if he or she is swaddled or heavily dressed; the cool air will help begin the waking process. Then try sitting baby up, one hand supporting the back and the other holding the chin, and rub his or her back gently. Massaging the arms and legs or dabbing a little cool water on the forehead may help, too. The moment he or she stirs, quickly adopt the nursing position. Or lay your sleeping baby on your bare chest. Babies have a keen sense of smell, and the aroma of breast milk may awaken him or her.

- Don't try to feed a screaming baby. Ideally, you should feed your baby when he or she first shows signs of hunger or interest in sucking, which might include mouthing the hands or rooting around for the nipple, or just being particularly alert. Crying is not a feeding cue, so try not to wait until frantic crying—a late indication of hunger—begins. But if crying has begun, do some rocking and soothing before you start nursing. Or offer your finger to suck on until baby calms down. After all, it's hard enough for an inexperienced suckler to find the nipple when calm; when your baby has worked up to a full-fledged frenzy, it may be impossible.

- Stay calm. Start out as relaxed as you can, and try to stay that way no matter how frustrating the nursing episode becomes. Send visitors packing fifteen minutes before feeding time, and use that time to clear your head of all sources of anxiety (including thoughts of your hospital bill). Do some relaxation exercises before you begin (see page 127) and tune in to some soft music, if you find it calming. Then try to keep your cool as you nurse and to keep in mind that it *will* get better. Tension not only hampers milk letdown (your breasts' way of making the milk your body has produced available for suckling), it can generate anxiety in your baby, and infants are extremely sensitive to their mother's moods. An anxious baby can't nurse effectively.

- Keep track—once your milk comes in. Until breastfeeding is well established, keep a running written record of baby's feedings (when they begin and end) as well as of wet and soiled diapers produced each day. That way you will have a good sense of how breastfeeding is going and will be able to report progress more accurately to your baby's doctor. Continue to strive for at least eight to twelve feedings in each twenty-four-hour period, but never force your baby to suckle. Though the length of feedings will vary considerably, once engorgement and nipple soreness have leveled off they should average about half an hour each, usually divided between both breasts (though sometimes a baby will turn away or fall asleep before latching on to breast number two, which is fine as long as number one has been emptied).[5] Your baby's weight gain and the condition of the diapers will give you an even clearer picture of baby's intake. There should be at least six

---

5. To be sure each breast gets a chance to be stimulated, use a reminder (such as a safety pin clipped to the outside of your bra, on the side from which your baby last fed first). Or jot down which side was first in your breastfeeding journal.

wet diapers (the urine should appear clear and not dark yellow) and at least three bowel movements over a twenty-four-hour period. No matter how long baby is suckling, if the output is satisfactory and weight gain is within the norm, you can assume that the intake is, too.

♦ If your baby has to be in the neonatal intensive care unit (NICU) for any reason and can't go home with you, don't give up on breastfeeding. Babies who are premature or have other problems do better on breast milk. Talk to your baby's neonatologist and the nurse in charge to see how you can best feed your baby in this situation. If you can't nurse directly, perhaps you can pump milk to be given to your baby via tube feeding or bottle. If even this isn't possible, see if you can keep pumping milk to keep your supply up until your baby is ready to feed from you directly.

ENGORGEMENT: WHEN THE MILK COMES IN

Just when you and your baby seem to be getting the hang of it, your milk comes in. Up to now, your baby has been getting tiny amounts of colostrum (premilk), and your breasts have been quite comfortable. Then a problem very commonly arises. Your breasts become swollen, hard, and painful—all within a few hours.[6] Nursing becomes difficult for the baby and agonizing for you. Fortunately, this period of engorgement is usually brief—often no more than

twenty-four to forty-eight hours, though sometimes as long as a week. While it lasts, there are a variety of ways of relieving it and the accompanying discomfort:

♦ Use heat briefly to help soften the areola and encourage letdown at the *beginning* of a nursing session. To do this, place a washcloth dipped in warm, not hot, water on just the areola, or lean into a bowl of warm water. You can also encourage milk flow by gently massaging the breast your baby is suckling.

♦ Use ice packs *after* nursing to reduce engorgement. And although it may sound a little strange and look even stranger, chilled cabbage leaves may also prove soothing (use large outer leaves and make an opening in the center of each for your nipple; rinse and pat dry before applying).

♦ Wear a well-fitting nursing bra (with wide straps and no plastic lining) around the clock. Pressure against your sore and engorged breasts can be painful, however, so make sure the bra is not too tight. And wear loose clothing that doesn't rub against your sensitive breasts.

♦ Don't be tempted to skip or skimp on a feeding because of pain. The less your baby sucks, the more engorged your breasts will become.

♦ Hand-express a bit of milk from each breast before nursing to lessen the engorgement. This will get your milk flowing, and soften the nipple so that your baby can get a better hold on it.

♦ Alter the position of your baby from one feeding to the next (try the football hold at one feeding, the cradle hold at the next; see page 400). This will ensure that all the milk ducts are being emptied and may help lessen the pain of engorgement.

---

6. A few lucky new mothers don't experience engorgement when their milk comes in, possibly because their babies were vigorous nursers from birth; there may also be less engorgement with subsequent babies than with the first.

THE BREASTFEEDING DIET

The quality of the breast milk you pro- duce isn't always directly related to the quality of what you eat. The levels of protein, fat, and carbohydrates in your breast milk aren't usually affected by the levels of these nutrients in your diet, though levels of some vitamins (A and B$_{12}$, for example) are. The quantity of milk, however, is a different story. Women whose diets are deficient in protein and/or calories, for example, may pro- duce milk of good composition but in in- adequate quantities. To make good breast milk, and plenty of it, continue taking your pregnancy (or pregnancy/lactation) vitamin-mineral supplement, and adhere to the Pregnancy Diet (see Chapter 4), with these modifications:

◆ Increase your caloric intake by about 500 calories per day over your *pre*preg- nancy requirements. This is flexible and, as during pregnancy, you can let your scale be your guide. If you have a lot of fat stores from pregnancy (or be- fore), you can take fewer calories, as the fat will be burned to produce milk (and you will lose weight). If you are underweight and accumulated little in the way of fat stores while you were pregnant, you may need more than 500 additional calories daily (the recom- mendation assumes some use of fat stores, which you don't have). No mat- ter what your weight, you may find that you need still more calories as the baby grows and demands more milk. Again, you will be able to determine this by checking your scale. If you start dropping pounds at a rapid rate, in- crease your daily intake. If you're not losing any weight at all or, worse, you're putting on pounds, cut back. Baby's scale can also clue you in on whether you're taking in enough calo- ries; if he or she is growing well, you can assume you're eating enough to produce sufficient milk.

◆ If you're a vegetarian, continue taking the supplements recommended in pregnancy.

◆ Increase your calcium requirement to five servings per day. Calcium-fortified juice and milk may make meeting that requirement less of a struggle. So can adding a calcium supplement.

◆ Drink at least eight glasses of fluids (milk, water, broths or soups, and juices); take more during hot weather and if you've been perspiring a lot. (Though it's all right to drink a cup or two of tea or coffee daily, and an oc- casional alcoholic beverage, don't count them as filling your fluid re- quirement, since they have a dehy- drating effect.) Excess is not best, however; flooding yourself with fluid (more than twelve glasses per day) can paradoxically slow milk production. Thirst and urinary output can help you gauge your needs.

◆ Continue to eat plenty of foods that are high in brain-building DHA (see page 91).

◆ Splurge occasionally. After nine months of careful diet watching, you're entitled to your just desserts. The key is moderation. Some sugar won't inter- fere with milk production, but a steady diet of sweets can, by dulling your ap- petite for necessary nutrients. Ditto for other nutritionally superfluous foods, such as potato chips, french fries, and white bread; eat them, if you want, to supplement your otherwise healthy diet, not as staples that stand in for nutritious fare.

◆ For severe pain, you might consider taking acetaminophen or another mild pain reliever prescribed by your practitioner.

SORE NIPPLES

Tender nipples can make nursing a miserable—and frustrating—experience. Most women, fortunately, don't suffer for long; their nipples toughen up quickly and breastfeeding soon becomes painless. But some women, particularly those whose babies are incorrectly positioned, and those who have "barracuda babies" (with a very vigorous suck), have continued trouble with soreness and cracking so painful they may come to dread each feeding. But there are routes to relief of the discomfort:

◆ Be sure your baby is correctly positioned, facing your breast (see box, page 400).

◆ Expose sore or cracked nipples to the air briefly after each feeding. Protect them from clothing and other irritations and surround them with a cushion of air by wearing breast shells (not shields). Change nursing pads often if leaking milk keeps them wet. Also, make sure the nursing pads don't have a plastic liner, which will only trap moisture.

◆ If you live in a humid climate, wave a blow dryer, set on warm, across the breast (about six to eight inches away) for two or three minutes (no more) after feedings. This is very comforting for many women. In a dry climate, moisture will be more helpful—let whatever milk is left on the breast after a feeding dry there. Or express a few drops of milk at the end of a feeding and rub it on your nipples, making sure to let your nipples dry before putting your bra back on.

◆ Nipples are naturally protected and lubricated by sweat glands and skin oils. But studies show that using a commercial preparation of modified lanolin can prevent and/or heal nipple cracking. After nursing, apply ultra-purified, medical grade lanolin, such as Lansinoh, but avoid petroleum-based products and petroleum jelly itself (Vaseline) and other oily products. Wash nipples only with water—never with soap, alcohol, tincture of benzoin, or premoistened towelettes—whether your nipples are sore or not: your baby is already protected from your germs, and the milk itself is clean.

◆ Wet regular tea bags with cool water and place them on your sore nipples. The properties in the tea may help to soothe and heal them.

◆ Vary your nursing position so a different part of the nipple will be compressed at each feeding; but always keep baby facing your breasts.

◆ Don't favor one breast because it is less sore or because the nipple isn't cracked; the only way to toughen up nipples is to use them. Try to use both breasts at every feeding, even if only for a few minutes—but nurse from the less sore one first, since the baby will suck more vigorously when hungry. If both nipples are equally sore, start off the feeding with the breast you used last.

◆ Relax for fifteen minutes or so before feeding. Relaxation will enhance the let-down of milk (which will mean that baby won't have to suck as hard), whereas tension will hinder it. If the pain is severe, ask your practitioner about taking an over-the-counter pain medication to relieve it, taken before nursing.

♦ If your nipples are cracked, be especially alert to signs of breast infection (see below), which can occur when germs enter a milk duct through a crack in the nipple.

OCCASIONAL COMPLICATIONS

Once nursing is established, it generally continues uneventfully until weaning. But once in a while, complications occur, among them:

Clogged milk ducts. Sometimes a milk duct clogs, causing milk to back up. Since this condition (characterized by a small, red, and tender lump on the breast) can lead to infection, it's important to try to remedy it quickly. The best way to do this is to offer the affected breast first at each feeding, and to let your baby empty it as completely as possible. If he or she doesn't do the job, any remaining milk should be expressed by hand or with a breast pump. Keep pressure off the duct by making sure your bra is not too tight (avoiding underwires may help), and by varying nursing positions to put pressure on different ducts. Applying hot packs or warm compresses before nursing and gentle massage may also be helpful (baby's chin, if correctly positioned, can provide a clogged duct with an excellent massage). Do not use this time to wean the baby; discontinuing nursing now will only compound your problem.

Breast infection. A more serious complication of breastfeeding is mastitis, or breast infection, which can occur in one or both breasts, most often between the 10th and 28th days postpartum (though it can start earlier or later), and more often in first-time mothers. The factors that can combine to cause mastitis are failure to empty breasts completely of milk at each nursing, germs gaining entrance into the milk ducts through a crack or fissure in the nipple (usually from the baby's mouth), and lowered resistance in the mother due to stress, fatigue, and inadequate nutrition.

The most common symptoms of mastitis are severe soreness or pain, hardness, redness, heat, and swelling of the breast, with flulike symptoms—generalized chills and a fever of about 101°F to 102°F. If you develop such symptoms, contact your doctor. Prompt medical treatment is necessary, and may include bed rest, antibiotics, pain relievers, increased fluid intake, and moist heat applications. During treatment you should continue to nurse. Since the baby's germs probably caused the infection in the first place, they won't be harmful. And emptying the breast will help to prevent clogged milk ducts. Nurse first on the infected breast, and empty whatever baby doesn't finish with a pump. If the pain is so excruciating that you can't nurse, try pumping your breasts while lying in a tub of warm water with your breasts floating comfortably. (Don't use an electric pump in the tub.)

MEDICATION AND LACTATION

Many medications are known to be safe for use while you're breastfeeding; others are known not to be; and the scientific jury's still out on the rest. But just as you did while you were expecting, check all medications (prescription or over-the-counter) with your practitioner and your baby's pediatrician before taking them—and be sure any physician who prescribes a new medication knows that you're nursing. Keep in mind that it's usually best to take medication just after a feeding, so that levels in your milk will be lowest when you nurse next time.

BREASTFEEDING TWINS

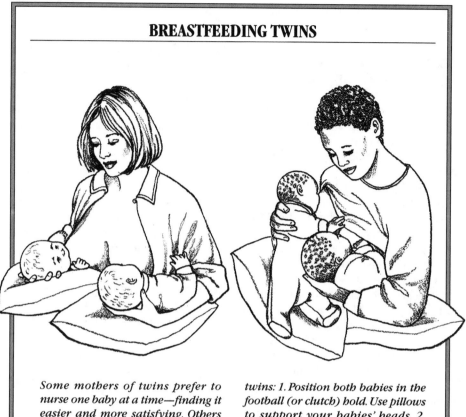

Some mothers of twins prefer to nurse one baby at a time—finding it easier and more satisfying. Others would rather not spend all day breastfeeding, and find that nursing both babies simultaneously saves time and works well. Here are two positions you can use while nursing twins: 1. Position both babies in the football (or clutch) hold. Use pillows to support your babies' heads. 2. Combine the cradle hold and the football hold, again using pillows for support and experimenting until both you and your babies are comfortable.

Delay in treating mastitis or discontinuing treatment too soon could lead to the development of a breast abscess, the symptoms of which include excruciating, throbbing pain; localized swelling, tenderness, and heat in the area of the abscess; and temperature swings between 100°F and 103°F. Treatment includes antibiotics and, generally, surgical drainage under anesthesia. The drain may stay in place after surgery. Breastfeeding can continue in most cases.

In rare instances, when mastitis is so severe that breastfeeding with the affected breast must be temporarily halted, a breast pump should be used regularly to empty it until healing is complete and breastfeeding can be resumed. In the meantime, nursing can continue on the unaffected breast.

Don't let breast and nursing problems with your first baby discourage you from nursing future babies. Engorgement and nipple soreness are far less common with subsequent births.

BREASTFEEDING AFTER A CESAREAN

How soon you can breastfeed your newborn after a surgical delivery will depend on how you feel and how your baby is doing. If you are both in good shape, you can probably introduce baby to breast in the delivery room after the surgery is completed, or in the recovery room shortly afterward. If you're groggy from general anesthesia or your baby needs immediate care in the nursery, you may have to wait. If after twelve hours you still haven't been able to get together with your baby, you probably should ask about using a pump to express milk (at this point it is actually premilk, or colostrum) to get lactation started.

You may find breastfeeding after a cesarean uncomfortable at first—most mothers do. It will be less so if you try to avoid putting pressure on the incision with one of these techniques: place a pillow on your lap under the baby; lie on your side; or use the football hold, again supported by a pillow, to nurse. Both the afterpains you experience as you nurse and the soreness at the site of the incision are normal and will lessen in the days ahead.

BREASTFEEDING TWINS

Breastfeeding, like just about every aspect of caring for newborn twins (or other multiples), seems as though it will be impossible until you fall into the rhythm of it. Once you have a routine established, it is not only possible but very rewarding. To nurse twins successfully, you should:

- Fulfill all the dietary recommendations for lactating mothers (see the Breastfeeding Diet, page 404), with these additions: 400 to 500 calories above your prepregnancy needs for each baby you are nursing (you may need to increase your caloric intake as the babies grow bigger and hungrier, or decrease it if you supplement nursing with formula and/or solids, or if you have considerable fat reserves you would like to burn); an additional serving of protein (for a total of four) and an additional serving of calcium (six total) or a calcium supplement.

- Drink eight to twelve glasses of fluid a day—but not more, because too much may suppress milk production.

- Get as much help as you can with housework, meal preparation, and infant care, in order to conserve your energy. Fatigue can reduce your milk supply.

- Explore the various feeding options. Nurse each separately (which can take a total of ten hours or more a day), or both together (see illustration, page 407). Combining individual and dual feedings, giving each infant at least one private feeding a day (while Dad or a baby-sitter feeds the other baby a bottle) is a good compromise that encourages mother-baby closeness. Relief bottles can be either formula or expressed milk.

- Recognize that the twins have different personalities, needs, and nursing patterns, and don't try to treat them identically. But do keep careful records to be sure both are fed at each feeding.

◆ ◆ ◆

CHAPTER 16

Postpartum: The First Six Weeks

B y now you're probably either set-tling into your new life as a fledg-ling mom or figuring out how to juggle new baby care with the demands of older children. Almost certainly, much of your daily—and nightly—attention is focused on that recently arrived little bundle. But that doesn't mean you should neglect yourself and your own needs. The first six weeks after the birth of a baby are still considered a "recovery" period, with your body and your psyche slowly getting back to a semblance of normal (whatever that is). In the meantime, though most of your questions and concerns are likely to be baby related, you're sure to have some that are a little more mommy-centric, too—from the state of your emotions ("Will I ever stop crying during insur-ance commercials?"), to the state of your sexual union ("Will I ever want to do 'it' again?"), to the state of your waist ("Will I ever be able to wear jeans that zip?"). The answer to most of these is yes; just give it time.

What You May Be Feeling

D uring the first six weeks postpar-tum, depending on the type of delivery you had (easy or diffi-cult, vaginal or cesarean), how much help you have at home, and other indi-vidual factors, you may experience all, or only some, of the following:

PHYSICALLY

◆ Continued periodlike vaginal discharge (lochia), dark red, pink, turning brownish, then yellowish white

◆ Fatigue

◆ Some continuing pain, discomfort, and numbness in the perineum, if you had a vaginal delivery (espe-cially if you had stitches) or labored before having a cesarean

- Diminishing incisional pain, continuing numbness, if you had a cesarean delivery (especially if it was your first)

- Continuing constipation (although this should be easing up in the first week postpartum)

- Gradual slimming of your abdomen as your uterus recedes into the pelvis (but only exercise will bring you fully back to prepregnancy shape)

- *Gradual* loss of weight

- Breast discomfort and nipple soreness until breastfeeding is well established

- Backache (from weak abdominal muscles and from carrying the baby)

- Joint pain (from joints loosened during pregnancy in preparation for delivery)

- Achiness in arms and neck (from carrying the baby)

- Hair loss

EMOTIONALLY

- Elation, depression, or swings between the two

- A sense of being overwhelmed, a growing feeling of confidence, or swings between the two

- Little interest in sex or, less commonly, increased desire

What You Can Expect at Your Postpartum Checkup

Your practitioner will probably schedule you for a checkup four to six weeks postpartum.[1] During that visit, you can expect the following to be checked, though the exact content of the visit will vary depending upon what your particular needs are and your practitioner's style of practice.

- Blood pressure

- Weight, which may possibly be down by about 17 to 20 pounds

- Your uterus, to see if it has returned to prepregnant shape, size, and location

- Your cervix, which will be on its way back to its prepregnant state, but will still be somewhat engorged

- Your vagina, which will have contracted and regained much of its muscle tone

- The episiotomy or laceration repair site, if any; or, if you had a cesarean delivery, the site of your incision

- Your breasts

- Hemorrhoids or varicose veins, if you have either

- Questions or problems you want to discuss—have a list ready

At this visit, the practitioner will also discuss with you the method of birth control that you will be using. If you plan on using a diaphragm and your cervix has recovered sufficiently, you will be fitted for one (your old one will no longer fit properly); if not, you may have to use condoms until you can be fitted. If you're

---

1. If you had a cesarean, you may be asked to come in at about three weeks postpartum to have your incision checked.

not breastfeeding and plan to take birth control pills, they may be prescribed now. There are birth control pills that have been shown to be safe for use during lactation, such as the "mini-Pill." If you are breastfeeding and would like to use the Pill for contraception, ask your practitioner about prescribing one of these.

What You May Be Concerned About

BABY BLUES AND DEPRESSION

"I have everything I have always wanted: a wonderful husband, a beautiful new baby—why do I feel so blue?"

Roughly 60 to 80 percent of all new mothers find themselves feeling at least a little blue at least occasionally during one of the happiest times of their lives. That's the paradox of "baby blues."

Hormones, so often the culprit fingered in the case of a woman's mood swings, may offer at least a partial rationale for baby blues, the symptoms of which may include sadness, crying, irritability, restlessness, and anxiety. Levels of estrogen and progesterone drop precipitously after childbirth, often taking a newly delivered woman's moods down with them. But why do all women experience the same hormonal fluctuations, but not all experience baby blues? Probably for the same reason that some women have PMS (premenstrual syndrome) and others never do—because sensitivity to hormonal fluctuations varies from woman to woman. Supporting that theory is the fact that women who are subject to pronounced PMS are more likely to experience both baby blues and postpartum depression.

But there is also a host of nonhormonal factors that probably contribute to the postpartum blues—which are most common around the third day after delivery and last usually no longer than two to three weeks. You may be surprised—and relieved—to find that so many of the feelings you're experiencing as you adjust to your new role are similar to those of most new mothers. Some of these feelings may include:

A sense of disappointment in the birth and/or in yourself. If unrealistic expectations of an idealized childbirth experience weren't realized (you wanted natural but you got cesarean, for example), you may feel that you've failed (though you haven't) or been cheated.

A sense of disappointment in the baby. He or she's so small, so red, so puffy, so unresponsive—not quite the all-smiles dimpled darling you'd pictured. Guilt about your feelings may add to your depression.

A feeling of anticlimax. Childbirth—the big event you'd schooled for and looked forward to for nine months—is over. Now what?

The shift from center stage to backstage. Your baby is now the star of the show. It starts in the hospital: visitors would rather run to the nursery than sit at your bedside inquiring after your health. It follows you home, with friends and family cooing over the cradle and barely noticing you. The pampered pregnant princess status you may have relished is probably a thing of the past. You may feel more like the postpartum Cinderella now, with no royal ball in sight—just the next midnight feeding.

Hospitalization. If you're still in the hospital, you may be frustrated by the lack of control you have over your life and your baby's.

Going home. It's normal to feel overwhelmed and overworked by the responsibilities that greet you (particularly if you have other children and no help).

Exhaustion. Fatigue from a strenuous labor and from too little sleep in the hospital is compounded by the round-the-clock rigors of caring for a newborn, and often contributes to the feeling that you don't have the strength to meet the demands of motherhood.

Feelings of inadequacy. Diapers, baths, cord care, feeding. As a first-time mother, there's so much you don't yet know, and so much you have to learn on the job—amid trial and plenty of error. Wasn't this mothering thing supposed to come naturally?

There may be plenty of moments of self-doubt, too, even if this is your second time around. How can you possibly handle the demands of a newborn and older child? Why is this one so different from the first? Why does what worked for number one not work for number two?

Breastfeeding difficulties. Painful engorgement, sore cracked nipples, fumbling and frustration on both sides of the breast—until nursing becomes second nature, you may have second thoughts about your native nurturing abilities.

A sense of mourning for the old you. Your carefree, possibly career-oriented, self has passed on (at least temporarily) with your baby's birth—and your new role as a mother doesn't yet fit. Who are you anyway?

Unhappiness over your looks. Before you were fat and pregnant; now you feel you're just fat. You can't stand wearing maternity clothes, but nothing else fits. And let's not get started on the bags under your eyes.

Relationship adjustments. The dynamics of your twosome are bound to experience some changes when baby makes three. Until you and your partner figure out how to balance the demands of the two most significant relationships in your lives (i.e., how to be a couple again, instead of just a couple of parents) your romantic life will probably be put on hold, which can put a stressful strain on your twosome.

Other possible triggers. Perhaps your pregnancy was unplanned or even unwanted; you have financial or work difficulties; you are going through a major life change (a distant move, a job change, a divorce, illness, or a death in the family).

Probably the only good thing that can be said about the baby blues (besides the fact that they're normal and very common) is that they don't last very long—about forty-eight hours for most women, and, occasionally, up to a couple of weeks. And though there's no cure other than the passage of time, there are ways to help yourself feel better:

♦ Drop the guilt. Being a new mother is a monumental challenge, and virtually everyone (pediatricians, baby nurses, and child development experts included) has a lot of on-the-job learning to do. And even once you learn, don't expect perfection. There's no such thing as a perfect parent or a perfect child. Accept that and life will be easier.

♦ If the blues arrive at the hospital, you might have your spouse bring in a special celebratory dinner for the two of you. Limit visitors if their chattering grates on your nerves, have more of them if they cheer you up. If it's the hospital that's getting you down, inquire about early discharge.

◆ Fight fatigue and that "overwhelmed" feeling by accepting (and, if necessary, asking for) help from others, by being less compulsive about doing things that can wait (like writing thank-you notes or organizing baby's wardrobe), by trying to squeeze in a nap or rest period when your baby is sleeping. Use feeding times as rest times, nursing or bottle-feeding in bed or in a comfortable chair with your feet up.

◆ Follow the Breastfeeding Diet (see page 404) to keep your strength up (minus 500 calories and three calcium servings if you're not breastfeeding). Avoid sugar (especially combined with chocolate) and alcohol, both of which can act as depressants.

◆ Cry, if you feel like it. But laugh, too. Watch favorite sitcoms or rent some comedies. Laughter is one of the best medicines for the baby blues and for many other things.

◆ Try meditation or other relaxation techniques to help you regain your calm when you start to lose it (see page 127).

◆ Find a baby-sitter and treat yourselves to dinner out, if possible. Even if you're breastfeeding, you should be able to squeeze in a couple of hours at a nearby restaurant. If not, make believe. Order dinner in (or let your spouse cook), dress up, create a restaurant ambiance with candlelight and soft music. And keep your sense of humor handy, in case the baby decides to interrupt your romantic interlude.

◆ Look good so you'll feel good. Walking around in a robe all day with unkempt hair is depressing to anyone. Shower before your spouse leaves in the morning (or you may not have a chance again); comb your hair; put on makeup if you ordinarily wear it. Buy an attractive new outfit (washable, of course) that fits loosely now but can be belted so that it continues to fit as you lose weight (which you will!).

◆ Get out of the house. Go for a walk with the baby or, if someone volunteers to sit, go out without the baby. Exercise (see Getting Back into Shape, page 426) helps chase away the baby blues and will help you get rid of any postpartum flab that might be adding to your depression.

◆ If you think your misery might like some company, get together with any new mothers you know, and share your feelings with them. If you don't have any newly delivered friends, make some. Approach other new mothers in the playground, or contact women who were in your childbirth class, possibly organizing a weekly after-birth reunion. Or join a new mom's support group or a postpartum exercise class. Or do your chatting on-line. Talking to your practitioner or your baby's doctor may also be helpful.

◆ If yours is the kind of sadness that would rather be by itself, indulge in some solitude. Though depression usually feeds on itself, some experts believe that this is not true of the postpartum variety. If going out with cheerful people, or having cheerful people visit, makes you feel worse, don't do it. But be sure you don't leave your spouse out in the cold. Communication in the immediate postpartum period is vital for you both. (Men, too, are susceptible to postpartum depression, and your spouse may need you as much as you need him.)

GETTING HELP FOR POSTPARTUM DEPRESSION

Until recently, postpartum depression was a condition that was largely swept under the rug of medical practice, much as premenstrual syndrome was. It was ignored by the public, minimally discussed by doctors, and suffered with unnecessarily in shame and silence by the women who experienced it. This mentality of denial has prevented women from learning about postpartum depression and the many effective therapies available to treat it. Worst of all, it has kept women from getting help they need when they need it.

Fortunately, thanks to some new efforts, there's been a slow shift in the way the medical community views and treats PPD. Public education campaigns are or soon will be under way in some states, requiring hospitals to send women home with educational material about PPD, so that new moms (and their spouses) will be more likely to spot the symptoms early and seek treatment. Practitioners are becoming better educated, too—learning how to look for risk factors during pregnancy that might predispose a woman to PPD, to screen routinely for the illness postpartum, and to treat it quickly, safely, and successfully. There are also several standardized tests (Edinburgh Postnatal Screening Scale and Cheryl Beck's Postpartum Depression Screening Scale) that have been shown to be effective in screening for PPD.

Postpartum depression is one of the most treatable forms of depression. So if it strikes you, don't suffer with it any longer than you have to. Speak up—and get the help you need *now*.

For more help contact *Postpartum Support International*, 927 N. Kellogg Avenue, Santa Barbara, CA 93111, (805) 967-7636, www.postpartum.net; *Postpartum Assistance for Mothers*, 390 Diablo Road, Suite 115, Danville, CA 94526, (925) 552-5127, www.postpartumassistance. com; *Depression After Delivery*, www. depressionafterdelivery.com.

◆ If you are single, enlist one or more relatives or friends to give you a hand when you need it. Going it alone is something no one should have to do.

"My baby is over a month old, and I still can't stop feeling depressed. Shouldn't I be feeling better by now?"

When the blues just won't fade, chances are postpartum depression is the problem. Though "baby blues" and "postpartum depression" are often used interchangeably, they're actually two different conditions. True postpartum depression (PPD) is less common (affecting about 10 to 20 percent of women) and much more enduring (lasting anywhere from a few weeks to a year or more). It may begin at birth, but more often not until a month or two later. Sometimes PPD is late onset; it doesn't start until a woman gets her first postpartum menstrual period or until she weans her nursing baby (and hormones fluctuate again). Women who have had PPD before, have a personal or family history of depression or severe PMS, spent a lot of time feeling down during pregnancy, and/or had a complicated pregnancy and delivery or have a sick or difficult baby are more susceptible to the illness.

The symptoms of PPD are similar to those of "baby blues," though much more pronounced. They include crying and irritability; sleep problems (not being able to sleep or wanting to sleep the day away); eating problems (having no appetite or an excessive one); persistent feelings of sadness, hopelessness, and helplessness; an inability (or lack of desire) to take care of yourself or your newborn; social withdrawal; excessive worry; feeling all alone; and memory loss.

If you haven't already tried the tips for fading the baby blues (see page 412), do try them now—some of them may be helpful in easing postpartum depression, too. But if symptoms have persisted for more than two or three weeks without any noticeable improvement, chances are your PPD won't go away without professional attention. Don't wait to see if it does. First, call your practitioner and ask for a thyroid test; since irregularities in thyroid hormone levels can lead to emotional instability, this is usually one of the first steps taken when evaluating postpartum depression (see page 417). If your thyroid levels check out normally, ask for a referral to a therapist who has a clinical background in the treatment of postpartum depression and make an appointment *promptly*. Antidepressants (there are several that are safe even if you're breastfeeding), combined with counseling, can help you feel better fast. Bright light therapy may also bring relief from the symptoms of PPD, and can be used instead of or in addition to medication. Whichever treatment route you and your therapist decide is right for you, keep in mind that swift intervention is critical. Without it, depression can prevent you from bonding with, caring for, and enjoying your baby. It can also have a devastating effect on the other relationships in your life (with your spouse, with other children), as well as on your own health and well-being.

Recent studies have shown that for women who are high-risk, taking antidepressants such as Paxil, Zoloft, or Prozac right after delivery can prevent postpartum depression. Some physicians will even prescribe low doses of antidepressants during the last trimester of preg-

nancy to women with a history of depression. If you decide to become pregnant again, it might be a good idea to discuss these options with your practitioner beforehand, so you can head PPD off before it starts.

Some women, instead of (or in addition to) feeling depressed postpartum, feel extremely anxious or fearful, sometimes experiencing panic attacks, including rapid heartbeat and breathing, hot or cold flashes, chest pain, dizziness, and shaking. These symptoms also require prompt treatment by a qualified therapist, which may include medication.

Much more rare and much more serious than PPD is postpartum psychosis. Its symptoms include loss of reality, hallucinations, and/or delusions. If you are experiencing suicidal, violent, or aggressive feelings, are hearing voices, seeing things, or have other signs of psychosis, call your doctor and go to the emergency room *immediately*. Don't underplay what you're feeling, and don't be put off by reassurances that such feelings are normal during the postpartum period—they're not. To be sure you don't act out any dangerous feelings while you're waiting for help, try to get a neighbor, relative, or friend to stay with you.

"I feel terrific, and have since the moment I delivered three weeks ago. Is all this good feeling building up to one terrific case of letdown?"

Baby blues are common, but they're by no means universal. And there's no reason to believe that you're in for an emotional crash just because you've been feeling buoyant. Since baby blues only occur within the first postpartum week, it's pretty safe to assume you've escaped them.

The fact that you're not suffering from postpartum depression, however, doesn't necessarily mean your family has escaped this problem completely. Studies show that while new fathers (who, believe it or not, also go through hormonal changes postpartum) are unlikely to be depressed when their wives are, their risk of falling into a postpartum slump increases dramatically when the new mother is feeling great. So be sure that your spouse isn't experiencing the baby blues; some new dads try to hide such feelings to avoid burdening their spouses (see page 446 for more).

RETURNING TO PREPREGNANCY WEIGHT AND SHAPE

"I knew I wouldn't be ready for a bikini right after delivery, but I still look six months pregnant a week later."

Though childbirth produces more rapid weight loss than any diet you'll find on the best-seller lists (an average of 12 pounds overnight), most women don't find it quite rapid enough. Particularly after they catch a glimpse of their postpartum silhouettes in the mirror, looking distressingly pregnant.

The fact is, no one comes out of the delivery room looking much slimmer than when they went in. Part of the reason for that protruding postpartum abdomen is the still-enlarged uterus, which will be reduced to prepregnancy size by the end of six weeks, reducing your abdominal girth in the process. Another reason for your bloated belly is leftover fluids, five pounds or so of which will flush out within a few days or so after delivery. But the rest of the problem is stretched-out abdominal muscles and skin, which may sag for a lifetime unless a concerted exercise effort is made. (See Getting Back into Shape, page 426.)

As hard as it might be to put it out of your mind, you shouldn't even think about the shape you're in during the first six weeks postpartum, especially if you're breastfeeding. This is a recovery period, during which ample nutrition is important for both energy and resistance to infection. Sticking to the Breastfeeding Diet if you're nursing (or to the Diet minus the 500 extra nursing calories and the extra calcium serving[2] if you're not) right now should start you on the way to slow, steady weight loss. If, after six weeks, you aren't losing any weight, you can start cutting back somewhat on calories. If you're nursing, don't go overboard. Eating fewer than 1,800 calories a day can reduce milk production, and burning fat too quickly can release toxins into the blood, which can end up in your breast milk. If you're not nursing, you can go on a sensible, well-balanced weight-loss diet six weeks postpartum.

Some women find that the extra pounds melt off while they're breastfeeding; others are dismayed to find the scale doesn't budge. If the latter turns out to be the case with you, don't despair; you should easily be able to shed any remaining excess poundage once you've weaned your baby.

How quickly you return to your prepregnant weight will also depend on how many pounds you put on during pregnancy. If you didn't gain much more than 25 pounds, you should be able to pack away those pregnancy jeans in a few months, without strenuous dieting. If you gained 35 or more pounds, you may find it takes more effort and more time— anywhere from ten months to two years—to return to prepregnancy weight.

---

2. Women who are not nursing should continue to get adequate calcium to prevent the development of osteoporosis later in life. If necessary, take a calcium supplement to get your intake up to 1,200 mg daily.

THYROIDITIS GOT YOU DOWN?

Nearly all new mothers feel run-down and tired. Most have trouble losing weight. Many suffer from some degree of depression and a certain amount of hair loss. It may not be a pretty picture, but for the majority of moms, it's a completely normal one in the postpartum period—and one that gradually begins to look better as the weeks pass. For the estimated 5 to 9 percent of women who suffer from postpartum thyroiditis, however, the picture may not improve with time. The problem is, because the symptoms of postpartum thyroiditis (PPT) are so similar to those weathered by *all* new mothers, the condition may go undiagnosed and untreated.

For most women, postpartum thyroiditis may start anywhere from one to three months after delivery with a brief episode of *hyper*thyroidism (probably due to the inflammation and breakdown of the thyroid gland due to an attack by antibodies, which stimulates leakage of thyroid hormone). This period of excess thyroid hormone circulating in the bloodstream may last a few weeks or longer. During this hyperthyroid period, a woman may be tired, irritable, and nervous, feel very warm, and experience increased sweating and insomnia—all of which are common in the immediate postpartum period anyway, making an easy diagnosis more elusive. Treatment isn't usually needed for this phase.

This period will generally be followed by one of *hypo*thyroidism, when the thyroid gland is underproducing because of damage done by the antibodies. (In some women, however, PPT ends with the hyperthyroid period because the damage done to the thyroid gland wasn't great enough to reduce thyroid hormone production.) With hypothyroidism, fatigue continues, along with depression (longer lasting and often more severe than typical "baby blues" or postpartum depression), muscle aches, hair loss, dry skin, cold intolerance, poor memory, and an inability to lose weight.

If your postpartum symptoms seem to be more pronounced and persistent than you would have expected, and especially if they are preventing you from eating, sleeping, and enjoying your new baby, check with your practitioner. Tests can determine whether PPT is the cause of your troubles. (Some endocrinologists believe that thyroiditis is such a common cause of postpartum depression that *all* women who suffer from it should have their thyroid function tested.) Be sure to mention any history of thyroid problems in your family, since there is a very strong genetic link.

Most women recover from postpartum thyroiditis within a year after delivery. In the meantime, treatment with supplementary thyroid hormone can help them feel much better much faster. About 25 percent of women, however, will remain hypothyroid, requiring lifetime treatment (which is as easy as taking a pill every day and having a yearly blood test). Even in those who recover spontaneously, thyroiditis is likely to recur during or after subsequent pregnancies. Some may develop hypothyroidism or Graves disease (hyperthyroidism) later in life. For this reason, it makes sense for women who have had PPT to have a yearly thyroid screening and, if they are planning another pregnancy, to be screened in the preconception period and during pregnancy.

BREAST MILK

"Does everything I eat, drink, or take get into my breast milk? Could any of it harm my baby when she nurses?"

Feeding your baby outside the womb doesn't require quite as many limitations as feeding her inside did. But as long as you're breastfeeding, a little extra attention to what goes into you will ensure that everything that goes into your baby is safe.

The basic fat-protein-carbohydrate composition of human milk isn't dependent on what a mother eats. If a mother doesn't eat enough calories and protein to produce milk, her body's stores will be tapped and the baby will be fed, at least until the stores run out. Some vitamin deficiencies in the mother's diet will, however, affect the vitamin content of her breast milk. So will excesses of some vitamins. A wide variety of substances, from medications to seasonings, can also show up in milk, with varying results.

To keep breast milk safe and healthful:

◆ Follow the Breastfeeding Diet (page 404).

◆ Avoid foods to which your baby seems sensitive. Garlic, onion, cabbage, dairy products, and chocolate are common offenders, causing bothersome gas in some, though by no means all, babies. One study found most babies loved the taste of breast milk after their mothers ate garlic (bring on the Caesar salad, Mom!), though some infants with finicky palates may be displeased by the flavor an unexpectedly strong seasoning may impart (but hold the curry!). Interestingly, such likes and dislikes may be tied to Mom's own preferences. Seasonings and foods that are familiar—because Mom ate plenty of them during pregnancy and/or since delivery—are often most preferred by a nursing baby. (Which means that moms who craved Indian food while they were expecting may have babies who relish that curry-flavored milk.) Such preferences may even continue later on in your child's life (a good reason to eat your vegetables now).

◆ Take a vitamin supplement especially formulated for pregnant and/or lactating mothers. Do not take any other vitamins or nutritional supplements without the advice of your physician.

◆ Do not smoke. Many of the toxic substances in tobacco enter the bloodstream, and eventually your milk. Besides, smoking near the baby can cause respiratory problems for her and increases the risk of SIDS (sudden infant death syndrome), or crib death. If you can't manage to give up smoking, however, don't feel that you must give up breastfeeding (see page 312).

◆ Do not take any medications (traditional or herbal) without consulting your physician. Although some medications are perfectly safe to take while you're nursing, some pass into the breast milk, and can be harmful to a tiny infant even in small doses. (Particularly dangerous are antithyroid, some anticancer, and some antihypertensive drugs; prescription painkillers; tranquilizers, barbiturates, and sedatives; lithium; radioactive iodine; bromides.) Often, safe substitutes can be found for a medication you must take; a medication can be given in a way that reduces risk;[3] or perhaps a particular medication can be discontinued for the duration of nursing. (Do make sure that any doctor who prescribes a medication for you is aware that you are breastfeeding.) All illicit drugs are dangerous during lactation and should be avoided.

◆ Limit alcohol. Have a single drink only occasionally. Heavy daily imbibing or binge drinking can make baby

---

3. For example, your physician may advise youu to take a certain medication right before a feeding or one hour before the next feeding to minimize the amount that will get into your breast milk.

drowsy and depress the nervous system, and may slow motor development as well as reduce your milk supply. If you do have a drink, have it right after nursing and try not to nurse again for at least two hours.

◆ Cut down on caffeine. One or two cups of caffeinated coffee or tea or caffeinated soft drinks a day probably won't affect your baby. But because babies store caffeine in their bodies, rather than eliminate it quickly, it's wise to avoid heavy intakes. Four or more cups could make her jittery and irritable and could interfere with sleep. (Some babies may be affected by one or two cups; if your baby seems jittery and has trouble sleeping, you may want to cut out the caffeine and see if it makes a difference.)

◆ Don't take laxatives to promote regularity (some of them will have a laxative effect on your baby); increase your fiber and fluid intakes.

◆ Seek safe relief from pain. Good options when you're nursing include acetaminophen and alternative treatments (see page 455 and the Appendix). Take aspirin or ibuprofen only with your practitioner's approval, but don't take more than the recommended dose, and don't take them frequently.

◆ Opt for foods that are as close to their natural state as possible. Read labels so you'll be able to steer clear of foods that contain many chemical additives, including artificial colors and flavorings (see page 146).

◆ Be smart about sweeteners. Avoid saccharin, since it passes into the breast milk and has been shown in animal studies to cause cancer. Sucralose (Splenda), on the other hand, is safe, and aspartame, which seems to

pass into the breast milk in only small quantities, appears to be safe in moderate quantities. But be sure that the foods you consume that contain sweeteners aren't full of a lot of other chemical additives. (For more on sweeteners, see page 65.)

◆ Minimize your ingestion of incidental pesticides. Peel vegetables and fruits or wash well; eat low-fat or fat-free dairy products, lean meats, white-meat poultry with the skin removed, and limited amounts of organ meats. (The pesticides ingested by animals are stored in fat, skin, and some organs.)

◆ Avoid eating any fish that might be contaminated. (The same rules for safe fish and seafood consumption that apply to pregnant women apply to lactating women; see page 147.) And since food poisoning is something you'd really like to avoid right now, also see the safe-eating tips on page 150.

◆ If you have high blood levels of lead (over 40 mcg per deciliter), you may have to stop breastfeeding, or halt it temporarily until levels can be lowered.

LEAKING MILK

"I seem to be leaking milk from my breasts all the time. Is this normal? Is it going to last?"

The first few weeks of nursing can be very wet ones. Milk may leak, drip, or even spray from your breasts, and it can happen at any time, anywhere, without warning. All of a sudden, you'll feel the tingle of let-down—and before you can grab a nursing pad or a sweater to cover up with, you'll look down to see the telltale circle of dampness that gives new meaning to the term "wet T-shirt."

Besides those inopportune and public

moments ("So that's why the bank teller was looking at me funny!"), you might find yourself springing spontaneous leaks when you're sleeping or taking a warm shower, when you hear your baby cry, when you think about or talk about your baby. Milk may drip from one breast while you nurse from the other, and if your baby has settled into a somewhat regular feeding schedule, your breasts may be dripping with anticipation before baby latches on.

Though it may be uncomfortable, unpleasant, and endlessly embarrassing, this side effect of breastfeeding is completely normal and very common, particularly in the early weeks. (Not leaking at all or leaking only a little can be just as normal, and in fact, many second-time mothers might notice that their breasts leak less than they did the first time around.) In most cases, as breastfeeding becomes established, the system eventually settles down and leaking lessens considerably. In the meantime, while you may not be able to turn off that leaky faucet, you may be able to make living with it a little less messy:

◆ Stock up on nursing pads. If you're a leaker, you'll find that in the first postpartum weeks, you'll be changing your nursing pads as often as you nurse—sometimes even more frequently. Keep in mind that, like a diaper, they should be changed whenever they become wet. Make sure you use pads that don't have a plastic or waterproof liner; they'll just trap moisture and lead to irritated nipples. Some women prefer the disposable variety, while others like the feel of the reusable cotton ones.

◆ Protect your bed. If you find you're leaking a lot at night, use extra nursing pads, or place a large towel under you while you sleep. The last thing you'll want to be doing now is changing your sheets every day or, worse, shopping for a new mattress.

◆ Don't pump to prevent leaking. Extra pumping will not control the leak; on the contrary, the more you stimulate your breasts, the more milk they'll produce, and the more leaking you'll have to contend with.

◆ Try to stop the overflow. Once nursing is well established and your milk production has leveled off, you can try to stop the leaking by pressing your nipples (though probably not in public) or holding your arms against your breasts. Don't, however, do this in the first few weeks, because it may inhibit milk letdown and can lead to a clogged milk duct.

LONG-TERM CESAREAN RECOVERY

"It's been a week since my c-section. What can I expect now?"

While you've definitely come a long way since you were wheeled into recovery, like every new mother you still have some recuperation ahead of you in the next few weeks. Keep in mind that the better you are about getting the rest you need now (as well as about following your practitioner's instructions), the shorter that recuperation time will ultimately be. In the meantime, you can expect:

You'll need plenty of help. Paid help is best for the first week at home, but if that's not possible, make sure someone (your spouse, mother, another relative, or a friend) is around to lend a hand. It's best not to do any lifting (including the baby) or any housework during this week. If you must lift the baby, lift from waist level, so you use your arms, not your abdomen. If you have to lift something from the floor, bend at the knees, not at the waist.

Little or no pain. Most of it should have dissipated by now. But if you do hurt, a mild pain reliever should help. Don't take any medication other than acetaminophen, however, if you're breastfeeding—unless it has been approved by your doctor.

Progressive improvement. Your scar will be sore and sensitive for a few weeks, but it will improve steadily. A light dressing may protect it from irritation, and you will probably be more comfortable wearing loose clothing that doesn't rub. Occasional sensations of pulling or twitching and other brief pains in the region of the scar are a normal part of healing and will eventually subside. Itchiness may follow—ask your practitioner to recommend an anti-itch ointment that you can apply. The numbness surrounding the scar will last longer, possibly several months. Lumpiness in the scar tissue will probably diminish (unless you tend to get that kind of scar), and the scar may turn pink or purple before it finally fades.

If pain becomes persistent, if the area around the incision turns an angry red, or if a brown, gray, green, or yellow discharge oozes from the wound, call your doctor. The incision may have become infected. (A small amount of clear fluid discharge may be normal, but report it to your physician anyway.)

A four-week wait (at least) for intercourse. The guidelines are pretty much the same for those who've delivered vaginally and those who've had a cesarean section (though how well your incision is healing will also be a consideration in determining how long you'll need to wait). See the next couple of pages for more.

To get moving. Once you're free of pain, you'll be able to begin exercising. Since the muscle tone of your perineum probably hasn't been compromised (unless you went through labor before your c-section), you may not need to do Kegel exercises, though they benefit anyone. Concentrate instead on those that tighten the abdominal muscles. (See Getting Back into Shape, page 426.) Make "slow and steady" your motto; get into a program gradually and continue it daily. Expect it to take several months before you're back to your old self.

RESUMING SEXUAL RELATIONS

"When can my husband and I start making love again?"

That's at least partly up to you. According to the recommendations of the American College of Obstetricians and Gynecologists, sex can, in most cases, be safely resumed when a woman feels ready—typically, about four weeks postpartum, though many nurse-midwives give the green light to intercourse as early as two weeks postpartum. In certain circumstances (for instance, if healing has been slow or there has been an infection or lochia is still being produced), your practitioner may recommend waiting longer—in which case it's wise to follow that advice. The six-week rule, once routinely applied to all women postpartum, regardless of condition, is still followed by some practitioners. If you think that may be the case with yours and you're feeling up to making love sooner, ask why he or she doesn't think this is wise. If there is no special reason, then ask if you can get started sooner. Should your health and safety require waiting the full six weeks, keep in mind that time flies when you're caring for a newborn. In the meantime, feel free to indulge in other forms of lovemaking.

LACK OF INTEREST IN MAKING LOVE

"I've gotten the go-ahead from my practitioner, but sex is the last thing I feel like right now."

Of all the things on a woman's must-do list postpartum, sex rarely makes the top ten, and for good reason. Sex takes energy, concentration, and time—all of which are in particularly short supply in the lives of new parents. Your libido, and your partner's, must regularly compete with sleepless nights, exhausting days, dirty diapers, and an endlessly demanding baby. Your body is still recuperating from the trauma of childbearing; your hormones are re-adjusting. Fears (of pain, of doing some damage internally, of not being the same, of becoming pregnant again too soon) may plague you. If you're breast-feeding, this may unconsciously be satisfying your need for intimacy. Or making love may stimulate uncomfortable— and unsexy—leakage of milk.

All in all, it's not surprising—and perfectly normal—if your sexual appetite, no matter how voracious it once was, is temporarily suppressed. (On the other hand, some women have strong sexual drives now, particularly in the immediate postpartum period, when there is engorgement of the genital region—and that's normal, too, though a little inconvenient if the green light for love-making hasn't been issued.)

If your problem is lack of interest, there are many ways to make sexuality appealing again. Which ones will work for you will depend on you, your spouse, and your situation:

Make time your ally. Give your body time to heal, especially if you had a difficult delivery or a cesarean. Your hormonal balance won't be back to normal until you start menstruating, and if you're breastfeeding, that may not be for many months. Even if the doctor's given you the go-ahead, don't feel obligated to make love if it doesn't feel good, emotionally or physically. And when you do, start slowly, possibly with cuddling, foreplay, mutual masturbation, and/or oral sex, but no penetration.

Don't be discouraged by pain. Many women are surprised and disheartened to find that postpartum intercourse can really hurt. If you've had an episiotomy or a laceration, there may be discomfort (ranging from slight to severe) for weeks, even months, after the stitches have healed. You may also have pain with intercourse, although it may be less severe, if you delivered with the perineum intact—and even if you've had a cesarean. (Though if you had a planned cesarean, without labor, you may have somewhat less discomfort.) Until the pain eases, you can try to minimize it in the ways described in the Easing Back into Sex box on the facing page.

Keep your expectations realistic. Don't expect a perfect experience, complete with simultaneous orgasms, the first time you make love after delivery. Some usually orgasmic women don't have orgasms at all for several weeks, or even longer. With love and patience, sex will eventually be as satisfying as ever—or more so.

Communicate. A really good sexual relationship must be built on trust, understanding, and communication. If, for instance, you're too wrapped up in motherhood one night to feel sexy, don't beg off with a headache. Be honest. A spouse who's been included in parenting since conception is most likely to understand. If intercourse is painful, don't be a martyr. Explain to your spouse what hurts, what feels good, what you'd rather put off until another time.

EASING BACK INTO SEX

Lubricate. Lowered hormone levels during the postpartum period (which may not rise in the nursing mother until her baby is either partially or totally weaned) can make the vagina uncomfortably dry and intercourse painful. Using lubrication such as K-Y jelly or Astroglide until your own natural secretions return can reduce pain and increase pleasure.

Medicate, if necessary. Your practitioner may prescribe an estrogen cream to lessen pain and tenderness.

Warm up. Think of foreplay as the appetizer that will whet your appetite for the main course. So indulge in plenty—time permitting, of course.

Loosen up. Try relaxation exercises (see page 127), a shower for two, a massage, or anything else that helps you unwind. If you aren't breastfeeding (or occasionally, even if you are), you can try a glass of wine or a cocktail—but be aware that too much alcohol can interfere with sexual desire and performance.

Set the mood. Dimmed lighting (think scented candles) is more romantic and may also be kinder and gentler to your not-quite-back-to-shape figure, which could make you feel self-conscious. (Keep in mind that your partner is not likely to be nearly as concerned about what you consider figure flaws as you are.) Play some mood music, too, and don't forget to let voice mail answer the phone.

Vary positions. Side-to-side or woman-on-top positions allow more control of penetration and put less pressure on an episiotomy site or a cesarean scar. Experiment to find what works best for you.

Find alternative means of gratification. If intercourse isn't pleasurable yet, seek sexual satisfaction through mutual masturbation or oral sex. Or if you're both too pooped to pop, find pleasure in just being together. There's absolutely nothing wrong (and everything right) about lying in bed together, cuddling, kissing, and swapping baby stories.

Fit it in when you can. When your twosome becomes a threesome, you can no longer make love when and where you want to. Instead, you'll have to either grab it when you can (if the baby is napping at three o'clock on Saturday afternoon, drop everything) or make a point of planning ahead. Don't feel that unspontaneous sex can't be fun. Instead, think of the advance planning as giving you the opportunity to build anticipation. ("The baby will be asleep at eight—can't wait!" Or "Let's drop her off at Grandma's and make a beeline back to the bedroom!") Accept interruptions—there will be many—with a sense of humor, and try to start again where you left off as soon as possible. And should sex turn out to be less frequent than before, strive for quality, not quantity.

Cut other corners. A lot of postpartum exhaustion is natural; learning to become parents is certainly taxing. But some of it is unnecessary, often caused by trying to do too much too soon. Forgo the dusting for now. Put your favorite take-out on speed dial. If you cut some dispensable corners, you may sometimes have energy left for loving.

Don't worry. Despite how you may be feeling now, you will live to love again, with as much passion and pleasure as ever. (And because shared parenthood can often bring couples closer together, you may find the flame not only rekindled, but burning brighter than before.) Worry now can only put an unnecessary damper on your sexual relationship.

BECOMING PREGNANT AGAIN

"I thought that breastfeeding was a form of birth control. Now I hear you can get pregnant while nursing, even before you get your period."

Unless you don't mind becoming pregnant again soon (probably not a good idea for either you or for your new baby), don't even think about relying on breastfeeding for contraception.

It's true that, on average, women who nurse resume normal menstrual cycles later than those who don't. In mothers who aren't nursing, menstruation usually begins somewhere between six and twelve weeks after delivery, whereas in nursing mothers the average is somewhere between four to six months. As usual, however, averages are deceptive. Women who are nursing have been known to begin menstruating as early as six weeks and as late as eighteen months postpartum. The problem is, there's no sure way to predict when *you* will get your first post-baby period, though several variables can influence the timing. For example, frequency of nursing (more than three times a day seems to suppress ovulation better), duration of nursing (the longer you nurse, the greater the delay in ovulation), and whether or not feedings are being supplemented (your baby's taking formula, solids, even water can interfere with the ovulation-suppressing effect of nursing).

Why worry about birth control before that first menstrual period? Because the point at which you ovulate for the first time after delivery is as unpredictable as when you menstruate. Some women have a sterile first period; that is, they don't ovulate during that cycle. Others ovulate before the period, and therefore can go from pregnancy to pregnancy without ever having had a menstrual period. Since you don't know which will come first, the period or the egg, contraceptive caution is highly advisable. For information on choosing birth control methods, see *What to Expect the First Year.*

Of course, accidents can happen. Medical science has yet to develop a method of contraception (with the possible exception of sterilization) that is 100 percent effective. So even if you've been using contraception—and especially if you haven't been—pregnancy is still a possibility. Unfortunately, the first symptom of pregnancy you would ordinarily look for (absence of menstruation) will not be apparent if you've been nursing and not yet menstruating. But because of hormonal changes (there are different sets of hormones in operation during pregnancy than during lactation), your milk supply would probably diminish noticeably soon after a new pregnancy is established. You might, in addition, experience any or all of the other symptoms of pregnancy. Of course, if you do have any suspicion that you might be pregnant, the best thing to do is take a pregnancy test and, if it is positive, visit your practitioner as soon as possible. If you do turn out to be pregnant, you can continue breastfeeding as long as you feel up to it. But you will need plenty of rest and good nutrition—including more calories and protein. And after delivery, the new baby should have nursing priority.

HAIR LOSS

"My hair seems to be falling out suddenly. Am I going bald?"

No need to stock up on hats. This hair fall is normal, and will stop well in advance of baldness. Ordinarily the average head sheds 100 hairs a day, which are being continually replaced. During pregnancy, the hormonal changes keep those hairs from falling out. But the reprieve is only temporary. Those hairs are slated to go, and they will, within three to six months of delivery. Some women who are breastfeeding exclusively find that hair fall doesn't begin until they wean their baby or supplement the nursing with formula or solids.

To keep your hair healthy, eat well, continue taking a vitamin supplement, and treat your hair with kindness. That means shampooing only when necessary, using a conditioner to reduce the need to untangle, using a wide-toothed comb if you do have to untangle, and avoiding the application of heat (with blow dryers or curling or straightening irons). It may also be a good idea to avoid further damage by postponing permanents, hair colorings, and hair-relaxing treatments until your tresses seem back to normal.

If hair loss is excessive, especially if you are also experiencing other symptoms of thyroid disease (see page 417), consult with your practitioner.

Just because you lost a lot of hair following this pregnancy doesn't mean you will if there's a next time. Your body's reaction to each pregnancy, as you are sure to find out, can be very different.

TAKING TUB BATHS

"I seem to be getting a lot of contradictory advice about whether or not tub baths are all right in the postpartum period. Are they?"

At one time, new mothers weren't permitted to set foot in a tub until at least one month after delivery, because of fear of infection from the bathwater. Today, because it's known that still bathwater does not enter the vagina, infection from bathing is no longer considered a threat. Some physicians, in fact, recommend tub baths in the hospital (when a tub is available) because they

believe bathing removes lochia from the perineum—and from between the folds of the labia—more efficiently than showering. In addition, the warm water is comforting to the episiotomy site, relieves soreness and edema in the area, and soothes hemorrhoids. (You can also take a sitz bath, with just a few inches of warm water, for these purposes.)

If you do bathe during the first week or two following delivery, be sure the tub is scrubbed meticulously before it's filled. (But be sure you're not the one who does the scrubbing.) And have help getting into and out of the tub during the first few postpartum days, when you're still likely to be shaky. If you're recovering from a cesarean, baths are usually permitted after the first week, but check with your doctor.

EXHAUSTION

"It's been nearly two months since I had the baby, but I feel more tired than ever. Could I be sick?"

Many a new mother has dragged herself into her doctor's office and complained of overwhelming chronic fatigue, convinced that she's fallen victim to some fatal malady. The nearly invariable diagnosis? A classic case of motherhood.

Rare is the mother who escapes this maternal fatigue syndrome, characterized by tiredness that never seems to ease up and an almost total lack of energy. And it's not surprising. There's no other job as emotionally and physically taxing as that of being a new mother. The strain and pressures are not, as in most other jobs, limited to eight hours a day or five days a week. (And mothers don't get lunch hours or coffee breaks, either.) Motherhood for first-timers also has the stress inherent in any new job: there's always something new to learn, mistakes to be made, problems to solve. If all this isn't enough, add the energy that goes into breastfeeding (especially before you and your baby get the hang of it), the strength sapped by toting around a rapidly growing infant and accompanying paraphernalia, and night after night of broken sleep. The fatigue may be even more pronounced in the stressed-out mothers who have a very low birthweight baby or a baby with other problems, and those with older children at home.

Check with your doctor to be sure there is no other physical cause responsible for your exhaustion (such as postpartum thyroiditis; see page 417). If you get a clean bill of health, be assured that time, experience, and your baby sleeping

through the night will gradually help relieve much of your fatigue. Your energy level should pick up a bit, too, as your body adjusts to the new demands of motherhood (including the sleep deprivation). Also make sure that you're not trying to do too much (if you are, cut back in the less important departments, such as housekeeping), that your spouse is fully sharing the load (both with the baby and with household chores), that you're taking every possible opportunity (as impossible as it may seem) to put your feet up and rest, and that you're eating regularly and well. In the meantime, try the tips for relieving the baby blues and postpartum blues (page 411), both of which are tied to fatigue.

What It's Important to Know: GETTING BACK INTO SHAPE

It's one thing to look six months pregnant when you *are* six months pregnant, and quite another to look it when you've already delivered. Yet most women can expect to come out of the birthing room not much trimmer than when they went in—with a little bundle in their arms and a sizable one still around their middles. As for the pencil-thin pants optimistically packed for the going-home trip, they're likely to stay packed, with maternity jeans the depressing substitute.

How soon after you become a new mother will you stop looking like a mother-to-be? The answer will depend primarily on three things: (1) How much weight you gained during pregnancy; (2) How well you control your intake of calories; (3) How much exercise you get.[4]

"Who needs exercise?" you may wonder. "I've been in perpetual motion since I got home from the hospital. Doesn't that count?"

Unfortunately, not much. Exhausting as it is, that kind of activity won't tighten up the perineal and abdominal muscles that have been stretched and left saggy by pregnancy and childbirth—only an exercise program will. And the right kind of postpartum exercise will do more than tone you up. It will help keep baby-toting backaches at bay, promote healing and hasten recovery from labor and delivery, help pregnancy-loosened joints tighten up, improve circulation, and reduce the risk of a variety of other unpleasant postpartum symptoms, from varicose veins to leg cramps. Kegel exercises, which target the perineal muscles, will help you avoid stress incontinence (the leaking of urine) and postpartum sexual problems. Finally, exercise can

---

4. It may also depend on your metabolism and heredity.

GROUND RULES FOR THE FIRST SIX WEEKS

♦ Wear a supportive bra and comfortable clothing.

♦ Try to divide your exercise schedule into two or three brief sessions, rather than doing one long session a day (this tones muscles better and will be easier on your recovering body—and you're more likely to be able to fit it in).

♦ Start each session with the exercise you find least strenuous.

♦ Do exercises slowly, and don't do a rapid series of repetitions. Instead, rest briefly between movements (the muscle buildup occurs then, not while you are in motion).

♦ As during pregnancy, it's necessary to avoid jerky, bouncy, erratic motions during the first six weeks postpartum. Also avoid knee-to-chest exercises, full sit-ups, and double-leg lifts during this period.

♦ Monitor your heart rate.

♦ Be sure to replenish fluids lost during exercise.

♦ Take it slowly and sensibly; "No pain, no gain" wasn't a motto created with new mothers in mind. Don't do more than recommended, even if you feel you can, and stop before you feel tired. If you overdo it, you probably won't feel it until the next day, by which time you may be so exhausted and achy that you won't be able to exercise at all.

♦ Don't let taking care of your baby stop you from taking care of yourself. Your baby will love lying on your chest as you go through your exercise paces.

have a profound psychological benefit; as exercise-released endorphins circulate in your system, improving your mood and your ability to cope, you'll find yourself much better equipped to handle the stresses of new parenthood.

And you can probably start sooner than you think. If your delivery was vaginal and uncomplicated and you don't have any other major health issue that might slow you down, you can begin your postpartum exercise program as early as twenty-four hours after delivery. (If you've had a surgical or a traumatic delivery, check with your doctor first.)

Don't even think about starting off with a bang, however; your still-recovering body needs to take it slowly and carefully. The following three-phase program will help guide you. You can supplement it by using a postpartum exercise book or video, joining a class for new mothers (the camaraderie helps with motivation, and many include infants in the fun), and making daily strolls with baby a part of your routine.

PHASE ONE: TWENTY-FOUR HOURS AFTER DELIVERY

Kegel exercises. You can resume these exercises immediately after delivery (see page 193 for directions, if you haven't done them before), though you won't be able to feel yourself doing them at first. Kegel exercises can be done in any comfortable position—lying down, standing up, while you're waiting on line at the supermarket, nursing, changing diapers, riding in the car, sitting in the tub, you name it. Work up to twenty-five repetitions four to six times a day and continue for the rest of your life

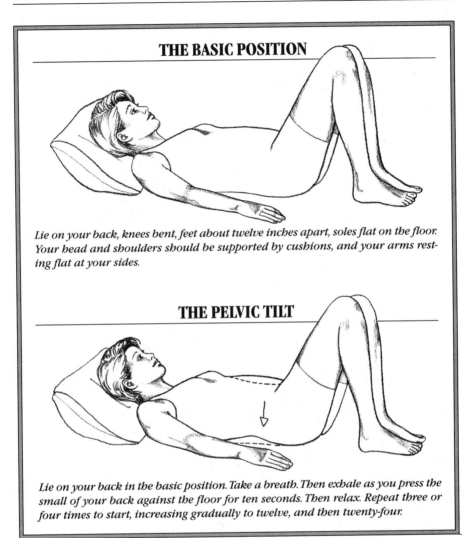

THE BASIC POSITION

Lie on your back, knees bent, feet about twelve inches apart, soles flat on the floor. Your head and shoulders should be supported by cushions, and your arms resting flat at your sides.

THE PELVIC TILT

Lie on your back in the basic position. Take a breath. Then exhale as you press the small of your back against the floor for ten seconds. Then relax. Repeat three or four times to start, increasing gradually to twelve, and then twenty-four.

for good pelvic health (and increased sexual pleasure!).

Deep diaphragmatic breathing. In the Basic Position (see box, above), place your hands on your abdomen so you can feel it rise as you inhale slowly through your nose; tighten the abdominal muscles as you exhale slowly through your mouth. Start with just two or three deep breaths at a time, to prevent hyperventilating. (Signs that you've overdone it are dizziness or faintness, tingling, or blurred vision.)

PHASE TWO: THREE DAYS AFTER DELIVERY

Three days after you deliver, you can move up another rung on the workout ladder and begin doing more strenuous exercises. But before you take that step, you should make sure that the pair of vertical muscles that form your abdominal wall have not separated during pregnancy. Fairly common, especially in women who have had several children,

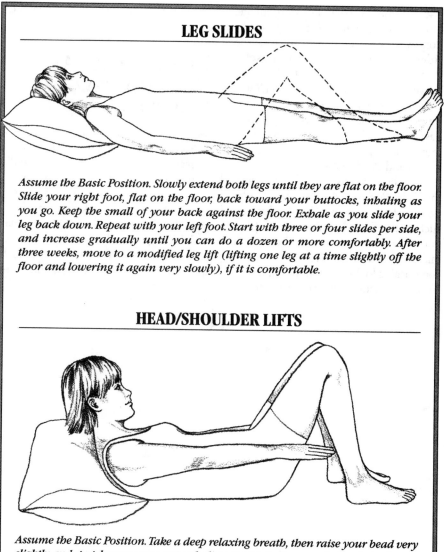

LEG SLIDES

Assume the Basic Position. Slowly extend both legs until they are flat on the floor. Slide your right foot, flat on the floor, back toward your buttocks, inhaling as you go. Keep the small of your back against the floor. Exhale as you slide your leg back down. Repeat with your left foot. Start with three or four slides per side, and increase gradually until you can do a dozen or more comfortably. After three weeks, move to a modified leg lift (lifting one leg at a time slightly off the floor and lowering it again very slowly), if it is comfortable.

HEAD/SHOULDER LIFTS

Assume the Basic Position. Take a deep relaxing breath, then raise your head very slightly and stretch your arms out, exhaling as you do. Lower your head slowly, and inhale. Raise your head a little more each day, gradually working up to lifting your shoulders slightly off the floor. Don't try full sit-ups for the first six weeks—and then only if you have always had very good abdominal muscle tone.

this separation will get worse if you do anything even mildly strenuous before it heals. Ask your nurse or practitioner to check the condition of the abdominal muscles, or examine them yourself this way: as you lie in the basic position, raise your head slightly with your arms extended forward; then feel for a soft lump below your navel. Such a lump indicates a separation.

If you do have a separation, you may be able to help correct it with this exercise: assume the Basic Position; inhale. Now cross your hands over your abdomen, using your fingers to draw the sides of your abdominal muscles together as you breathe out while raising your head slowly. Inhale as you lower your head slowly. Repeat three or four times, twice a day. When the separation has closed, or if you've never had one, move on to Head/Shoulder Lifts, Leg Slides, and Pelvic Tilts.

All these exercises should be done in the Basic Position. At first, they can be done in bed, then on a harder surface, such as the floor. (An exercise mat is a good investment, not only because it makes these exercises easier and more comfortable to do now, but because your baby can practice rolling over and try his or her first tentative crawls on it later on in the year.)

Phase Three: After Your Postpartum Checkup

Now, with your practitioner's permission, you can resume a more active exercise schedule. You can gradually return to, or begin, a program that includes walking, running, bicycling, swimming, water workouts, aerobics, yoga, Pilates, weight training, or similar activities. Or enroll in a postpartum exercise class. But don't try to do too much too soon. As always, let your body be your guide.

◆ ◆ ◆

CHAPTER 17

Fathers Are Expectant, Too

Though it's certainly true—future medical breakthroughs and Hollywood movies notwithstanding—that only women can become pregnant, it's just as true that fathers are expectant, too. Not only are dads-to-be essential members of the baby-making team, but by caring for and supporting their pregnant spouses, they are also invaluable nurturers of the unborn. As an expectant father, you'll participate fully in the process, the excitement, the responsibility—and, of course, the worry—of pregnancy. Some concerns will overlap with those of the expectant mother; others will be uniquely yours. And just like your mate, you're entitled to your share of reassurance, not just during the pregnancy and the birth, but in the postpartum period as well.

And so this chapter—dedicated to the equal, but often neglected, partner-in-reproduction. Keep in mind, however, that the pages that follow aren't intended for your eyes only, any more than the rest of the book is intended only for the mother-to-be. Your spouse can gain some valuable insights into what you're feeling, fearing, and hoping by reading this chapter; you can better understand the physical and emotional challenges she will undergo during pregnancy, childbirth, and postpartum—and at the same time better prepare yourself for your own role in the unfolding drama—by reading the rest of this book.

What You May Be Concerned About

FEELING LEFT OUT

"So much attention has been focused on my wife since she became pregnant that I hardly feel I have anything to do with the pregnancy—beyond taking part in conception."

In generations past, a male's involvement in the reproductive process

GET READY, GET SET . . . THEN GO

Giving your baby the best start in life can start even before sperm meets egg. If your partner isn't yet pregnant, you both have time to get yourselves into optimal baby-making shape first. Read Chapter 21, and follow all the suggestions for the pre-conception period. If you're already expecting, don't worry about what you haven't done—just start taking good care of yourselves and each other now.

ended once his sperm had fertilized his partner's ovum. Fathers-to-be watched pregnancy from afar, and childbirth not at all.

Great strides have undeniably been made in the past few decades for fathers' rights. Today's father doesn't just watch pregnancy and childbirth, he participates in them. Still, social reeducation can't change the fact that pregnancy takes place within a woman's body. Or the fact that some fathers are lost in what is still largely considered a woman's shuffle and end up feeling forgotten, left out, and even jealous of their wives.

Sometimes the woman is unwittingly responsible, sometimes the man is. And, of course, sometimes both contribute to this problem. Either way, it's vital that the father's feelings are resolved before resentment grows and is allowed to spoil what should be one of the most wonderful experiences of *both* parents' lives. The best way to accomplish this is for you to get involved in as many aspects of your wife's pregnancy as you can.

Talk it out. Your spouse may be leaving you out unintentionally; she may not even be aware that you'd like to be more involved. It's very likely that she'd be as

happy to include you in the pregnancy proceedings as you would be to be included in them. Airing your feelings is likely to have an added benefit: improved communication during a time in your relationship when such sharing becomes more important than ever.

See an obstetrician (or nurse-midwife)—as often as your partner does, if possible. Virtually all practitioners encourage fathers to attend prenatal checkups. If your schedule won't permit a monthly visit, perhaps you can arrange to come along for the landmark appointments (when the heartbeat is expected to be heard for the first time, for instance) and prenatal tests (including the ultrasound, when you'll actually see an image of the baby).

Act pregnant. You don't have to show up for work in maternity clothes or start sporting a milk mustache. But you can do your partner's pregnancy exercise routine with her; cut back on junk food for nine months (at least when you're around her); quit smoking, if you're a smoker. And when someone offers you a drink, you can join her in a sparkling water.

Get an education. Even dads with advanced degrees (including some with MDs) have a lot to learn when it comes to pregnancy and childbirth. Read as many books and articles as you can. Attend childbirth classes together; attend classes for fathers, if they are available locally. Chat up friends and colleagues who've become new fathers recently or chat with other pregnant dads online.

Make contact with your baby. A pregnant woman may have the edge in bonding with the unborn baby because it's comfortably ensconced in her uterus, but that doesn't mean that you can't start getting to know the new family member, too. Talk, read, sing to your baby frequently; a fetus can hear voices from about the end of the sixth month on, and hearing yours often now will help your newborn recognize it after delivery. Enjoy baby's kicks and squirms by resting your hand or your cheek on your wife's naked abdomen for a few minutes each night—it's a nice way to share intimacy with her, too.

Shop for a layette. And a crib, and a stroller—with your partner. Decorate the nursery together. Buy and scan baby name books. Attend consultations with prospective baby doctors. In general, become active in every aspect of planning and preparing for the baby's arrival.

CHANGES IN ATTITUDES TOWARD SEX

"Now that we're pregnant, I just don't seem very interested in sex. Is this normal?"

Expectant fathers, like expectant mothers, can experience a wide range of reactions when it comes to interest in sex during pregnancy—all of them "normal." And there are plenty of good reasons why your sex drive may be in a slump now. Perhaps you and your spouse worked so conscientiously at conception that sex suddenly feels too much like hard work. Maybe you're so focused on the baby and on becoming a father that your sexual side is taking a backseat. Or the changes in your spouse's body are taking some getting used to (especially because they're an ever-present reminder of how your life and relationship are also changing). Or fear that you'll hurt your wife or your baby during sex (you won't) has sent your libido into hiding.

Just as normal can be sexual apathy on your pregnant partner's part—for all the same reasons. Compounding these for her may be some physical factors: nausea, urinary frequency, fatigue, and painfully tender breasts don't only hamper desire but overpower the potential for pleasure.

Confusing these conflicted feelings even more could be miscommunication between partners: he thinks she's not interested, so he subconsciously puts his urges on ice. She thinks he's not interested, so she douses her own desires.

The frequency of sexual intercourse is far less important right now than the quality of your intimacy. You may actually find that increased intimacy of other kinds—cuddling with and confiding in each other, for example—can lead to increased sexual activity. Though a sexual slowdown is fine—and temporary (though frequency may not be what it once was, at least until baby's sleeping through the night)—try not to let the nurturing of your baby interfere with the care and feeding of your relationship. Make romance a priority (surprise her with flowers, light candles at dinner, bring massage oil to bed), open up those lines of communication (don't hesitate to share your feelings and fears, and encourage her to share hers), and keep the hugs and kisses coming (and coming . . . and coming . . .), and your passions will live to ignite again.

For more tips on enjoying sex more when you're doing it less, see Making Love During Pregnancy, page 233.

A PARTNER IN PARENTING BY ANY NAME

Most of the tips in this chapter also apply to the partner in a nontraditional family. Pick and choose questions and answers that fit your situation or can be applied to it.

"I find my wife incredibly sexy now. But she hasn't been in the mood since the day we found out we were pregnant."

Even couples who have always been in sexual sync can find themselves suddenly out of step in bed once they're expecting. That's because so many factors, both physical and emotional, can affect sexual desire, pleasure, and performance during pregnancy. It may be as simple as your liking what you see; many men find the roundness and fullness of the pregnant form surprisingly sensual, even erotic. Your more powerful lust may also be fueled by affection; the fact that you're expecting a baby together may have deepened your already strong feelings for your wife, arousing even greater passions.

But just as your increased sexual interest is both understandable and normal, so is her decreased interest. It could be that pregnancy symptoms, particularly nausea, vomiting, and lack of energy, have leveled her libido. Or that she's as turned off by her new roundness as you are turned on by it. Or that she's preoccupied with all things baby, and/or having a hard time blending the roles of mother and lover.

RESOURCES FOR DADS

Expectant fathers are just as hungry for reassurance, support, information, and empathy as expectant mothers. Here are some places you can turn to, both during pregnancy and once you're a full-fledged dad:

Fathering Magazine:
www.fathermag.com

Fathering Forum Online:
www.fathersforum.com

Boot Camp for New Dads:
www.dadsworld.com

Whatever's causing your current sexual incompatibility, don't worry—it's likely only temporary. Most women find that slacked-off sexual interest picks up again in the second trimester, thanks to increased blood flow to their sexual organs and breasts. Even if it doesn't, or if it drops off again in the third trimester (because of an increase in fatigue or in back pain or because of that growing watermelon tummy) or in the postpartum period (which it almost certainly will for both of you), nurturing the nonsexual aspects of your relationship in the interim will ensure that you'll eventually be able to pick up where you left off sexually.

In the meantime, don't push your sexual agenda, but do increase the romance, communication, and cuddling. Not only will these bring you closer together, but, because they're powerful aphrodisiacs for women, they may just bring you what you're craving. When one thing does lead to another, make sure you spend plenty of time warming her up with foreplay before you start your own engine. And be sure to ask what feels good and what doesn't, since the roadmap is sure to have changed since conception. It may also help to try to find positions that make intercourse more comfortable for both of you. When intercourse isn't on the calendar, consider alternate forms of "pleasuring," such as masturbation, oral sex, and massage.

And don't forget to tell your partner—often—how sexy and attractive you find the pregnant her. Women may be intuitive, but they're not mind readers.

SAFETY OF SEX IN PREGNANCY

"Even though the doctor has assured us that sex is safe throughout pregnancy, I often have trouble following through for fear of hurting my wife or the baby."

Never is sex more a mind-over-matter situation—for both partners—than during pregnancy. This is true particularly as gestation advances and the mind (and libido) must confront a very sizable matter: the expanding pregnant belly and its precious contents.

Fortunately, you can put your mind to rest. As vulnerable as mother and baby may seem to an anxious father contemplating intercourse, in a normally progressing low-risk pregnancy, neither one is. (There are a few caveats, particularly in the last two months, detailed in Making Love During Pregnancy, page 233.)

Orgasm (with or without intercourse) may stimulate contractions, but not the kind that triggers premature labor in a normal pregnancy. In fact, research shows that low-risk women who stay sexually active during pregnancy actually are less likely to deliver preterm (finally—some good news!). And not only can making love to your wife not do her any harm (assuming the caveats are observed), but it can do her a world of good by filling her increased needs for physical and emotional closeness, and letting her know that she's desired at a time when she may be feeling less than desirable.

As for your baby, he or she is well cushioned and protected by fluid and muscle in a snug uterine home sealed off by the cervical mucous plug (which effectively prevents bacteria and semen from entering).[1] Oblivious to the proceedings, your baby can't see you having sex and certainly will have no memory of it. If anything, he or she will be pacified by the gentle rocking motion of intercourse and of the contracting uterus during orgasm.

---

1. However, if deep penetration causes pain, it should be avoided.

PREGNANCY DREAMS

"I've had more dreams about sex lately than I've ever had before, even though sex is the last thing on my mind during the day right now. Why would that be?"

For expectant mothers and fathers, pregnancy is a time of intense feelings, feelings that run the roller coaster from joyful anticipation to panic-struck anxiety and back again. It's not surprising that many of these feelings find their way into dreams, where the subconscious can act them out and work them through safely. Dreams about sex (particularly when it's with a different partner) is your subconscious telling you what you probably already know—that you're worried about how being pregnant and having a baby is affecting and is going to affect your sex life. Not only are such fears normal, they're valid. Acknowledging that your relationship is in for some changes now that baby's making three is the first step in making sure that your twosome stays cozy.

Sexual dreams are most common in early pregnancy. They taper off later on, only to be replaced by dreams about family. You may dream about your parents or grandparents; this is your subconscious way of linking past generations to the future one. You may dream about being a child again yourself, which may express an understandable fear of the responsibilities to come and a longing for the carefree years of the past. You may even dream about being pregnant yourself, which may express sympathy for the load your spouse is carrying, jealousy of the attention she's getting, or just a desire to connect with your unborn baby. Or because you worry deep down that becoming a nurturer may in some way diminish your manliness, you may find yourself dreaming uncharacteristically "macho" dreams—of making a touchdown or driving in the Indianapolis 500, for instance. The flip side of your subconscious may also get equal time (sometimes even in the same night); dreaming about taking care of your wife or of your baby helps the "nurturing you" prepare for your new role. Dreams about loneliness and being left out are extremely common; these speak to those feelings of exclusion experienced by so many expectant fathers.

Not all of your dreams will express anxiety. Some dreams—of being handed or finding a baby, of christenings or baby-naming ceremonies or family strolls through the park—show how excited you are about the imminent arrival.

One thing is for sure: you're not dreaming alone. Expectant mothers (for hormonal reasons) are even more subject to strange and vivid dreams than fathers are. Sharing dreams with each other in the morning can be an intimate and therapeutic ritual, as long as both of you understand that the dreams represent subconscious feelings, not reality.

IMPATIENCE WITH YOUR WIFE'S MOOD SWINGS

"I know it's not her fault that my wife's hormonal changes are making her so weepy and volatile. But I don't know how much longer I can be patient."

If patience is a virtue, you'll have to be very virtuous for the rest of this pregnancy. Although the stabilization of hormone levels by the fourth month eases the pronounced premenstrual-like weepiness and moodiness of early pregnancy, the stresses of being pregnant continue. And many women continue to be subject to sudden bursts of emotion and feelings of vulnerability right up to—and during—delivery. It doubtless won't

be easy, and at times you may find it close to impossible. But there's also little doubt that your efforts will pay off. Touchiness met with understanding will dissipate faster than touchiness met with anger and frustration; a shoulder offered to your wife for a fifteen-minute cry won't have to carry around the weight of her unvented angst for days at a time.

Also try to keep in mind that pregnancy is *not* a permanent condition, and that the changes in your wife's emotional status are as transient as the changes in her figure.

MOODINESS— HIS AND HERS

"Ever since we got the positive pregnancy test, my wife and I seem to be going through opposite mood swings. When she's feeling good, I'm feeling down, and vice versa."

More attention has been focused on the "pregnant" father recently as studies have shown that he can experience many of the prenatal symptoms that are common in pregnant women. In fact, one recent study showed that men's hormone concentrations shift significantly throughout the course of their wives' pregnancies and after the baby is born. Depression is one of those symptoms men also experience. Although in about 1 in 10 cases both parents succumb simultaneously to depression, most often the depression occurs in just one partner at a time. This may be because signs of depression in a loved one can summon up the inner strength needed to rise above your own feelings and become supportive. As soon as your loved one's mood has picked up, you let yourself drop down.

The best way to banish mild pregnancy depression—which is common among expectant fathers and likely to be self-limiting—is to vent. Talk your feelings over with your wife (open communications will benefit both your moods, so make a point of sharing daily), with a friend who recently became a father, or even with your own father. Avoid alcohol and other drugs, which can aggravate depression and mood swings. Stay busy (prepare for the baby both mentally and practically by participating in shopping, painting the nursery, arranging your finances). Keeping physically active and getting those endorphins flowing will also help. The couple that exercises together (with the practitioner's okay, of course) generally stays happier together. Even a nightly walk before or after dinner can help.

You can also try some of the other tips recommended for mothers experiencing prenatal depression, including relaxation techniques (see page 127). If nothing works, and your depression deepens and begins to interfere with your work and other aspects of your life, then seek professional help from your physician, a therapist, a psychiatrist, or a member of the clergy.

Be aware, too, that *postpartum* depression can also afflict dads; see page 446 for more.

SYMPATHY SYMPTOMS

"It's my wife who's pregnant, so why am I having morning sickness?"

Women may have a corner on the pregnancy market, but not on pregnancy symptoms. As many as half, or even more (depending on the study), of expectant fathers suffer from some degree of couvade syndrome or "sympathetic pregnancy" during their wives' gestation. The symptoms of couvade (which comes from the French "to hatch") most often appear in the third month and again at delivery, and can mimic virtually all the normal symptoms of pregnancy—including nausea and vomiting, abdominal pain, appetite changes, weight gain, food cravings, constipation, leg cramps, dizziness, fatigue, and mood swings.

Many theories have been suggested to explain couvade—all, some, or none of which may be appropriate to you: sympathy for and identification with the pregnant wife; jealousy over being left out, and a resultant desire for attention; stress from living with a woman who's become irritable, moody, and possibly off-limits sexually; guilt over being responsible for putting your wife in such an uncomfortable situation; or anxiety over the impending addition to the family. Some men seem to have an increase in female hormones during this time (and after the birth of the baby as well), which may also explain the symptoms—and which may be nature's way of bringing the nurturer out in the male.

Since your symptoms could also indicate illness, it's a good idea to check with a doctor. But if an examination uncovers no physical problem, couvade is a likely diagnosis. The underlying cause, if you can identify it, may offer a clue to the cure. For instance, if it's sympathy that's making you queasy, finding other ways of expressing your concern—bringing your spouse breakfast in bed, doing the shopping and vacuuming while she gets some extra rest—may bring you both relief. If the trigger is jealousy, becoming more involved in your wife's pregnancy may relieve your symptoms. Or if it's anxiety over handling a newborn for the first time, taking a course in infant care, reading a copy of *What to Expect the First Year,* or spending some time with a friend's baby might prove helpful.

Even if you can't put your finger on any one cause for your symptoms, talking out your feelings about pregnancy, childbirth, and parenthood with your wife may alleviate your sympathy pains. So might discussing them with other expectant or new parents. Should none of this help, be assured that your reactions are normal, and that all symptoms that don't go away during pregnancy will disappear soon after delivery.

Equally normal, of course, is the father who doesn't have a sick day during his wife's pregnancy. Not suffering from morning sickness or not putting on weight doesn't mean an expectant father doesn't empathize and identify with his wife, just that he's found other ways to express his feelings.

ANXIETY OVER YOUR WIFE'S HEALTH

"I know pregnancy and childbirth are safer today than ever in history, yet I still can't stop worrying that something will happen to my wife."

There's something undeniably vulnerable about a pregnant woman, and something very natural about your desire, as a loving husband, to want to protect your wife from any possible harm. But you can relax—she is in virtually no danger. Women in developed countries very, very rarely die as a result of pregnancy or childbirth anymore—and the vast majority of the very few who do haven't had the benefits of prenatal care or adequate nourishment.

But just because the risks are minimal doesn't mean you can't help her reduce them even further and help make pregnancy a safer and more comfortable experience by making sure she gets the best medical care possible and that she eats the best possible diet (see Chapter 4); exercising with her (with the approval of her practitioner); letting her get extra

rest while you do the laundry, make dinner, or clean the house; and by giving her the kind of emotional support she can't get from anyone else. (No matter how far obstetrical science advances, pregnant women will always be *emotionally* vulnerable.)

Being well informed about pregnancy (by reading this book and anything else you can get your hands on) will also help you feel more confident and comfortable—which will greatly reduce your level of anxiety.

ANXIETY OVER THE BABY'S HEALTH

"I'm so afraid that something will be wrong with the baby, I can't even sleep at night."

Mothers-to-be by no means have a monopoly on worry. Like almost every expectant mother, virtually every expectant father worries about his unborn baby's health and well-being. Happily, nearly all such worry is needless. The chances that your baby will be born both alive and completely well are overwhelming—far better than ever before.

Happily, too, you don't have to just sit back and hope for the best. You can actually take some steps to help ensure your baby's good health:

♦ Be sure your wife gets good medical care right from the start; be sure she keeps all her prenatal appointments and follows her practitioner's advice. Ideally, attend appointments with her and take notes for her on what is discussed. Speak up, if either of you has any specific concerns.

♦ Since both physical and emotional stress can affect pregnancy, reduce these in her life as much as possible.

Help around the house, take over some of the chores that have traditionally been hers, encourage her to reduce her workload if her life is too frenetic. If your social calendar is usually filled to overflowing, see that it's cut back and that more evenings are spent at home relaxing. If they work for both of you, try doing some relaxation exercises (see page 127) together.

♦ Encourage her to eat well. If you make nutrition a priority yourself—cutting down on the junk food you eat, taking seconds on salad, munching fruit for a snack—she'll have a much easier time feeding herself and the baby well. But remember, there's a fine line between encouraging and nagging; for best results, don't cross it.

♦ If she's having trouble giving up alcohol, drugs, or tobacco, help her. Research shows you can be most convincing if you abstain yourself, at least when you're with her. So sip club soda with her at parties, forgo wine with dinner, and if you're smokers, quit together. (Not using tobacco in front of her can directly impact your baby's chances of being born healthy, since secondhand smoke is linked to pregnancy problems.)

♦ Share your fears with your wife, and let her share hers with you. This will serve to unburden you both, or at least make your burden of worries easier to carry.

Of course, even the most reassuring statistics and the best preventive measures probably won't be able to banish all your worries; only the birth of a healthy baby will do that. But knowing how overwhelmingly good the odds are, and that you're doing all you can

to contribute to that important end, will make the waiting—and the sleeping—a little easier.

ANXIETY OVER LIFE CHANGES

"Ever since I saw him on ultrasound, I've been looking forward to our son's birth. But I've also been worrying about what kind of father I will be—and whether I'll like being a father."

You and probably every first-time father-to-be in history. At least as much, and possibly even more, than the expectant mother, the expectant father worries about impending parenthood and about the effect it will have on his life. The most common worries include:

Will I be a good father? Few men are born "good" fathers (or women good mothers, for that matter). They learn to meet the challenge in time through on-the-job training, persistence, and love. But if you feel you'll be more comfortable with the tasks at hand if you're formally prepared, by all means take a parenting class to learn how to diaper, bathe, feed, hold, dress, and play with your baby. Classes are proliferating across the country, but if a class isn't available in your area, or if you have an endless appetite for such preparation, start reading *What to Expect the First Year* now. If you have friends who have recently arrived infants, turn to them for some hands-on instruction. Ask them to let you hold, diaper, and play with their babies.

Will our husband-wife relationship change? Every set of new parents finds that their relationship undergoes some change after childbirth. Anticipating this change during pregnancy is an important first step in dealing with it postpartum. No longer will being alone together be as simple as closing the blinds and taking the phone off the hook; from the moment baby comes home from the hospital, spontaneous intimacy and complete privacy will be precious, and often unattainable, commodities. Romance may have to be planned (for the hour Grandpa's taken baby to the park, for instance) rather than spur of the moment, and interruptions may be the rule (you can't take a baby off the hook). But as long as you both take the trouble to make time for each other—whether that means skipping your favorite television show so that you can share a late dinner after baby's in bed, or giving up Saturday golf with the guys so you can make love during baby's morning nap—your relationship will weather the changes well. Many couples, in fact, find that becoming a threesome ultimately deepens, strengthens, and improves their twosome.

How will we divide the child care? This wasn't an issue for fathers a generation or two ago, when child care was widely considered woman's work. But most of today's fathers are aware that parenting is a two-person job (at least when there are two parents), although they're not exactly sure what the division of labor should be. Don't wait until baby needs his first midnight diaper change or his first bath to decide this question. Start divvying up duties now. Some details of your plan may change once you really start operating as parents (she had signed up for baths, but you turn out to be the better bather), but exploring the options in theory now will make you feel more confident about how baby care is going to work in practice later.

Can I continue my work schedule and still be a good father? That depends on your work schedule. If you currently work long hours with little time off, you may need to make some serious changes in order to make fatherhood the priority

in your life that it should be. And don't wait until you officially become a father. Take time off now for doctor's visits, as well as to help your exhausted spouse with baby preparations. Start weaning yourself off those work-until-midnight days and resist the temptation to continue your day at the office at home. Avoid trips and a heavy workload during the two months before and after your baby's E.T.A. And if it's at all possible, consider taking a leave of absence in the early weeks of baby's life.

Will we have to give up our social lives? You probably won't have to toss out your social calendar after baby is born, but you should expect to trim it down quite a bit. A new baby does, and should, take center stage, pushing some old lifestyle habits at least temporarily aside. Parties, movies, and shows may be tricky to fit in between feedings; cozy dinners for two in your favorite bistro may become noisy meals for three in "family" restaurants that tolerate squirming infants. Your circle of friends may change, too; you may suddenly find yourself gravitating toward fellow stroller-pushers for empathetic companionship. Try thinking of life with baby as a new world to explore—with some room for the best parts of your old life as well as plenty of uncharted pleasures still to discover.

Can I afford a larger family? Especially today, when child-rearing costs are going through the roof (as are the costs of maintaining or enlarging that roof), many fathers-to-be lose sleep over this very legitimate question. But once the baby comes, they often find that the alteration of priorities makes available the money that's needed for the newborn. Opting for breastfeeding over bottle-feeding, accepting all hand-me-downs that are offered (new clothes start to look like hand-me-downs after a few spitting-up episodes, anyway), letting

BEING THERE

The very best way to start off your new life as a father is at home with your spouse and baby. So if it's possible and financially feasible, do consider taking off as much time as you can right after delivery—either through the Family and Medical Leave Act (which allows for twelve weeks unpaid leave for mothers and fathers; see page 111), the policy at your company (ask ahead of time what it is), or by taking a chunk of vacation time (the beach will be there next year, but your baby will be a newborn only once). Or, if that's impossible (or not your preference), try to arrange to work part-time for a few weeks, or do some work from home.

Should none of these possibilities prove practical, and your job duties call, make the most of your time. Make sure you're home as much as you can be; learn to say no to long hours, early or late meetings, and business trips that can be put off until another time. Especially in the postpartum period, when the new mom is still recovering from labor and delivery, try to do more than your share of household chores and baby care whenever you're home. Keep in mind that no matter how physically or emotionally stressful your occupation, there is no more demanding job than being a full-time parent.

While you should make bonding with your child a priority, don't forget to devote some time to nurturing your spouse as well. Pamper her when you're home, and let her know you're thinking of her when you're at work. Call her with messages of support and empathy (and so she can complain as much as she needs to); surprise her with flowers or takeout from a favorite restaurant.

---

friends and family know which gifts you really need rather than allowing them to fill baby's shelves with silver spoons and other dust gatherers can all help reduce the cost of caring for the new arrival. If either the mom or you is planning to take extra time off from work (or to put career plans on hold during baby's formative years) and this concerns you from a financial standpoint, recognize that weighed against the costs of quality child care, refurbishing a business wardrobe, and commuting, the amount of income lost may really be minimal.

FALLING APART DURING LABOR

"I'm not sure I can handle watching the labor. I'm afraid I'll fall apart."

Few fathers enter the birthing room without fear. Even obstetricians who've assisted at births of thousands of other people's babies can experience a sudden loss of self-confidence when confronted with their own baby's delivery.

Yet very few of these fears—of freezing, falling apart, fainting, or becoming sick to the stomach while watching the delivery—are ever realized. And though being prepared for the birth (by taking childbirth education classes, for instance) generally makes the experience more satisfying, even most unprepared fathers come through labor and delivery better than they thought they would.

But, like anything new and unfamiliar, childbirth becomes less frightening and intimidating if you know what to expect. So become an expert on the subject. Read the entire chapter on labor and delivery, beginning on page 337. Attend childbirth education classes, watching the labor and delivery films with your eyes wide open. Visit the hospital ahead of time so that you'll be acquainted with the technology that's used in labor and delivery rooms. Talk to friends who have recently become first-time parents. You will probably find they had the same anxieties beforehand but came through feeling terrific.

Though it's important to get an education, it's also important to remember that childbirth isn't the final exam in your childbirth education course. Don't feel that you (or your wife) must perform perfectly at the delivery. Nobody does. Nurses and doctors won't be evaluating your every move or comparing you to the coach next door. More important, neither will your wife. She won't care if you forget every coaching technique you learned in class. Your being beside her, holding her hand, urging her on, and providing the comfort of a familiar face and touch will do her more good than having Dr. Lamaze himself at her bedside.

Some couples find, however, that having a doula present during birth helps them *both* to get through labor and delivery with less stress and discomfort. See page 296 for information on hiring a doula.

"The sight of blood makes me queasy, so I'm worried about being at the delivery."

Most expectant fathers—and mothers—worry about how they'll cope with seeing blood at delivery. But few ever actually end up being aware of the blood, never mind being bothered by it—for a couple of reasons. First of all, there typically isn't very much blood to see. Second, the excitement of watching their baby emerge usually preoccupies parents (as do the efforts of birthing).

If at first glance the blood does bother you, keep your eyes focused on your spouse's face as you coach her through those last pushes. You'll probably want to turn back to the main event for that momentous moment; at that point, blood is going to be the last thing you'll notice.

"My wife is having a planned cesarean. Hospital regulations won't allow me to be there, and I'm afraid that our new family won't get off to the best start."

Don't give up—at least not without a civilized fight. With the support of your wife's obstetrician (if such support is forthcoming), try first to persuade hospital officials to bend—or even change—the regulations. (It may help to remind them that a majority of hospitals allow fathers to be present at nonemergency surgical deliveries.) If your campaign is unsuccessful (or if a hasty delivery precludes your presence), you have every right to be disappointed—but not to let that disappointment take the joy out of the birth of your child. Your not being at the birth can't threaten your relationship with your baby unless you let it, by harboring feelings of guilt, resentment, or frustration.

FATHERING FEARS

"I want to be a good father, but the thought is terrifying. I've never even seen or held a newborn, much less taken care of one."

First of all, keep in mind that not only do most dads-to-be feel the way you do, many moms-to-be do, too. That's because though parental love comes naturally, parental skills must be learned. And learning the basic child care techniques in advance—diapering, bathing, holding, burping, soothing, first aid—will definitely make you feel more competent and confident.

Fortunately, classes for expectant and new fathers that teach these important skills are finding their way into communities across the country. There are "boot camps" for new dads and other preparatory classes in many hospitals and community centers. Ask about them at the next prenatal appointment, check into them at the hospital or birthing center you'll be delivering at, or do some research on-line. If there are no formal classes available locally, ask the hospital staff if you can observe and learn from their baby care techniques.

And remember, too, that just as mothers have different parenting techniques, so do dads. Relax, trust your instincts (surprise . . . fathers have them, too!), and feel free to find the style that works for both you and your baby. Before you know it, you'll be fathering with the best of them.

THE GRANDPARENT ISSUE

"My wife and I keep debating whether or not we should have her parents stay with us after the baby's born. They just want to be helpful, but I'm not sure their being around will be."

Having the support and advice of those older and wiser (or at least more experienced) to guide you through those early days with baby sounds like a good idea. And, in fact, having your parents around to show you the ropes of parenting—and the finer points of diapering and bathing newborns—does have its benefits, especially if they're also willing to cook and clean.

However, the arrangement can also have its drawbacks. First of all, three generations can be a crowd—a crowd that can interfere with what should be an intimate bonding experience between parents and baby. Too much support and advice from well-intentioned grandparents can also prevent you from finding your own parental way. And though their help might keep you from making mistakes, it'll also keep you from learning from those mistakes, an important step in building your confidence as a parent. (Of course, if their advice is outdated, which it's likely to be, it might actually lead you to make some mistakes—such as putting a newborn on a feeding "schedule" or down to sleep on his or her stomach.) Another potential problem: having houseguests can add to postpartum exhaustion, especially for the newly delivered mother. Even if they're thoughtful guests (i.e., the kind that clean up messes, rather than making them), you and your wife may feel compelled to entertain them, which can be draining at a time when you'll already be drained.

A good compromise for long-distance grandparents might be for you to wait a few weeks before inviting them to make that first visit. By that time the two of you will be feeling more comfortable in your new roles, your wife will have recovered from many of her postpartum symptoms, and, as a bonus for those who crave a good coo and some good photos, the baby will be more alert and responsive to company and cameras.

If the grandparents are local, you can suggest that they come by for short, scheduled visits—long enough to get their baby fix (and even to let the two of you slip out for a quick walk or bite or even a movie) but not so long or so frequent that they crowd your threesome or cramp your fledgling parenting style.

Be firm but loving as you put a positive spin on the visitation limitations ("We hope to be as good at this parenting thing as you, but to do that, we'll need to figure things out for ourselves"), and your parents are bound to understand why they need to give the three of you some time and space to get to know each other.

For those couples who feel overwhelmed and who really need some help in the early days—with housework, laundry, cooking, or an older child—and are comfortable having their parents around, that's fine, too. But help should be mostly confined to these chores, rather than to new baby care.

EXCLUSION DURING BREASTFEEDING

"My wife is thinking about breastfeeding our new baby, but I'm not sure I can handle it."

For a newborn, there is no more perfect food than breast milk and no more perfect food delivery system than a breast. As long and as hard as formula companies formulate, chances are they'll never be able to duplicate Mother Nature's time-honored recipe. Breastfeeding offers an overwhelming number of health benefits for a baby (from preventing allergies, obesity, and illness to promoting brain development) and for its mother (nursing is linked to a speedier recovery postpartum and possibly a reduced risk of breast cancer later on in life).

Clearly, your wife's decision to choose the breast over the bottle can make a dramatic difference in your child's life—and in hers. And you can help make that difference. Studies show that when fathers are supportive of breastfeeding, moms are much more likely to succeed at it.

Talking to other fathers whose wives have breastfed may help you feel more comfortable with the idea; reading more about breastfeeding (see page 308) will reinforce its importance. Keeping in mind that it is a natural process, one that has sustained young lives since the first mother nursed the first baby, may also help. If you're having trouble coming to terms with your wife's breasts being used for such a practical purpose, see page 447.

"My wife is breastfeeding our son. There's a closeness between them that I can't seem to share, and I feel left out."

There are certain immutable biological aspects of parenting that exclude the father: he can't be pregnant, he can't labor and deliver, and he can't breastfeed. But, as millions of new fathers discover each year, a man's natural physical limitations don't have to relegate him to spectator status. You can share in nearly all the joys, expectations, trials, and tribulations of your wife's pregnancy, labor, and delivery—from the first kick to the last push—as an active, supportive participant. And though you'll never be able to put your baby to the breast (at least not with the kind of results the baby's looking for), you *can* share in the feeding process:

Be your baby's supplementary feeder. Once breastfeeding is established, there's more than one way to feed a baby. And though you can't nurse, you can be the one to give any supplementary bottles. Not only will your being the supplementary feeder give your wife a break (whether in the middle of the night or in the middle of dinner), it will give you extra opportunities for closeness with your baby. Don't waste the opportunity by propping the bottle up to the baby's mouth. Strike a nursing position, with the bottle where your wife's breast would be and your baby snuggled close to you. Opening up your shirt, which allows for skin-to-skin contact, will enhance the experience for both of you.

Don't sleep through the night until your baby does. Sharing in the joys of feeding also means sharing in the sleepless nights. Even if you're not giving supplementary bottles, you can become a part of night-time feeding rituals. You can be the one to take the baby out of the crib, do any necessary diaper changing, deliver him to your wife for his feeding, and return him to bed once he has fallen asleep again.

Watch in wonder, and appreciate. There can be enormous satisfaction in simply watching the miracle of breast-feeding, as there is in watching the miracle of birth. Instead of feeling left out, feel privileged to be a witness to the love that passes between your wife and your baby as they nurse.

Participate in all other daily rituals. Nursing is the *only* daily chore limited to mothers. Dads can bathe, diaper, and rock with the best of moms, given the chance. And chances are that if you make as many other chores as possible your responsibility, you'll be too busy to be jealous.

BONDING

"I'm so excited about my new daughter that I'm afraid I'm almost overdoing the attention."

Some things in life you can overdo—but not loving and caring for your baby. Not only do infants thrive on attention from their fathers, there is no better way to cement your relationship with your new offspring. All the time you're spending with the baby will also help your spouse bond better with the baby (a mother who carries the load of baby care alone may find herself too exhausted and resentful to bond well).

And if you're surprised by your enthusiasm for your daughter, don't be. Recent studies have found that males in both the human and animal kingdoms experience a surge in female hormones when their babies arrive. Nurturing, long thought the province of mothers, apparently comes naturally to dads, too.

As you're busy nurturing your newborn, however, don't forget that there's another relationship that needs attention (and that's ultimately even more significant): the one with your spouse. Make sure she knows how much you care about her, too. And make sure that she gets her share of cuddles.

"My wife had a last-minute cesarean, and I wasn't allowed to be with her. I didn't hold the baby for twenty-four hours, and I'm afraid I didn't bond with him."

Until the 1960s, few fathers ever witnessed the birth of their children, and since the word *bonding* originated only in the 1970s, none knew what they were missing—or even that there was anything to miss—in that department. But such a lack of enlightenment didn't prevent generations of loving father-child relationships from developing. Conversely, every father from this era who attends his child's birth and is allowed to "bond" with him or her immediately afterward isn't instantly cementing a lifetime of closeness. Bonding, for all its benefits, doesn't perform like Super Glue; the kind of relationship that lasts a lifetime takes time and effort to nurture and grow. Being with your wife during delivery is ideal. And being deprived of that opportunity is reason for disappointment, particularly if you spent months preparing for childbirth. But it's no reason to fear for your future with your son. What will really bond you with your baby is caring for him now—changing diapers, giving baths, feeding, cuddling, lullabying, and rocking. Making eye contact and skin contact (open your shirt and hold him against your chest as you sing him to sleep) as you carry this out can enhance the closeness and tighten the bond. (This kind of contact will also, according to research, speed his brain development—so it's good for both of you.)

If you find that your wife is monopolizing the baby care (she may do this without even being aware that she's doing it), let her know that you'd like to take on at least your share. Volunteering to spend time alone with the baby whenever possible—while your wife takes an exercise class, meets a friend for coffee, or just soaks in a tub with a good book—will guarantee that maternal good intentions won't interfere with you and your son getting to know each other. And don't feel you have to spend your quality time with your son at home. Newborns are highly portable, so feel free to pack a diaper bag, strap him into a stroller, car seat, or baby sling, and take a stroll or run an errand with baby in tow.

And don't let regret or guilt spoil your baby's first months. Instead, start taking advantage of the lifetime of fathering that lies ahead. Not having been there for the moment of your son's birth won't ever have an impact on him—but not being there from now on could.

YOUR BABY BLUES

"I'm so happy to be a father, and I'm thrilled to have a daughter. So why do I feel so down?"

Just as expectant fathers aren't immune to pregnancy mood slumps, new fathers aren't immune to postpartum variety blues. Many of the triggers for baby blues in moms apply to dads, too, at least in a modified form—from feeling overwhelmed and underprepared, to being endlessly exhausted, to concern over shifting family dynamics and lifestyle adjustments. Even hormones play a role for many men; it has been shown that surges in female hormones before and after birth can generate a variety of symptoms in fathers—including depression. Not surprisingly, many of the same tips that can help pull a new mother out of a postpartum slump can also help a new father. Especially helpful are exercise (the endorphins released in a workout are nature's finest mood elevators) and communication (talking your feelings out with your partner, as well as with other fathers who know how you feel). So, typically, is the passage of time (the more comfortable you begin to feel with your new life, the happier you'll be with it). See pages 411–416 for more.

In many cases, new mothers and fathers don't suffer from baby blues concurrently; more often, they take turns feeling down. Either way, taking depression-fighting steps together can help you both feel better, while helping to prevent future blues attacks.

If blues persist, or depression deepens, especially if it interferes with your work, your relationship with your baby or your spouse, or your sleeping or eating, be sure to seek professional help.

FEELING UNSEXY AFTER DELIVERY

"The delivery was absolutely miraculous to watch. But seeing our little girl come out of my wife's vagina seems to have turned me off sexually."

Human sexual response, compared to that of other animals, is extremely delicate. It's at the mercy not only of the body but of the mind as well. And the mind can, at times, play merciless havoc with it. One of those times, as you probably already know, is during pregnancy. Another, as you're discovering, is during the postpartum period.

It's very possible that the cause of your sudden sexual ambivalence has nothing to do with having seen your baby delivered. Most brand-new fathers find both the spirit and the flesh somewhat less willing after delivery (although there's nothing abnormal about those who don't) for many very understandable reasons: fatigue, especially if the baby still isn't sleeping through the night; fear that she will awake crying at the first caress (particularly if she is sharing your room); concern that you may hurt your wife by having intercourse before her body is thoroughly healed; and, finally, a general physical and mental preoccupation with your newborn, which sensibly concentrates your energies where they are most needed at this stage of your lives. Your feelings may also be influenced by the temporary increase in female hormones that many new fathers experience—since it's the male hormones, in both women and men, that spark desire.

In other words, it's probably just as well that you aren't feeling sexually motivated, particularly if your wife (like many women in the immediate postpartum period) isn't feeling emotionally or physically up to it, either. Just how long it will take for your interest, and hers, to return is impossible to predict. As with all matters sexual, there is a wide range of what is "normal." For some couples, desire will precede even the practitioner's go-ahead—which, depending on the circumstances, may be anywhere from two to six weeks. For others, six months can pass before *l'amour* and *le bébé* begin to coexist harmoniously in the same home. (Some women find desire somewhat lacking until they stop breastfeeding, but that doesn't mean they can't enjoy the intimacy of intercourse.)

Some fathers, even if they've been prepared for the childbirth experience, do come out of it feeling that their "territory" has been "violated"—that the

special place meant for loving has suddenly taken on a practical purpose. But as the days pass, that feeling usually does, too. The father begins to realize that the vagina has two functions, equally important and miraculous. Neither excludes the other, and, in fact, they are very much interconnected. He also comes to recognize that the vagina is a vehicle for childbirth only briefly, while it is a source of pleasure for himself and his wife for a lifetime.

If the sexual urge doesn't return and its absence begins to cause tension, professional counseling is probably needed.

"Before the baby, my wife's breasts were a focus of sexual pleasure—for both of us. Now that she's breastfeeding, they seem too functional to be sexy."

Like the vagina, breasts were designed to serve both a practical and a sexual purpose (which, from a strictly procreative standpoint, is also practical). And though these purposes aren't mutually exclusive in the long run, they can conflict temporarily during lactation.

Some couples find breastfeeding a sexual turn-on, especially if breasts are full for the first time. Others, for esthetic reasons (leaking milk, for instance) or because they feel uncomfortable about using the baby's source of nourishment for their sexual pleasure, find it a very definite turn-off. They may find this effect wears off, however, as breastfeeding becomes more second nature for all concerned.

Whatever turns you on—or off—is what is normal for you. If you feel that your wife's breasts are too functional to be sexy now, focus foreplay elsewhere until you've become more comfortable sharing them with baby (or until baby has been weaned). Be sure, however, to be open and honest with your wife; taking a sudden, unexplained hands-off approach to her breasts could leave her feeling unappealing. Be careful, also, not to harbor any resentment against the baby for using "your" breasts; try to think of nursing as a temporary "loan" instead. And enjoy the "interest" that comes with the loan— a healthy, well-fed newborn.

NEW DADS AND HORMONES

Think just because you're a guy you're immune to the hormonal swings usually reserved for the female of the species? Think again. Researchers have found that expectant and new dads experience a drop in their testosterone levels and an increase in the hormone estradiol—a female sex hormone. Experts believe that the shift in hormones infuses an extra dose of tenderness in a new father that helps in parenting. It may also keep dad's libido in check (a good thing, since a raging sex drive can be inconvenient—to say the least—when there's a new baby in the house). Hormone levels typically return to normal within three to six months, bringing with them a return to libido business as usual (though not necessarily to sex life as usual until baby's sleeping through the night).

◆ ◆ ◆

Part 4

OF SPECIAL CONCERN

If You Get Sick

E very woman expects to succumb to at least a few of the less pleasant pregnancy symptoms during her nine-month stint—morning sickness and leg cramps, for instance, or indigestion and exhaustion. But it's easy to forget that you're also susceptible to symptoms that have nothing at all to do with pregnancy: those associated with such "civilian" sicknesses as colds, flu, and gastroenteritis.

Fortunately, though such illnesses may affect the way you feel, most will not affect your pregnancy. Prevention is, of course, the best way to avoid falling ill and to keep that healthy glow of pregnancy going strong. But when it fails, quick treatment, in most cases under the supervision of your practitioner, can help you feel better fast.

What You May Be Concerned About

THE COMMON COLD

"I have a terrible cold, and I'm worried about it affecting my baby."

M ost pregnant women come down with a cold at least once during their nine months. Fortunately, even a bad cold won't hurt your baby, though you may feel miserable, uncomfortable, and eager for relief. *Un*fortunately, the medications and supplements that you're probably accustomed to reaching for in order to find that relief (or to prevent a cold), including aspirin and ibuprofen, megadoses of vitamin C and zinc, and most herbs, are not recommended. So do not take any of these without your

practitioner's approval. He or she should be able to steer you toward cold treatments that are considered safe in pregnancy as well as those that will work best in your case. None will cure a cold, but some may help relieve its symptoms and make you feel more comfortable. (See page 456 for information on taking medication during pregnancy.)

If you've already taken a few doses of a medication that isn't recommended for use during pregnancy, don't worry. But do check with your practitioner if you need extra reassurance.

Thankfully, some of the most effective cold remedies are also the safest for both you and your baby. These tips can help nip a cold in the bud, before it blossoms into a nasty case of sinusitis or another secondary infection, while helping you to feel better faster. At the very first sneeze or tickle in the throat:

♦ Rest, if you feel the need to. Taking a cold to bed doesn't necessarily shorten its duration, but if your body is begging for some rest, be sure to listen. On the other hand, if you feel up to it (and you're not running a fever or coughing), light to moderate exercise can help you feel better faster.

♦ Don't starve your cold, fever—*or* baby. Eat as nutritiously as you can, given how crummy you feel and how little appetite you probably have. Choose foods that appeal to you or at least don't turn you off completely. Be sure to have some citrus fruit or juice (oranges, tangerines, grapefruit) as well as plenty of other vitamin-C-rich fruits and vegetables (see page 96) every day, but don't take extra vitamin C supplements (beyond what comes in your pregnancy vitamin supplement) without medical approval. The same holds true for zinc (in the form of tablets or lozenges). Echinacea, believed to be effective in preventing or reducing the severity of colds, is probably safe to use during pregnancy but is still not recommended because no large study has been done to prove its safety.

♦ Flood yourself with fluids. Fever, sneezes, and a runny nose will cause your body to lose fluids that you and your baby need. Keep a thermos of hot diluted grapefruit or orange juice (½ cup unsweetened frozen juice concentrate to 1 quart of hot water) next to your bed, and try to drink at least one cupful an hour. If too much citrus upsets your stomach, switch between the juice mixture and plain or spark-ling water. Also try the "Jewish penicillin": chicken soup. Medical researchers have proven that it not only replaces fluids but also helps make cold sufferers more comfortable. Other juices and soups can also help fill your fluid requirements.

♦ When you're lying down or sleeping, use a couple of pillows to keep your head elevated. This will make it easier for you to breathe through a stuffy nose. Nasal strips (which gently pull your nasal passages open, making breathing easier) may help, too. They're sold over the counter, and are completely drug-free.

♦ Keep your nasal passages moist with a humidifier and by spraying the inside of your nose with saline nose drops (which are also drug-free).

♦ If your throat is sore or scratchy, or if you're coughing, gargle with salt water (¼ teaspoon of salt to 8 ounces of water) at the temperature of hot, but not scalding, tea.

♦ Bring down a fever promptly. For more on fever treatment, see page 454.

♦ Don't put off calling the doctor or refuse to take a medication he or she prescribes because you think *all* drugs are harmful in pregnancy. Many are not. But do be sure the prescribing doctor knows you are expecting.

Unfortunately, colds tend to last longer during pregnancy, possibly because the immune system slows down a bit in order to protect the baby (a foreign body) from immunological rejection. If your cold is severe enough to interfere with eating or sleeping, if you're coughing up greenish or yellowish sputum, if you have a cough with chest pain or wheezing, if your sinuses are throbbing (see the next question), or if symptoms last more than a week, call your doctor. Prescribed medication may be needed for your safety and your baby's.

SINUSITIS

"I've had a cold for about a week. Now my forehead and cheeks are starting to really hurt. Is this related, and what should I do?"

Sounds as though your cold has turned into sinusitis. Signs of sinusitis include pain and often tenderness in the forehead and/or one or both cheeks (beneath the eye), and possibly around the teeth (pain usually worsens when you bend over or shake your head) and thickened and darkened (greenish or yellowish) mucus.

Sinusitis following a cold is fairly common, but is even more common among pregnant women, since their hormones tend to swell mucous membranes (such as those leading to and in the sinuses), causing blockages that allow germs to build up and multiply in the sinuses. These germs tend to linger longer in the sinuses since immune cells, which destroy invading germs, have difficulty reaching their deep recesses. As a result, sinus infections that aren't treated can persist for weeks—or even become chronic. Treatment of them with antibiotics and decongestants can bring relief quickly, so call your doctor and take care of the problem now.

INFLUENZA, OR "FLU"

"It's flu season, and I'm wondering if I should get a flu shot. Is it safe during pregnancy?"

A flu shot is definitely your best line of defense during flu season. In fact, the Centers for Disease Control recommends that any woman who will be pregnant during flu season (generally October through March) be given the flu shot.

The flu vaccine must be taken prior to *each* flu season—or at least early in the season—for best protection. It's not 100 percent effective, since it protects only against the flu virus that is expected to cause the most problems in a particular year. Still, it greatly increases the chance that you will escape the season flu-free. And even when it doesn't prevent infection, it usually reduces the severity of symptoms. Side effects occur

---

IS IT THE FLU OR A COLD?

Here's how to tell which has you down:

A cold, even a bad one, is milder than the flu. It's usually heralded by a sore or scratchy throat (which lasts only a day or two) followed by the gradual appearance of symptoms. These include a runny, and later stuffy, nose; lots of sneezing; and possibly slight achiness and mild fatigue. There is little or no fever (usually less than 100°F). Coughing may develop, particularly near the cold's end, and may continue for a week or more after other symptoms have subsided.

Influenza (or the flu) is more severe and comes on more suddenly. Symptoms include fever (usually 102°F to 104°F); headache; sore throat (generally worsens by second or third day); often intense muscle soreness; and general weakness and fatigue (which can last a couple of weeks or longer). There may also be occasional sneezing and often a cough that can become severe. In some cases, nausea or vomiting may also occur—but don't confuse this with what is often called "stomach flu"—see page 459.

infrequently and are generally mild. Pregnant women should not buy Flumist, the nasal spray flu vaccine. That vaccine, unlike the flu shot, is made from live flu virus, and could actually give you a mild case of the flu.

If you suspect you might have the flu (see symptoms in box on the facing page), call your doctor immediately so that you can be treated. (In the meantime, take steps to bring down the fever; see page 454.) This is particularly important in the last trimester, when untreated flu can become severe in the expectant mother and may lead to pneumonia or even premature delivery. Treatment is typically symptomatic— aimed at reducing fever, aches and pains, and nasal stuffiness. Most important: rest and plenty of fluids, essential for preventing dehydration.

URINARY TRACT INFECTION

"I'm afraid I have a urinary tract infection."

Urinary tract infections (UTIs) are so common in pregnancy that 10 percent of pregnant women can expect to develop at least one, and those who have already had one have a 1 in 3 chance of an encore. Most often it takes the form of cystitis, a simple bladder infection. In some women, cystitis is "silent" (without symptoms) and is diagnosed only after a routine urine culture. In others, symptoms can range from mild to quite uncomfortable (an urge to urinate frequently, pain or a burning sensation when urine—sometimes only a drop or two—is passed, pressure or sharp pain in the lower abdominal area). The urine may also be foul smelling and cloudy and possibly contain some blood.

Regardless of whether there are symptoms or not, once an infection is diagnosed it should be treated promptly by a physician, with an antibiotic approved for use during pregnancy.[1] Don't be tempted to discontinue treatment once you're feeling better; finishing the prescription is vital to preventing a recurrence.

In 20 to 40 percent of cases, *untreated* bladder infection during pregnancy progresses to kidney infection, which is more of a threat to mother and baby. This occurs most often in the last trimester, and can lead to preterm labor. The symptoms are the same as those of cystitis but are frequently accompanied by fever (often as high as 103°F), chills, blood in the urine, backache (in the mid-back on one or both sides), and nausea and vomiting. Should you experience these symptoms, notify your doctor immediately. Antibiotics can generally cure a kidney infection, but hospitalization may be necessary so that the drugs can be administered intravenously.

Many physicians today try to head off kidney infection by screening pregnant women, at their first visit, for susceptibility. If a culture of the urine turns up bacteria (and it does in about 7 to 10 percent of pregnant women),[2] precautionary antibiotics are administered to prevent the development of cystitis or kidney infection.

There are some home remedies and preventives that may also help ward off UTI; used in conjunction with medical treatment, they may help speed recovery when infection occurs.

◆ Drink plenty of fluids, especially water, which can help flush out any

---

1. Do not take a medication previously prescribed for you or for anyone else, even if it was prescribed for a urinary tract infection.

2. A urine specimen can be taken at your practitioner's office or you can ask about a home testing kit that has been approved by the FDA.

bacteria. Cranberry juice may also be beneficial, possibly because the tannins it contains keep bacteria from adhering to the walls of the urinary tract. Avoid coffee and tea (even decaffeinated varieties) and alcohol, which may increase risk of infection.

♦ Wash your vaginal area well and empty your bladder just before and after intercourse.

♦ Every time you urinate, take the time to empty your bladder thoroughly. Leaning forward on the toilet will help accomplish this. It sometimes also helps to "double void"—after you urinate, wait five minutes, then try to urinate again. And don't put off the urge when you have it; regularly "holding it in" increases susceptibility to infection.

♦ To give your perineal area "breathing space," wear cotton-crotch underwear and panty hose, avoid wearing tight pants, don't wear panty hose under slacks, and sleep without panties or pajama bottoms on.

♦ Keep the vaginal and perineal areas meticulously clean and irritation-free. Wipe front to back after using the toilet to keep fecal bacteria from entering the vagina or urethra (the short tube through which urine is excreted from the bladder). Wash daily (shower rather than bathe) and avoid bubble bath and perfumed powders, soaps, sprays, detergents, and toilet tissue. Also avoid pools that aren't properly chlorinated.

♦ Eat unsweetened yogurt or frozen yogurt that contains active cultures when taking antibiotics, to help restore the balance of bacteria. If you can't tolerate or just don't like yogurt, ask your practitioner about taking *Lactobacillus acidophilus, L. bulgaricus,* or *Streptococcus thermophilus* in tablet or capsule form.

♦ Keep your resistance high by eating a nutritious diet, getting adequate rest and exercise, not working to the point of fatigue, and not letting your life get too stressful.

FEVER

"I'm running a fever. Should I take aspirin to bring it down?"

During most of your life, fever needn't be feared or fought. In fact, it is one of the body's most powerful allies in the war against infection. During pregnancy, however, a significant and sustained increase in body temperature can occasionally cause birth defects—particularly during weeks 3 to 7. Exactly at what temperature risk occurs isn't entirely clear, though some suggest anything over 102°F could be a problem. So bringing a fever down promptly, rather than letting it run its course, is the safest way to go. Since fever is usually a sign of infection, and some types of infection have been linked to pregnancy complications, the infection itself may also need to be treated.

How best to bring a fever down will depend on how high it has gone up, and on your practitioner's recommendations. Call your practitioner the same day if you're running a fever of between 100°F and 102°F; call right away if it's 102°F or higher. While you're waiting to speak to the doctor, take two acetaminophen tablets to start reducing the fever. Taking a tepid bath or shower, drinking cool beverages, and keeping clothing and covers light will also help bring your temperature down. (Such home remedies may be effective enough in reducing a low-grade fever that's under 100°F; in that case, medication won't be necessary.) For a higher temperature related to a bacterial infection, acetaminophen teamed with an antibiotic (there are several that are considered safe for use during pregnancy) will probably be prescribed. Aspirin or ibuprofen should not be routinely taken for fever (see below).

If you had a high fever earlier in pregnancy and did not report it to the practitioner, you should do so now. Though the chances that it caused any problem are low, as always, the more information the practitioner has, the better care you and your baby will receive.

TAKING ASPIRIN AND NONASPIRIN

"Last week I took two aspirins for a pounding headache, and now I read that it can cause bleeding in pregnancy. I'm a nervous wreck."

Of the millions of Americans who opened their medicine cabinets today and reached for a bottle of pain reliever, few thought twice—or even once—about its safety. And for most people, occasional aspirin or ibuprofen use is helpful and perfectly harmless. But during pregnancy, there is concern that these pain relievers, like many other ordinarily innocuous over-the-counter remedies, may be potentially harmful.

If you've unwittingly taken one or two aspirin or ibuprofen on one or even a few occasions in the first two trimesters, don't worry—there is no evidence they will hurt your baby. For the rest of your pregnancy, however, it's advisable to treat pain relievers as you would any other drug, taking them only when necessary and only when recommended by a practitioner who knows you're pregnant.

Aspirin use is most risky in the third trimester, when even one typical dose can interfere with fetal growth and cause other problems.[3] Because it is an antiprostaglandin, and prostaglandins are involved in the mechanism of labor, aspirin can prolong both pregnancy and labor and lead to other complications during delivery. And since it interferes with blood-clotting, aspirin taken during the two weeks before delivery can increase the risk of hemorrhage at delivery and even of bleeding problems in the newborn.

But indiscriminately popping aspirin substitutes in place of aspirin isn't a good idea, either. Though the moderate use of acetaminophen (such as Tylenol) in pregnancy appears to pose no problem, it, too, should be taken only when necessary. Check with your practitioner for guidelines in taking acetaminophen.

Ibuprofen (examples are Advil and Motrin) should be used with caution in pregnancy. Similar to aspirin in some ways, it may trigger a cross reaction in those sensitive to aspirin. Because its use in the last trimester can result in problems in the unborn child, a prolonged pregnancy, a prolonged labor, and/or bleeding problems, don't use ibuprofen at all in the last three months of pregnancy. Use it earlier only if recommended by a physician who knows you are pregnant and only for short periods. (But don't worry about the ibuprofen you took before you found out you were pregnant.)

Ketoprofen (Actron and Orudis KT) and naproxen (Aleve), both nonsteroidal anti-inflammatory drugs (NSAIDs), are not recommended for use in pregnancy at all. Besides having antiprostaglandin properties, they can cause other severe side effects.

While caution is wise in considering the use of antipain or antifever medica-

---

3. Low-dose aspirin therapy for the prevention of preeclampsia in certain high-risk women is considered safe through the 36th week.

tions, there's no reason to avoid their use entirely. There are times when pain cannot be relieved or a fever brought down in any other way. The most sensible course in pregnancy is first to try to use nondrug remedies (see Appendix, page 547) for pain or low-grade fever. Then, if those methods fail (or if fever is higher), it makes sense to turn to nonaspirin acetaminophen products—under medical supervision.

TAKING MEDICATIONS

"How do I know which medicines, if any, are safe to take during pregnancy, and which aren't?"

No drug, prescription or over-the-counter, traditional or herbal, is 100 percent safe for 100 percent of the people 100 percent of the time. And when you're pregnant, every time you take a drug there is the health and well-being of two individuals, one very small and vulnerable, to consider. Although a few drugs have been shown to be particularly harmful to a developing fetus, many drugs have been used safely during pregnancy, and there are situations in which medication is absolutely essential to life and/or health. Whether you will take a particular medication at a particular time during pregnancy is something you and your practitioner will have to decide by weighing the drug's potential risks against the benefits it offers. In any case, the general rule should be: take medication only on the advice of a practitioner who knows you are pregnant, and only when it is absolutely necessary.[4]

Which drug you take in a specific situation will depend on the latest information available on drug safety in

---

4. If you are a diabetic, have other chronic health problems, or take any kind of medication regularly, be sure to inform your doctor of this as well, since many medicines that might be safe for others may not be safe for you.

ON-LINE DRUG SHOPPING

Too busy or exhausted to run to your pharmacy? Thinking of shopping for your medications on-line instead? Before you do, there are some important things to keep in mind. While there are some on-line pharmacies that provide legitimate prescription services, there are others that make buying on-line risky. To ensure that your on-line pharmacy purchase is a legal and safe one:

◆ Only buy medications that have been prescribed by *your* doctor. Don't purchase from sites that don't require prescriptions (which, by the way, is illegal).

◆ Make sure the on-line pharmacy verifies each prescription before dispensing the medication. (A written verification policy is usually posted on the site.)

◆ Make sure you're buying from a licensed pharmacy. Look for the NABP VIPPS (National Association of Boards of Pharmacies Verified Internet Pharmacy Practice Sites) seal on the Web site. This certification ensures that the on-line pharmacy meets all applicable state and federal regulations, complies with the patient's right to privacy, verifies all prescription orders, and adheres to a quality assurance policy. To find out which on-line pharmacies have been approved, go to www.nabp.net/vipps/consumer/listall.asp.

---

pregnancy. The many lists of safe, possibly safe, possibly unsafe, and definitely unsafe drugs may provide some assistance, but most are outdated and unreliable by the time they're published. Package inserts and labels are of limited use, since most warn not to use the product during pregnancy without a physician's orders, even when the product is believed safe. Your best sources of information will be:

♦ A well-informed physician (not all are familiar with drug safety in pregnancy); a maternal-fetal medicine specialist may be particularly helpful in some cases.

♦ The Food and Drug Administration—contact your regional office or write to the Public Health Service, FDA, Parklawn Building, 5600 Fishers Lane, Rockville, MD 20857, or visit www.fda.gov.

♦ The March of Dimes—try your local office first, or contact the March of Dimes Resource Center at (888) MODIMES or (888-663-4637); www.modimes.org.

If you do need some kind of medication during pregnancy, follow these steps for increased benefit and reduced risk:

♦ Discuss with your physician the possibility of taking the medication in the smallest effective doses for the shortest possible time.

♦ Take the medication when it's going to benefit you the most—a cold medication at night, for instance, so it will help you sleep.

KEEPING MOIST

Hot, dry air can contribute to dry skin, coughing, and possibly to an increase in colds and other respiratory ailments. Adding moisture to your home can help reduce this problem, but how you do this can make a difference. Sometimes the suggested cure can do more harm than good.

Vaporizers and humidifiers, for example, have to be chosen and used with caution. Steam vaporizers manufactured since the 1970s are safe and effective, although if young children are around, the vaporizer must be carefully positioned out of reach. Cold-mist humidifiers, which became popular because they didn't present a burn hazard, encourage bacterial growth and spread germs, and should not be used at all. Ultrasonic humidifiers spew tiny particles of bacteria and other impurities from the water into the air and can cause allergic reactions or illness if they are not cleaned daily and if plain tap water (rather than unfiltered or undistilled water) is used in them. Pans of water on radiators can add small amounts of moisture to the air but, again, could be a burn risk for small children. A steaming kettle under a tented towel also presents a burn problem and should be used with care for brief periods only.

Manufacturers have been attempting to produce safer humidifiers. Warm-mist humidifiers (which boil the water before mixing it with cool water to produce a mist) and wicking humidifiers (which use wicks to remove impurities) appear to release fewer germs than older cool-mist units. All humidifiers should be drained and cleaned before storing, and should be thoroughly cleaned before being used again.

No matter which method you use to add humidity to your home, limit the time of operation. Don't humidify around the clock—among other things, this can encourage the growth of molds on plants and furniture. Instead, try not to let the air in your home become dry and overheated in the first place. To do this, keep the indoor temperature under 68°F in cold weather. And don't make your home totally airtight—allow some leakage through windows or doors. (This will also minimize indoor pollutants, such as radon.)

◆ Follow directions carefully. Some medications must be taken on an empty stomach; some should be taken with food or milk. If your physician hasn't given you any instructions, ask your pharmacist for particulars— most provide handouts with full directions and information (including possible side effects) on each prescription drug they sell.

◆ Explore nondrug remedies, and use them, as appropriate, to supplement the drug therapy—for instance, eliminating as many offending allergens from your home as you can, so your physician can reduce the amount of prescribed antihistamine you take.

◆ Make sure the medication gets where it's supposed to by taking a sip of water before you swallow a capsule or tablet, to make it go down more easily, and by drinking a full glass afterward, to ensure that it is washed speedily down to where it will be absorbed. Taking the medication while sitting or standing, rather than lying down or propped up, may also help speed its passage.

◆ For additional safety, try to get all your prescriptions at the same pharmacy. The pharmacist will have you and all your prescriptions on the computer and should be able to warn you of potential drug interactions. Also be sure you've gotten the right prescription (or over-the-counter medication, or herbal preparation). Check the name and dosage on the bottle to be sure it's the one specified by your doctor (many drug names are similar). For additional reassurance, ask the pharmacist what the drug is meant to treat. If you know you were supposed to get an antihistamine for your allergies and the drug you are handed is for hypertension, you've got the wrong medication.

◆ Ask about possible side effects and which ones should be reported to your doctor. Antihistamines (including garlic pills), for example, can occasionally cause nighttime urination problems such as pain, burning, and difficulty urinating.

Once you've made certain that a prescribed drug is considered safe for use during pregnancy, don't hesitate to take it because you're still afraid it might somehow harm your baby. It won't—but delaying treatment might.

HERBAL CURES

"I wouldn't think of taking any drugs during pregnancy. But would it be all right to substitute medicinal herbs?"

Medicinal herbs *are* drugs—often very powerful ones. Some (such as foxglove) are so powerful that they're used in laboratories to produce prescription medicines (digitalis, for example). Others have been used for generations in some societies to induce abortions, and some have been linked to miscarriage. Even in a seemingly soothing cup of tea, some herbs are capable of producing such symptoms as diarrhea, vomiting, and heart palpitations. Plus, the use of herbal medicines presents a risk that isn't present in traditional medicines. Thanks to lax governmental controls, they are not made under quality-controlled conditions, and may be dangerously strong or impotently weak. They may also contain harmful contaminants, including allergens such as insect parts, pollens, and molds, and even toxic agents such as lead or arsenic.

So treat medicinal herbs as you would any drugs during pregnancy. Do not take them except on the advice of your doctor. If you are experiencing any symptoms that need treatment, check with your practitioner instead of trying to self-treat. If you are already taking an herbal medication, tell your practitioner, so that he or she can assess its safety. And if your practitioner prescribes an herbal medication, purchase a brand produced in Germany, which does oversee manufacture of these preparations, or by a major pharmaceutical company in the United States that claims the product is "standardized."

Nutritional supplements—also not government regulated—can be risky during pregnancy, unless prescribed by your practitioner.

As for traditional medicines, don't rule them out. They may often be necessary for your health or that of your developing baby (see previous question).

GASTROINTESTINAL ILLS

"I've got a stomach bug, and I can't keep anything down. Will this hurt my baby?"

Fortunately, gastroenteritis (an inflammation of the stomach and intestines) usually has a limited life span—often no longer than twenty-four hours, very rarely longer than seventy-two. And as long as you manage to take in enough fluids to replace those lost through vomiting and/or diarrhea, even complete lack of solid nourishment for a day or two won't harm your baby.

But just because the virus isn't affecting your baby's health doesn't mean you should ignore it. Take these steps to increase your comfort and speed your recovery while you're waiting for your bug to bug off:

Consult with your practitioner. Discuss all of your symptoms—just in case they're the result of something more serious than a stomach bug. In addition to vomiting and diarrhea, you may experience fever;

mucus, blood, or worms in your stool; persistent abdominal pain; or infrequent urination or dark yellow urine (signs of dehydration). Inform the doctor if others who have eaten with you recently become sick at the same time and/or if you have eaten potentially contaminated food (particularly unpasteurized dairy products or juices; undercooked or raw meats, fish, poultry, or eggs; or alfalfa sprouts) in the last few weeks; in that event, you may have food poisoning and, if it's a bad case, may require medical care. Also report any recent travels to an exotic destination, in which case parasites or other indigenous infectious organisms may be responsible for your distress; such infections might also require treatment.

Follow your doctor's recommendations for treating the bug. Call again as instructed, and/or if symptoms last more than forty-eight hours; additional treatment may be needed. But do not take any medications—including over-the-counter preparations—without your doctor's recommendations. In some cases (as when there is a bacterial infection or parasites), it's best to allow the diarrhea to continue, so that it can cleanse the intestines of the disease-causing organisms; trying to stop the flow with medication may only prolong the illness. Here are some other tips:

Take your bug to your bed, if possible. Bed rest, particularly in a dark, quiet room, seems to reduce the symptoms.

Replenish lost fluids. Diarrhea and vomiting remove great quantities of fluid from the body and are therefore extremely dehydrating. That's why fluid intake is more important than solid intake for the short term, and why it's essential to keep the clear liquids coming, in whatever form is palatable to you. Try taking small sips every fifteen minutes or so of still or sparkling water, weak decaffeinated tea, orange juice diluted with an equal quantity of water, diluted white grape juice, or diluted apple juice (but only if diarrhea isn't a problem). If symptoms are severe, your practitioner may recommend a rehydration fluid. Beef or chicken broth may also be helpful. If you can't even keep these down, suck on ice pops,[5] ice chips, or ice cubes. Avoid the traditional cure of sugary soft drinks, such as ginger ale or colas—they will only prolong your symptoms. Milk may, too. And skip anything with caffeine (including colas, coffee, and tea), since caffeine increases the loss of fluids from the body, worsening dehydration.

Modify your diet. Traditional wisdom says that unless you're really hungry, it's probably better to eat nothing for the first twelve hours or so when you have a stomach virus. More recent research, however, suggests that continuing solids may actually be preferable to semi-starvation. Check with your practitioner for advice. Whether you continue solids or wait twelve to twenty-four hours before digging in, keep your diet simple and easily digestible. At first stick to diluted fruit juices, clear broth, or bouillon; thinned cream of wheat or cream of rice; unbuttered white toast (this is one time when whole wheat's not your best bet); boiled or steamed converted white rice; boiled, baked, or mashed potato without the skin; bananas, applesauce, gelatin desserts (make these with unflavored gelatin and fruit juice instead of sugary mixes). Gradually add, as they become appealing to you, low-fat cottage cheese, yogurt, chicken, fish, then cooked vegetables and fruit, before returning to your normal diet. Listen to your body—and eat accordingly.

Supplement when you can. Getting your vitamin insurance is an especially

good idea now, so try to take your supplement when it's least likely to come back up. Don't worry, however, if you can't manage to keep it down for a few days or so; no harm done.

Of course, even better than trying to get rid of a stomach bug is preventing it in the first place. So always observe the prevention tips on pages 150 and 468.

LISTERIOSIS

"A friend who is pregnant said to stay away from unpasteurized dairy products because they can make you sick when you're expecting. Is this true?"

More bad news for adventurous eaters. Unpasteurized milk and cheeses made from unpasteurized milk (including some mozzarella, blue cheese, Mexican cheeses, Brie, Camembert, and feta) can make you sick anytime, but particularly when you're expecting. These foods, along with raw or undercooked meat, fish, shellfish, poultry, eggs, unwashed raw vegetables, and deli meats can contain listeria, bacteria that can cause serious illness (listeriosis), especially in high-risk individuals, including young children, the elderly, those with compromised immune systems, and pregnant women, whose immune systems are also somewhat suppressed. Listeria, unlike many other germs, enters the bloodstream directly and can therefore get to the baby quickly through the placenta (other food contaminants generally stay in the digestive tract and may only cause problems if they get into the amniotic fluid).

Listeriosis is hard to detect. This is partly because symptoms can appear anytime between twelve hours and thirty days after contaminated food is eaten and partly because the symptoms—headache, fever, fatigue, muscle aches, and occa-

---

5. Rehydration ice pops for children are available in drugstores, and it might make sense to keep a pack in your own freezer, just in case.

sionally nausea and diarrhea—are similar to those of flu, and some can even be mistaken for pregnancy side effects. In more serious cases, infection can lead to bloodstream infection or spread to the nervous system and cause meningitis (with accompanying stiff neck, severe headaches, confusion, and loss of balance). Antibiotics are needed to treat and cure listeriosis. If the illness is not treated, convulsions and even death can occur. In an expectant mother, infection can also lead to premature labor, miscarriage or stillbirth, or infection of the fetus.

So, clearly, it's important to prevent infection in the first place by staying away from the risky foods that carry listeria, especially now. See page 150 for more tips on food safety and the prevention of food-borne diseases.

TOXOPLASMOSIS

"Though I've given all the cat-care chores over to my husband, just the very fact that I live with cats makes me worry about toxoplasmosis. How would I know if I came down with the disease?"

Chances are you wouldn't. Most people who are infected show no symptoms at all, though some do notice mild malaise, slight fever, and swollen glands two or three weeks after exposure, followed by a rash a day or two later.

But chances are, too, that you wouldn't come down with the disease in the first place. If you've lived with cats for a long time, it's very likely that you've already become infected and have developed antibodies to the virus that causes toxoplasmosis. Unfortunately, determining whether or not you have those antibodies is an imprecise science. Though a blood test for antibodies to *Toxoplasma gondii* is available, it won't be useful unless you were tested before you conceived. That's because the tests are not sensitive enough to show whether a woman who was never tested before has a new infection or simply has antibodies from an old infection.

Check with your practitioner to see if you were tested before pregnancy. If you had antibodies then—very likely if you've been living with cats—you're immune and needn't worry about developing an infection now. If you had no antibodies, you are not immune. In the unlikely event that you are not immune and you do experience the symptoms of toxoplasmosis, you may be tested at that point. (Don't try to test yourself, however, since home tests for toxoplasmosis are highly unreliable.)

If a new infection *is* detected, the point in your pregnancy at which the infection occurs is an important factor to consider. The risk of a fetus becoming infected in the first trimester is relatively small, probably less than 15 percent, but the risk of serious damage to the fetus is high. In the second trimester, the likelihood of infection is a little higher, but the risk of fetal damage somewhat smaller. In the last trimester, the baby is most likely to be infected, but the risk of serious damage is smallest. Only 1 baby in 10,000 is born with severe congenital toxoplasmosis.

Recent advances have made it possible to test fetal blood and/or amniotic fluid to learn whether or not the fetus itself has actually become infected, though not usually before 20 to 22 weeks. If no fetal infection is detected, the fetus is probably fine.

In the rare case that a pregnant woman and her fetus both show an infection, a thorough discussion of the options with the doctor, a maternal-fetal medicine specialist, or possibly with a genetic counselor should be the next step. If she wishes to continue her pregnancy, it's recommended that she be treated with special antibiotics, possibly for several months. Such treatment appears to greatly reduce the risk of a baby being born with severe problems. Treating an infected baby immediately after birth can also reduce complications and may improve the prognosis for such children.

The best "treatment" of toxoplasmosis (as with most diseases), however, is prevention. See page 67 for tips on how to avoid infection.

CYTOMEGALOVIRUS (CMV)

"My doctor told me that I should take a leave of absence from my teaching job at a nursery school because I could contract CMV, which she says could harm my baby."

It's true that the chances of exposure to CMV (cytomegalovirus) are greatest with a job like yours, because somewhere between 25 and 60 percent of all preschoolers carry the virus and can excrete it in saliva, urine, and feces for months or even years. But it's also true that the chances of picking up the infection from your young charges and passing it on to your baby are very small. First of all, the virus is not extremely contagious—at least for adults. Second, a majority of adults were infected in childhood, and if you are among that majority, you can't "catch" CMV now. (Your CMV could become *reactivated,* but in that case, the risks to your baby are even smaller than if you have a new infection during pregnancy.) Third, though roughly 1 in 200 babies is born with the virus (about half of infected moms bear infected infants), only a small percentage of these actually show any of the ill effects commonly associated with CMV infection in utero.

Still, some physicians, like yours, suggest that unless a woman knows for sure that she has already been infected (most women don't have this information unless they are tested prenatally,

since CMV usually comes and goes with no obvious symptoms), it's a good idea to take a leave of absence from any job that puts her in daily contact with large numbers of preschoolers, at least for the first 24 weeks of pregnancy, during which the potential risks to the fetus are the greatest. Others recommend wearing gloves on the job, washing up carefully after changing diapers (which you should do anyway), and resisting kissing the toddlers in your care or nibbling on their leftovers. (Pregnant women with toddlers of their own needn't worry about catching CMV; the possibility is extremely remote. That doesn't mean, of course, that good hygiene in the home should be ignored—it should be practiced whether you're worried about CMV or not.)

Should you come down with fever, fatigue, swollen lymph glands, and sore throat, however, do check with your doctor. Whether these symptoms signal CMV or another illness (such as flu, strep throat, or mononucleosis), you need treatment. If CMV is diagnosed, this treatment may include CMV immunoglobulin, which may help to prevent your fetus from getting infected. It is also likely that the doctor will recommend testing the amniotic fluid or a fetal blood sample (after 21 weeks gestation and 7 weeks after your own illness is diagnosed) to see if your child has contracted the disease.[6] If the test is positive, another test should be taken in two weeks. If that, too, is positive, you will need to discuss the options with your doctor.

FIFTH DISEASE

"I was told that a disease I had never even heard of before—fifth disease—could cause problems in pregnancy."

6. While these tests will provide an accurate diagnosis, ultrasound—which is sometimes recommended—probably will not.

Fifth disease is the fifth of a group of six diseases that cause fever and rash in children. But unlike its sister diseases (such as measles and chicken pox), fifth disease isn't widely known because its symptoms are mild and can go unnoticed—or may even be totally absent. Fever is present in only 15 to 30 percent of cases. The rash—which for the first few days gives the cheeks the appearance of having been slapped, then spreads in a lacy pattern to trunk, buttocks, and thighs, recurring on and off (usually in response to heat from the sun or a warm bath) for one to three weeks—is often confused with the rash of rubella and other childhood illnesses or even a sunburn. Fifth disease is not highly contagious, so it's not likely to be passed on through casual contact. Concentrated exposure from caring for a child sick with fifth disease or from teaching at a school where it is epidemic does, however, increase the risk of contracting the illness.

But since most women of childbearing age had fifth disease during childhood and are already immune, infection is not common among pregnant women. Current or previous exposure to parvovirus B$_{19}$, the cause of fifth disease, can easily be detected by testing the blood for parvovirus antibodies. If a blood test shows that you once had the infection, it means you can't "catch" it again or pass it on to your baby. Even if the test reveals you have had a more recent infection, the chances that you might transmit the infection to your baby are quite small—perhaps less than 1 percent, according to recent studies.

If tests show you are *not* immune and not infected, the odds of your developing an infection are still remote. As a precaution, if your job requires you to care for young children, it might be wise to take a leave of absence should an epidemic of fifth disease develop. Should your own child become sick with the disease, take the appropriate steps to avoid infection (see page 468).

Recently fifth disease has been linked to a very slightly increased risk (1 or 2 percent) of miscarriage in women who contract it. If the disease does cause a miscarriage in one pregnancy, however, a repeat miscarriage due to parvovirus is not likely.

Very rarely, fifth disease later in pregnancy may lead to an unusual form of fetal anemia, similar to that in Rh disease. For that reason, women who have fifth disease during pregnancy are generally examined periodically with ultrasound to look for the swelling (resulting from fluid retention) in the fetus that is characteristic of this kind of anemia; if it is found, treatment will probably be necessary.

CHICKEN POX (VARICELLA)

"My toddler was exposed to chicken pox at her day care center — by a child who wasn't immunized. If she comes down with it, could the baby I'm now carrying be hurt?"

Not likely. Well insulated from the rest of the world, the fetus can't contract chicken pox, or varicella, from a third party—only from its mother. And you would have to catch it first, which may very well be impossible. First of all, your child isn't likely to catch it and bring it home if she was immunized with the varicella vaccine. Second of all, it's very likely you had the infection as a child (85 to 95 percent of today's adult population has had it) and are already immune. Ask your parents or check your health records to find out whether you have had chicken pox. If you can't find out for sure, ask your practitioner to run a test now to see if you are immune.

Though the chances of your becoming infected are slim if you aren't immune, an injection of varicella-zoster immune globulin (VZIG) within ninety-six hours of a documented personal exposure may be recommended. It isn't clear whether or not this will protect the baby should you come down with chicken pox anyway, but it should minimize complications for you, which is significant, since this mild childhood disease can be quite severe in adults, sometimes causing varicella pneumonia. If you should be hit with a severe case, you may be given an antiviral drug to further reduce the risk of complications.

There is some risk of damage to the fetus when the mother is infected, but it is a small one. Even if a fetus is exposed when most vulnerable—during the first half of pregnancy—recent research shows that there's only a 2 percent chance of its developing the defects typical of congenital varicella syndrome. When the exposure occurs in the second half of pregnancy, fetal damage is extremely rare.

Chicken pox becomes more of a concern close to term, when a maternal infection can lead to a baby being born with neonatal varicella. If a mother develops chicken pox within one week of delivery, there's a 15 to 30 percent chance her newborn will arrive infected and will develop the characteristic rash within a week or so. Since neonatal varicella can be extremely serious, VZIG is usually given to the baby. The risk of the newborn being infected is small if maternal infection occurs between seven and twenty-one days before delivery, which gives the mother's body a chance to develop antibodies and pass them onto the fetus through the placenta.

Incidentally, shingles, or herpes zoster, which is a reactivation of the chicken pox virus in someone who had the disease earlier, does not appear to be harmful to a developing fetus, probably because the mother and thus the baby already have antibodies to the virus.

If you are not immune and escape infection this time, ask your doctor about getting immunized after delivery, to protect any future pregnancies. Immunization should take place at least a month before any new conception.

LYME DISEASE

"I know I live in an area that's high-risk for Lyme disease. Is Lyme dangerous when you're pregnant?"

Lyme disease—which got its name from Lyme, Connecticut, where it was first diagnosed in the United States —is most common among those who spend time in woods frequented by deer, mice, or other animals carrying deer ticks, but it can also be picked up in forest-free cities via greenery brought from the country or purchased at a farmer's market. Lyme disease can be passed on to the fetus, but whether or not the fetus can suffer permanent harm isn't entirely clear. It is suspected, but not proven, that the disease may be linked to heart defects in the babies of infected mothers.

The best way to protect your baby as well as yourself is by taking preventive measures. If you are out in woodsy or grassy areas, or if you are handling greenery grown in such areas, wear long pants tucked into boots or socks, and long sleeves; use an insect repellent effective for Lyme ticks on your clothing, but not on your skin. When you return home, check your skin carefully for ticks (removing them shortly after they attach—or at least within twenty-four hours—almost entirely eliminates the possibility of infection) and shower thoroughly to remove any repellent that might have gotten on your skin, as well as to clean out any bite marks. Before a future pregnancy, you may want to check with your doctor about the Lyme vaccine, which may prevent an infection.

If you've been bitten by a tick, see your doctor immediately; a blood test can determine instantly whether you are infected with Lyme. (Early symptoms may include a blotchy bull's-eye rash at the bite site, fatigue, headache, stiff neck, fever and chills, generalized achiness, swollen glands near the site of the bite; later symptoms may include arthritis-like pain and memory loss.) Prompt treatment may prevent your passing the infection on to your baby, and your becoming seriously ill.

MEASLES

"I'm a teacher, so I'm worried about all the childhood diseases I might become exposed to. Should I be immunized against measles?"

No. Measles vaccine is not given during pregnancy because of the theoretical risk to the fetus from the vaccine, though there have been no reports of problems among newborns whose mothers were inadvertently vaccinated. Besides, the chances are good that you are already immune to measles, since most women of childbearing age either had the disease or were vaccinated against it as children. If your medical history doesn't include this information and your parents can't recall it, your doctor can run a test to determine whether you are immune. If you're not, the risk that you will contract measles is still quite small since most, if not all, of the children in your class have been vaccinated against it and are themselves highly unlikely to come down with the disease.[7] Also reassuring is the fact that measles, unlike German measles (rubella) does not appear to cause birth defects, though it *may* be linked to an increased risk of miscarriage or premature labor.

In the very unlikely event that you are exposed *directly* to someone with measles and are not immune, your doctor may administer gamma globulin during the incubation period—between exposure and the start of symptoms—to decrease the severity of the illness should you come down with it. If you were to contract measles near your due date, there is a risk that your newborn might catch the infection from you, which could be serious. Again, gamma globulin may be administered to reduce the severity of such an infection. Keep in mind that all this is pretty much theoretical, since measles has virtually been wiped out in the United States. For more on immunization safety during pregnancy, see page 40.

MUMPS

"A co-worker of mine came down with a bad case of the mumps. Should I get immunized so I don't get it myself?"

Your co-worker is a pretty rare case— only about six hundred Americans contract mumps each year—thanks to immunization. Immunization against mumps during pregnancy, however, is not recommended because it might harm the fetus. But chances are good that you were vaccinated against the mumps with the MMR (measles, mumps, rubella) vaccine or had the disease as a child, which means you can't catch it now. Check for this information with your parents or the doctor who cared for you as a child, if that's possible.[8] But even if you aren't

7. In fact, the risk is almost nonexistent. In recent years, fewer than 100 cases of measles have been reported in the United States, and the great majority of those occurred among immigrants from foreign countries.

8. Keep a record of all immunizations and illnesses so that your child will have this information available as an adult, and pass that record along when he or she leaves home.

immune, the risk of contracting mumps is very low, since it isn't highly contagious through casual contact. However, because the disease appears to trigger uterine contractions and is associated with an increased risk of miscarriage in the first trimester or preterm labor later, you should be alert for the first symptoms of the disease (possibly vague pain, fever, and loss of appetite before the salivary glands become swollen; then ear pain and pain on chewing or on taking acidic or sour food or drink). Notify your doctor of such symptoms immediately, because prompt treatment can reduce the chance of problems developing. You might also want to consider the MMR vaccine before deciding to get pregnant again, just to be on the safe side.

GERMAN MEASLES (RUBELLA)

"I was exposed to German measles on a trip out of the country. Should I be worried?"

Happily, 6 out of 7 pregnant women are immune to German measles, also known as rubella, either because they contracted it at some other time in their lives (usually during childhood) or because they were vaccinated against it (usually in early adolescence or when they were about to be married). So the odds are good that you can't catch German measles and, consequently, have nothing to worry about. If you're not sure whether or not you are immune, you can find out with a simple test—a rubella antibody titer—which measures the level of antibodies to the virus in your blood and is performed routinely at the first prenatal visit by most practitioners. If this test was not performed earlier, it should be now.

In the unlikely event you turn out not to be immune, you still needn't consider drastic measures immediately. Exposure alone cannot harm your baby. For the virus to do its damage, you have to actually come down with the illness. The symptoms, which show up two or three weeks after exposure, are usually mild (malaise, slight fever, and swollen glands, followed by a slight rash a day or two later) and may sometimes pass unnoticed. A blood test during that time, however, can show whether or not you have an active infection. By 22 weeks it's possible to test a fetus to see if it has been infected (earlier, the infection may not show up), but this testing is rarely needed.

Unfortunately, there is no way of absolutely preventing an exposed woman with no immunity from coming down with rubella. Gamma globulin shots were once given routinely, but they have been found to be inconsistent in preventing infection. Should you come down with rubella, you will need to discuss with your doctor all the possible risks to your fetus before making a decision about terminating your pregnancy. It's important to understand that the risks involved decrease as a pregnancy progresses. If a woman is infected in the first month, the chance of her baby developing a serious birth defect is high, about 35 percent. By the third month, the risk is down to 10 to 15 percent. After that the risk is very slight.

Fortunately, the chance of being exposed to rubella in this country is very small. Because immunization has become routine in the United States, the disease has been eliminated in this country. In recent years, fewer than 10 people per year contracted the disease and all those cases have been traceable to foreigners. Still, if you aren't immune and don't contract the disease this time around, avoid the concern entirely in subsequent pregnancies by having your doctor vaccinate you after this delivery. As a precaution, you will be instructed not to become pregnant for three months following vaccination. But should you conceive accidentally during this time, or if you were vaccinated early in this pregnancy, before you knew you had conceived, don't worry. Though there is a theoretical risk of fetal damage, there have been no reported cases of birth defects of the type associated with congenital rubella in babies whose mothers were inadvertently vaccinated early in pregnancy or conceived soon after vaccination.

HEPATITIS

"One of the toddlers in the day care center where I work was just diagnosed as having hepatitis A. If I get it, could it affect my pregnancy?"

Hepatitis A is very common (nearly 1 in 3 children comes down with it before the age of five), is almost always a mild disease (often with no notable symptoms), and is not known to be passed on to a fetus or newborn. So even if you did catch it, it should not affect your pregnancy. Still, you're better off not contracting an infection of any kind. Since hepatitis A is passed by the fecal-oral route, be sure to wash your hands after changing diapers or taking your young charges to the bathroom, as well as before eating. You might also ask your physician about immunization against hepatitis A.

"Is hepatitis B contagious? My husband came down with a case of it, which is strange because he isn't in a high-risk category."

It's not really so strange. While about 6 in 10 hepatitis B victims fall into the so-called high-risk categories,[9] 1 in 3

9. At highest risk of hepatitis B, which is transmitted through blood and body fluids, are IV drug users, homosexual men, and heterosexuals with more than one partner in a six-month period. Also at risk are health care workers and immigrants from China, Southeast Asia, and other high-prevalence areas. Vaccination is available and is recommended for these groups.

cases occur in those with no known risk factors. These cases may be caused by eating contaminated food, swimming in contaminated water, or by other means unrelated to high-risk behaviors.

Since this liver infection, which is most common during the childbearing years of fifteen to thirty-nine, can be passed from mother to fetus, it's of concern to expectant parents. And since it can be transmitted through the kind of contact husbands and wives typically share (including the sexual kind), it's of particular concern to you. The first thing you want to find out is whether or not you have already been infected. Since hepatitis B may be so mild that no symptoms are noted, or only nausea and vomiting, which are common in pregnancy anyway (other possible symptoms include yellowing of the skin or whites of the eyes, light clay-colored stools, extreme fatigue, abdominal pain, and loss of appetite), you probably won't be able to ascertain this without testing. It is recommended that all pregnant women be tested for hepatitis B. If you haven't been, or if you were tested before your husband's illness was diagnosed, you should be now.

If you test negative, it's time for you and your partner to take precautions against your becoming infected: no sharing of drinks, toothbrushes, razors, or other personal items, and no sexual intercourse (condoms are not completely protective). And ask your doctor about immunization, which is safe during pregnancy—but since the vaccine doesn't provide complete protection immediately, you'll need to take the other precautions, too. If there are unimmunized older children or other adults living in your household, they, too, may be given preventive shots to forestall infection.

If you test positive, treatment consisting of bed rest and a nutritious diet (high in protein and calories, with no alcoholic beverages) will be started. Your blood will be checked periodically to monitor the progress of the disease. In 95 percent of cases, full recovery can be expected.

Since hepatitis B is passed on to the baby during delivery, it is important to take prompt steps to protect your child if the virus is present in your system at that time. Bathing the newborn as soon as possible to remove all traces of your blood as well as other secretions, and administering hepatitis B vaccine (which is routine at birth anyway) and immune globulin within twelve hours of birth, usually prevent the infection from taking

hold in the baby. Vaccination is repeated at one or two months and then again at six months, and the child is usually tested at twelve to fifteen months to be sure that the therapy has been effective.

Other forms of hepatitis may also be a problem. Hepatitis C can be transmitted from infected mother to child, probably in the uterus rather than during delivery. The rate of transmission is low—about 3 to 4 percent. And since hep C is usually transmitted via blood (for instance, through illegal drug injections or past transfusions), most women are unlikely to be infected. The infection, if diagnosed, can often be treated.

What It's Important to Know: STAYING WELL

In pregnancy, because of the potentially harmful effects of both illness and some medications on the unborn baby, the proverbial ounce of prevention is worth far more than a pound of cure. The following suggestions will increase your odds of staying well, whether you're pregnant or not.

Immunize. See page 40.

Keep your resistance up. Eat the best diet possible; get enough sleep and adequate exercise; and don't run yourself down by running yourself ragged. Reducing stress in your life as much as you can will also help keep your immune system in tiptop shape.

Avoid sick people. Try to stay away from anyone who has a cold, flu, stomach virus, or anything else noticeably contagious. Distance yourself from coughers on the bus, avoid lunching with a colleague who's complaining of a sore throat, and evade the handshake of a

friend with a runny nose (germs as well as greetings can be exchanged in a handshake). Also avoid crowded or cramped indoor spaces when you can.

Wash your hands. Hands are the major spreader of infections, so wash them often and thoroughly with soap and warm water for ten to twenty seconds, particularly after exposure to someone you know is sick, and after spending time in public places or riding on public transportation. Handwashing is especially important before eating. Keep a waterless hand sanitizer in your handbag so that you can wash up when there's no sink in sight.

Keep your distance. At home, limit contact with sick children or a sick spouse as much as possible (have other family members, a sitter, or a nonpregnant friend play nursemaid). Avoid finishing up their lunches, drinking from their cups, and kissing them on the face. Wash your hands after any contact with the patients, their linens, or soiled tissues, especially before touching your own eyes, nose, or mouth. See that they wash their hands frequently, too, and try to get them to cover their mouths when they cough or sneeze. Use disinfectant spray or wipes, such as Lysol, on telephones and other surfaces they handle. Isolate contaminated toothbrushes.

If your own child or a child you regularly spend time with develops a rash of any kind, avoid close contact and call your doctor at once unless you already know that you are immune to rubella (German measles), chicken pox, fifth disease, and CMV (cytomegalovirus).

Be pet wise. Keep pets in good health, updating their immunizations as necessary. If you have a cat, take the precautions to avoid toxoplasmosis (page 67).

Watch out for Lyme. Avoid outdoor areas where Lyme disease is prevalent, or be sure to protect yourself adequately (see page 464).

Don't share. That includes toothbrushes or other personal items. Use disposable cups for rinsing in the bathroom.

Eat safe. To avoid food-borne illnesses, practice safe food preparation and storage habits (see page 150).

◆ ◆ ◆

CHAPTER 19

Coping with a Chronic Condition

Anyone who's lived with a chronic condition knows that life can get pretty complicated, what with special diets, medications, and medical monitoring. Anyone who's lived with a chronic condition while being pregnant knows that those complications can double, with the special diet needing to be modified, medications altered, and medical monitoring stepped up.

In the past there was another complication for women with chronic conditions who became pregnant: major risk to themselves and their babies. Today,

happily, that complication is much less common. Thanks to many scientific advances, most chronic conditions are now completely compatible with pregnancy. Still, special precautions are necessary on the part of both the mother-to-be and her medical providers. This chapter outlines those precautions for the most common chronic conditions. Where the recommendations in this chapter differ from those issued by your doctor, be sure to follow doctor's orders, since they probably have been tailored to your personal needs.

What You May Be Concerned About

ASTHMA

"I've been an asthmatic since childhood. I'm concerned that the attacks and the drugs I take for them might harm my baby."

While it's true that a severe asthmatic condition does put a pregnancy at

higher risk, studies have shown that this risk can be almost completely eliminated. Asthmatics who are under close, expert medical supervision (preferably by their internist and/or allergist in collaboration with their obstetrician) throughout their pregnancies have about as good a chance of having normal pregnancies and healthy babies as nonasthmatics. But while asthma, if well controlled, has only a minimal effect on pregnancy, pregnancy can have an effect on asthma—though the effect varies from woman to woman. For about one-third of pregnant asthmatics, the effect is positive—their asthma improves. For another third, their condition stays about the same. For the remaining third (usually those with the most severe disease), the asthma worsens, generally after the 24th week of pregnancy. If you've been pregnant before, you're likely to find that your asthma behaves the same way in this pregnancy as it did in earlier ones.

Whether your asthma is mild or severe, you and your baby will benefit if you get the condition under control before conception or at least early in pregnancy. The following steps will help:

♦ If you smoke, quit immediately. See page 61 for how-to tips.

♦ Identify environmental triggers. Allergies are the major cause of asthma in the peak childbearing years. (See Allergies, page 188, for tips on avoiding allergens.) If you were started on allergy shots before pregnancy, this treatment will probably be continued. If necessary, this type of therapy may be initiated during pregnancy. The most common asthma-triggering offenders are pollens, animal danders (you may need to board your pet at a friend's), dust, and molds. Tobacco smoke, household cleaning products, and perfumes can also provoke a reaction, and it's a good idea to steer clear of them. Attacks can also be brought on by exercise; these can usually be prevented by taking prescribed medication before your workout or any other kind of exertion.

♦ Try to avoid colds, flu, and other respiratory infections, which are also asthma triggers. Your doctor may give you medication to ward off an asthma attack at the beginning of a cold, and will probably want to treat any but the most minor respiratory infections with antibiotics. You should also be immunized against influenza and pneumococcal infections.

♦ If you suffer from sinusitis or gastroesophageal reflux, both of which are more common in pregnancy, be sure these conditions are treated, since they can interfere with the management of your asthma.

♦ Monitor your breathing with a peak-flow meter, according to your physician's directions.

♦ Use only medications that have been prescribed by your physician during your pregnancy, and take them only as prescribed for pregnancy use. If your symptoms are mild, you may not require medication. If they are moderate to severe, there are several medications that are considered "probably safe" for the fetus. In most cases, inhaled medications appear to be safer than those taken by mouth. The risks, if any, of taking these medications are quite small compared to the benefits: a good supply of oxygen for you and your baby.

♦ If you have an asthma attack, treat it immediately with your prescribed medication, to avoid depriving the fetus of oxygen. If the medication doesn't help, call your doctor or head for the nearest emergency room immediately.

An asthma attack may trigger early uterine contractions, but the contractions usually stop when the attack does. If the contractions continue, you will receive prompt treatment to try to stop them.

Because of your history of breathing problems, you may find the normal breathlessness that afflicts a majority of women in late pregnancy (see page 286) alarming. But be assured that it is not dangerous. However, in the last trimester, as breathing becomes more labored because of the enlarged uterus crowding the lungs, you may notice a worsening of asthmatic flare-ups. Prompt treatment is especially important during such attacks.

Most women with asthma seem to be able to handle the breathing techniques of Lamaze and other childbirth education methods. While asthma flare-ups during delivery are rare, it is usually recommended that you continue your regular medications when you're in labor; if your asthma has been serious enough to require oral steroids or cortisone-type medications, you may also require IV steroids to help you handle the stress of labor and delivery. Your oxygenation will be checked when you are admitted to the hospital, and if it is low, preventive medications may be given. An epidural may be administered, since it reduces oxygen consumption; narcotic analgesia will probably be avoided because it may stimulate histamine release and thus an asthma attack. Though some babies of moms with asthma experience rapid breathing after delivery, the condition is only temporary.

The tendency toward allergies and asthma is inherited, and so it would be wise for you to postpone exposing your baby, once he or she arrives, to potential food allergens by breastfeeding *exclusively*—without adding formula or solids—for at least six months.[1] This may delay the onset of allergic sensitization in your child and possibly reduce the long-term risk of allergy.

As for your asthma, chances are you'll find your symptoms will return to the way they were prepregnancy (whether that's for the better or the worse) within three months of delivery.

DIABETES

"I'm a diabetic. How will that affect my baby?"

A generation ago, getting pregnant was a risky business for the diabetic woman, and even riskier for her unborn baby. Today, with expert medical care and guidance *and* scrupulous self-care, the diabetic woman has the same excellent chances of having a successful pregnancy and a healthy baby as any other pregnant woman does. In fact, diabetic women in one study took such good care of themselves throughout their pregnancies that they and their babies had even fewer problems than their nondiabetic counterparts.

Research has proven that the key to successfully managing a diabetic pregnancy—whether the diabetes is type 1 or type 2—is achieving normal blood glucose levels before conception and maintaining them throughout the nine months following it. The availability in the past few years of home monitoring, split-dose administration of insulin, and even under-the-skin insulin pumps has made this increasingly possible.

Whether you came into pregnancy diabetic or developed gestational diabetes along the way, all of the following considerations will be important in working toward a safe pregnancy and a healthy baby:

The right doctor. The doctor who supervises your pregnancy should have plenty of experience and past success caring for diabetic mothers-to-be, and should work together with the doctor who has been in charge of your diabetes.

---

1. Continue to breastfeed for at least a year, if possible.

Additional support. Your treatment is likely to be most successful if a nutritionist and a nurse educator join your pregnancy team, both for the information they can offer and for the support they can provide. Support can also come from your spouse, other children (if any), friends, and extended family.

Doctor's orders. You will probably see your obstetrician (as well as your internist or endocrinologist) more often than other expectant moms do. You'll have more doctor's orders to follow, too, and you will have to be far more scrupulous in following them.

Good diet. A diet geared to your personal requirements should be carefully planned with your physician, a nutritionist, and/or a nurse-practitioner with expertise in diabetes. The diet will probably be high in complex carbohydrates, particularly beans (about half your daily calories should be from carbohydrates), moderate in protein (20 percent of caloric intake), low in cholesterol and fat (30 percent of caloric intake, no more than 10 percent saturated), and contain few or no sugary sweets. Plenty of dietary fiber will be important (40 to 70 grams daily are recommended), since some studies show that fiber may reduce insulin requirements in diabetic pregnancies. Your caloric requirement, like that of other pregnant women, will increase by about 300 a day over what you needed prepregnancy (unless you're overweight, in which case your doctor may recommend that you increase it somewhat less).

Carbohydrate regulation is typically not as rigid as it used to be, since fast-acting insulin can be adjusted if you go over your limit at one meal or another. Still, the extent of your carbohydrate restriction will depend on the way your body reacts to particular foods. Some women can handle fruit and fruit juices; others get sharp blood sugar increases

from them, in which case they have to get more of their carbohydrates from vegetable, grain, and legume sources than from fruits. To maintain normal blood sugar levels, you will have to be particularly careful to get enough carbohydrates in the morning. Snacks will also be important, and ideally they should include both a complex carbohydrate (such as whole-grain bread) and a protein (such as beans or cheese or meat). Skipping meals or snacks can dangerously lower blood sugar, so be sure to eat on schedule, even if morning sickness or other pregnancy miseries are putting a damper on your appetite. Eating six to eight mini-meals a day, regularly spaced, carefully planned, and supplemented as needed by healthy snacks, is your best bet.

Perfecting dietary control in a diabetic pregnancy is so important that many specialists recommend in-hospital training for diabetic women prior to conception or early in pregnancy. In some cases, in-hospital training may also be recommended for women who develop diabetes as pregnancy progresses (see Gestational Diabetes, page 499).

Sensible weight gain. It's best to try to reach your ideal weight before conception (something to remember if you plan another pregnancy). But if you start your pregnancy overweight, don't plan on using the gestational period for slimming down. Getting sufficient calories is vital to your baby's well-being. Weight gain should progress according to the guidelines set by your physician. Sometimes babies of diabetics grow very large, even if their mothers don't gain excessively. Your baby's growth will be carefully monitored using ultrasound.

Exercise. A moderate exercise program, especially for women with type 2 diabetes, will give you more energy, aid in regulating your blood sugar, and help you get in shape for delivery. But it must be planned in conjunction with your medication schedule and diet plan by, or with the help of, your medical team. If you experience no other medical or pregnancy complications and are physically fit, moderate exercise such as brisk walking, swimming, and light stationary biking (but not jogging) will likely be suggested. Chances are only very light exercise (such as leisurely walking) will be allowed if you were out of condition prior to pregnancy or if there are any signs of problems with your diabetes, your pregnancy, or your baby's growth.

Precautions you may be asked to observe when exercising include taking a snack, such as milk, before your workout; not allowing your heart rate (pulse) during exercise to exceed 70 percent of the maximum safe heart rate for your age (see box on the facing page); and never exercising in a warm environment (80°F or higher). If you are on insulin, you will probably be advised to avoid injecting insulin into the parts of the body being exercised (your legs, for example, if you're walking) and not to reduce your insulin intake prior to exercise.

Rest. Especially in the third trimester, adequate rest is very important. Avoid overtaxing your energies, and try to take some time off during the middle of the day for putting your feet up or napping. If you have a job, especially a demanding one, your doctor may recommend that you begin your maternity leave early.

Medication regulation. If diet and exercise alone do not control your blood sugar, you will probably be put on insulin. If you had been taking oral medication for diabetes prior to conception, you might be switched to injected insulin or an under-the-skin insulin pump for the duration of your pregnancy. If you need insulin for the first time, you may be hospitalized briefly so that your blood

sugar can be stabilized under close medical supervision. Since levels of the pregnancy hormones that work against insulin increase as pregnancy progresses, your insulin dose may have to be adjusted upward periodically. The dose may also have to be recalculated as you and your baby gain weight, if you are ill or under emotional strain, or if you overdo your carbs. New studies show that the oral drug glyburide is an effective alternative to insulin therapy during pregnancy.

In addition to being sure your diabetes medication is on target, you will want to be extremely careful about any other medications you take. A great many over-the-counter drugs can affect your insulin levels—and some may not be safe in pregnancy—so do not take *any* until you check with both the physician who is overseeing your diabetes and the one taking care of your pregnancy.

Blood sugar regulation. You may have to test your blood sugar (with a simple finger-prick method) at least four or as often as ten times a day (possibly before and after meals) to be sure it is remaining at safe levels. Your blood may also be tested for "glycosylated hemoglobin" (hemoglobin A1c), since research has indicated that high levels of this substance are a sign of poorly controlled sugar levels. To maintain normal blood glucose levels, you will have to eat regularly (again, no meal skipping), adjust your diet and exercise as needed, and, if necessary, take medication. If you were insulin dependent before pregnancy, you may be more subject to low blood sugar episodes (hypoglycemia) than when you were not pregnant, especially in the first trimester—and so careful monitoring is a must.

In the future, another approach to normalizing blood sugar may become standard therapy in pregnancy: transplantation of pancreatic islet cells.

Urine monitoring. Since your body may produce ketones—acidic substances that may result when the body breaks down fat—during this close regulation of your diabetes, your urine may be checked for these regularly.

Careful monitoring. Don't be concerned if your physician orders a great many tests for you (in and out of the hospital), especially during the third trimester, or even suggests hospitalization for the final weeks of your pregnancy. This doesn't mean something is wrong, only that he or she wants to be sure that everything stays right. The tests will primarily be directed toward regular evaluation of your condition and of your baby, in order to determine the optimal time for delivery and whether any other intervention is needed.

You will probably have regular eye exams to check the condition of your retinas and blood tests to evaluate your kidneys (retinal and kidney problems tend to worsen during pregnancy, but usually return to prepregnancy status after delivery). The condition of your baby and the placenta will probably be evaluated through stress and/or nonstress tests (see page 324), biophysical profiles, amniocentesis (to determine lung maturity and readiness for delivery), and ultrasound (to size up your baby to be sure it's growing as it should be and so that delivery can be accomplished before he or she is too big for vaginal delivery).

After the 28th week, you may be asked to monitor fetal movements yourself three times a day (see page 243 for one way to do this, or follow your doctor's recommendation). If you don't feel movement during any test period, call your doctor immediately.

Because there is a higher risk of preeclampsia for diabetics, it is also important to be aware of the symptoms of this condition (see page 500) and to report them to the doctor immediately if you experience any of them.

Elective early delivery. Because babies of many diabetics tend to grow too large for full-term vaginal delivery (particularly when normal blood sugar levels have not been maintained throughout pregnancy); because their placentas often begin to deteriorate early (robbing the fetus of vital nutrients and oxygen during the last weeks); and because they are subject to acidosis (abnormal acid-base balance in the blood) and other problems, they are often delivered a week or two before term, generally at about 38 or 39 weeks. The various tests mentioned above help the physician decide when to induce labor or perform a cesarean—late enough so that the fetal lungs are sufficiently mature to function outside the womb, not so late that fetal safety has been jeopardized. Women who developed gestational diabetes, as well as women with preexisting

SAFE EXERCISE HEART RATE FOR DIABETIC PREGNANCIES

Exercise is generally safe and healthful if you're a pregnant diabetic, as long as you're careful not to overdo. It's usually recommended that pregnant women with diabetes not exercise beyond 70 percent of the maximum safe heart rate for their age group. You can determine this rate by subtracting your age from 220, then multiplying the result by .70. If you're 30, for example, you would figure it this way: $220 - 30 = 190$; then $190 \times .70 = 133$. This means that 133 beats per minute would be your upper safe limit of exercise intensity, the level you should not exceed.

mild diabetes and sometimes even those with very well controlled moderate disease, can often carry to term safely.

Don't worry if your baby is placed in a neonatal intensive care unit immediately after delivery. This is routine procedure in most hospitals for infants of diabetic mothers. Your baby will be observed for respiratory problems (which are unlikely if the lungs were tested and found to be mature enough for delivery) and for hypoglycemia (which, though more common in babies of diabetics, responds quickly and completely to treatment).

CHRONIC HYPERTENSION

"I've had hypertension for years. How will my high blood pressure affect my pregnancy?"

Since increasing numbers of women are choosing to conceive in their thirties and forties, and hypertension (high blood pressure) is more common as one gets older, the condition is showing up in more and more pregnant women. (And for reasons not completely understood, it's even more common in African American women.) So you're not alone. Still, yours is considered a high-risk pregnancy, which means that you will be seeing your doctor or doctors more often (preferably beginning with prepregnancy counseling), and will have to follow their advice more faithfully. But assuming that your blood pressure remains under control, with good medical and self-care it is very likely that both you and your baby will come through pregnancy well.

All of the following can help increase the odds of a successful pregnancy:

The right doctors. The doctor who supervises your pregnancy should have plenty of experience caring for mothers-to-be with chronic hypertension, and should be joined on your pregnancy care team by the doctor who has been in charge of your hypertension.

Relaxation. Pay more than just passing attention to the kinds of relaxation exercises mentioned on page 127. Studies have shown that relaxation can help lower high blood pressure.

Other alternative approaches. Try any that are recommended by your physician, such as biofeedback.

Blood pressure monitoring. You may be advised to take your own blood pressure daily, using a home blood pressure kit. Take it when you are most rested and relaxed.

Good diet. The Pregnancy Diet should be modified with the help of your physician to fit your needs. Moderating your sodium intake and eating plenty of fruits and vegetables, low-fat or no-fat dairy products, and grains may be especially helpful in keeping your blood pressure down.

Adequate fluid. Though your first impulse on experiencing a slight swelling of your feet and ankles may be to cut down on your fluid intake, it's wise to do just the opposite. Drinking more water (up to a gallon a day), rather than less, will help flush out the excess. (But don't drink more than 2 cups—16 ounces—at a time.) In most cases, a diuretic (a drug that draws fluid from the body) is not recommended during pregnancy.

Plenty of rest. Take rest breaks, preferably with your feet up, both morning and afternoon. If you work at a high-stress job, consider giving it up or cutting down on hours or responsibilities until after the baby arrives. If you have your hands full at home with other children, get help, paid or volunteer.

Prescribed medication. If you have been taking medication to control your blood pressure, your physician may okay your continuing it, or may prescribe one that is considered to be safer in pregnancy. There are several blood-pressure-regulating drugs that appear to be safe when taken as directed and others that are not recommended.

Attention to your body. Be alert to signs of a pregnancy problem (see page 130), and contact your physician immediately if you experience any of them.

Close medical monitoring. Your physician will probably schedule more frequent visits for you than for other expectant mothers, and may subject you to many more tests. Recent studies show that even those hypertensive women who have some kidney impairment can usually have successful pregnancies, assuming that good medical care is in place. But protein in the urine early in pregnancy and the development of preeclampsia (see page 500) are predictors of possible complications for both mother and baby.

If your blood pressure is very high and remains high in spite of medication, and/or you have serious side effects, such as retinal hemorrhages, severely impaired kidney function, or an enlarged heart, the risks of an unfavorable outcome to your pregnancy increase. In such a case, you may, in consultation with your physicians, have to weigh risks against benefits before deciding to attempt a pregnancy or continue with one already under way.

CORONARY ARTERY DISEASE (CAD)

"My doctor warned me not to get pregnant because I have coronary artery disease. But I did accidentally, and I don't want to abort. My husband and I want this baby more than anything."

Your situation isn't as unique as it once might have been. Coronary artery disease (CAD), which is seen more often as women grow older, is becoming more common in pregnancy as more women opt to have their babies at a later age.

Whether or not it's safe for you to continue your pregnancy depends on the nature of your condition. If the disease is mild (you have no limitations on physical activity, and ordinary activity doesn't cause undue fatigue, palpitations, breathlessness, or angina) or moderate (you have slight limitations on physical activity, are completely comfortable at rest, but do experience symptoms with ordinary physical activity), chances are good that you can, under very close medical supervision, safely carry a pregnancy to term. If your disease is severe (you have marked limitations on physical activity, and even very light activity causes symptoms, though you are comfortable at rest) or very severe (any physical activity causes discomfort, and symptoms are noted even at rest), your doctor will probably tell you that carrying this baby will put your life at risk.

If your cardiologist believes you can weather pregnancy safely, you will probably be given some very strict instructions. They will vary depending on your condition, but you may be told to:

◆ Avoid physical and emotional stress. You may be asked to limit your activities for the duration of your pregnancy, possibly even go on bed rest.

◆ Take your medications faithfully (you'll be switched to ones that are safe for your baby; many are).

◆ Watch your diet carefully so that you don't gain excess weight, which can put additional strain on your heart.

♦ Eat a low-cholesterol, low-saturated-fat, low-overall-fat diet if your condition requires it, but not a fat-free diet; some fat is essential for healthy fetal development. Moderate sodium restriction (about 2,000 milligrams a day) is usually recommended, but greater restriction is not. An iron supplement is generally prescribed.

♦ Wear pressure-graded support panty hose, to help reduce the pooling of blood in your legs.

♦ Quit smoking—a recommendation for all pregnant women.

Toward the end of your pregnancy, you are likely to undergo frequent ultrasound scans and nonstress tests, so that the physician can keep a close eye on your baby's condition. The tests will also help assure you that everything is okay.

If you pass through pregnancy without heart or lung complications, you're not likely to encounter problems during labor and delivery. Nor are you more likely to need a cesarean than other mothers.

THYROID DISEASE

"I was diagnosed as being hypothyroid when I was a teenager and am still taking thyroid hormone. Is this safe for the baby I'm carrying?"

It's not only safe, it's crucial to continue taking your medication One reason is that women with untreated hypothyroidism (a condition in which the thyroid gland does not produce adequate amounts of the hormone thyroxine) are more likely to miscarry. Another reason is that thyroid hormones are necessary for fetal brain development; babies who don't get enough of these hormones in

utero can be born with problems such as retardation, brain damage, and, possibly, deafness (if there is inadequate thyroxine before hearing is developed in the fetus). Your dose, however, may need to be adjusted, since pregnancy affects the function of the thyroid gland. Check with your endocrinologist and your obstetrician to be sure your dose is appropriate.

Iodine deficiency, which is becoming more common among women of childbearing age in the United States, can interfere with the production of thyroid hormone, so be sure you are getting adequate amounts of this trace mineral. It's most commonly found in iodized salt and seafood.

"I have Graves disease. Is this a problem for my pregnancy?"

Graves disease is the most common form of *hyper*thyroidism, a condition in which the thyroid gland produces excessive amounts of thyroid hormones. Hyperthyroidism can also be caused by growths on the thyroid gland or an enlarged thyroid gland (goiter), excessive thyroid medication or iodine excess (since the thyroid gland uses iodine to produce hormones), and thyroiditis (a temporary inflammation of the thyroid gland). Sometimes, human chorionic gonadotropin (hCG), a hormone produced in large quantities early in pregnancy, can trigger mild hyperthyroidism, which may not need to be treated.

Mild cases of hyperthyroidism sometimes improve during pregnancy, since the pregnant body requires more thyroid hormone than usual. But moderate to severe hyperthyroidism is a different story. Left untreated, these conditions could lead to serious complications for both you and your baby, so appropriate treatment is necessary. For the unpregnant, there are three forms of treatment for Graves disease: surgery to reduce the thyroid (thyroidectomy), the use of radioactive iodine, and the administration of antithyroid medications. For the pregnant woman, the treatment of choice is the antithyroid medication propylthiouracil (PTU) in the lowest effective dose. If a woman is allergic to PTU, methimazole (Tapazole) may be used. If neither drug can be used, then surgery may be needed. Radioactive iodine is not safe during pregnancy, but organic iodine might be helpful for a short period of time just prior to surgery, to slow the production of thyroxine. In addition to treatment, you should be certain not to smoke (see page 61 if you need help quitting) and to try to minimize stress (see page 125), since both smoking and stress are risk factors for Graves disease.

AN EATING DISORDER

"I've been fighting bulimia for the last ten years. I thought I'd be able to stop the bingeing/purging cycle now that I'm pregnant, but I can't seem to. Will it hurt my baby?"

Not if you get help right away. The fact that you've been bulimic (or anorexic) for a number of years puts your baby and your body at a disadvantage right off the bat—your nutritional reserves are probably low. Fortunately, early in pregnancy the need for nourishment is less than it will be later on, so you have the chance to make up for the abuse done to your body before it can hurt your baby.

There has been very little research in the area of eating disorders and pregnancy, partly because these disorders cause disrupted menstrual cycles, reducing the number of women who suffer with these problems becoming pregnant in the first place. But the studies that have been done suggest the following:

- A pregnant woman with an eating disorder *who gets help with getting it under control* is as likely as anyone else to have a healthy baby, all other things being equal.

- It is critical that the practitioner who is caring for the pregnancy be informed of the eating disorder.

- Counseling from a professional who is experienced in treating eating disorders is advisable for anyone who suffers from such a problem, but it is essential for the woman who is pregnant. Support groups may also be helpful.

- The laxatives, diuretics, and other drugs taken by bulimics are harmful to a developing fetus if the mother continues taking them once she learns she's pregnant. They draw off nutrients and fluids from the mother's body before they can be utilized to nourish her baby (and later to produce milk); and they may lead to fetal abnormality if used on a regular basis. These medications, like all others, should not be used by any pregnant woman unless prescribed by a physician who is aware of the pregnancy.

It is also clear that it is necessary for you, and anyone else with an eating disorder, to understand the dynamics of weight gain in pregnancy. Keep in mind:

- The pregnant shape is healthy and beautiful. Pregnancy weight gain is vital to your baby's growth and well-being as well as to your own health.

- Gaining a moderate amount of weight each week in the second and third trimesters of pregnancy is not only normal, it's necessary (see page 169). If you stay within the recommended guidelines (which are higher in those who begin pregnancy underweight; check with your practitioner if you are underweight), you will be able to lose all the weight easily after the baby arrives.

◆ If the weight is gained on high-quality foods, as recommended in the Pregnancy Diet, the chances of having a healthy baby increase considerably, as do the chances that you'll recover your figure faster postpartum.

◆ Exercise can help avoid excessive weight gain, and can ensure that the pounds added end up in the right places—but it should be exercise that is appropriate for a pregnant woman (see page 190).

◆ All of the weight gain of pregnancy won't drop off in the first few days after delivery. With sensible eating, the average woman returns to *close* to—but does not hit—her prepregnancy weight about six weeks after delivery. Getting *all* the weight off and getting back into shape (which requires exercise) can take much longer. For this reason, many women with eating disorders find that negative feelings about their body image causes them to slip back into bingeing and purging or starving during the postpartum period.

This is particularly common with women who had an unplanned pregnancy, gestational diabetes, or postpartum depression. Since this kind of behavior could interfere with your ability to recover from childbirth, to parent effectively, and to produce milk if you choose to breastfeed, it's important that you continue professional counseling postpartum with someone experienced in the treatment of eating disorders or get help if you hadn't previously.

If you can't seem to refrain from bingeing, vomiting, using diuretics or laxatives, or practicing semi-starvation during pregnancy, you should discuss with your physician the possibility of hospitalization until you get your disease under control.

SYSTEMIC LUPUS ERYTHEMATOSUS (SLE)

"My lupus has been pretty quiet lately. I just became pregnant. Is this likely to bring on a flare-up? Will my baby get lupus?"

There's a lot that's still unknown about systemic lupus erythematosus (SLE), an autoimmune disease that affects primarily women between the ages of fifteen and sixty-four, black women more often than white. The studies that have been done seem to indicate that pregnancy doesn't affect the long-term course of lupus. During pregnancy itself, some women find that their condition improves, other women find it worsens. More confusing still, what happens in one pregnancy doesn't necessarily predict what will happen in subsequent ones. In the postpartum period, there does appear to be an increased risk of flare-ups across the board.

Whether and how SLE affects pregnancy, however, isn't absolutely clear. It does seem that the women who do best are those who, like you, conceive during a quiet period in their disease. Though their risk of pregnancy loss is slightly increased, their chances of having a healthy baby are excellent. Those with the poorest prognosis are women with SLE who have severe kidney impairment (ideally, kidney function should be stable for at least six months before conception) or who have what is called the "lupus anticoagulant" in their blood. No matter what the severity of a pregnant woman's lupus, it is extremely unlikely that her baby would be born with the disease.

If needed for arthritic symptoms or by women with the lupus anticoagulant, and if taken at the lowest effective doses, both daily doses of aspirin and the steroid prednisone seem to be helpful. Many other steroids are also safe to use in pregnancy—some because they don't cross the placenta. Even some that do cross the placenta are safe, and some may actually benefit the fetus by hastening lung maturity.

Because of your lupus, your pregnancy care will be more complicated than most, with more, and more frequent, tests and possibly more limitations. But if you, your obstetrician or maternal-fetal medicine specialist, and the physician who treats your lupus all work together, the odds are very much in favor of a happy outcome that will make it all worthwhile.

RHEUMATOID ARTHRITIS

"I have rheumatoid arthritis. How will this affect my pregnancy?"

Your condition isn't likely to affect your pregnancy very much, but pregnancy is likely to affect your condition—and for the better. Many women with rheumatoid arthritis notice a significant decrease in the pain and swelling in their joints during pregnancy, though there is also a somewhat greater risk of symptom flare-up in the postpartum period.

The greatest change you may experience while you're pregnant is in the management of your condition. Since some of the medicines used to treat rheumatoid arthritis (such as ibuprofen and naproxen) are not safe for use during pregnancy, your physician will need to switch you over to treatments that are safe, such as steroids. Women who use steroids during pregnancy will

be given IV steroids during labor and delivery.

During labor and delivery, it will be important to choose positions that do not put undue stress or strain on affected joints. Discuss with the physician who manages your arthritis as well as with your practitioner which positions might work best.

MULTIPLE SCLEROSIS (MS)

"I was diagnosed several years ago as having multiple sclerosis. I've only had two episodes of MS, and they were relatively mild. Will the MS affect my pregnancy? Will my pregnancy affect my MS?"

The news is good for you and your baby. Multiple sclerosis appears to have little, if any, effect on pregnancy. Still, early and regular prenatal care, coupled with regular visits to your neurologist, is a must. Some extra precautions will be necessary, too. Iron supplements will probably be prescribed to prevent anemia and, if needed, stool softeners to combat constipation. Because urinary tract infections are more common in pregnancy, and because they could cause MS symptoms to flare, you may be given antibiotics as a preventive measure if you have a history of UTIs. Labor and delivery are not usually affected by MS, either. Epidural anesthesia, if needed and desired, appears to be safe for use during both.

Also, pregnancy doesn't seem to have much effect on MS, particularly over the long term. In general, there are fewer relapses during pregnancy, followed by an increased risk of relapse postpartum, then a return to the prepregnancy level after about three to six months. Some women with gait problems, however, find that as weight gain increases during pregnancy, walking becomes more difficult. Avoiding excessive weight gain may help minimize this problem.

Though the risk of relapse postpartum doesn't appear to affect the overall lifetime relapse rate or the extent of ultimate disability, it's possible to reduce the risk even further. To do this, take your iron supplements as prescribed, try to minimize stress, and get adequate rest. Also try to avoid infection of any kind and the fever that often accompanies it, and avoid raising your temperature in other ways (through strenuous exercise or in a hot tub, for example). Going back to work early in the postpartum period may increase both exhaustion and stress, so discuss this possibility with your doctor before deciding when to return.

Pregnancy can, however, affect MS treatment. While low to moderate doses of prednisone are considered safe to use, some other medications used for MS may not be. Be sure to have your doctor check out the safety for use in pregnancy of any medication before you take it. Women who take significant doses of prednisone prenatally may need to be given steroids in labor to best handle the stress of delivery. After delivery, breastfeeding will be possible, even if you occasionally need to take steroid medication; in small doses, very little of the drug passes into the breast milk. An added benefit: It appears that breastfeeding does not increase attacks. If you have to take large doses temporarily, you can pump your milk and discard it, giving your baby formula or previously pumped milk until the drug is gone from your milk. If breastfeeding is stressful for you, and you have to switch to bottle feeding partially or completely, don't feel guilty about your decision. Babies can thrive on a good formula and always do best when Mom's feeling well.

Most MS mothers manage to stay active for twenty-five years or more after the condition is diagnosed, and are able to carry out parenting without difficulty.

However, if MS does interfere with your functioning while your child is young, see the next question for tips on baby care for parents with disabilities.[2]

PHYSICAL DISABILITY

"I'm a paraplegic because of a spinal cord injury, and I'm confined to a wheelchair. My husband and I have wanted a baby for a long while, and I've finally become pregnant. Now what?"

Like every pregnant woman, you'll need to deal with first things first: selecting a practitioner. And as for every pregnant woman who falls into a high-risk category, your practitioner should ideally be an obstetrician or maternal-fetal medicine specialist who has experience dealing with women who face the same challenges as you do. That may be easier to find than you'd think, since a growing number of hospitals are developing special programs to provide women with physical limitations better prenatal and obstetrical care. If such a program or practitioner isn't available in your area, you need a doctor who is willing to learn "on the job," and who is able to offer the wholehearted support you and your spouse will need. Toward the end of your pregnancy you will also have to start looking for a pediatrician or family doctor who will be supportive of you as a physically challenged parent.

Just which special measures will be necessary to make your pregnancy successful will depend on your physical limitations. In any case, restricting your

---

2. Many women with MS are concerned about passing the disease on to their children. Though there is a genetic component to the disease, placing these children at increased risk of being affected as adults, the risk is really quite small. Between 90 and 95 percent of children of MS mothers remain MS free. If you are concerned nevertheless, see a genetic counselor.

weight gain to within the recommended range (25 to 35 pounds) will help to minimize the stress on your body. Eating the best possible diet will improve your general physical well-being and decrease the likelihood of pregnancy complications. And keeping up your physical therapy will help ensure that you have maximum strength and mobility when the baby arrives; water therapy may be particularly helpful and safe.

It should be reassuring to know that, though pregnancy may be more difficult for you than for other pregnant women, it should not be any more stressful for your baby. And there is no evidence of an increase in fetal abnormality among babies of women with spinal cord injury (or of those with other physical disabilities not related to hereditary or systemic disease). Women with spinal cord injuries, however, are more susceptible to such pregnancy problems as kidney infections and bladder difficulties, palpitations and sweating, anemia, and muscle spasms. Childbirth, too, may pose special problems, though in most cases a vaginal delivery will be possible. Because uterine contractions will probably be painless, you will have to be instructed to note other signs of impending labor—such as rupture of the membranes—or you may be asked to palpate your uterus periodically to see if contractions have begun.

Long before your due date, devise a fail-safe plan for getting to the hospital, one that takes into account the fact that you may be home alone when labor strikes (you may want to plan to leave for the hospital early in labor to avoid any problems caused by delays en route). You'll also want to be sure the hospital staff is prepared for your special needs.

Parenting is always a challenge, particularly in the early weeks. It will be even more so for you and your husband. Planning ahead will help you meet this challenge more successfully. Make any necessary modifications to your home to make child care easier; sign on help (paid or otherwise) to at least get you started; enlist your spouse in the preparations for your baby's arrival, and divide up the household chores and baby care tasks for when baby comes home. Be creative. You don't have to do things "by the book"— do them in the way that works best for you. Breastfeeding, if it's possible, will make life simpler; you won't have to rush off to the kitchen to prepare a bottle when baby starts to cry, or shop for formula. A diaper service (they can deliver cloth or disposable diapers) will also save effort and time. The changing table should be tailored for you to use from your wheelchair, and the crib should have a drop side so you can take baby in and out easily. If you are going to be able to bathe baby, you will have to arrange a baby tub on an accessible table. Since daily tub baths aren't a must, you can sponge baby on the changing table or on your lap on alternate days. Or Dad can handle the baby bathing. A baby carrier may be a convenient way for you to tote your baby around, leaving your hands free to control your chair—though you may need help getting it on. (It may be helpful to have your spouse put it on you in the morning, which will allow you to take baby in and out of it as needed.) Joining a support group of parents with disabilities can be not only a source of comfort and strength but also a gold mine of ideas and advice.[3]

---

3. For more help, see *Mother-to-Be: A Guide to Pregnancy and Birth for Women with Disabilities,* by Judith Rogers and Maureen Matsumura (Demos Press). For preparing for baby, see *Adaptive Baby Care Equipment: Guidelines, Prototypes & Resources,* by Kris Vens, Judith Rogers, Christi Tuleja, and Anitra DeMoss (Through the Looking Glass). For parenting advice, call Through the Looking Glass at (800) 644-2666 (voice) or (800) 804-1616 (TTY) or online at www.lookingglass.org.

It won't be easy, for you or for your husband, who may have to be a more-than-equal partner in parenting. But knowing that you're not the first to do it—and that the vast majority of those who have done it before you have reported that the satisfactions are more than worth the struggles—should be reassuring.

EPILEPSY

"I'm epileptic, and I want desperately to have a baby. Is it safe to conceive?"

With the right precautions, your chances of having a healthy baby are excellent. Seeing an obstetrician now and getting your condition under the best control possible before conception is the first step. (For those who have already conceived, seeing the doctor as early in pregnancy as possible is, of course, crucial.) If you haven't already done so, inform the physician who cares for your epilepsy of your pregnancy plans; close supervision of your condition, and possibly frequent adjustment of medication levels, will be necessary, as will communication between your doctors.

Though mothers-to-be with epilepsy may be slightly more likely to experience excessive nausea and vomiting (hyperemesis), they aren't at higher risk for any serious complications of pregnancy and childbirth. There seems to be a slight increase in the incidence of certain birth defects in the children of epileptic mothers, but these appear to be more often caused by the use of certain anticonvulsant medications during pregnancy, rather than by the epilepsy itself. Discuss with your doctor ahead of time the possibility of being weaned from your medications prior to conception. This may be possible if you've been seizure-free for a period of time. If you have been having seizures, it's important to try to

get them under control, preferably immediately. You will need medication to do this, but it may be possible to switch to a less risky drug than the one you've been taking. Taking one drug appears to cause fewer problems in pregnancy than multidrug therapy, and is the preferred way to go. And it's important not to stop taking a necessary medication for fear of hurting your baby; not taking it—and having frequent seizures—may be more dangerous to your unborn child.[4]

Since the greatest risk of abnormalities developing exists during the first three months, there is less reason to worry about the effects of medication after that. Sometimes ultrasound or alpha-fetoprotein tests can determine early in pregnancy whether the fetus has been affected. If you've been taking valproic acid (Depakene), the doctor may want to look specifically for neural tube defects, such as spina bifida.

Important for all pregnant women with epilepsy is getting plenty of sleep and the best nutrition, and maintaining adequate fluid levels. Even with a good diet, however, women with epilepsy often develop folate-deficiency anemia (which research shows may be why their babies are at a slightly higher risk of developing neural tube defects). Taking a pregnancy supplement that contains folic acid will reduce that risk dramatically (though it may also occasionally increase the frequency of seizures in some women); ideally, the supplement should be started three months before conception. (Or if a surprise conception

---

4. To help future moms with epilepsy or yourself, ask your doctor about registering with the Antiepileptic Drug Pregnancy Registry (800) 233-2334 or on-line at aeregistry@helix.mgh. harvard.edu/aed/registry.nclk. Their goal is to determine which therapies are associated with an increased risk. You will also receive a packet of information about preconception planning and prenatal care.

made that impossible, as soon as you discover you're pregnant.) Vitamin D supplementation may also be recommended, since some medications can interfere with metabolism of the vitamin. During the last four weeks of pregnancy, a vitamin K supplement may be prescribed to reduce the risk of hemorrhage, another condition that babies of epileptic moms are at slightly greater risk for. Or, alternatively, the baby will be given an injection of the vitamin at birth.

Most women find that pregnancy does not exacerbate their epilepsy. Half experience no change in their disease, and a smaller percentage find that seizures become less frequent and milder. A few discover, however, that their seizures become more frequent and severe. This may be because of individual differences, or because medication has been vomited or overly diluted in the normally high fluid levels of pregnancy. Taking a time-release anticonvulsant before going to bed, which allows medication to build up in the system before vomiting begins in the morning, can often minimize the problem of losing medication via vomiting. If the problem is overdilution of the medication, a readjustment of the dosage may do the trick.

Labor and delivery aren't likely to be more complicated for you, though it is important that anticonvulsant medication continue to be administered during labor to minimize the risk of a seizure during delivery. Epidural anesthesia can be used to ease pain.

Breastfeeding your baby shouldn't be a problem, either. Most epilepsy medications pass into the breast milk in such low doses that they are unlikely to affect a nursing baby. But do check with your baby's doctor to be sure the specific medications you are taking are okay. And if your baby becomes unusually sleepy after nursing, report this to the doctor. A change in medication may be necessary.

PHENYLKETONURIA (PKU)

"I was born with PKU. My doctor let me get off a low-phenylalanine diet when I was in my teens, and I was fine. But when I discussed getting pregnant, my obstetrician said I should go back on the diet three months before conception and stay on it for my entire pregnancy. Should I take her advice even though I feel perfectly fine on a regular diet?"

Not only should you take her advice, you should thank her for it. Pregnant women with phenylketonuria (PKU) who are not on a low-phenylalanine diet put their babies at great risk for a variety of problems, including mental retardation. Ideally, as your doctor recommended, the special diet should be resumed three months before conception and blood levels of phenylalanine kept low through delivery. (Even starting the diet early in pregnancy can reduce the seriousness of developmental delay in children of PKU mothers.) The phenylalanine-free milk substitute and measured amounts of other foods permitted on this diet should be augmented with a pregnancy vitamin-mineral supplement containing such micronutrients as zinc and copper, which might otherwise be absent. And, of course, all foods sweetened with aspartame (Equal or NutraSweet) are *absolutely* off-limits.

Though this diet isn't appealing and is understandably difficult to stick with, most mothers feel it's clearly worth the sacrifice to protect their developing babies from harm. If in spite of this incentive you find yourself slipping off the diet, try to get some professional help from a therapist who is familiar with your type of problem. A support group of other PKU mothers may be even more helpful; the misery of such dietary deprivation definitely benefits from the company of those similarly deprived. If you are finding it impossible to stick to the diet, discuss options with your doctor.

SICKLE-CELL ANEMIA

"I have sickle-cell disease, and I just found out that I'm pregnant. Will my baby be okay?"

Not too many years ago, the answer would not have been reassuring. Today, however, thanks to major medical advances, women with sickle-cell disease have a good chance of coming through childbirth safely and of winding up with a healthy baby. Even those women with such sickle-cell complications as heart or kidney disease are often able to have a successful pregnancy.

Pregnancy for the woman with sickle-cell anemia, however, is usually classified as high-risk. The added physical stress of pregnancy increases her chances of having a sickle-cell crisis, while the added stress of sickle-cell disease increases the risks of certain pregnancy complications, such as miscarriage, preterm delivery, and fetal growth restriction. Preeclampsia is also more common in women with sickle-cell anemia, but it isn't clear whether this is because of the sickle cell or because of race. (Women with sickle-cell disease are usually African American, and African Americans are more subject to hypertension.)

The prognosis for both you and your baby will be best if you receive state-of-the-art medical care. You should have prenatal checkups more frequently than other pregnant patients—possibly every two to three weeks up to the 32nd week, and every week thereafter. Your care should be multidisciplinary; your obstetrician should be familiar with sickle-cell disease and should work closely with a knowledgeable hematologist. And possibly at least once (usually in early labor or just prior to delivery), or even periodically throughout pregnancy (though whether or not this treatment is beneficial is controversial), you will be given a blood transfusion. You are as likely as other mothers to have a vaginal delivery. Postpartum, you may be given antibiotics to prevent infection.

If both parents carry a gene for sickle-cell anemia, the risk that their baby will inherit a serious form of the disease is increased. Early in your pregnancy (if not prior to conception), your spouse should be screened for the sickle-cell trait. If he turns out to be a carrier, you may want to see a genetic counselor, and possibly undergo prenatal diagnosis (see page 46) to see if your fetus is affected.

CYSTIC FIBROSIS

"I have cystic fibrosis, and I know that makes pregnancy complicated—but how complicated?"

As someone who's lived with cystic fibrosis for her whole life, you're already used to the challenges that the condition can pose. And the challenges do increase somewhat with pregnancy.

The first challenge may be gaining enough weight, something you'll have to work closely with your doctors (and possibly a nutritionist) to overcome, so that your baby can grow properly. Pulmonary care will be especially important, too—particularly as the increasing size of the uterus makes lung expansion more difficult. If you have severe lung disease, your illness may become exacerbated during pregnancy. All pregnant women with CF will be monitored closely for pulmonary infection.

Your pregnancy will, like your pulmonary health, be watched closely, and you will have more frequent prenatal visits. Activity may be limited, and since you'll be at higher risk for premature delivery, steps will be taken to lower that risk. It's also possible that periodic hospitalization may be required. Genetic counseling is recom-mended to screen for CF in the fetus.

Pregnancy is never easy, and it's cer-tainly more challenging for women with CF. Still, the joys of bringing a child into the world can make all the challenges you'll face more than worthwhile.

What It's Important to Know: LIVING WITH THE HIGH-RISK OR PROBLEM PREGNANCY

Pregnancy is a normal process to be experienced, not a condition to be treated—so the popular ges-tational dogma goes these days. But if yours is a high-risk pregnancy, you're all too aware that this adage is not univer-sally true. Though you may experience plenty of the joy and anticipation "nor-mal" expectant couples do, you and your spouse may also live with:

Anxiety. While other parents-to-be are excitedly preparing for impending parent-hood, you may be too busy worrying about the day-to-day well-being of you and your fetus to think about life with baby.

Resentment. Especially if your activities are limited, you may resent all the re-strictions your high-risk pregnancy places on you ("Why me? Why do I have to give up my job? Why do I have to stay in bed?"). The anger may be aimed at your baby, at your spouse, or elsewhere. The father-to-be may, of course, have his own share of resentments ("Why do I have to do all the work? Does she really have to stay in bed? Do I have to stay home with her every evening?"). There may be unspoken resentments on both sides about the high cost of medical care, all the doctor's appointments and moni-toring, and the lack of lovemaking, if it's off-limits. Both of you may also resent your own feelings of resentment, and your inability to control them.

Guilt. You may agonize over what you might have done to make this a high-risk pregnancy or to lose previous pregnan-cies, even though, in the vast majority of cases, your actions aren't the cause at all. You may feel less valuable as a person if you have to stay in bed or leave your job early. You may fear that your restrictions are putting a strain on your relationship with your spouse or with your other chil-dren. Dad may feel guilty, too—guilty that you're doing all the suffering, or guilty about resentments he may be harboring.

Feelings of inadequacy. If you can't have a "normal" pregnancy, you may consider yourself somehow lacking ("Why can't I be like everyone else?").

Constant pressure. As a high-risk ex-pectant parent, you'll have to keep your pregnancy and its requirements in mind every moment of every day, pausing al-most constantly to ask yourself, "Can I do this? Is that allowed? When is my next test? Did I take my meds?"

Marital stress. Any kind of crisis puts stress on a marriage, but a high-risk preg-nancy often adds the strain of limited or prohibited sexual intercourse, which may make it hard for you to achieve satisfying intimacy. There may be added stress from the high cost of your high-risk pregnancy (much of which may not be totally reimbursed by insurance) and from a loss of income if you can't continue working.

The stress of being alone. If you're single and in a high-risk pregnancy, the stress can be enormous. You'll have to turn to others for help more often than you'd like. You may have no one to hold your hand when waiting to hear the results of the latest test—and no one to talk to about the consequences. You may be forced to spend many lonely nights taking it easy—or may have to take to bed, with no one to help you. You may even wonder why you got yourself into this situation in the first place.

Though the ultimate rewards are sure to make all the efforts more than worthwhile, the next nine months may be rough for you and your spouse. The following may help make the going a little easier:

Financial planning. As other parents save for college, you'll need to save for your baby's safe delivery. (Knowing in advance that yours will be a high-risk, and thus an expensive, pregnancy is ideal, but it isn't always possible, at least not the first time.) If you know there are going to be high costs ahead, it makes sense to shop around for the best available insurance plan, and to budget well so you can sock away some of the needed cash before the pregnancy begins. If you don't know in advance, start taking belt-tightening steps as soon as you discover your belt will be expanding.

Social planning. If your pregnancy requires bed rest, partial or complete, don't resign yourselves to the hermit's life. Invite your best friends to supper in the bedroom (order pizza in and have someone whip up some Mock Sangrias), to play Monopoly, Scrabble, or cards, or to watch a movie that's just come out on video. If you have to miss an important family event, a friend's wedding, or your company's annual party, have your spouse or a friend or relative attend and record (in his head, on audiotape, on video, or with a camera) the goings-on so he can share them with you later. If your sister is getting married a thousand miles away and the doctor has vetoed traveling, videotape a message of love to her, or write a special poem to be read at the reception. Ask her to videotape the ceremony so you can share it.

Filling time. Months—or even a few weeks—in bed may sound like a life sentence. Perhaps you can view it as a time to do all the things you haven't had time for in your hectic life. Read those best-sellers everyone's been talking about, or some of the old classics that you never got around to enjoying. Start subscribing to parenting magazines—you may never again have so much free time to read them. Join a video club that offers a good selection and good prices (how many other people have the time to take advantage of those "two-films-for-the-price-of-one" offers?). Study a foreign language, listen to a good book if you're tired of reading, or cultivate a new interest via audiotapes. Learn to knit or crochet or embroider—and make something for yourself, your spouse, your mom, or your doctor if you're too superstitious to make something for your baby. If you're permitted to sit up, get a laptop computer and organize your financial life or surf the Net and learn more about pregnancy and parenting. Keep a journal of your thoughts, both the good and the bad, as a way both to pass the time and to work out your resentments. Collect some of the best catalogs, and do your shopping by phone. Or become an on-line shopper.

Best of all, do something for others. Nothing makes one feel better than that. Make phone calls for a charity, seal and stamp letters for an organization you'd like to help, write cheery letters to elderly friends and relatives.

Childbirth preparation. If you can't go to Lamaze classes, ask your coach to go and tape them, or to take notes and report on them verbally. If your bedroom is large and the class is small, ask if the others would mind holding at least one session at your home. Though you may feel that learning about normal childbirth may jinx your chances of having one, it will be important for you to be as well informed as possible. Read what you can on the subject in books and on-line; view a childbirth preparation course on video. And though you may feel that you'd rather not know, learn all you can, too, about what delivery is like for someone with your particular problem—from your doctor as well as from books.

Mutual support. A high-risk pregnancy, particularly when there are a lot of restrictions, is a real test of a relationship. You'll be going through a period of months where many of the normal pleasures are missing (sex, dinners out, and weekend trips, for example) and where even the joy of expecting a baby is marred and muddled. To be sure you end up with a healthy baby and a healthy relationship, each of you will have to think about the other's needs. As the expectant mother, yours will be most obvious. You'll need support in

---

MOMS HELPING MOMS

Often a woman who has a high-risk or difficult pregnancy, or who has experienced a pregnancy loss, feels left out and alone; she is acutely aware of how different her pregnancy experience is from those of her "normal" friends. If you feel this way, you may find comfort, empathy, and support in a group of women who have had experiences similar to yours.

Discussions at support-group meetings may cover such topics as feeling guilty or inadequate over not being able to have a normal pregnancy; coping with being confined at home or in the hospital; coping with being a single parent in a high-risk pregnancy; concern over subsequent pregnancies; grieving over the loss of a baby; finding sources of emotional support; dealing with feelings of alienation. A lot of practical advice is also exchanged at support groups—for instance, how to manage your household when confined to bed; keep your family going when you have a baby in intensive care; get the best care for a particular disorder. Continuing with such a group even after you start to feel better (or after you deliver) also helps you bring your own experience full circle, and helps with your healing while you support other women in need.

If you think you might benefit from a support group, try to find out if there is one in your area that meets your particular needs (check with your hospital, doctors, midwives, nurses). If there isn't and you have the energy, consider collecting the names of women in similar situations and starting a group yourself.

If you are stuck in bed and can't attend a support group, try on-line chats with other expectant mothers in bed, hold a meeting at your home occasionally, or subscribe to "LeftSide Lines," the newsletter for women with complicated pregnancies (Sidelines National Support Network, PO Box 1808, Laguna Beach, CA 92652; [949] 497-2265; and visit their very useful Web site at www. sidelines.org.

everything, from sticking to a restricted diet to staying away from restricted activities. But the needs of your spouse, who must be providing a lot of this support, may be neglected as a result. Even from your bedridden or otherwise depressingly restricted position, you should try to acknowledge your partner's feelings and let him know how truly important he is in all that is going on. Though realistically it won't always be easy, make time for romance whenever you can—a weekly candlelit dinner in bed (order in, unless your spouse prefers to cook) can help rekindle your relationship.

Sexual sublimating. Making love doesn't always have to mean sexual intercourse. There are plenty of ways to achieve intimacy in pregnancy even when the doctor says "no sex" (page 237).

Spiritual support. Relaxation exercises, meditation, visualization, or prayer can help you weather this difficult time—not just emotionally, but often physically as well. Such complementary techniques have been shown to boost immune system function, reduce pain, and improve the way patients with medical problems feel.

Outside support. As with so many of life's crises, being able to talk to others in the same boat can help immeasurably. This is especially important for the single mother. See the box on page 489 for tips that can help.

◆ ◆ ◆

BETTER BED REST

For most hard-working women, the idea of spending weeks on end lounging around in bed sounds like a daydream come true . . . until it's actually prescribed, in the form of pregnancy bed rest. If you've been banished to bed by your practitioner, mover over—you've got company. More than one in five expectant moms are assigned to a week or more of bed rest at some point in pregnancy. And while the benefits of bed rest have not been well documented in clinical studies, many practitioners continue to prescribe it in certain high-risk situations, in the hope that it will prevent preterm labor and a variety of other pregnancy complications.

Although the jury's still out on the benefits of bed rest, the drawbacks are clear. Paradoxically, lying around can be exhausting and debilitating—and women on prolonged bed rest can suffer backaches, hip and muscle pain, headaches, dry skin, increased fatigue, muscle loss— the list goes on, depending how long a stay is prescribed.

Fortunately, many of the side effects of bed rest can be minimized if you keep moving—at least, as much as you're allowed. Shift positions often—going from your left side to your right side (but not on your back). Do simple exercises to keep your muscle tone (as they say, if you don't use it, you lose it) and enhance blood flow: Point and flex your toes, rotate your hands and feet, lift your arms and legs, roll your head side to side, up and down, tense and relax the arm and leg muscles. Keep a jar of lotion—and a large bottle of water—by your bed so that you can keep yourself hydrated inside and out. Avoid sleeping too much during the day, which can trigger headaches and worsen fatigue.

Of course, losing muscle tone may be less of a concern when you're stuck between the sheets than losing your mind. For tips on keeping yourself busy while on bed rest, see page 488.

CHAPTER 20

When There's a Problem

Considering the incredibly intricate processes that are involved in the creation of a baby, from the impeccably precise divisions of a fertilized egg to the dramatic transformation of a shapeless bundle of cells into a tiny human form, it's nothing short of miraculous that all goes perfectly most of the time. And it's not surprising that very occasionally something goes wrong. Modern medicine, modern sanitation, and an understanding of the significance of diet and lifestyle have all overwhelmingly improved the chances that a pregnancy (and the labor and delivery that follow) will be completed successfully and safely, without problems of any kind. Fortunately, with today's technology on our side, even when a complication does crop up, early diagnosis and treatment can usually resolve it, allowing the pregnancy story to have a happy ending.[1]

Most women go through pregnancy and childbirth without any complications. If you've had no complications, then this chapter, which describes the most common ones and their symptoms and treatments, *is not for you.* Skip it, and save yourself some unneeded anxiety.

Pregnancy Complications

The following conditions, though more common than some pregnancy complications, are still quite unlikely to be experienced by the average pregnant woman. So read this chapter only if you've been diagnosed with a complication or you're experiencing symptoms that might indicate a complication. If you are diagnosed with one, use the discussion of the condition

---

1. Most complications that can occur during the postpartum period are covered in *What to Expect the First Year.*

in this section as a general overview—so you know what you're dealing with—but expect to receive more specific (and possibly different) advice from your doctor.

EARLY MISCARRIAGE

What is it? A miscarriage (also called a spontaneous abortion) is the spontaneous expulsion of an embryo or fetus from the uterus before it is able to live on the outside. Such a loss in the first trimester is referred to as an *early* miscarriage. Early miscarriage is very common (many doctors believe that virtually every woman will have at least one sometime in her reproductive years), occurring in as many as 40 to 65 percent of conceptions. More than half of these occur so early that pregnancy is not even suspected yet (which is why the miscarriage rate among diagnosed pregnancies is much lower); so these miscarriages often go unnoticed, passing for a normal or sometimes heavier period. The vast majority of women who experience miscarriage will go on to have a normal pregnancy in the future.

Early miscarriage is usually related to a chromosomal or other genetic abnormality in the embryo. In many cases, it will be triggered by an embryo or fetus that is no longer living. It can also be caused by the mother's body failing to produce an adequate supply of pregnancy hormones; inadequate levels of thyroid hormone or too little iodine intake; an immune reaction to the embryo; or, possibly, too much of the hormone prolactin. Environmental factors—such as poor nutrition, infection, smoking, alcohol, and so on—may play a role, too. In a normal pregnancy, miscarriage is *not* caused by exercise, having sex, working hard, or lifting heavy objects. Nausea and vomiting, even severe, will not cause a miscarriage. In fact, there is some evidence that women who have these symptoms are *less likely* to miscarry. It

is also unlikely that a fall, a blow, or a sudden fright can cause a miscarriage.

Signs and symptoms. Most often, there is bleeding with cramps or pain in the center of the lower abdomen or back. Sometimes, there is severe or persistent pain that lasts twenty-four hours or more and is unaccompanied by bleeding; heavy bleeding (like a menstrual period) without pain; persistent light staining (that continues for three days or more). Clots or grayish matter may be passed as the miscarriage actually begins.

Treatment. When there is bleeding or cramps, the situation is called a threatened abortion; miscarriage will not necessarily happen, but there is a chance that it might. If, on examination, the practitioner finds that the cervix is dilated, and/or the membranes surrounding the fetus have broken, it is assumed that a miscarriage has occurred or is in progress. In such a case, nothing can be done to prevent the loss. If fetal tissue has been passed, it is likely the miscarriage has already occurred.

On the other hand, if the fetus is shown to be alive through either ultrasound or Doppler and there is no dilation, the chances are very good that the threatened miscarriage will not occur. If the fetus is not alive but has not yet passed out of the mother's body, it is called a missed miscarriage.

In threatened abortions, the practitioner will probably impose bed rest and restrictions on activities, including sexual intercourse, and possibly prescribe pain medication until the bleeding or pain has passed. Other physicians will suggest no particular treatment on the theory that a doomed pregnancy will end (therapy or no) and a healthy pregnancy will hang in there (also with or without therapy). Hormones, once given routinely for early bleeding, are now rarely used because there is doubt about their effectiveness and concern over the effect they might

BLEEDING IN EARLY PREGNANCY

Bleeding in early pregnancy can be scary, but, fortunately, it doesn't usually signal a problem. The two most common causes of first-trimester bleeding—*neither of which is an indication of trouble*—are:

Normal implantation of the pregnancy in the uterine wall. Such bleeding, which sometimes occurs when the fertilized egg attaches itself to the wall of the uterus (two to five days after conception), is brief and light, lasting a day or two. Implantation normally occurs around five to ten days after conception.

Hormonal changes at the time menstruation would ordinarily have occurred. Bleeding is usually light, though occasionally can seem like an actual period.

Often the actual cause can't be pinpointed, but the bleeding stops spontaneously, and as in the above situations, the pregnancy continues to a happy conclusion. As a precaution, however, *any* bleeding should always be reported to your practitioner so it can be evaluated. Be precise in describing the bleeding: Is it intermittent or persistent? When did it start? Is the color bright or dark red, brownish or pink? Is it heavy enough to soak a sanitary pad in an hour, just occasional spotting, or somewhere in between? Is there any unusual odor? Do any tissue fragments (bits of solid material) seem to have been passed with the blood? (If so, try to save them in a jar or plastic bag.) Be sure to report, too, any accompanying symptoms, such as excessive nausea and vomiting, cramps or pain of any kind, fever, weakness, and so on.

Slight spotting or staining that is not accompanied by other symptoms is not considered an emergency situation; if it begins in the middle of the night, you can wait until morning to call the doctor. It could be a subchorionic bleed, a common occurrence in which a small blood clot forms at the edge of the placenta. Such bleeding usually stops on its own and is not usually cause for concern. Nevertheless, your practitioner will likely want to monitor the bleeding with ultrasounds to assure the clot has resolved. Any other kind of bleeding suggests a prompt call or, if the doctor is unavailable, a trip to the ER, since it might indicate a less common, but more worrisome, cause of early bleeding such as:

Miscarriage. When a miscarriage is threatened, there is usually light bleeding, which becomes heavy and is accompanied by crampy lower abdominal pain, which may come and go. When a miscarriage is actually taking place, there is generally the passage of embryonic material in the blood. A brownish discharge may indicate a missed miscarriage (see facing page). Sometimes, when the fertilized egg (ovum) doesn't develop (a blighted ovum), the sac is empty and no embryonic material is passed.

Ectopic pregnancy. Signs include brown vaginal spotting or light bleeding, intermittent or persistent, accompanied by abdominal and/or shoulder pain, which can often be quite severe (see page 498).

Molar pregnancy. A continuous brownish discharge is the prime symptom of this rare problem (see page 513).

have on the fetus if the pregnancy continues. In very unusual cases, however, patients with a history of miscarriages who appear to be producing too little progesterone may benefit from taking the hormone. In recurrent miscarriages, when excess prolactin is the cause, medication to reduce prolactin levels in the mother's blood may allow a pregnancy to proceed to term.

Sometimes, when a miscarriage does occur, it isn't complete—only parts of the placenta, sac, and embryo are expelled. If you've had or believe you've had a miscarriage, and bleeding and/or pain continue, phone your doctor im-

WHEN A MISCARRIAGE IS INEVITABLE

When parents are given the terrible news that a miscarriage is under way or inevitable, they are also sometimes offered two options: to let nature take its course (otherwise known as "expectant management") or to intervene with a D & C. If this happens to you, here are some factors that you and your practitioner can consider in making that decision:

◆ How far along the miscarriage is. If bleeding and cramping are already heavy, the miscarriage is probably already well under way. In that case, allowing it to progress naturally may be preferable to a D & C. On the other hand, if it has been determined through ultrasound that the fetus has died, but there has been little or no bleeding (as in a missed miscarriage), a D & C is probably the better alternative.

◆ How far along the pregnancy is. The more fetal tissue there is, the more likely it will be that a D & C will be necessary to completely clean the uterus out.

◆ Your emotional and physical state. Waiting a miscarriage out (which can take as long as three to four weeks in some cases) can be emotionally and physically debilitating for a woman, as well as for her spouse. It's likely that the necessary process of coming to terms with, and grieving for, your loss cannot be completed, either, while the pregnancy is still inside you.

◆ Risks and benefits. Because a D & C is invasive, it carries a slightly higher (though still very low) risk, most commonly of infection (a 0 to 10 percent chance). The benefit of having the miscarriage complete sooner, however, may greatly outweigh that small risk for most women. With a naturally occurring miscarriage, there is also the risk that it won't completely empty the uterus, in which case a D & C may be necessary to finish what nature has started.

◆ Evaluation of the miscarriage. When a D & C is performed, evaluating the cause of the miscarriage through an examination of the fetal tissue will be easier.

No matter what course is taken, and whether the ordeal is over sooner or later, the loss will be difficult for you. See pages 497 and 526 for help in coping.

---

mediately. A D & C (dilation and curettage)[2] may be required to reduce the bleeding. It's a simple procedure in which the cervix is dilated and any remaining fetal or placental tissue is scraped or suctioned out. Or your doctor may just take a wait-and-see approach, known as "expectant management." This seems to be as effective as the surgical D & C approach when a woman

has no fever, has stable blood pressure and heart rate, and no excess bleeding or severe pain. In most cases, the uterus will naturally expel whatever remnants are left inside it without intervention. (If possible, try to save such material in a clean jar. Your physician may want to evaluate it for clues to the cause of the miscarriage.) The use of medications to expel the remnants of the pregnancy seems to be less effective than either a D & C or expectant management. See the box above for more.

---

2. Later in pregnancy, the procedure may be called D & E, or dilation and evacuation.

If your pain from the miscarriage is severe, your doctor may recommend or prescribe a pain reliever. Don't hesitate to ask for relief if you need it.

Prevention. Most miscarriages are a result of a defect in the embryo or fetus and can't be prevented. There are steps you can take, however, to reduce miscarriage *risk,* including checking thyroid levels prepregnancy or early in pregnancy and using iodized salt in or on your food; getting chronic conditions under control before conception; possibly avoiding excessive physical stress (such as heavy exercise or lifting extremely heavy objects) around the time your fertilized egg is implanting (usually between days five to ten after the estimated date of ovulation); avoiding lifestyle practices that increase the risk of miscarriage, such as alcohol use and smoking; and embracing a pre- *and* postconception lifestyle that is good for both you and the baby you hope to have. Such a lifestyle should include:

◆ Good nutrition

◆ Nutritional supplementation appropriate for pregnant women, which includes folic acid and other B vitamins. New research has shown that some

---

BLEEDING IN MID- OR LATE PREGNANCY

Light or spotty bleeding in the second or third trimester is generally *not a cause for concern.* It is often the result of trauma to the increasingly sensitive cervix during an internal exam or sexual intercourse, or simply of causes unknown. Occasionally, however, bleeding is a sign that immediate medical attention is needed. Since only your practitioner can determine the cause, he or she should be notified if you experience *any* bleeding—*immediately* if bleeding is heavy or accompanied by pain or discomfort, *the same day* even if it is only spotty and there are no accompanying symptoms. Ultrasound examination can often determine whether or not a problem exists.

The most common causes of serious bleeding in the second or third trimester are:

Placenta previa, or low-lying placenta. Bleeding is usually bright red and painless. It most often starts spontaneously, though coughing, straining, or sexual intercourse can also trigger it. It can be light or heavy, and it usually stops, only to recur later on in pregnancy. See page 505 for further information.

Abruptio placenta, or premature separation of the placenta. Bleeding may be as light as a light menstrual flow, as heavy as a heavy one, or much heavier, depending on the degree of separation. The discharge may or may not contain clots. The intensity of the accompanying cramping, pain, and abdominal tenderness will also depend on the degree of separation. With a major separation, signs of shock from blood loss may be evident. See page 516.

Other possible causes of bleeding. Occasionally, the uterine lining may tear, causing heavy bleeding—as any cut might. There may also be crampy pain involved, due to the accumulation of blood near the cervix. Bed rest will usually allow the tear to heal.

Late miscarriage. When miscarriage is threatening, the discharge may at first be pink or brown; when bleeding is heavy and accompanied by pain, a miscarriage may be imminent. See page 496.

Premature labor. Labor is considered premature when it begins after the 20th week but before the 37th. A bloody mucousy discharge accompanied by contractions could signal preterm labor. See page 508.

women have trouble conceiving and/or sustaining a pregnancy because of a vitamin B_{12} deficiency. Once these women begin B_{12} supplementation, they are able to conceive and carry to term.

♦ Weight control (you should try to be neither extremely overweight nor extremely underweight when you conceive)

♦ Caution in the use of medications (taking only those that are okayed by a doctor who knows you are pregnant and avoiding those that are known to be risky for the expectant mother)

♦ Steps to avoid infections, such as sexually transmitted diseases or gum infection[3]

If you've had two or more miscarriages, you should have tests to try to determine the probable cause so future pregnancy losses can be prevented. Some factors that might be related to recurrent miscarriage include a thyroid problem; abnormalities in the production of other endocrine hormones; immune or autoimmune problems (in which the mother's immune system attacks the embryo); or a misshapen uterus. There are now many tests that may pick up risk factors for pregnancy loss (such as antithyroid antibodies or a vitamin B_{12} deficiency) and suggest possible ways of preventing such loss. Some are still in the research stage, others are already believed to be effective.

LATE MISCARRIAGE

What is it? Any spontaneous expulsion of a fetus between the end of the first trimester and the 20th week is termed a late miscarriage. After the 20th week, when the fetus may be able to live outside the uterus—even if only with a lot of help from the neonatal nursery staff and high-tech equipment—the event is labeled a preterm birth.[4]

The cause of late miscarriage is usually related to the mother's health, the condition of her cervix or uterus, her exposure to certain drugs or other toxic substances, or to problems of the placenta.

Signs and symptoms. A pink discharge for several days, or a scant brown discharge for several weeks, indicates a *threatened* miscarriage. Heavier bleeding, especially when accompanied by cramping, often means a miscarriage is *inevitable,* especially if the cervix is dilated. (There may be other causes of heavy bleeding, however, such as a tear in the uterine lining; see box, page 495.)

Treatment. For a threatened late miscarriage, bed rest is often prescribed. If the spotting stops, this is taken as an indication that it wasn't related to miscarriage, and a resumption of normal activity is usually permitted. If the cervix has started to dilate, a diagnosis of incompetent cervix may be made and cerclage (stitching the cervix closed; see page 35) may prevent miscarriage.

Once the heavy bleeding and cramping that signal a miscarriage begin, treatment is aimed at protecting the mother's health. Hospitalization may be required to prevent hemorrhaging. If cramping and bleeding continue following a miscarriage, a D & C may be necessary to remove any remnants of the pregnancy.

Prevention. If the cause of a late miscarriage can be determined, it may be pos-

---

3. Inflammations from infections can cause the production of such substances as prostaglandins, which can stimulate labor.

4. When a baby is born dead after the 20th week, it's usually described as a stillbirth rather than a miscarriage. The definitions of late miscarriage and stillbirth may vary from state to state.

IF YOU'VE HAD A MISCARRIAGE

Though it is hard for parents to accept it at the time, when an early miscarriage occurs it is usually because the condition of the embryo or fetus is incompatible with normal life. Early miscarriage is generally a natural selection process in which a defective embryo or fetus (defective because of genetic abnormality; because of environmental factors, such as radiation or drugs; because of poor implantation in the uterus; because of maternal infection, random accident, or other unknown reasons) is lost because it is incapable of survival or is overwhelmingly malformed.

All that said, losing a baby, even this early, is tragic and traumatic. But don't let guilt compound your misery—*a miscarriage is not your fault.* Do allow yourself to grieve, a necessary step in the healing process. Expect to be sad, even depressed for a while. Sharing your feelings with your spouse, your practitioner, a relative, or a friend will help. So will joining or forming a support group for couples or singles who have experienced pregnancy loss. Ask your practitioner if he or she knows of one in your area, or inquire at your hospital. This sharing with others who *truly* know how you feel may be especially important if you've experienced more than one pregnancy loss. For more suggestions on coping with your loss, see page 526.

For some women, the best therapy is getting pregnant again as soon as it is safe. But before you do, discuss possible causes of the miscarriage with your doctor. Most often, miscarriage is simply a random one-time occurrence caused by chromosomal abnormality, infection, chemical or other teratogenic exposure, or chance, and is not likely to recur. Repeat miscarriages (more than two) may be related to hormonal abnormalities in the mother or to the mother's immune system rejecting a "foreign" intruder, the embryo. In both these situations, treatment when you conceive again, or even before, can often prevent a recurrence. Rarely, repeated miscarriages are due to genetic factors that are detectable by prepregnancy chromosome tests of both parents. Check with your doctor about whether such tests are indicated in your case.

Whatever the cause of your miscarriage, some practitioners suggest waiting two to three months before trying to conceive again, though sexual relations can often be resumed after six weeks. Other practitioners let Mother Nature take over; they tell their patients that their bodies will know when it's time to conceive again. Some studies have shown that women actually have a higher than normal fertility rate in the first three cycles following a first trimester loss. If your practitioner does recommend a waiting period, however, use reliable contraception, preferably of the barrier type—condom, diaphragm—until the waiting time is up. Take advantage of this waiting period—spend it improving your diet and your health habits (if there's room for improvement) and generally getting your body into tiptop baby-making shape (see Chapter 21). Happily, the chances are excellent that next time around you'll have a normal pregnancy and a healthy baby. Most women who have had one miscarriage do not miscarry again. In fact, a miscarriage is an assurance that you're capable of conceiving, and the great majority of women who lose a pregnancy this way go on to complete a normal one.

sible to prevent a repeat of the tragedy. If a previously undiagnosed incompetent cervix was responsible, future miscarriages can be prevented by cerclage early in pregnancy, before the cervix begins to dilate. If hormonal insufficiency was to blame, hormone replacement may allow future pregnancies to progress to term. If chronic disease, such as diabetes or hypertension, is responsible, the condition should be brought under control prior to any future pregnancy. Acute infection can be prevented or treated. And an abnormally shaped uterus or one that is distorted by the growth of fibroids or other benign tumors can, in some instances, be corrected by surgery.

ECTOPIC PREGNANCY

What is it? An ectopic pregnancy is one that implants outside the uterus, most often in a fallopian tube, usually due to a condition (such as scarring from a past infection) that obstructs or slows the passage of the fertilized egg. Women at risk include those with a history of pelvic inflammatory disease, endometriosis, prior ectopic pregnancy, or tubal

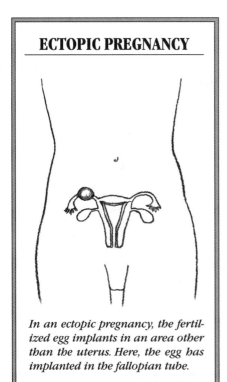

ECTOPIC PREGNANCY

In an ectopic pregnancy, the fertilized egg implants in an area other than the uterus. Here, the egg has implanted in the fallopian tube.

surgery, as well as smokers. Early diagnosis of and treatment for ectopic pregnancy are very effective. Without them, the pregnancy will continue to grow in the tube, which will eventually burst, destroying its ability in the future to carry fertilized eggs on their way to the uterus. An uncared-for ruptured tube could also threaten the mother's life.

Signs and symptoms. The first sign may be a dull ache that progresses to colicky (spasmodic), crampy pain with tenderness, starting on one side and often spreading throughout the abdomen; pain may worsen on straining of bowels, coughing, or moving. Often there is brown vaginal spotting or light bleeding, intermittent or continuous, which may precede pain by several days or weeks. Sometimes there is nausea and vomiting, dizziness or weakness, shoulder pain, and/or rectal pressure. If the tube ruptures, heavy bleeding may begin, signs of shock (rapid, weak pulse, clammy skin, and fainting) are common, and pain becomes very sharp and steady for a short time before diffusing throughout the pelvic region.

Treatment. Getting to the hospital immediately is important. New techniques for early diagnosis and treatment of tubal pregnancy have removed most of the risk for the mother while greatly improving the chances of preserving her fertility.

Diagnosis is usually made through a combination of three procedures: (1) a pelvic examination; (2) a series of highly sensitive pregnancy tests that track the level of the hormone hCG in the mother's blood (if the levels of hCG fall or fail to rise as the pregnancy progresses, an abnormal pregnancy, possibly in a fallopian tube, is suspected); and (3) high-resolution ultrasound to visualize the uterus and the fallopian tubes (an empty uterus[5] and, though this isn't always visible, a pregnancy developing in a fallopian tube are signs of ectopic pregnancy). If there is any doubt, confirmation is most often made by viewing the tubes directly, by means of a tiny viewing instrument (a laparoscope) inserted through the navel. High-tech diagnostic tools such as these have made early diagnosis of ectopic pregnancies possible, catching 80 percent of them before a rupture.

Successful treatment of an ectopic pregnancy is also dependent on high-tech medicine. Laparoscopy is usually the surgical method of choice because it allows for a much shorter hospital stay and more rapid recovery. In this procedure, two tiny incisions are made, one in the navel for the insertion of the viewing instrument, the laparoscope, and another lower in the abdomen for the surgical instruments. Depending on the circumstances, lasers or electrocautery may be used to remove the pregnancy from the fallopian tube. As an alternative to surgery, a single dose of the drug methotrexate[6] and/or misoprostol—which destroy the misplaced embryo by halting cell growth—may be used. A major advantage: these drugs do not damage the tubes as surgery may. In some cases, it can be determined that the ectopic pregnancy is no longer developing and can be expected to disappear over time, which would also eliminate the need for surgery.

---

5. In women who were given fertility treatment gonadotropins (Clomid, Perganol) to stimulate the release of multiple eggs by the ovaries, it may rarely happen that one fertilized egg made its way down to the uterus while another remained in a fallopian tube. So it makes sense for the doctor to check for this possibility on ultrasound.

6. There is a very, very slight chance that treatment with methotrexate could lead to a serious form of pneumonia; report to the doctor any coughing and/or breathlessness following treatment.

Since residual material from a pregnancy left in the tube could damage it, a follow-up test of hCG levels is performed to be sure that the entire tubal pregnancy was removed or has disappeared. Unless the fallopian tube has been irreparably damaged, it is usually possible to save it, improving the chances of a successful pregnancy in the future.

The majority of women treated for ectopic pregnancy will be able to conceive and have a normal pregnancy within one year after it.

Prevention. Seeking immediate treatment for sexually transmitted diseases (STDs), and prevention of STDs (through the practice of safe sex) can help reduce the risk of an ectopic pregnancy, as can quitting smoking.

GESTATIONAL DIABETES

What is it? Gestational diabetes is a temporary form of diabetes in which the body does not produce adequate amounts of insulin to deal with the increased blood sugar of pregnancy. Women are routinely tested for gestational diabetes around the 28th week of pregnancy because that is when the placenta begins producing large amounts of hormones that can cause insulin resistance. This type of diabetes is more common in older moms-to-be and almost always goes away after delivery.

Diabetes, both the kind that begins in pregnancy and the kind that started before conception, is generally not dangerous for either the fetus or the mother—*if* it is controlled. But if excessive sugar is allowed to circulate in a mother's blood, and thus to enter the fetal circulation through the placenta, potential problems for both mother and baby are serious. Women who have uncontrolled gestational diabetes are at risk for having a too large baby, as well as for developing preeclampsia (pregnancy-induced hypertension).

Signs and symptoms. The first sign may be sugar in the urine (when tested in your practitioner's office), but there may also be unusual thirst, frequent and very copious urination (as distinguished from the also frequent but usually light voiding of early pregnancy), and fatigue (which may be difficult to differentiate from pregnancy fatigue).

Treatment. Fortunately, virtually all of the potential risks associated with diabetes in pregnancy can be eliminated through the scrupulous control of blood sugar levels achieved by good medical and self-care. If the doctor's instructions are followed (see page 472 for recommended care), the diabetic mother and her baby will have as good a chance to come through pregnancy and childbirth well as any other mother and baby. Even when tests for sugar are borderline, treating the condition, rather than waiting for it to worsen, seems to improve outcome. If you developed gestational diabetes, you should be checked a few months after delivery to be sure blood sugar levels have returned to normal. You should also always be on the lookout for signs and symptoms of late onset adult type 2 diabetes (such as frequent urination, persistent thirst, and increased sugar in blood and urine), which you are at somewhat increased risk of developing later in life.

Prevention. Good diet, weight control, and regular exercise will reduce the risk. Obese women who exercise cut their risk of gestational diabetes by half.

PREGNANCY-INDUCED HYPERTENSION OR PREECLAMPSIA

What is it? Pregnancy-induced hypertension (PIH), or preeclampsia,[7] also called toxemia, is a high blood pressure–related condition that begins during pregnancy. It is characterized by swelling, high blood pressure, and protein in the urine. Preeclampsia occurs in about 5 to 10 percent of pregnancies.

Those at greatest risk are women carrying multiple fetuses, women over forty, diabetics, and women who already have chronic high blood pressure; the condition is also somewhat more likely to occur in first, rather than subsequent, pregnancies, and in African American women. No one knows for sure what causes preeclampsia, though there does seem to be a genetic link. Researchers hypothesize that the genetic makeup of the fetus could be one of the factors that predisposes a pregnancy to preeclampsia; if your mother or your spouse's mother had preeclampsia during their pregnancies with either of you, you are more likely to have preeclampsia during your pregnancies.

Increasingly, too, research links some cases of preeclampsia to gum disease as well as to poor nutrition, including deficiencies in vitamins C and E and magnesium. Women with preeclampsia are also more likely to have high levels of triglycerides, which can result from a high-sugar diet. Another theory researchers are looking into is that some women with preeclampsia may have a defect in their blood vessels that causes them to constrict during pregnancy instead of widen (as usually happens). As a result, there is a drop in the blood supply to organs like the kidney and liver.

---

7. These terms are used interchangeably.

In addition, it's theorized that preeclampsia may be an immune response to a foreign intruder—the baby. This means that the woman's body becomes "allergic" to the baby and placenta. This "allergy" causes a reaction in the mother's body that can damage her blood and blood vessels. Further research into this theory and others may lead to better ways of dealing with the condition.

Signs and symptoms. Preeclampsia is diagnosed when, after the 20th week of pregnancy, blood pressure rises to 140/90 or more in a woman who has never before had high blood pressure. With mild preeclampsia there is swelling of hands and face with sudden excessive weight gain (both related to water retention), swelling of the ankles that doesn't go away after twelve hours of rest, and protein in the urine. If untreated, the condition can progress quickly to severe preeclampsia, characterized by a further increase in blood pressure (usually to 160/110 or higher), increased quantities of protein in the urine, blurred vision, headaches, fever, rapid heartbeat, confusion, scanty urine output, severe pain in the upper abdomen, exaggerated reflex reactions, restlessness and twitching, and/or abnormal kidney function. There may also be growth restriction in the fetus and inadequate quantities of amniotic fluid in the uterus. Pregnant women with this condition may have any or all of the signs and symptoms.

Fortunately, in women who are receiving regular medical care, preeclampsia is almost invariably caught early on and managed successfully. If it goes untreated, it could progress to eclampsia, a much more serious condition (see page 515).

Occasionally, preeclampsia does not appear until labor and delivery, or even until the postpartum period. A sudden increase in blood pressure at these times may be merely a reaction to stress or may be true preeclampsia. Therefore, women who exhibit elevated blood pressure at any point are watched very carefully, with frequent checks not just of their blood pressure, but also of their urine (for protein), their reflexes, and their blood chemistry.

Treatment. The ultimate treatment in most cases is delivery. There are medications and treatments to keep preeclampsia from progressing into a more serious condition, but the only "cure" is delivery.

With mild preeclampsia, the treatment is aimed at lowering blood pressure. Options include diet, exercise, stress reduction, and, if needed, medication. If the woman is near term and her cervix is ripe (softened and thinned), she is usually induced and her baby delivered without delay. The woman who isn't ready for delivery is generally hospitalized for complete bed rest (lying on the left side is best) and close observation. In some very mild cases, bed rest at home may be permitted once blood pressure is normalized. If you are allowed to go home with preeclampsia, you must be monitored by a visiting nurse or a home care service and must make frequent visits to the doctor's office. You should be alert to the danger signs—severe headache, visual disturbances, rapid heartbeat, or upper right or mid-abdominal pain—which may warn you that your condition is worsening, and you should seek emergency medical attention immediately should you experience any of them.

The baby's condition will be assessed regularly: fetal movements will be checked daily, and stress or non-stress tests, ultrasound, amniocentesis, and other procedures will be performed as needed. If at any point the mother's condition worsens or the tests of the fetus indicate the baby would be better off outside the uterus, the situation will be evaluated to determine the best mode of delivery. If the cervix is ripe and ready, and the baby is not in acute distress, labor will probably be induced. Otherwise, a cesarean is recommended. Generally, a woman with preeclampsia will not be allowed to go past her due date, since post-term the environment in the uterus begins to deteriorate more rapidly in these pregnancies than in normal ones.

With appropriate treatment, a woman with mild preeclampsia has virtually the same excellent chance of having a positive pregnancy outcome as a woman with normal blood pressure.

With severe preeclampsia, the treatment is usually more aggressive. Intravenous magnesium sulfate is begun promptly because it almost always prevents progression to eclampsia. (The side effects of this treatment are uncomfortable, but not usually serious.) If the fetus is close to term, and/or if its lungs are determined to be mature, immediate delivery is usually the recommended route. If the fetus is preterm, but at least 28 weeks old, many doctors will still choose to deliver immediately because they believe it is best for both mother (in order to normalize her blood pressure and improve her general condition) and baby (who will be better off continuing growth in a neonatal intensive care unit than in the less than hospitable environment in its mother's uterus). Some doctors will administer steroids to the fetus to try to speed fetal lung maturity before delivery.

Between 24 and 28 weeks, virtually all physicians try conservative management of preeclampsia, even when it's severe, in order to give the fetus a little more time in the uterus. Before 24 weeks (when the fetus is rarely able to live outside of the uterus and when severe preeclampsia is fortunately uncommon), delivering the pregnancy is sometimes necessary to reverse the preeclamptic process, even though the baby has little or no chance of survival. Women with such severe disease are best delivered in a major medical center, where optimum maternal support as well as neonatal care for the premature infant are available.

In 97 percent of the women with preeclampsia who do not also have chronic hypertension, blood pressure returns to normal following delivery. The drop takes place for the majority of new mothers within the first twenty-four hours after childbirth, and for most of the others within the first week. If blood pressure doesn't return to normal by the six-week checkup, the doctor will look for underlying disease.

With appropriate and prompt medical care of severe preeclampsia, the chances that the mother and, except in rare instances, her baby will come through fine are very good.

Prevention. Recent research has suggested that daily low-dose aspirin therapy may prevent preeclampsia in certain high-risk women, and can be used safely through the 36th week. Though calcium supplements do not seem to reduce the risk of preeclampsia in women with adequate calcium intakes, there is some evidence that it might be helpful in those who don't get enough. Good nutrition, which ensures adequate intakes of antioxidants, magnesium, vitamins, (especiall C), and minerals, may reduce risk. Minimizing stress can also reduce risk, as can proper dental care.

INTRAUTERINE GROWTH RESTRICTION (IUGR)

What is it? Sometimes when the uterine environment is not ideal—because of maternal illness, maternal lifestyle, placental inadequacy, or other factors—the fetus doesn't grow as rapidly as it should. Without intervention, that baby will be

REPEAT LOW-BIRTHWEIGHT BABIES

A mother who has already had a low-birthweight baby has only a slightly increased risk of having another one—and, to her advantage, statistics show that each subsequent baby is actually likely to be a bit heavier than the preceding one. Whether or not her subsequent babies will be small depends to a great extent on the reason her first baby was small and whether or not the same factor, or factors, exist the next time she conceives.

If the cause of her previous baby's IUGR is known, and it is reversible, steps should be taken to remedy the problem as soon as possible. Any woman who has had an IUGR baby and who is pregnant again or is planning to become pregnant should pay extra attention to all the factors that can reduce the risk this time around.

born, whether prematurely or at term, small for gestational age (SGA), also called "small for date" (generally considered to be under five pounds). But if IUGR is diagnosed prenatally, as it often is when a mother is receiving regular medical care, steps may be taken that may reverse it.

IUGR appears to occur in about 2.5 to 3 percent of pregnancies. It is somewhat more common in first pregnancies and in fifth and subsequent ones, as well as among women who are under seventeen or over thirty-five. Fortunately, more than 90 percent of babies who are born small for date do fine, catching up with their larger counterparts in the first couple of years of life. Still, it is important to remedy IUGR when it is discovered prenatally, because a small percentage of the children who are born undersized have trouble catching up, both in size and development.

Signs and symptoms. Carrying small is *not* usually a tip-off to IUGR—just as carrying large or having gained a lot of weight is not necessarily a sign that the baby is big. In fact, there are rarely any obvious symptoms that might alert a mother to the fact that her fetus isn't growing as it should. Usually, the practitioner uncovers the problem during a prenatal checkup, when routine measurement and palpation of the abdomen indicate that the uterus or fetus may be small for date. The diagnosis can be confirmed, or ruled out, with an ultrasound examination and sometimes a variety of other tests.

Treatment. When measures to prevent or control certain conditions or factors that might lead to a baby failing to thrive (see below for a list of these) fail, and IUGR is diagnosed, a variety of approaches may be tried to deal with the problem, depending on the suspected cause. Among the procedures that may be beneficial are bed rest in the hospital, especially if the home environment is less than ideal, intravenous feedings if necessary; medications to improve placental blood flow or to correct a diagnosed problem that may be contributing to the IUGR; and, finally, prompt delivery of the fetus if the intrauterine environment is very poor and can't be improved, and the baby's lungs are known to be mature.

Prevention. Since most babies who are delivered early are small (though they may be an appropriate size for their gestational age and don't necessarily suffer from IUGR), altering the factors that lead to premature labor and halting premature labor when it begins or is anticipated (see page 508) can have a major impact on the risk of having a low-birthweight baby.

Controlling certain maternal conditions that contribute to poor fetal growth, preferably beginning before conception, can help prevent IUGR, correct it, or minimize its effects. These conditions include chronic illness (diabetes, high blood pressure, lung or kidney disease); illnesses related to pregnancy (anemia, preeclampsia); and acute illnesses not related to pregnancy (such as urinary tract infections). To learn how these are treated in pregnancy, see the specific conditions.

Other risk factors can also be modified or eliminated before pregnancy begins or, in many cases, even when it's under way (some changes can dramatically improve the quality of uterine life and, with it, baby's growth). These include inadequate prenatal care (finding a practitioner early and having regular prenatal visits can reduce the risk considerably); poor diet, low maternal weight and/or inadequate weight gain (a well-balanced pregnancy diet, with enough protein, calories, and iron, such

as the Pregnancy Diet, and/or treatment for severe morning sickness can help remedy both of these problems); excessive caffeine intake; cigarette smoking (the sooner a mother quits, the better her baby's chances of being born at a healthy weight); alcohol or other substance abuse; a short time between pregnancies (less than six months between the end of one pregnancy and the beginning of the next may shortchange the new pregnancy, although excellent nutrition, lots of rest, and top-notch medical care will go a long way toward improving uterine conditions if such a pregnancy has already begun); a malformed uterus or other problems with reproductive or urinary organs (surgery or other therapy may remedy these); exposure to toxic substances or environments, including occupational hazards (see page 76).

Recent research has turned up a variety of additional factors that may be involved in producing a too small baby. These include physical stress (including chronic lack of rest) and possibly *excessive* psychological stress; inadequate increase in the mother's blood plasma volume (volume is supposed to increase during pregnancy, but sometimes doesn't); and

LOWERING THE RISKS FOR THE BABY AT RISK

If there is any reason to believe that a baby may be less than perfectly healthy at birth, it is important to be sure that he or she comes into the world under the best of all possible conditions. In most cases, this means being delivered in a major medical center (also known as a tertiary medical center), one that is equipped to handle the most serious of maternal or newborn emergencies. (Studies show that this is preferable to moving a sick baby after birth.) If yours is a high-risk pregnancy that puts your baby at serious risk,

talk to your doctor about arranging delivery in a major medical center. If the medical center is far from home, you will also need to make the necessary arrangements to ensure that you'll be able to get there when the time comes. Specially equipped ambulances or even helicopters may be available to transport you in a hurry, if need be.

Be sure, too, that a specialist (or specialists) familiar with your condition and that of your baby is on hand at the delivery.

progesterone deficiency and possibly deficiency of other hormones. Turning these factors around may also reduce the risk of having a small baby.

Some factors that make a woman somewhat more likely to have a baby who does not grow well are difficult or impossible to alter. These include being poor and/or uneducated (probably because it is less likely that a woman in these circumstances will receive optimum nourishment and prenatal care); DES exposure before her own birth (page 43); living at a high altitude (though risk is only very slightly increased); having had a previous low-birthweight baby, a baby who has a birth defect, or multiple miscarriages; carrying multiples; having first- or second-trimester bleeding, placental problems (such as placenta previa or abruptio placenta), or very severe nausea and vomiting that continues after the third month and *doesn't* respond to treatment; having too much or too little amniotic fluid, abnormal hemoglobin, or premature rupture of the membranes; or Rh isoimmunization (see page 29). Having been small at birth yourself also puts you at an increased risk of having a small baby and the risk is even higher if the baby's father was also born small. But in almost every instance, optimum nutrition and the elimination of any other existing risk factors can improve the chances for normal fetal growth.

Even when prevention and treatment are unsuccessful and a baby is born smaller than normal, the chances that he or she will do well are increasingly good thanks to the many advances in neonatal (newborn) care.

PLACENTA PREVIA

What is it? Placenta previa sounds like a disease of the placenta, but it isn't that at all. It refers to the position of the placenta, not its condition. In placenta previa, the placenta is attached in the lower half of the uterus, covering, partially covering, or touching the edge of the cervical os, the opening of the uterus. In early pregnancy, a low-lying placenta is fairly common; but as pregnancy progresses and the uterus grows, the placenta usually moves upward.[8] Even when it doesn't move up, it is unlikely to cause a serious problem unless it actually touches the cervical opening. In the small percentage of cases in which it does touch, it can trigger bleeding late in pregnancy and at delivery. The closer to the cervix the placenta is situated, the greater the possibility of bleeding. When the placenta blocks the cervix partially or completely, safe vaginal delivery is usually impossible.

The risk of having placenta previa is higher in women who have scarring of the uterine wall from cesareans, uterine surgery, or D & Cs following miscarriage. The need for greater placental surface area due to an increased need for oxygen or nutrients on behalf of the fetus (because of smoking, living at a high altitude, or carrying more than one fetus) may also increase the risk of placenta previa.

Signs and symptoms. Painless bleeding as the placenta pulls away from the stretching lower portion of the uterus (occasionally before the 28th week but most often between the 34th and 38th) is the most common sign of placenta previa, though an estimated 7 to 30 percent of women with low-lying placentas don't bleed at all before delivery. The bleeding is usually bright red, not associated with significant abdominal pain or tenderness, and usually appears without any obvious cause, though it can also be triggered by coughing, straining, or sexual intercourse. It can be light or heavy, and often stops for a

---

8. Even low-lying placentas fairly late in pregnancy may occasionally continue to move upward, allowing for a normal delivery at term.

while, only to recur later. When bleeding is present and placenta previa suspected, diagnosis is usually made by ultrasound. Because the placenta is blocking their way, fetuses with low-lying placentas do not usually "drop" into the pelvis in preparation for delivery.

In women who have no symptoms, the condition may be discovered during a routine ultrasound exam or may not be found until delivery.

Treatment. Because most early cases of low-lying placenta correct themselves long before delivery and never cause a problem, the condition doesn't require treatment before the 20th week. If a woman doesn't have any bleeding but is diagnosed with placenta previa via ultrasound, there is usually no need for her to change her activity level. She should, however, be alert for any bleeding. If a woman diagnosed with placenta previa does experience some bleeding, she will be put on bed rest, be told to refrain from

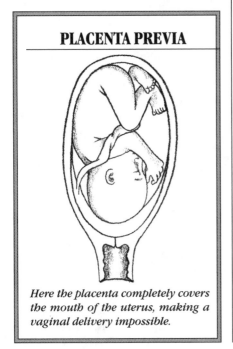

PLACENTA PREVIA

Here the placenta completely covers the mouth of the uterus, making a vaginal delivery impossible.

sexual intercourse, and be monitored more closely by her practitioner. If there is a lot of bleeding, hospitalization is usually needed to evaluate the condition of mother and baby, and, if necessary, to try to stabilize them. If the bleeding stops or becomes very light, conservative treatment is usually recommended, including careful monitoring and supplementation with iron and possibly vitamin C. If bleeding is very heavy, transfusions may be necessary until the fetus is mature enough for delivery. If the pregnancy is less than 34 weeks along, steroid injections may be used to speed fetal lung maturity. A high-fiber diet with stool softeners may be prescribed to reduce the need to strain at the toilet. Occasionally a mother who has had no bleeding for a week, has easy access to the hospital (within fifteen minutes' travel time), can be relied upon to stay in bed, and can find an adult relative or friend or a home health worker who can be with her twenty-four hours a day (and, if necessary, drive her to the hospital in a hurry) may be allowed to go home and follow a similar restricted regimen. There are also, in some areas, home care services that provide nursing care and equipment for such home stays.

The goal is to try to keep the pregnancy going until at least 36 weeks. At that point, if testing finds the fetal lungs are mature, the baby may be delivered by cesarean to reduce the risk of massive hemorrhage. Of course, if before that time the mother and/or her baby are endangered by the bleeding, delivery will not be postponed, even if this means the baby will be premature. Thanks to the skill and caring of top-notch neonatal intensive care units, most of these babies will do much better connected to lifesaving equipment in the NICU than connected to a bleeding placenta in the uterus.

Roughly 3 in 4 women with diagnosed placenta previa will be delivered by cesarean section before labor starts. Rarely, if the condition isn't discovered until labor has begun, bleeding is mild, and the placenta is not blocking the cervix, vaginal delivery may be attempted. In either case, results are usually excellent; though placenta previa once posed a very serious threat, nearly 99 percent of mothers today come through it okay, as do almost as many of their babies.

CHORIOAMNIONITIS

What is it? Chorioamnionitis is an infection of the amniotic fluid and fetal membranes. It is diagnosed in 1 in 100 pregnancies, though it is suspected that the true incidence may be higher. The infection is believed to be a major cause of preterm premature rupture of the membranes as well as of premature labor.

Signs and symptoms. In some cases, chorioamnionitis has no symptoms, particularly at first. Diagnosis is complicated by the fact that there is no simple test that can confirm the presence of infection. Often, the first sign of chorioamnionitis is rapid heartbeat (tachycardia) in the mother. (Tachycardia may also be caused by dehydration, medication, low blood pressure, or anxiety, but should in any case be reported to the practitioner.) Then a fever over 100.4°F develops, and in many cases there is uterine tenderness. If the membranes have ruptured, there may also be a foul odor from the amniotic fluid; if they are intact, there may be an unpleasant-smelling vaginal discharge, originating in the cervix. Lab tests will reveal an increased white blood count (a sign that the body is fighting an infection). The fetus may score low on a biophysical profile (see page 324), indicating some distress. The newborn is at risk for infection (which can be treated with antibiotics) and possibly for low APGAR scores, but usually not for any long-term problems.

Treatment. Chorioamnionitis can be caused by a wide range of microorganisms, and the treatment will depend on the particular organism involved as well as on the condition of the mother and the fetus. Usually, before treatment is begun, other reasons for the symptoms will be ruled out, lab tests to determine the type of infectious organism involved will be ordered, and the fetus will be monitored. If the pregnancy is near term and the membranes have ruptured, and/or if the fetus or mother is in trouble, a prompt delivery is generally the preferred course. If the fetus is extremely immature, large amounts of antibiotics that can also reach and protect the baby are given, while the situation is carefully monitored. Delivery is postponed, if possible, until the fetus is more mature.

Prevention. Recent medical advances allowing for more rapid diagnosis and treatment have greatly reduced the risk of chorioamnionitis to both mother and baby; further improvement of diagnostic tools teamed with a better understanding of how to prevent such infections in the first place will reduce these risks even further.

PRETERM PREMATURE RUPTURE OF THE MEMBRANES (PPROM)

What is it? PPROM refers to the rupture of the membranes (or "bag of waters"), which cradles the fetus in the uterus, before 37 weeks. The major risk of PPROM is a premature birth; other risks include infection of the amniotic fluid (and possibly the fetus); prolapse or compression of the umbilical cord; and abruptio placenta. (Premature rupture of the membranes that isn't

preterm—that is, takes place after 37 weeks, but before labor begins—is discussed on page 338.)

Signs and symptoms. One sign is leaking or gushing of fluid from the vagina; the flow is heavier when the woman is lying down. An examination of the vagina reveals fluid that is alkaline coming from the cervix, rather than acid, as would be the case with a vaginal discharge or with urine coming from the urethra. Various tests may be used to diagnose PPROM.

Treatment. Most doctors agree that initially, for anywhere from a few hours to a full day, the expectant mother whose membranes rupture preterm should be closely observed. During this initial evaluation, she will probably be admitted to the hospital for bed rest and carefully monitored to see if contractions are beginning; the baby's condition is also evaluated. The mother's temperature and white blood count will be checked periodically so that doctors can take action immediately should infection, which can lead to premature delivery, develop. A culture from the cervix may also be taken to check for infection, and in many cases intravenous antibiotics will be given even before the results of the culture are in to prevent any infection from moving into the now open amniotic sac. Antibiotics appear to lengthen the time to delivery in PPROM, improving the outcome for the fetus. Steroids may be given to help the fetal lungs mature and, possibly, prevent other complications in the newborn.

If contractions begin and the fetus is believed to be too immature for delivery, medication may be given to try to halt them. As long as both mother and baby are all right, this conservative course may be continued until the baby is deemed mature enough for safe delivery. If at any point mother or baby is thought to be in danger, delivery will be carried out promptly. Rarely, the break in the membranes heals and the leakage of amniotic fluid stops on its own. If that happens, the mother may be allowed to go home and resume her normal routine while remaining on the alert for signs of further leakage.

Some doctors will try to delay delivery until 33 or 34 weeks of pregnancy, at which point they will induce labor. Others will try to postpone induction until 37 weeks. (To help them decide whether or not to induce labor, some doctors will perform amniocentesis or check the amniotic fluid in the vagina to determine the maturity of the baby's lungs.)

With the right treatment of PPROM, both mother and baby should be fine, though if the birth is premature, there may be a long stay in the neonatal intensive care unit for baby.

Prevention. Studies have shown that preterm premature rupture of the membranes is sometimes related to poor nutrition, particularly a deficiency in vitamin C, so eating a well balanced diet rich in vitamin C may help to avoid this complication. Vaginal infections, particularly bacterial vaginosis, can also lead to PPROM; therefore, watching out for and treating these infections can be effective in preventing PPROM.

PRETERM OR PREMATURE LABOR

What is it? Labor is preterm when it begins after the age of viability (20 weeks in most states) and before the 37th week (after which the baby is considered full term). About 12 percent of babies are born preterm in the United States. There is a wide range of risk factors associated with preterm labor, including maternal age under eighteen or over forty; inadequate prenatal care; smoking; cocaine use; a history of multiple induced abortions; a history or family history of preterm births; the mother's exposure to DES in the uterus; very low prepregnancy weight; a malformed uterus; incompetent cervix; uterine fibroids; vaginal, amniotic fluid, urinary tract, and other infections (including those of the gums); early production of the hormone oxytocin; hypertension or other chronic illness in the mother; excessive amniotic fluid; PPROM; placenta previa; second-trimester bleeding; carrying twins or more; extreme physical stress on the job (especially walking or standing for more than five hours a day during the third trimester); or physical abuse by a partner.

Preterm births are also more common among disadvantaged women, and among teenage and single mothers, most likely because they have a high level of other risk factors, particularly that they are less likely to receive good medical care and support during pregnancy. Still, there is much more to be learned about what causes labor to begin early; at least half of the women who go into preterm labor have no known risk factors.

Signs and symptoms. These consist of menstrual-like cramps, with or without diarrhea, nausea, or indigestion; lower back pain or pressure; an achiness or pressure in the pelvis, thighs, or groin; a watery or pinkish or brownish discharge, possibly preceded by the passage of a thick, gelatinous mucous plug; and/or a trickle or flow of amniotic fluid from the vagina, actual contractions, or uterine tightening. If testing finds high levels of fetal fibronectin (FFN, a form of protein found in body fluids; see box on page 510) in the cervical or vaginal fluids— even when there are no symptoms— there may be an increased risk for preterm delivery. Changes in the cervix (thinning, opening, or shortening as measured by ultrasound) will indicate whether or not preterm labor is actually beginning or about to begin.

Treatment. Prompt medical attention to the above symptoms is important, since treatment can occasionally halt or postpone premature labor, and each day a baby remains in the uterus, the better its chances of survival become.

Postponement or prevention of the onset of premature labor can often be achieved through limitations on sexual intercourse and other physical activities, partial to complete bed rest, home nurse contact weekly, and, if necessary, hospitalization. Home uterine monitoring, once recommended, has been shown not to be effective. In about half the cases of women who have early strong contractions but no bleeding, hospitalized bed rest alone, without medication, will halt contractions. If the membranes are also intact and the cervix has not effaced or dilated, 3 out of 4 of these women will carry to term. Tocolytic agents (drugs, such as nifedipine, indomethacin, ritodrine, terbutaline, and magnesium sulfate, which relax the uterus and have the potential to halt contractions) may be administered to stop contractions, if it is deemed necessary.[9] Risk and benefit, however, will be considered in each case, and the safest tocolytic should be given for the shortest amount of time. Long-term use of these drugs is not currently recommended. Although they can stop contractions and halt labor temporarily, tocolytic drugs alone have not been shown to improve the condition of the baby around birth or afterward and can have adverse effects on the mother. Newer drugs are under study and perhaps will turn out to be more effective and safer.

When the mother and/or child is in imminent danger from illness or other problems (as is the case in about 1 in 4 preterm deliveries), no attempt is made

9. It may be inappropriate to use tocolytics when there is vaginal bleeding, PPROM, or advanced dilation of the cervix.

OF SPECIAL CONCERN

PREDICTING PRETERM LABOR

Even among women who are at high risk for preterm labor, most will carry to term. One way to predict preterm labor is the examination of cervical or vaginal secretions for what is known as fetal fibronectin (FFN). Studies show that some women who test positive for FFN stand a good chance of going into preterm labor within one to two weeks of the test. The test, however, is better at diagnosing women who are *not* at risk for going into preterm labor (by detecting no FFN) than as an accurate predictor of women who *are* at risk.* When FFN is detected, steps should be taken to reduce the chances of preterm labor. The test is not widely available, is expensive, and is usually reserved for high-risk women only. If you are not considered high risk for preterm birth, you *do not* need to be tested for FFN.

---

*False positives occur if there was a vaginal exam performed, or if intercourse or other manipulation of the cervix occurred in the twenty-four hours before the test was administered.

to postpone delivery. Sometimes, when it's deemed safe, delivery may be delayed for twenty-four hours or so to allow the administration of a steroid to help improve fetal lung maturity. Antibiotics may be given, especially if infection is believed to have triggered labor. Delivery in a medical center with a neonatal intensive care unit (NICU) can improve the outlook for the newborn and justifies moving the mother with the baby in utero to the center before birth if she is stable for a safe transport.

Prevention. Not all preterm births can be avoided, since not all are due to

preventable risk factors. However, all the following measures reduce the risk of preterm delivery: getting early and good prenatal care; getting good dental care; avoiding smoking, cocaine, alcohol, and other drugs not prescribed by your doctor; getting tested for and, if necessary, treated for any infections, particularly those of the genital tract; following your practitioner's recommendations as to limitations on strenuous activity, including sexual intercourse and hours spent standing or walking on the job, especially if you have had previous preterm deliveries; for those at high risk, possibly receiving a weekly injection of a drug derived from the hormone progesterone.

VENOUS THROMBOSIS

What is it? It's a blood clot that develops in a vein, usually in a leg. Women are more susceptible to clots during pregnancy, delivery, and *particularly* in the postpartum period. This happens because nature, wisely worried about too much bleeding at childbirth, tends to increase the blood's clotting ability—occasionally too much—and because the enlarged uterus makes it difficult for blood in the lower body to return to the heart. Clots in superficial veins near the surface (thrombophlebitis) occur in about 1 or 2 out of 100 pregnancies. Deep vein thrombosis (in a vein deep in a limb), which if untreated can result in the clot moving to the lungs and threatening the patient's life, is fortunately much less common. Women who are at a somewhat increased risk of developing clots are those who have a family history of clots; have had previous clots themselves; are over thirty; have had three or more previous deliveries; have been confined to bed for long periods; are overweight, anemic, or have varicose veins; or have undergone midforceps or cesarean delivery in the past.

Signs and symptoms. In superficial thrombophlebitis, there is usually a tender, reddened area that runs in a line over a vein near the surface in the thigh or calf.

In deep vein thrombosis (DVT), the leg may feel heavy or painful, there may be tenderness in the calf or thigh, swelling (ranging from slight to severe), distention of the superficial veins, and calf pain on flexing the foot (turning the toes up toward the chin). Any such symptoms, as well as any other unusual leg symptoms, unexplained fever, or speeded-up heartbeat, should be reported to the practitioner. Ultrasound, phlebography (using an instrument for making a tracing of the venous pulse), or other methods may be used to diagnose the blood clot. If the blood clot has moved to the lungs (a pulmonary embolus), there may be chest pain, coughing with frothy, bloodstained sputum, speeded-up heartbeat and breathing rate, blueness of lips and fingertips, and fever. These symptoms require *immediate* medical attention.

Treatment. After diagnosis, treatment will depend on the degree and type of clot. A superficial clot will be treated with rest, leg elevation, local ointments, moist heat, an elastic compression stocking, and possibly, postpartum, with aspirin. *Prenatally*, with deep vein thrombosis, an anticoagulant drug (almost always heparin) is given, usually intravenously for a week or ten days, then under the skin until labor starts, at which point the drug is discontinued. Several hours after delivery it is resumed once more, and continued for the first few weeks postpartum. Rarely, a filter may be inserted in the inferior vena cava, a vein that receives blood from the lower limbs and the pelvic and abdominal organs and empties it into the heart, to help prevent the clot from moving to the lungs. With a clot that reaches the lungs, drugs *and* surgery may be needed, as well as treatment for any accompanying side effects. *Postpartum* treatment is basically the same, but, obviously, there's no interruption for labor and delivery.

Prevention. The best treatment is prevention: wear support hose if you are prone to blood clots or are in a high-risk category; avoid sitting for more than an hour or so without walking about and stretching your legs; exercise your legs as recommended by your practitioner if you are confined to bed; and don't sleep or exercise while lying flat on your back.

Uncommon Pregnancy Complications

The following complications of pregnancy are, for the most part, rare. The average pregnant woman is extremely unlikely to encounter any of them. So, again (and this deserves repeating), read this section only if you need to—and even then, read just what applies to you. If you are diagnosed with any of these complications during your pregnancy, use the information here to learn about the condition and its treatment (as well as how to prevent it in future pregnancies), but realize that your doctor's protocol for treating you may be different.

HYPEREMESIS GRAVIDARUM

What is it? An exaggerated form of morning sickness, hyperemesis gravidarum is characterized by excessive vomiting, which probably occurs in fewer than 1 in 200 pregnancies. It is more common in first-time mothers, in young mothers, in obese women, in women who are carrying multiple fetuses, and in women who suffered from the condition during a past pregnancy. Sensitivity of the vomiting center in the brain, which seems to vary from person to person, is one factor; psychological stress may also occasionally play a role. Excessive intake of saturated fat may also be a factor, as may endocrine imbalances, vitamin B deficiency, and *H. pylori* infection.

Signs and symptoms. The nausea and vomiting of early pregnancy is unusually frequent and severe (it may be impossible to keep anything down), and lingers longer (sometimes for the full nine months). Other symptoms include infrequent urination and urine that is dark yellow (signs of dehydration from loss of fluids through vomiting); weight loss of greater than 5 percent of original body weight; and/or blood in the vomited material. If untreated, the frequent vomiting can lead to malnutrition, dehydration, and possibly harm to the health of mother or baby, so any of these symptoms should be reported to your practitioner. Severe abdominal pain along with morning sickness (with or without other symptoms) could signal a gallbladder or pancreatic problem and requires prompt medical attention.

Very rarely, nausea and vomiting begin in the third trimester and are accompanied by upper abdominal pain and, later, confusion. These symptoms, most likely to occur in women with a metabolic disorder, may be a sign of preeclampsia or acute liver disease, and, again, require immediate medical attention.

Treatment. Milder cases may be controlled at home with dietary measures, rest, acupressure bands (Sea Bands or the battery-operated Relief Bands), antacids, and antivomiting (antiemetic) medication.[10] In some cases, medication administered through a pump may be possible. This is usually effective, but some women experience side effects severe enough to make them want to quit the therapy. Complementary and alternative therapies (such as acupuncture, biofeedback, meditation, and hypnosis) can also bring some relief; see page 246. Eating small amounts frequently may help, too, with lots of fluids between meals. Along with alcohol and tobacco (off-limits for *all* pregnant women), caffeine, carbonated beverages, and high-fat foods should be avoided. If vomiting continues and a significant amount of weight is lost, hospitalization may be necessary.

Further tests may be run to rule out nonpregnancy-related causes of vomiting, such as gastritis, an intestinal blockage, gallstones, or an ulcer. A darkened room and limitations on visitors reduce stimulation; counseling or psychotherapy may be given in an effort to reduce tension, which can exacerbate symptoms. If necessary, intravenous feeding may be given, along with an antiemetic and an electrolyte solution. When fluid levels and electrolyte balance are

---

10. Do not take any antivomiting/antiemetic medication (traditional or herbal) without your doctor's approval. Since some of these drugs interact adversely with other drugs, be sure to let your doctor know about any medication you are presently taking before an antiemetic is prescribed.

restored (usually within twenty-four to forty-eight hours), a clear liquid diet is begun. If this is tolerated, the mother will graduate to six small meals a day. If she still can't keep food down, intravenous feeding may be continued, though some food by mouth will still be encouraged. Occasionally, when the problem persists long enough to threaten the proper nutrition of the mother or fetus, special nutrients are added to the intravenous fluids to keep both fed while allowing the gastrointestinal tract to rest for a matter of weeks. This is known as "IV hyperalimentation." This almost always allows the pregnancy to continue without harm to mother or child. The good news is that, as miserable as the condition makes the expectant mother feel, it is unlikely to affect her baby. Most studies show that there is no health or other difference between infants of women who experience hyperemesis gravidarum and those who do not.

MOLAR PREGNANCY

What is it? In roughly 1 in 2,000 pregnancies in the United States—more often in women over forty-five than in younger mothers—an abnormal mass, instead of a normal embryo, forms inside the uterus after fertilization. The trophoblast—the layer of cells that line the gestational sac—converts into a clump of clear tapioca-like vesicles instead of the beginnings of a healthy placenta. Without a placental support system, the fertilized egg deteriorates. Also known as trophoblastic disease or hydatidiform mole, a molar pregnancy is probably caused by a chromosomal abnormality in the fertilized egg.

Signs and symptoms. The first sign of a molar pregnancy is usually an intermittent, though sometimes continuous, brownish discharge. Frequently, the normal morning sickness of pregnancy becomes abnormally severe. There may also be excessive levels of thyroid hormone in the mother's system, probably triggered by high levels of human chorionic gonadotropin (hCG). As the pregnancy progresses, 1 in 5 women may pass a few of these tiny vesicles through the vagina. The uterus is larger than expected and feels doughy rather than firm; no fetal heartbeat can be detected. Preeclampsia (with its elevated blood pressure, excessive swelling, and protein in the urine), or in some cases loss of weight and other indications of increased thyroid activity, may also be seen. The definitive diagnosis will depend on an ultrasound exam, which will show the absence of embryonic or fetal tissue and the uterus distended with these small vesicles. The ovaries may also be enlarged because of the accompanying high levels of hCG.

Treatment. The cervix is dilated and the contents of the uterus are carefully emptied, via a D & C. Follow-up is important, since about 10 to 15 percent of molar pregnancies don't stop growing immediately. If blood hCG levels fail to return to normal, another D & C is performed. In the rare instances that hCG levels remain elevated after a second procedure, the physician will check for a new pregnancy or for spread of the molar tissue to the vagina or lungs, which may be treated with chemotherapy. Very rarely, a molar pregnancy becomes malignant (see Choriocarcinoma, page 515), so close medical follow-up is especially important, since this condition is very curable with early diagnosis and treatment.

It is now generally recommended that attempts to conceive again following a molar pregnancy be postponed for a year; research has shown that such pregnancies usually turn out well. Careful

WHEN A SERIOUS FETAL DEFECT IS DETECTED

It's the nightmare of everyone who undergoes any kind of prenatal diagnosis: something actually does turn out to be wrong, so wrong that termination of the pregnancy may have to be considered. The fact that such a nightmare becomes a reality only rarely is no consolation to the couples who receive that dreaded abnormal report.

Before you do consider terminating your pregnancy, you should be sure that the diagnosis is correct. Ask your doctor if there are other tests that can confirm the first results. Then get a second opinion and a clear picture of your options, preferably from a genetic counselor or a specialist in maternal-fetal medicine.

If the pregnancy is to be terminated, you may find that comfort is hard to come by. Well-meaning friends and relatives may not understand what you're going through and may underplay what you view as a tragedy with comments like "It's for the best" or "You can try again." Professional support—from your doctor, a therapist, a social worker, or a genetic counselor—or support from a group of parents who have gone through the same experience may be necessary to help you cope. Accepting your loss won't be easy. You'll probably go through all or most of the stages of grieving—denial, anger, bargaining, and depression—before you reach acceptance.

Often, couples who get bad news saddle themselves with an added, and unnecessary, burden: guilt. It's important to realize that birth defects are most often a matter of chance. You wouldn't knowingly hurt your baby, and if you did so unknowingly, you aren't to blame. See page 526 for additional help on dealing with the loss of a baby.

If you decide to terminate, it may help you to keep in mind that if this diagnosis were not made prenatally, you would have carried your baby, getting to know and love it, for nine months, only to lose it shortly after birth. Or you would have delivered a baby who lingered for months or years, but with no semblance of life as we know it. Instead, by the time your due date rolls around you may have had the opportunity to become pregnant once again—this time, hopefully, with a healthy baby. That in no way, of course, takes away your right to mourn for the loss of this one—which is very important to do.

If, despite a hopeless prognosis, you opt (because of religious or other beliefs) to continue your pregnancy, you will need at least as much support, possibly more—not only from couples who have made the same choice, but from your medical team. A caring practitioner who is willing to support you through the rest of your pregnancy, through childbirth and beyond, will make a tremendous difference during a very difficult time.

---

monitoring of any new pregnancy is vital because of the possibility of another mole developing.

Prevention. Since there is some very tentative evidence that links trophoblastic disease to an inadequate intake of animal protein and vitamin A, getting plenty of both (see the Protein and Green Leafy and Yellow Vegetables and Yellow Fruit requirements of the Preg-

nancy Diet) is a good idea before conceiving again, and throughout any subsequent pregnancy.

PARTIAL MOLAR PREGNANCY

What is it? In a partial molar pregnancy, as in a complete molar pregnancy (page 513), there is abnormal development of the trophoblast. With a partial mole, however, identifiable embryonic or fetal tissue is present. If the fetus survives, it may be growth-restricted and have a variety of congenital abnormalities, such as webbed (or connected) fingers and toes and water on the brain (hydrocephalus). If a normal baby is born, it usually turns out that it was part of a multiple pregnancy, with the partial mole belonging to a twin that had deteriorated.

Signs and symptoms. These are similar to those of an incomplete or missed abortion. There is usually irregular vaginal bleeding, no fetal heartbeat, and a uterus that is either small or normal for the length of the pregnancy. Only a small percentage of women with partial molar pregnancies have an enlarged uterus, as is common in a complete molar pregnancy. Ultrasound and hCG levels are used to diagnose the condition.

Treatment. If the fetus is living and appears on ultrasound to be in good condition, the pregnancy will probably be allowed to continue. If not, follow-up and treatment are similar to that for a complete molar pregnancy, and a new pregnancy is not recommended until hCG levels have been normal for one year.

Prevention. Most women can have healthy babies after having had a partial molar pregnancy, but since the risk of a repeat exists, early ultrasound examination is important in future pregnancies to rule out that possibility.

CHORIOCARCINOMA

What is it? Choriocarcinoma is an extremely rare cancer related directly to pregnancy. About half the cases develop when there is a molar pregnancy (page 513), 30 to 40 percent following a miscarriage, and 10 to 20 percent after a normal pregnancy.

Signs and symptoms. The signs of the disease include intermittent bleeding following a miscarriage, a pregnancy, or the removal of a mole, along with elevated hCG levels and a tumor in the vagina, uterus, or lungs.

Treatment. Chemotherapy. With early diagnosis and treatment, survival is the norm and fertility is unaffected, though it is usually recommended that pregnancy be deferred for two years after treatment is complete and there is no evidence of residual disease.

ECLAMPSIA

What is it? Eclampsia occurs when preeclampsia (see page 500) progresses to involve the central nervous system, leading to seizures (convulsions) and sometimes coma. Eclampsia is a very serious but *extremely rare* condition that, if untreated, may be fatal for both mother and baby. Very few women receiving proper medical care ever progress from the manageable preeclampsia to the more serious eclampsia.

Signs and symptoms. Eclampsia is characterized by seizures. The seizures can develop without warning and usually occur during or close to delivery. Postpartum seizures can also occur, with the majority happening within the first forty-eight hours after delivery, but they may occur as late as three weeks postpartum.

Treatment. The woman is prevented from injuring herself during the convulsions. Oxygen and drugs to arrest the seizures are administered; the woman's environment is kept as free of stimuli, such as light and noise, as possible. Labor will generally be induced or a cesarean performed when the woman is stable. With optimum care the survival rate is 98 percent, and the majority of women rapidly return to normal after delivery, though careful follow-up is necessary to be certain blood pressure doesn't stay up and seizures don't continue.

Prevention. Proper management of preeclampsia can successfully prevent the progression of the condition to eclampsia. Postpartum follow-up is critical.

HELLP Syndrome

What is it? HELLP (Hemolysis, Elevated Liver enzymes, and Low Platelet count) syndrome is a condition that can occur on its own or in association with preeclampsia. HELLP is characterized by liver and blood platelet abnormalities (thrombocytopenia) and severe upper-right abdominal pain (from a distended liver), nausea, and possibly vomiting. When HELLP develops, there is a higher risk of health complications for the mother, leading to permanent damage of her nervous system, blood vessels, lungs, kidneys, and other organs, and growth restriction (because of a reduced blood supply through the placenta) or oxygen deprivation in the baby.

Signs and symptoms. Symptoms are very vague, consisting of generalized malaise, gastrointestinal pain, nausea, vomiting, headaches, and other viral-type illnesses in the third trimester. There may also be allover itching, and most women have severe tenderness and pain in the upper right side of the abdomen. Blood tests will reveal a low platelet count, elevated liver enzymes, and hemolysis (the breakdown of red blood cells). Liver function rapidly deteriorates in women with HELLP, so treatment is critical.

Treatment. With HELLP syndrome, immediate delivery on diagnosis is usually considered a must, but it may be postponed if the fetus is very premature (usually under 26 weeks). Waiting even a couple of days—while administering steroids—seems to help mature the fetal lungs and improve the mother's condition at the same time. But this is usually recommended only at a major medical center. Immediately following diagnosis, while awaiting the decision to deliver, women with HELLP are put on complete bed rest (lying on their left sides) and given magnesium sulfate, to prevent seizures, along with blood pressure medication and fluids, as needed. The fetal condition will also be monitored.

Prevention. Because a woman who has had HELLP in a previous pregnancy is likely to have it again, close monitoring will be necessary in any subsequent pregnancy.

Abruptio Placenta

What is it? In abruptio placenta, the placenta separates, or abrupts, from the uterus prematurely. The condition is responsible for roughly 1 in 4 cases of late-pregnancy bleeding. It is more likely to occur in older mothers who have had babies before, and in women who smoke, use illegal drugs such as cocaine, have hypertension (chronic or pregnancy-induced), have been taking aspirin late in pregnancy, or have had a previous premature separation of the placenta. A short umbilical cord or trauma due to an accident is occasionally the cause of an abruption.

Signs and symptoms. With a *slight* separation, bleeding may be as light as a light menstrual flow or as heavy as a heavy one, and may or may not contain clots. There may also be cramping or a mild ache in the abdomen, and uterine tenderness. Occasionally, particularly when there has been trauma to the abdomen, there may be no bleeding at all.

With a *moderate* separation, bleeding is heavier, the abdomen is tender and firm, and abdominal pain may be more severe, stemming in part from strong uterine contractions. Both mother and baby may show signs of blood loss.

With *severe* separation, when more than half of the placenta separates from the uterine wall, an emergency situation exists for both mother and baby. The symptoms are similar to those for a moderate separation, but more extreme.

The diagnosis is made using patient history, physical examination, and observation of uterine contractions and the fetal response to them. Ultrasound may be helpful, but only about half of abruptions can actually be seen on ultrasound.

Treatment. When the separation is *slight,* bed rest often stops the bleeding, and you can usually resume your normal routine, with some restriction on activity, a few days later. Though it's not usual, there is the possibility of a repeat bleeding episode or even of a hemorrhage, so it's necessary for the mother-to-be to remain alert to symptoms and for the rest of her pregnancy to be closely monitored. If signs of separation recur and the baby is near term, prompt delivery may be the chosen course.

In most cases, a *moderate* separation also responds to bed rest. But sometimes transfusions and other emergency treatment may also be needed. Careful monitoring of both mother and baby is necessary, and if either shows signs of distress, delivery without delay may be essential.

When a *severe* separation occurs, prompt medical action, including transfusions and immediate delivery, is imperative.

At one time the outlook was bleak for both mothers and their babies when a placenta separated prematurely. Today, with expert and prompt medical care, virtually all the mothers with placental abruption and almost all their babies will survive the crisis.

PLACENTA ACCRETA

What is it? In this very rare condition, the placenta grows into the deeper layers of the uterine wall and becomes firmly attached to it. Depending on how deeply the placental cells invade, the condition may also be called placenta percreta or placenta increta. This condition is most common in women who have scarring of the uterine wall from previous surgeries or cesarean deliveries and in those with placenta previa. Sometimes it may be diagnosed by transabdominal color Doppler sonography, a form of ultrasound, and the results can help in deciding on treatment.

Signs and symptoms. There may be no apparent symptoms, so unless placenta accreta is diagnosed earlier by ultrasound, it may not be recognized until the third stage of childbirth, when the placenta unexpectedly does not separate from the uterine wall. Rarely, placenta accreta may be severe enough to rupture or partially rupture the uterus. In that case, there will be severe pain and bleeding.

Treatment. In most cases, the placenta must be removed surgically after delivery to stop the bleeding. Very rarely, when the bleeding cannot be controlled by tying off the exposed blood vessels, removal of the entire uterus may be necessary.

OLIGOHYDRAMNIOS

What is it? Oligohydramnios is a condition in which there is too little amniotic fluid in the uterus. The majority of women diagnosed with oligohydramnios will have a completely normal pregnancy. But, occasionally, the condition can lead to or signal potential problems. In early

WHEN MULTIPLE FETUSES AREN'T THRIVING

Since the initiation of fertility treatments, otherwise known as assisted reproductive technology (ART), the number of twin, triplet, quadruplet, and other multiple births has greatly increased. Because the risks to both mother and babies can multiply with multiple pregnancies, the American College of Obstetricians and Gynecologists recommends that efforts be made during fertility treatment to reduce the possibility of multiple births. To this end, using in vitro fertilization (joining egg and sperm in a test tube and then inserting into the mother's uterus the fertilized egg or eggs—generally, three for women under thirty-five, four for women ages thirty-five to thirty-nine, and five for those over forty) instead of hormone treatment (to stimulate the release of many eggs by the mother, many of which may be fertilized) is considered the best way to go. Other techniques are under study, including letting the embryos develop outside the uterus for a couple of extra days, so that the healthiest can be transferred, increasing the chances of a successful pregnancy and reducing the need to use so many of the embryos.

If, thanks to nature or technology, you do end up with more than one fetus, the chances are good that your babies will do well. However, since multiples are more prone to poor fetal growth than singletons, especially in the third trimester, multiple pregnancies are followed closely with a series of ultrasound checks from the 20th week on. If one or more of the babies are not growing as well as they should, intensive surveillance, usually in the hospital, will be needed. The babies will be delivered promptly either when it is determined that the lungs of the larger (or largest) fetus are mature or when it becomes risky for the smaller fetus to continue to remain in the uterus. Fortunately, such circumstances arise *very* infrequently.

Nature often attends to such situations on her own. It's believed that each year thousands more multiple births are conceived than are born. Because the mother's body is unable to support so many fetuses, generally all but one die early in these pregnancies, often leaving no visible evidence that they ever existed. Sometimes, however, the multiple fetuses continue to struggle on together, all of them suffering, none of them doing well enough to survive. When nature hasn't taken the initiative, another option may be considered: using multifetal pregnancy reduction (MFPR) to save one or more of the babies, rather than letting them all perish.

Recently, it's been recommended that nonselective reduction of multiple embryos be considered early in pregnancy, before they begin showing signs of doing poorly. Some physicians reserve such pregnancy reduction for situations where there are four or more fetuses; others are willing to reduce triplets as well, when it seems appropriate. Reduction is usually performed at or after the 9th week, with a drug injected into the vicinity of the fetal heart. Some doctors, however, believe that since up until the end of the first trimester nature may still spon-

pregnancy, there is the slight risk of umbilical cord constriction or the development of a club foot in the fetus who doesn't have enough room in the womb. Later in pregnancy, it can be a sign of fetal distress. Oligohydramnios also can accompany some types of fetal defects, such as problems in the fetus's digestive or urinary system. The baby's urine is part of the makeup of amniotic fluid, and if the baby is not excreting it properly, oligohydramnios may occur. The condition may also be caused by placental insufficiency.

Signs and symptoms. There are no symp-

taneously reduce the number of fetuses, it's best to wait until the end of this period to consider a procedure.

If nonselective reduction early in pregnancy wasn't attempted, and tests show that one or more of the fetuses are not thriving as the pregnancy progresses, then selective reduction later in pregnancy may be considered. That means removing one or more fetuses (those doing least well) in order to give the others a chance to survive and thrive. This procedure may also be recommended if one of the fetuses is seriously malformed (lacking part of the brain, for example) or there is serious maternal bleeding.

Though pregnancy reduction is a difficult procedure for doctors to perform, it's certainly even more difficult for parents to contemplate. If at any time in your pregnancy a reduction is suggested, the decision will be a painful one to make. Before you decide, you should get a second opinion to be sure that the evaluation of the tests on your fetuses is accurate. Then you should discuss the risks of the procedure—including the risk that all the fetuses may be lost—with your physician. This risk is lower, of course, when the surgeon has had a great deal of experience and success with pregnancy reduction. In general, it seems that when a pregnancy with four or more fetuses is reduced, more babies are likely to survive than would if reduction were not performed.

Finally, if religion plays an important part in your life, getting advice from spiritual as well as medical advisers is a good idea. It will probably also be helpful to talk to a specialist in medical ethics (check with your local hospital), a genetic counselor, a maternal-fetal medicine specialist, or another counselor familiar with this issue. In these discussions, you will probably find that most ethicists (even some conservative theologians) believe that trying to save one baby is preferable to taking the chance that all will die.

Reading "When a Serious Fetal Defect Is Detected" (page 514) and "Coping with Pregnancy Loss" (page 526) may also provide some insight. So might talking to other parents who are going through, or have gone through, a similar challenge (try finding a support group or individuals you can talk to through your doctor or hospital, or on-line).

In the end, however, the decision will rest with you and your partner. No one else can know how you feel, and no one else can better assess what's right in your situation. If you are definitely opposed to the procedure on philosophical or religious grounds, and opt to continue carrying all of the fetuses no matter what the risks to them or to you, you will need to be in the care of a physician who is ready to support your decision (and not just carry it out) without reservation. Similarly, if you choose reduction, you'll need to have a physician who wholeheartedly supports that decision.

Once you've made your decision, try not to second-guess it. Accept that it was the best one you could make—and that you made it with the best of intentions. But recognize, too, that feelings of guilt, blame, or anger may be inevitable—and that you may need help overcoming them.

---

toms in the mother other than a uterus that measures smaller than it should (though a small uterus can also just mean that her due date has been miscalculated). Oligohydramnios is usually detected through ultrasound. Signs of the condition include decreased fetal movement and possibly IUGR (slowed growth).

During labor there is an increased risk for a slowdown in the fetal heart rate.

Treatment. Some practitioners feel that replacing the fluid through amnioinfusion is a good idea. Maternal oral and IV hydration may also help to correct the condition. If oligohydramnios is detected in a term or postterm pregnancy, many practitioners will induce labor. It's important for women with oligohydramnios to eat well, rest more, and avoid smoking, as well as to report any signs of preterm labor to their practitioner.

HYDRAMNIOS (OR POLYHYDRAMNIOS)

What is it? Hydramnios is when there is too much amniotic fluid in the uterus. Most cases of hydramnios are mild and transient, simply the result of a temporary change in the normal balance of the amniotic fluid production. Far fewer cases are linked to a fetal defect, either in the central nervous system or in the baby's bladder and kidneys, or to a swallowing problem (as might be caused by a gastrointestinal obstruction, such as esophageal stenosis or pyloric stenosis, or a facial deformity, such as cleft lip or palate). It can also be related to untreated diabetes in the mother and is more likely to occur when there are multiple fetuses.

Signs and symptoms. Hydramnios is usually detected by a routine or diagnostic ultrasound. The uterus may measure larger than it should. The condition can cause abdominal discomfort, indigestion, swelling in the legs, breathlessness, or hemorrhoids, and may put the pregnancy at high risk for breech position, preterm labor, placental abruption, or cord prolapse.

Treatment. If the hydramnios is advanced, amniocentesis may be performed to remove some fluid. Medications may also be used sometimes. When hydramnios exists, the practitioner usually will not artificially rupture the membranes during labor because of the risk of cord prolapse with the large gush of fluid. Some will rupture the membranes very slowly, with a small pinprick, to allow the water to trickle out slowly in a controlled setting. If membranes break naturally, there is increased risk for cord prolapse, so call your practitioner immediately if you have been diagnosed with hydramnios and your water breaks.

KNOTS AND TANGLES IN THE CORD

What are they? Once in a while, the umbilical cord becomes knotted or tangled or wrapped around a fetus, often at the neck (when it is known as a "nuchal cord"). Some knots form during delivery; others form during pregnancy when the baby moves around. As long as the knot remains loose, it generally does not harm the baby. Sometimes, however, the knot can be pulled tight, slowing or stopping the flow of blood to the fetus. A stoppage of blood flow can be fatal to the fetus, so action must be taken immediately if such a cord problem is suspected.

FIRST AID FOR THE FETUS

In late pregnancy, absence of fetal activity could be a sign that something is wrong (for a home test, see page 243). Since diminishing activity (generally judged to mean fewer than ten movements in a two-hour period) is often noted while there is still time to help the fetus, it should be reported immediately to your practitioner. If he or she is not available, have someone take you to the emergency room or the labor and delivery area of your local hospital immediately. With prompt action it is very often possible to save a fetus in trouble.

Signs and symptoms. Studies have shown that the most frequent sign is a significant decrease in fetal activity after 37 weeks. (If you're testing regularly for fetal movement—see page 243—it will be easy to note such a change.) If you experience these symptoms or any other unexpected change in fetal behavior, call your practitioner at once and ask to have the condition of your fetus checked. If you're in labor, and the fetus is being monitored, the cord problem may show up in abnormal fetal heart tracings. An ultrasound can be used to uncover a problem with the cord.

Treatment. If there is a cord problem, immediate delivery, usually by cesarean, is the best approach.

CORD PROLAPSE

What is it? The umbilical cord is a baby's lifeline in the uterus. Rarely, when the amniotic membranes rupture, the cord slips, or prolapses, through the cervix or even well into the vaginal canal, carried by the rush of amniotic fluid. It then becomes vulnerable to compression by the baby's presenting part as it presses through the cervix and down the canal during delivery. If the cord does become compressed, the vital supply of oxygen to the fetus can be reduced or even cut off. Prolapse is most common in premature labors (because the presenting part of the fetus is so small it doesn't completely fill the pelvis)

or when a part other than the head, especially a foot, presents first (because a foot, for example, takes up less space than a head, allowing the cord to slip down). Prolapse is also more common when the membranes rupture before labor begins or if there is excess amniotic fluid (hydramnios).

Signs and symptoms. An umbilical cord can prolapse so far that it may be seen hanging from the vagina, or it may just be felt as "something in there." If it becomes compressed, any distress is likely to show up on the fetal monitor or other tests of fetal well-being.

Treatment. If you should actually see or feel your baby's umbilical cord in your vagina, or you suspect it might have prolapsed, get on your hands and knees to reduce pressure on the cord. If the cord protrudes, support it gently (don't press or squeeze) with warm wet gauze pads or a clean towel or diaper. Have someone rush you to the hospital, or call 911 or your local medical emergency service.

At the hospital, a saline solution may be injected into your bladder to cushion the cord; a cord that is outside the vagina may be tucked back in and held in place by a special sterile tampon; and drugs may be given to stop labor while you are readied for an emergency cesarean. With prompt and appropriate medical care, the outcome is usually very good.

Childbirth and Postpartum Complications

Many of the following conditions can't be anticipated prior to labor and delivery—and there's no need to read up on them (and start

worrying) ahead of time, since the chances that any of them will occur during or after *your* childbirth are very small. They are included here so that in the unlikely event you experience one, you can learn about it after the fact, or in some cases, learn how you can prevent it from happening in your next labor and delivery.

FETAL DISTRESS

What is it? The term "fetal distress" is used to describe a situation in which the fetus is believed to be in jeopardy, most often because of decreased oxygen flow. The distress may be caused by a variety of problems, including the mother's position putting pressure on major blood vessels; maternal illness (anemia, hypertension, heart disease, abnormally low blood pressure, or shock); a placenta that is no longer functioning well or has separated prematurely from the uterus; umbilical cord compression or entanglement; prolonged or excessive uterine activity; or fetal infection, malformation, hemorrhage, or anemia.

Signs and symptoms. The precise signals sent by the fetus vary with the cause of the distress. The mother may notice a change in fetal movement patterns or an absence of movement. The practitioner may pick up heartbeat changes typical of fetal distress with a Doppler or get a nonreassuring response on the fetal monitor (see page 327). Additional tests may then be performed.

Treatment. When fetal distress is confirmed, immediate delivery is usually indicated. If vaginal delivery is not imminent, then an emergency cesarean is usually performed. In some cases, the physician may elect to resuscitate the baby in the uterus before doing a cesarean delivery, to decrease the risk that it will suffer from oxygen deprivation. This is usually done by giving the mother medication to slow contractions (which will increase oxygen to the fetus) and to dilate her blood vessels and raise her heart rate (which will also enhance blood flow).

SHOULDER DYSTOCIA

What is it? Dystocia is labor that doesn't progress; in shoulder dystocia, labor doesn't progress because the baby's shoulders become stuck on their way through the birth canal after the head has been delivered.

Signs and symptoms. Delivery stalls after the head emerges and before the shoulders are out. This can occur unexpectedly in a labor that has progressed normally up to that point.

Treatment. A variety of approaches may be used to rescue the baby whose shoulder is lodged in the pelvis, including performing an extra-large episiotomy; trying to rotate the baby and maneuver the back shoulder out first; hyperflexing the mother's knees up on her abdomen; applying moderate pressure just above the brim of the pelvis; attempting various other maneuvers to force the shoulders out, including, if other measures fail, breaking the baby's collarbone. If possible (and rarely is it so), it may be preferable to tuck the baby's head back into the vagina and perform a cesarean.

Prevention. To make sure your baby doesn't get too big to maneuver through the birth canal, it's important to keep weight gain to recommended levels during pregnancy through good diet and sensible exercise. (Though a mother's weight gain doesn't always correlate with baby's size, too many pounds for mom sometimes means too many pounds for baby.) Diabetics need to be extremely careful in controlling their condition (see page 472) in order to avoid an overly large baby.

Uterine Rupture

What is it? A rupture or tear of the uterus during pregnancy (rare) or during labor (somewhat less rare). A scar in the uterine wall is the largest single cause of rupture. The scar may be the result of a prior cesarean section (especially if the incision made was a classic, or up-and-down one); a repaired uterine rupture; uterine surgery (to correct its shape or remove fibroids); or previous uterine perforation or trauma (as from a knife or bullet wound). Abnormalities related to the placenta (such as placenta previa, a placenta that separates prematurely, or placenta accreta, a placenta that is attached deeply in the uterine wall) or to fetal position (such as a fetus lying crosswise) can also increase the risk of uterine rupture. Extremely violent labor contractions (spontaneous or, more often, induced) can also lead to rupture; but this is *very* rare, particularly in a first pregnancy when there is no predisposing scar. Uterine rupture is more common in women who have already had six or more children, have a very distended uterus (because of multiple fetuses or excess amniotic fluid), have had a difficult labor previously, or are experiencing difficulties in their present delivery (particularly shoulder dystocia, see facing page; or a forceps delivery). Being induced during a VBAC trial of labor also greatly increases the risk of rupture.

Signs and symptoms. Women who are at increased risk—small though it may be—of rupture, because of a scarred uterus or any of the other factors above, should know the possible warning signs, just in case. The first sign of actual rupture is usually a searing pain in the abdomen, accompanied by a feeling that something inside is "ripping." This is generally followed by a brief period of relief, then diffuse abdominal pain and tenderness. Unless the rupture is in the lower segment of the uterus, contractions will generally cease. There may or may not be vaginal bleeding. The fetus, with part of the protective wrapping of the uterus torn away, will be more easily felt through the abdomen and may show signs of distress. (If the fetus is being monitored, sudden fetal heart abnormalities may show up.) If you experience such symptoms, which are more severe when the rupture is in the upper half of the uterus, seek immediate emergency medical attention.

Treatment. Immediate cesarean delivery is necessary, followed by repair of the uterus, if possible. If damage is extensive, a hysterectomy may be required. Sometimes a rupture isn't recognized until hemorrhaging occurs after delivery. Again, the uterus may be repaired or, if necessary, removed.

After a rupture, the mother is closely monitored to be sure complications don't occur, and antibiotics may be given to prevent infection. Depending on the situation, she may be allowed out of bed in as few as six hours or not for several days.

Prevention. Evaluating the condition of the uterus prior to delivery, through the use of transvaginal ultrasound, in women who have had a previous cesarean or other surgery or trauma to the uterus. If the uterus seems thinned in places, another cesarean should be planned. A repeat cesarean may also be considered in women who have had two or more previous cesarean deliveries, since they have a greater risk of uterine rupture than women with only one previous cesarean. Again, checking the uterus for thinning may help in making a decision. Women who are trying for a VBAC delivery should *not* be induced.

UTERINE INVERSION (INVERTED UTERUS)

What is it? An inverted uterus occurs when the placenta doesn't detach completely after delivery of a baby; when it emerges, it pulls the top, or fundus, of the uterus with it—in effect very much like a sock being pulled inside out. Women at slightly higher risk for this very rare complication are those who have had a previous inversion, many prior births, or a prolonged labor (over twenty-four hours) this time around; those with a placenta implanted across the top (fundus) of the uterus or abnormally attached to it; and those who were given magnesium sulfate, which relaxes the uterus, during labor. The uterus may also invert if it is overly relaxed or if the fundus isn't held in place while the placenta is coaxed out in the third stage of childbirth. Immediate treatment of the inverted uterus is important to protect the mother from serious hemorrhage and shock.

Signs and symptoms. Early diagnosis is critical in the case of an inverted uterus. Symptoms of uterine inversion include abdominal pain, excessive bleeding, and signs of shock in the mother. The practitioner, pressing down on the abdomen, will not be able to feel the uterus; in a complete inversion, part of the uterus will be visible in the vagina.

Treatment. In most cases, the uterus can be pushed back into place by hand, usually under general anesthesia, though sometimes other techniques, such as hydrostatic pressure (in which the uterus is filled with a salt water solution to push it back into place), are used. Intravenous fluids and blood transfusions may be needed if blood loss has been great. Drugs (such as magnesium sulfate or nitroglycerin) may be given to relax the uterus even further in order to facilitate the replace-ment. If fragments of placenta remain in the uterus, they may be removed before or after the uterus is replaced. In very rare cases, the uterus can't be replaced manually through the vagina, and abdominal surgery is necessary.

After replacement, pressure will usually be kept on the abdomen to keep the uterus in place, and oxytocin or other drugs given to firm it so it won't reinvert. Antibiotics may be given to prevent infection.

Prevention. Since a woman who has had one uterine inversion is at an increased risk for another, your practitioner should be informed if you've had an inversion in the past.

VAGINAL AND CERVICAL LACERATIONS

What are they? These are tears or lacerations in the perineal area around the vagina, in the vagina, and/or in the cervix, which can range from minor to extensive.

Signs and symptoms. Excessive bleeding may be the most obvious symptom, though the lacerations, especially if they are external, may also be evident to the practitioner after the delivery.

Treatment. Generally, all lacerations that are longer than 2 centimeters (about 1 inch) or that continue to bleed heavily are stitched. A local anesthetic may be given first, if one wasn't administered during delivery.

Prevention. Perineal massage and Kegel exercises (see pages 193 and 330), done for six to eight weeks before delivery, may help make the perineal area more flexible and reduce the risk of lacerations.

POSTPARTUM HEMORRHAGE

What is it? Postpartum hemorrhage is heavy bleeding that is difficult to stem. It is a very serious but extremely uncommon complication. And, when treated promptly, it is rarely the life-threatening situation it once was. Excessive bleeding may occur if the uterus is too relaxed and doesn't contract, due to a long, exhausting labor; a traumatic delivery; a uterus that was overdistended because of multiple births, a large baby, or excess amniotic fluid; an oddly shaped placenta, or one that separated prematurely; fibroids that prevent symmetrical contraction of the uterus; or a generally weakened condition of the mother at the time of delivery (due to, for example, anemia, preeclampsia, or extreme fatigue).

Hemorrhage can also occur immediately postpartum because of unrepaired lacerations to the uterus, cervix, vagina, or somewhere else in the pelvis or because the uterus has ruptured or inverted (been turned inside out). It can occur up to a week or two after delivery when fragments of the placenta are retained in, or adhere to, the uterus. Infection can also cause postpartum hemorrhage, right after delivery or weeks later. Postpartum hemorrhage occurs more frequently in women who had placenta previa or abruptio placenta prior to delivery. It can also be caused by the use of aspirin, ibuprofen, gingko biloba, large doses of vitamin E, or other drugs, herbs, or supplements that can interfere with blood clotting. Rarely, the cause of the hemorrhage is a previously undiagnosed bleeding disorder in the mother that is genetic.

Signs and symptoms. These consist of abnormal bleeding after delivery: bleeding that saturates more than one pad an hour for more than a few hours or is extremely bright red anytime after the first postpartum week, especially if it doesn't slow down when you do; a foul smell to your vaginal discharge (lochia); large blood clots (lemon-size or larger) in the discharge; pain and/or swelling in the lower abdominal area beyond the first few days after delivery.

Treatment. Depending on the cause of the hemorrhage, the physician may try one or more of the following to stem the bleeding: uterine massage to encourage the uterus to contract; the administration of drugs (such as oxytocin) to promote the contraction of the uterus; searching for and repairing any lacerations; removing any retained placental fragments. If bleeding isn't quickly arrested, further measures will be taken: intravenous fluids and, if necessary, transfusion; the administration of blood-clotting agents if failure of the blood to coagulate is the problem, and of antibiotics to prevent infection. Rarely, packing of the uterus with gauze to stem bleeding for six to twenty-four hours or the ligation, or tying off or blocking, of the major artery in the uterus will be needed. If these procedures fail, a new approach—the use of an intrauterine inflated balloon as a "tampon"—gives excellent results and can help avoid invasive procedures. When all attempts to stop the bleeding fail, the removal of the uterus may be necessary.

However, in most cases, the odds are very good that treatment of postpartum hemorrhage will be successful, and that the new mother will recover quickly.

Prevention. It is best to avoid any supplement or medication that may interfere with blood clotting (see Treatment, above), especially in the last trimester and the immediate postpartum period.

POSTPARTUM INFECTION

What is it? This is an infection related to childbirth, rare in women who are receiving good medical care and have had an uncomplicated vaginal delivery. The most common postpartum infection is endometritis, an infection of the lining of the uterus (the endometrium), which is vulnerable after the detachment of the placenta. Endometritis is more likely to occur after a cesarean section that followed a prolonged labor or early rupture of the membranes. It is also more likely to occur if a fragment of the placenta has been retained in the uterus. A laceration to the cervix, vagina, or vulva, or an episiotomy site, can also become infected postpartum.

Signs and symptoms. These vary according to the site of origin. A slight fever, vague lower abdominal pain, and sometimes a foul-smelling vaginal discharge characterize an infection of the endometrium. With infection of a laceration or an episiotomy site, there will usually be pain and tenderness in the area; sometimes a foul-smelling, thick discharge; abdominal or side pain; or difficult urination. In certain types of infection, the fever spikes as high as 105°F, and there are chills, headache, and malaise. On occasion, there are no obvious symptoms but fever. For this reason, any postpartum fever should be reported to your doctor.

Treatment. Treatment with antibiotics is very effective, but it should begin quickly. A culture may be taken to determine the organism that is causing the infection, so that the right antibiotic can be prescribed.

Prevention. Meticulous attention should be given to cleanliness during labor, delivery, and postpartum. Always wash your hands before touching the perineal area, wipe from front to back, don't use tampons for postpartum bleeding, and be sure maxi pads you use are clean.

Coping with Pregnancy Loss

No matter when you've lost a baby—early in pregnancy, later on during delivery, or after birth—the hurt is deep and the effect on your life profound.

Miscarriage. Just because it takes place early in pregnancy doesn't mean that miscarriage is any less painful for expectant parents. A miscarriage often brings shock, despair, depression, and a sense of failure, especially when the pregnancy is wanted. In fact, coping with early pregnancy loss may be, at least in certain ways, just as difficult as coping with the loss of a baby later on. First of all, because so many couples plan to refrain from spreading the word about their pregnancy until the third month has passed, even close friends and family may not have been told yet—which can mean that support may be hard to come by. Even those who knew about the pregnancy and/or are told about the miscarriage may offer less support than they would have had the pregnancy been further along. They may minimize the significance of the loss with a "Don't worry, you can try again." They fail to realize that the loss of a baby, no matter how early in pregnancy it occurs, can be devastating. Second, the fact that there is no possibility of holding the baby, taking a photo, having a funeral and burial—rituals of grieving that can all help offer some closure for parents of stillborn infants—also complicates the recovery process.

Still, if you've suffered a miscarriage (or an ectopic or molar pregnancy), it's important to remember that you have a right and a need to grieve. Finding a way to express your grief will honor the child you've lost, as well as help you cope and, eventually, move on. You might consider holding a small memorial service, just for very close friends and family. Even if a small service is too public for such private pain, you might hold a symbolic ceremony for just the two of you in a place you find comforting—for instance, sharing your thoughts about your baby as the sun rises over a quiet lake. You can also share your feelings—individually, through a support group, or online—with others who have experienced early miscarriage. Since so many women suffer a miscarriage at least once during the reproductive years, you may be surprised to find how many others you know have had the same experience but never talked about it with you, or perhaps never talked about it at all. Many of the tips for those who have later pregnancy losses may also be helpful for you. Also see Stages of Grief (see box on page 532).

Accept that you will always have a place in your heart for the pregnancy you lost, and that you may feel sad or depressed on the anniversary of the due date of your lost baby or on the anniversary of the miscarriage itself, even years later. It may help to plan to do something special at that time—at least for the first few years—that will be cheering yet allow you to remember: planting some new flowers or a tree, having a quiet picnic in the park, sharing a commemorative dinner with your spouse.

While it's normal and necessary to mourn your loss, you should start to feel gradually better as time passes. If you don't or if you have continued trouble coping with everyday life—you're not eating or sleeping, you're not able to focus at work, you're becoming isolated from family and friends—seek professional counseling to help with your recovery.

A miscarriage often means never again taking for granted that a pregnancy will lead to a baby. Recognize also that your next pregnancy will be less innocent. On the one hand, you'll try not to think about the baby too much for fear that you might miscarry again. On the other hand, you'll be extra attuned to every pregnancy symptom—twinges, aches, tender breasts—as a sign that the baby is still thriving.

Death in the uterus. When you don't hear from your baby for several hours or more, it's natural to fear the worst. And the worst, of course, is that your unborn baby has died. Fortunately, that's rarely the case. But when it does happen, it is devastating.

You are likely to be in a fog of disbelief and grief after being told that your baby's heartbeat can't be located and that he or she has died in the uterus. It may be difficult or even impossible for you to carry on with your normal life while carrying around a fetus that is no longer living, and studies show that a woman is much more likely to suffer severe depression after the delivery of a stillborn if the delivery is delayed more than three days after the death is diagnosed. For this reason, your mental state will be taken into account while doctors decide what to do next. If labor is imminent, or has already started, your stillborn baby will probably be delivered normally. If labor isn't clearly about to

LOSS OF ONE TWIN

The parent who loses one twin (or more babies, in the case of triplets or quads) has to face celebrating a birth (or births) and mourning a death (or deaths) at the same time. If this happens, you may feel too depressed and conflicted to either mourn your lost child or enjoy your living one—both vitally important processes. Understanding why you feel the way you do may help you to feel better.

◆ You've lost a baby. The fact that you have another doesn't minimize your loss. You're entitled to mourn that loss. In fact, you need to; otherwise you will have difficulty coming to terms with it. Take the steps for grieving parents described in this section, so that you can more easily accept your baby's death as a reality.

◆ You've lost the excitement of being the parent of twins (or triplets, or more). Even if you didn't know in advance that you were expecting more than one baby, you may feel cheated. Don't feel guilty if you do; your disappointment is normal. Let yourself mourn this loss as well as the loss of your baby.

◆ You're afraid it will be difficult and awkward to explain that you only have one baby to friends and family who have been eagerly awaiting the twins with you. To ease this burden, enlist a friend or relative to spread the word. When you first go out of the house with the baby, take someone with you who can help explain the situation to people you may run into, if you don't feel up to it.

◆ You may feel inadequate because you lost one of your babies, particularly if they were conceived through the use of fertility agents or IVF or GIFT (gamete intrafallopian transfer). But what happened had nothing to do with your value as a woman or mother.

◆ You feel you are somehow being punished—because you really didn't think you could have taken care of two children, or because you wanted a boy more than a girl (or vice versa), or because you really didn't want twins. Though such guilt is common in parents who experience a pregnancy loss, it is completely unwarranted.

◆ You are concerned that as your surviving infant grows—at birthdays, the first step, the first "mama" and "dada"—you will be reminded of the lost child and of what could have been. And it's true that you will be. It will help if you and your spouse share your feelings with each other on these occasions, and don't try to suppress them.

◆ You worry that your child, as he or she grows older, will be tormented by the loss. However, your child is not likely to suffer because of the loss unless you make an issue of it. Providing lots of love

start, the decision whether or not to induce it immediately, or to allow you to return home until it begins spontaneously, will depend on how far you are from your due date, and on your physical as well as your mental state.

The grieving process you will go through if your fetus has died in utero will probably be very similar to that of parents whose baby has died during or after birth, and it is important to try to follow the same paths, including, when possible and practical, holding your baby in your arms and having a funeral or memorial service.

Death during or after birth. Sometimes the death occurs during labor or delivery, sometimes just after delivery. Either way, your world comes crashing down. You've waited for this baby for nearly nine months—and now you're going

and attention will help ensure that he or she will grow up secure and happy.

♦ In trying to help, friends and family may overdo the fanfare when welcoming your living child and maintain a polite silence on the topic of your dead one. Or they may tell you to forget the lost child and appreciate your living one. These insensitive attitudes (well-intentioned though they may be) can anger and upset you. Try not to lash out, but do tell people how you feel. Let them know that you need to grieve for the lost baby as well as rejoice in the living one.

♦ You believe that to enjoy your surviving baby is somehow being disloyal to your dead one. Though it's a natural feeling, it's one you need to shake. Loving the sibling that your lost baby spent all those months cuddled up with in your uterus is a way of honoring that child. On the other hand, idealizing the dead baby and making the living one compete with this idealized image could be quite damaging. If you are uncomfortable about having a christening or a circumcision or other baby-welcoming event for the surviving baby, consider holding a memorial ceremony or farewell for the dead baby first or at the same time.

♦ You're experiencing postpartum depression. It's normal, whether you've lost a child or not, for hormones in chaos to make everything harder to deal with and feelings more conflicted. See page 414 for tips on dealing with postpartum depression.

♦ You're afraid that the loss you've experienced and your consequent depression will damage your relationship as a couple. This is very unlikely if you share feelings, both positive and negative, with each other. One study showed that fully 90 percent of parents who have gone through this experience have found that their marriage was strengthened by helping each other pull through the mourning period.

♦ You feel guilty that your ambivalence toward your surviving baby is making it difficult for you to care for your baby. Remind yourself that you have no reason to feel guilty about having feelings that are completely normal. Do, however, make sure that your baby's needs—both physical and emotional—are met. Seek help if you and your spouse are having trouble meeting these needs because of lingering depression or conflicted feelings.

♦ You feel alone in your pain. Getting support from others who know what you're going through can help immeasurably. Find it in a local support group or online. You can contact Centers for Loss in Multiple Birth (CLIMB), Inc., at www.climb-support.org.

Most of all, give yourself some time. Chances are that you'll feel progressively better and, if you let yourself, will soon be able to begin truly enjoying your new baby.

home empty-handed.

There's probably no greater pain than that inflicted by the loss of a child. And though nothing can banish the hurt you're feeling, there are steps you can take now to make the future more bearable, and to lessen the inevitable depression that follows such a tragedy—depression that may be more severe when there are no other children, when there have been recurrent pregnancy losses, when you're older and fear that another pregnancy won't happen.

♦ See your baby, hold your baby, name your baby. Grieving is a vital step in accepting and recovering from your loss, and it's difficult to grieve for a nameless child you've never seen. Even if your child is malformed, experts advise that it is better to see him or her than not to, because what is imagined is usually worse than the reality. Holding and naming your baby will make the death more real to you, and ultimately easier to recover from. So will arranging for a funeral and burial or a memorial service, which will give you another opportunity to say good-bye. If there is a burial, the grave will provide a permanent site where you can visit your baby in future years.

◆ If possible, ask not to be sedated in the hours after you hear the news. Though it will ease your pain momentarily, sedation will tend to blur your recollections and the reality of what happened. This makes it harder to get on with your grieving, as well as depriving you and your spouse of the chance to support each other.

◆ Discuss autopsy findings and other details with the doctor to harden the reality of what happened and to aid you in the grieving process. You may have been given a lot of details in the delivery room, but medications, your hormonal status, and the shock you felt probably prevented you from fully understanding them.

◆ Expect your breasts to be engorged and ask the nurses for help with lactation suppression. Milk production should stop on its own within a few days.

◆ Keep in mind that the grieving process usually has many steps, including denial and isolation; anger; depression; and acceptance (see page 532). Don't be surprised if you feel these emotions, though not necessarily in this order. And don't be surprised if you don't feel all of them or if you experience other emotions instead or in addition. Everyone is different and everyone reacts differently even in similar situations.

◆ Save a photo (many hospitals take them) or other mementos (a lock of hair, a handprint), so that you'll have some tangible reminders to cherish when you think about your lost baby in the future. As morbid as this may sound, experts say it helps. Try to focus on positive attributes—big eyes and long lashes, beautiful hands and delicate fingers, a headful of hair.

◆ Ask friends or relatives to leave the preparations you made for baby at home. Coming home to a house that looks as though a baby was never expected will only add to any tendency to deny what has happened.

◆ Cry—for as long and as often as you feel you need to. If you don't cry now, it will remain unfinished business that you may find you have to attend to later.

◆ Limit the use of tranquilizers and sedatives. Although they may seem helpful at first, they can interfere with the grieving process—and can also make you dependent on them. Also avoid using alcohol to drown your grief. Alcohol is a depressant; though its numbing effect may be welcome at first, once it wears off, you'll feel the sadness even more keenly.

◆ Expect a difficult time. For a while you may feel depressed, empty, or stressed; experience intense sadness; have trouble sleeping; fight with your spouse and neglect your other children; perhaps imagine you hear your baby crying in the middle of the night. You will probably feel the need to be a child yourself, to be loved, coddled, and cared for. All this is normal.

◆ Recognize that fathers grieve, too. Their grief may in some cases be or appear to be shorter-lived and/or less intense, partly because, unlike mothers, they haven't carried their baby inside them for so many months. But that doesn't make the pain any less real, or the process of mourning any less vital to healing. Sometimes fathers may have trouble expressing their grief. They may bottle up their emotions in an effort to be strong for their wives, or because they feel uncomfortable crying. Unfortunately, the pain may then come out in other, more destructive and self-destructive ways—in bad temper, loss of interest in life, detachment from family, alcohol abuse. Talking the pain out—with their partners, a counselor, another father who has been through such a loss—can help. Other positive ways of releasing and processing grief include exercise and volunteering, perhaps in a Big Brother program that teams boys in need of a father figure with men who can benefit from filling that role.

◆ Take care of each other. Grief can be very self-absorbing. You and your spouse may find yourselves so consumed by your own pain that you don't have the emotional reserves left to comfort each other. Unfortunately, marital problems can sometimes result when you shut your partner out that way, making recovering from the ordeal even more difficult. Although there will almost certainly be times when you'll want to be alone with your thoughts, you should also make time for sharing them with your spouse. Consider seeking grief counseling together, too, or joining a couples support group. It may not only help you both find solace, but may help preserve—and even deepen—your relationship.

◆ Don't face the world alone. If you're putting off getting back into circulation because you dread the friendly faces asking, "So, did you have a boy or a girl?" take a friend who can field the questions for you on the first several trips to the supermarket, bank, and so on. Be sure that those at work, at your place of worship, at other organizations in which you're active are informed before you return so you don't have to do any more difficult explaining than is absolutely necessary.

◆ Realize that some friends and family may not know what to do or say. Some may be so uncomfortable that they withdraw during the mourning period. Others may say things that hurt more than help: "I know just how you feel" or "Oh, you can have another baby" or "It's a good thing the baby died before you became attached to it." Though they certainly mean well, they may not understand that no one who hasn't lost a baby can know how it feels, that another baby can never take the place of the one you lost, or that parents can become attached to a baby long before birth, sometimes even before conception. If you are hearing such comments frequently, ask a close friend or relative to explain your feelings and to let others know that you would rather they just say they are sorry about your loss.

◆ Look for support from those who've been there. Like many other parents, you may derive strength from joining a support group for parents who have lost infants. But beware of letting such a group become a way of sustaining, rather than letting go of, your rage or grief. If after a year you're still having problems coming to terms with your loss (sooner, if you're having trouble functioning), you should seek individual therapy.

◆ Take care of yourself. In the face of so much emotional pain, your physical needs may be the last thing on your mind. They shouldn't be. Eating right, getting enough sleep, and exercising are vital not just in maintaining your health, but also in aiding your recovery. Make a conscious effort to sit down for meals, even if you're not feeling very much like eating. Take a warm bath or do some relaxation exercises to help you unwind before bed, so that you'll sleep better at night. Try to build some physical activity into your day, even if it's just a walk before dinner. And let yourself take a break from grieving once in a while. See a movie, accept an invitation to visit friends, take a weekend in the country—and enjoy yourself without feeling guilty. For life to go on, after all, you need to go on living.

◆ Remember your child by doing something for other children—setting up a scholarship fund, if you can afford it; donating books to a day care center that serves needy children; volunteering at a home for unwed mothers (once you feel strong enough to face pregnant women and babies). Or devise another memorial that has meaning for you. For example, plant a tree or a new flower bed at a nursery school or in your own backyard as a memorial to your child.

◆ Turn to religion, if you find it comforting. Some bereaved parents feel too angry with God to do this, but for many, faith is a great solace. So is understanding that God is not responsible for such tragedies, that they simply happen as part of the imperfect world in which we live.

◆ Don't expect that having another

STAGES OF GRIEF

Whether the loss of a baby comes early in pregnancy, near term, or at delivery, you will experience many feelings and reactions. While you can't wish them away, understanding them will eventually help you come to terms with your loss. Most people who suffer a loss go through a number of steps on their road to emotional healing. These steps are common, though the order in which they occur may vary; so, too, may the feelings you experience.

◆ Shock and denial. There may be numbness and disbelief, the feeling that "this couldn't have happened to me." This is a mental mechanism designed to protect your psyche from the trauma of the loss.

◆ Guilt and anger. Desperate to pin the blame for such a senseless tragedy on something, many parents blame it on themselves ("I must have done something wrong to cause the miscarriage" or "If I'd wanted the baby more, it would still be alive today"). There may also be feelings of rage at the unfairness of it all—perhaps targeted against God, or against your practitioner (even if he or she isn't at fault). There may be envy of others who are pregnant or who are parents, and even fleeting feelings of hatred for them.

◆ Depression and despair. You may find yourself feeling sad most or all of the time, crying constantly, unable to eat, sleep, be interested in anything, or otherwise function. You may also fear "I'll never be able to carry a baby to term."

◆ Acceptance. Finally, you'll come to terms with the loss. Keep in mind that this doesn't mean you'll forget the loss —just that you'll be able to accept it and get back to the business of life.

WHY?

The painful question "Why?" may never be answered.* But it is usually helpful to the grieving parents to attach some reality to the tragedy by learning about the physical causes of the death of a fetus or newborn. Often the baby looks perfectly normal, and the only way to uncover the cause of death is to carefully examine the history of the pregnancy and do a complete examination of the fetus or baby. If the fetus died in utero or was stillborn, histological examination of the placenta by a pathologist is also important. At first it may not seem that knowing the cause of death will make acceptance of the loss easier, but in the long run it will. Knowing what happened doesn't really tell you why it happened to you and your baby, but it helps put a closure on the event, and it will help you prepare for a future pregnancy.

Of course sometimes it's impossible to determine what went wrong, and in that case the grieving couple has to accept the event in light of their own personal philosophy. They may look upon it as God's will, or as a random occurrence over which humans have no control. In any case, the loss of a baby should never be viewed as punishment.

*For help in thinking about this question, see *When Bad Things Happen to Good People* by Harold S. Kushner.

---

baby will resolve any unresolved grief. Do become pregnant again, if that's what you want—first observing whatever waiting period the doctor recommends. But don't try to conceive in order to feel better, assuage guilt or anger, or gain peace of mind. It won't work, and it could put an unfair burden on any new arrival. Any decision about your future fertility—either to have another baby or to undergo sterilization—should be postponed until the period of deepest sorrow has passed.

♦ Expect your pain to lessen over time. At first there will be only bad days, then a few good days among them; eventually there will be more good days than bad. But be prepared for the possibility that remnants of the pain may last a lot longer. The grieving process, with nightmares and intrusive recollections, is often not fully completed for as long as two years, but the worst is usually over in three to six months after the loss. If after six to nine months your grief remains the center of your universe, if you lose interest in everything else and can't seem to function, seek help. Also seek help if, from the beginning, you haven't been able to grieve at all.

♦ Recognize that guilt can compound grief and make adjusting to a loss more difficult. If you feel that the loss of your baby was your punishment for having been ambivalent about your pregnancy, or for lacking the nurturing or other qualities necessary for motherhood, or for any other reason, seek professional support to help you understand that you are *in no way* responsible for your loss. Seek help, too, if you feel insecure about your womanhood and now believe your doubts have been confirmed (you couldn't produce a live baby), or if you feel you have failed your family and friends. If you feel guilty even thinking about getting your life back to normal because you sense it would be disloyal to your dead child, it may help to ask your baby, in spirit, for forgiveness or for permission to enjoy life again. You might try doing it in a "letter," in which you express all your feelings, hopes, and dreams.

♦ If there is a possibility or even a certainty that you won't be able to conceive again and/or carry a pregnancy to a healthy conclusion, don't despair. There are so many beautiful children greatly in need of loving parents. Yours will be ready when you are. Adoption may not seem what you want now, but as millions of adoptive parents can assure you, the child you adopt becomes yours every bit as much as the one you carry in your uterus.

♦ ♦ ♦

Part 5

THE NEXT BABY

Preparing for the Next Baby

I n the best of all possible worlds, we would be able to plan life to our precise specifications. In the real world, where most of us live, the best-laid plans often give way to the unexpected twists and turns of fate over which we have precious little control, leaving us to accept, and to make the best of, what comes our way.

To assure the best of all possible pregnancies, we would know in advance when we will be conceiving—and before we did we'd make all the changes and adjustments in our lifestyle necessary to help ensure the best possible outcome. But such advance planning is a luxury that many women—because of menstrual irregularity and/or the fallibility of contraception (or that of a couple winging it) —may never be able to indulge in. And as has been stressed throughout this book, what a woman does before she realizes she's pregnant rarely does anything to affect her pregnancy and her baby's health. Few women act pregnant from the moment of conception, and yet almost all give birth to normal, healthy babies.

But it would be remiss not to outline a plan for the best of all possible pregnancies—because the possibility does exist for an increasing number of women,

as family planning techniques become more reliable, to plan ahead. The plan is appropriate whether you've already begun trying to conceive or you're just in the thinking stage. Although it's never too late to start taking care of your body, it's also never too early. And, in fact, your good prepregnancy care will benefit not only your own children but your children's children.

There are a great many ways that both the prospective mother *and* the prospective father can enhance their fertility while ensuring the best chances for a safe pregnancy and for optimum health for the baby to come once sperm does meet egg. (Keep in mind, however, that if you are already pregnant, there's no need to worry if you didn't take all these precautions before you conceived. Simply start this book at Chapter 1, and make the very best of every day of pregnancy you have ahead of you.)

PRECONCEPTION PREP FOR MOTHERS

Get a thorough physical. See your internist or family doctor. An exam will pick up any problems that need to be corrected beforehand, or that will need to be monitored during pregnancy.

See your dentist. Make an appointment for a thorough examination and cleaning. Have any necessary work, including X rays, fillings, and dental surgery, completed now so that it won't have to be done during pregnancy. You should also be sure that your gums are in good shape—recent research has shown that gum (periodontal) disease can increase the risk of preterm birth. Follow up at home with good preventive care; if you don't already, start brushing and flossing regularly.

Select a practitioner—and have a prepregnancy exam. It's easier to choose a practitioner now, when you're not in a hurry, than when that first prenatal checkup is hanging over your head. So ask around, scout around, and take your time in picking the practitioner who's right for you. Then schedule a prepregnancy exam. Even if you plan on using a certified nurse-midwife during your pregnancy, you should still have an obstetrician-gynecologist or family practitioner whose medical opinion you respect perform this preconception examination to screen your planned pregnancy for high-risk potential. If your history and/or the exam does not suggest the possibility of a high-risk pregnancy, you can choose any practitioner you like (see Chapter 1 for your options). If a high-risk pregnancy is possible or inevitable, you will need the care of an obstetrician or even a maternal-fetal medicine specialist during your pregnancy.

Take a look at your pregnancy history. If you've had a previous pregnancy problem, such as a miscarriage, a premature delivery, or other pregnancy complication, talk to your practitioner about the measures that can be taken to head off a repeat.

Check your mother's pregnancy history. If you know, or suspect, that your mother took the drug diethylstilbestrol (DES) when she was pregnant with you, tell the doctor. The drug, which was prescribed up until 1971 to prevent miscarriage, caused damage to the reproductive organs in some females exposed to it in the uterus. If you were a DES baby, and haven't been examined previously, your doctor will probably want to take a look at your vagina and cervix with colposcopy (which allows a clear view of these organs).

Get tested. Tests that may be recommended before you conceive include those for:

♦ Hemoglobin or hematocrit, to test for anemia.

♦ Rh factor, to see if you are positive or negative. If you are negative, your partner should be tested to see if he is positive. (If you're both negative, there is no need to give Rh another thought; see page 29.)

♦ Rubella titer, to check for immunity to rubella (German measles).

♦ Varicella titer, to check for immunity to varicella (chicken pox).

♦ Urine, to screen for diabetes.

♦ Tuberculosis—this test is needed if you live in a high-incidence area.

♦ Hepatitis B—if you are in a high-risk category, such as being a health care worker, and have not been immunized.

♦ Cytomegalovirus antibodies, to determine whether or not you are immune to CMV (see page 462). If you have been diagnosed with CMV, it's generally recommended you wait six months—when antibodies appear in the blood—before trying to conceive.

♦ Toxoplasmosis titer, if you have a cat, regularly eat raw or rare meat, drink unpasteurized milk, or garden without gloves. If you turn out to be immune, you needn't worry about toxoplasmosis now or ever. If you're not, start taking the precautions on page 67 now.

♦ Thyroid function. Since thyroid function can seriously affect pregnancy and possibly even a child's IQ down the line, it's a good idea for *everyone* to be screened for this before conception. This is especially important if you have ever had thyroid problems or have them now or if you have a family history of thyroid disease (see page 478).

♦ Sexually transmitted disease. It is now recommended that *all* pregnant women be tested for *all* STDs, including syphilis, gonorrhea, chlamydia, herpes, human papilloma virus, bacterial vaginosis, Gardnerella vaginitis, and HIV. Having these tests before conception is even better; even if you're sure you couldn't have an STD, ask to be tested, just to be on the safe side.

Get treated. If any test turns up a condition that requires treatment, make sure you take care of it before trying to conceive. Also attend to minor elective surgery and anything else medical or dental—major or minor—that you've been putting off. Now is also the time to be treated for any gynecological conditions that might interfere with pregnancy, including:

♦ Uterine polyps, fibroids, cysts, or benign tumors

♦ Endometriosis (when the cells that ordinarily line the uterus spread elsewhere in the body)

♦ Pelvic inflammatory disease

♦ Recurrent urinary tract infections

♦ A sexually transmitted disease

If dealing with any of these conditions requires laser surgery, wait six months following surgery before conceiving.

Update immunizations. If you haven't had a tetanus-diphtheria booster in the past ten years, have one now. If you know you've never had rubella (German measles) or been immunized against it, or if testing showed you are not immune to the disease, get vaccinated now with the measles, mumps, and rubella (MMR) vaccine and then wait three months before attempting to conceive (but don't worry if you accidentally conceive earlier—any risk is purely theoretical). If testing shows you've never had chicken pox (varicella), or are at high risk for hepatitis B, immunization for these diseases is also recommended now, before conception.

Get chronic illnesses under control. If you have diabetes, asthma, a heart condition, epilepsy, or any other chronic illness, be sure that you have your doctor's okay to become pregnant, that your condition is *under control* before you conceive,[1] and that you start taking optimum care of yourself now (see Chapter 19). If you were a PKU baby (ask your mother if you aren't sure, or check your medical records), then begin a phenylalanine-free diet (distasteful as it may be) before conceiving (see page 485) and continue it through pregnancy.

If you need allergy shots, take care of them now. (If you start allergy desensitization now, you will probably be able

---

1. Ideally, you should try to keep these conditions under control all of the time, just in case you conceive unexpectedly.

to continue once you conceive.) Since depression can interfere with conception, it should also be treated before you begin your big adventure.

Have a genetic screening. If either you or your partner has any genetic disorders (such as Tay-Sachs, sickle cell, thalassemia, hemophilia, cystic fibrosis, muscular dystrophy, Huntington's chorea, fragile X syndrome) or other birth defects (such as Down syndrome) in your personal history or among blood relatives, or if there is mental retardation in the family (which could be genetic), see a genetic counselor or a maternal-fetal medicine specialist. You should also ask your practitioner about being tested for any genetic disease common to your ethnic background: cystic fibrosis if you're both Caucasian; Tay-Sachs disease if either of you is of Jewish-European (Ashkenazi), French Canadian, Irish American, or Louisiana Cajun descent; sickle-cell trait if you are of African descent; one of the thalassemias if you are of Greek, Italian, Southeast Asian, or Philippine origin. Previous obstetrical difficulties (such as two or more miscarriages, a stillbirth, a long period of infertility, or a child with a birth defect) or being married to a cousin or other blood relative are also reasons to seek genetic counseling.

Evaluate your birth control method. If you are using a method of birth control that might present some risk (however slight) to a future pregnancy, change it before you start trying to conceive. Birth control pills should be discontinued several months before conception, if possible, to allow your reproductive system to go through at least two normal cycles before you begin your baby-making efforts. In some cases, it may take even longer for your cycles to become normal—you'll need to be patient. If you use an IUD, it should be removed before you begin trying. Wait three to six months after stopping Depo-Provera (medroxyprogesterone) shots to try to conceive. If you use Norplant, you should wait two to three cycles before trying to conceive. Playing it extra safe also means discontinuing the use of spermicides (alone or with a diaphragm or condom) one month to six weeks before you want to become pregnant. The birth control method to switch to for the interim: the condom (used with care and without spermicide).

Improve your diet. First, and most important of all, be sure you are getting enough folic acid. Studies show that adequate intake of this vitamin in a woman's diet before she conceives and early in her pregnancy can dramatically reduce the risk of neural tube defects (such as spina bifida) in her developing infant. Folic acid is found naturally in whole grains and green leafy vegetables, and, by law, is now also added to most refined grains. But taking a pregnancy supplement containing folic acid is also important (see page 93).

Also start cutting back on junk food and refined sugars in your diet, and increasing whole grains, fruits, vegetables (especially green leafies and yellows), and low-fat dairy products (important for bone strength). And cut down on saturated fat, high intakes of which appear to increase the risk of severe pregnancy nausea and vomiting (hyperemesis gravidarum). You can use the Pregnancy Diet (Chapter 4) for a good basic food plan, but you will need only two protein servings and three calcium servings daily until you conceive.

If you have any unhealthy dietary habits (such as periodic fasting or a taste for laundry starch or clay), suffer or have suffered from an eating disorder (such as anorexia nervosa or bulimia), or are on a special diet (vegan, macrobiotic, diabetic, or any other), tell your practitioner.

Get as close to your ideal weight as possible. Being *very* overweight or *very* underweight not only reduces the chances of conception but, if you do conceive, weight problems can increase the risk of pregnancy complications. So add or cut calories in the preconception period as needed. If you're trying to lose weight, be sure to do so slowly and sensibly even if it means putting off conception for another couple of months. Strenuous or nutritionally unbalanced dieting (including low-carbohydrate, high-protein diets) can make conception elusive and can result in a nutritional deficit, which is no way to start your pregnancy. If you've been on a crash diet recently, start eating normally and give your body a few months to get back into balance before you try to conceive.

Take a vitamin-mineral supplement formulated for pregnancy. Even if you're eating plenty of foods high in folic acid, it's still recommended that you take a pregnancy supplement containing 400 mcg of the vitamin, preferably starting two months before you start trying to conceive.[2] Another good reason to start taking a prenatal supplement preconception: research indicates that women who take a daily multivitamin containing at least 10 milligrams of vitamin B6 before becoming pregnant or during the first weeks of pregnancy experienced fewer episodes of vomiting and nausea during pregnancy (once morning sickness started, it was usually too late). The supplement should also contain 15 mg of zinc, which may improve fertility. Stop taking other nutritional supplements before conceiving, however, since excesses of certain nutrients can be hazardous.

Shape up, but keep cool. An exercise program will tone and strengthen your muscles as well as improve your conditioning in preparation for the challenging tasks of carrying and delivering your baby-to-be. It will also help you take off excess weight. Avoid becoming overheated during workouts, however, when you begin trying to conceive, since this can lead to an increase in body temperature, which could interfere with conception. (Avoid hot tubs and direct exposure to heating pads and electric blankets for the same reason.) Keep in mind, too, that while exercise is good for you, you can get too much of a good thing. Excessive exercise can interfere with ovulation—and if you don't ovulate, you can't conceive.

Avoid illicit drugs. All so-called recreational drugs, including cocaine, crack, marijuana, and heroin, can be dangerous to your pregnancy. To varying degrees they can prevent your conceiving, and then if you do succeed, they are potentially harmful to the fetus and also increase the risks of miscarriage, prematurity, and stillbirths. If you use drugs, casually or regularly, stop all use immediately. If you can't stop, seek help before trying to conceive.[3]

Limit your intake of over-the-counter drugs. Since most nonprescription medications carry warnings about use in pregnancy, consult your physician before taking them once you start trying to conceive. Don't douche, since douching can actually interfere with conception.

Check the safety of your prescription drugs. Some (but *not* all) medications used in the treatment of certain chronic illnesses or disorders are linked with the development of birth defects; if you're taking *any* medication now, consult with

---

2. Ideally, every woman of childbearing age should take a supplement containing 400 mcg of folic acid, just in case she should become pregnant unexpectedly.

3. Also see *The Recovery Book* for help.

your physician. Potentially harmful drugs should be discontinued at least a month (for some, three to six months) before you begin trying to have a baby, with a safe alternative therapy standing in until pregnancy is over (or the baby is weaned, if the drug also poses a threat to the nursing infant). Sometimes a reduction in dosage will do the trick.

Accutane poses an extremely serious risk during pregnancy; if you have been taking this drug, you must discontinue it for a least one month before you start trying to become pregnant. In the interim, be extra careful that you don't conceive.

Be wary of herbal or other alternative medications. Herbs are natural, but natural doesn't necessarily mean safe. Such popular herbs as echinacea, ginkgo biloba, or St. John's wort, for example, can interfere with conception. Do not take any such products, supplements, or nutriceuticals without the approval of a doctor familiar with herbals and alternative medicines.

Cut back on caffeine. Moderating your intake of coffee, tea, and colas now will spare you the symptoms of withdrawal later, if you decide to abstain or cut back once you're pregnant (see page 63). Another reason to make fewer trips to the coffee bar, at least for espresso-based drinks: some research has linked heavy caffeine consumption (more than three cups a day) to decreased fertility. Whether this is because caffeine has a biological effect on fertility or because caffeine use is often part of the type of high-stress lifestyle that can compromise a couple's chances of conceiving (or both) is unclear. Regardless, it's a good idea to cut down if you're a big caffeine drinker.

Cut down on alcohol consumption. Although a daily drink will not be harmful in your pregnancy-preparation phase, avoid heavy drinking, which can interfere with fertility by disrupting your menstrual cycle. Once you start trying to conceive, stop drinking altogether (see page 56).

Quit smoking. Tobacco not only is hazardous to your pregnancy (see page 58) and increases the risk of SIDS and possibly cancer in the baby, but it can also reduce fertility, foiling attempts to conceive. A smoke-free environment is one of the best prebirth gifts you can give your baby.

Avoid unnecessary exposure to radiation. If X rays are necessary for medical reasons, be sure that your reproductive organs are protected (unless they are being targeted) and that the lowest doses possible are used. Once you start trying to conceive, keep in mind that you might have succeeded at any point. Inform any physician treating you with radiation, or technicians taking X rays, that you could be pregnant, and ask them to take all necessary precautions. Only radiation exposure that is absolutely required for your health or the baby's should be permitted once your efforts to become parents begin (see page 70).

Avoid excessive exposure to hazardous chemicals. Some chemicals (though far from all and usually only in very large doses) are potentially harmful to your eggs before conception, and later to a developing embryo or fetus. Though the risk is in most cases slight, you should play it safe by avoiding potentially hazardous exposure on the job. Special care should be taken in certain fields (medicine and dentistry, art, photography, transportation, farming and landscaping, construction, hairdressing and cosmetology, dry cleaning, and some factory work). Contact the Occupational Safety and Health Administration for the latest information on job safety and pregnancy; also see page 76. In some cases, it may be wise to ask for a transfer to another position, change jobs, or take special precautions before trying to conceive.

Because elevated lead levels when you conceive could pose problems for your baby, you should be tested if you have been exposed to lead in the workplace or elsewhere, such as in your water supply or your home (see page 71). If your blood levels are high, experts recommend chelation therapy to remove the lead from the blood (the lead is "trapped" by a chelating agent that is infused via an IV, then later secreted in urine), and then reduced exposure before conception is attempted. Avoid, too, excessive exposure to other household toxins.

Get fiscally fit. Having a baby can be expensive. So reevaluate your budget and begin creating a sound financial plan. As part of your plan, find out if your health insurance pays for the cost of prenatal care, birth, and well-baby care. If coverage will not start until a certain date, consider delaying your pregnancy until then. Or if you plan to switch policies, do so before you become pregnant. Some policies consider pregnancy a preexisting condition. Find out how much time your employer allows for maternity leave (see page 110) or any other maternity benefits you might be entitled to. And if you don't have a will yet, now is the time to draw one up.

Start keeping track. Once you've taken all the preparatory steps, it's time to get down to business. Your chances of conceiving will be much greater if you have intercourse during the fertile part of your cycle, around ovulation. To keep track, note the first day of each menstrual period on a handy calendar or diary; also try to note when you ovulate. Ovulation may occur at the midpoint of the cycle (on day 14 of a 28-day cycle, for instance), but is less easy to predict in women with irregular cycles. In fact, recent studies show that only 30 percent of women actually ovulate in the middle of their cycle. Most women have their window of fertility anywhere from before day 10 of the cycle to after day 17. The physical signs of ovulation are readily apparent to some women, more elusive to others. During ovulation your vaginal mucus is clear, egg white–like in consistency, and can be pulled into a long stretchy string, and you may experience mittelschmerz—a brief period of pain on one side of your back or lower abdomen. Another sign you wouldn't notice unless you were keeping track is a change in basal temperature (your base temperature at rest). To look for this change, purchase a special highly sensitive BBT thermometer, and take your temperature each morning before you get out of bed (shake the thermometer down before you go to bed so you won't affect your basal temperature with that movement). The basal temperature will reach its low point of the month the day before the ovulation cycle begins, then rise sharply (indicating that ovulation is imminent) and stay elevated until just before your period. If you have trouble identifying ovulation, appear to be ovulating irregularly (more likely if your periods are irregular), are having trouble conceiving, or just want to use an easier and more effective method, home ovulation predictor kits are available to help you pinpoint ovulation. Keeping track of when you have intercourse will also help you pinpoint conception later on, which will make calculating an estimated date of delivery easier.

Relax. This is perhaps the most important step of all. Getting tense and uptight about conception could prevent you from conceiving. Learn to do relaxation exercises, to meditate, and to cut down as much as possible on stress in your daily life (see page 125).

Give it time. Keep in mind that it takes an average of six months for a normal, healthy twenty-five-year-old woman to conceive, and longer for women who are older. It may also take longer if your partner is older. So stay calm if the miracle doesn't happen right away. Just keep on having fun trying, and give yourselves at least a year before consulting a doctor and, if needed, a fertility specialist. If you're over thirty-five, you may want to see a doctor after six months of trying.

PRECONCEPTION PREP FOR DADS

See your doctor. Get a thorough physical exam to be sure you have no medical condition (such as undescended testicles, testicular cysts or tumors, or depression) that might interfere with conception or a healthy pregnancy for your partner. Also ask about the sexual side effects of any prescription, over-the-counter, or herbal drugs you are taking. Some can cause fertility problems and lower sperm counts—something you don't want now.

Get a genetic screening, if needed. Because of family history, some couples should see a genetic counselor for testing and discussion before trying to conceive. See page 46 to see if that will be important for you and your partner.

Switch birth control methods, if necessary. If you've been relying on birth control pills for contraception, it's necessary for your partner to get off them at least a couple of menstrual cycles before you try conceiving. To play it safe while you wait, use condoms—*without* spermicide.

Improve your diet. The better your

nutrition, the healthier your sperm and the more easily you'll conceive. Your diet should mirror your partner's prepregnancy diet (see page 539), with caloric intake adjusted to accommodate your size and activity. To be sure you get adequate amounts of the most important nutrients (especially vitamin C, vitamin E, zinc, calcium, and vitamin D, all of which appear to affect fertility or the health of sperm), take a vitamin-mineral supplement while you are attempting to conceive. Make sure the supplement contains folic acid; a low intake of this nutrient in fathers-to-be has been linked to decreased fertility, as well as to birth defects. If you're a diabetic, you should get your blood sugar under control.

Change your lifestyle. All the answers are not yet in, but research is beginning to show that the use of drugs (including excessive amounts of alcohol) by the male partner prior to conception could prevent pregnancy or lead to a poor pregnancy outcome. The mechanisms aren't clear, but drug use and daily heavy drinking can apparently damage sperm as well as reduce their number and can alter testicular function and reduce testosterone levels. In addition, the substances may be excreted in the semen, which could cause birth defects. Heavy drinking (equivalent to two drinks a day or five on any one day) during the month prior to conception could also affect your baby's birthweight. Keep in mind, too, that if you cut down or cut out alcohol, it will be much easier for your partner to do likewise. If you are unable to quit drugs or reduce your alcohol intake, seek help now.

Kick the butt habit. Smoking reduces the number of sperm in males and makes conceiving more difficult. In addition, quitting now will improve the health of everyone in your family, since secondhand smoke is nearly as dangerous to them as firsthand smoke is to you. It can, in fact, increase your baby-to-be's risk of dying of SIDS.

Don't get zapped. High lead levels, as well as some organic solvents (such as are found in paints, glues, varnishes, and metal degreasers), pesticides, or other chemicals can interfere with a male's fertility, so it's important to avoid these or limit your exposure as much as possible in preparation for conception.

Keep 'em cool. Sperm production is impaired when the testicles become overheated. In fact, they prefer to be a couple of degrees cooler than the rest of the body. So avoid hot tubs and hot baths, saunas, and snug clothing, such as tight jeans and briefs (switch to boxers). Also avoid synthetic pants and underwear, which can overheat you in hot weather. And keep your laptop off your lap, since the heat from the device can raise your scrotal temperature and reduce your sperm count. Until you conceive, treat it like a desktop.

Keep 'em safe. If you play any rough sports (including football, soccer, basketball, hockey, baseball, horseback riding), wear protective gear to prevent injury to the genitals, which can damage fertility. Even too much bicycling has the potential to cause problems. The constant pressure on the genitals by a bicycle seat may, according to some experts, interfere with conception by damaging arteries and nerves. If you experience genital numbness, and changing seats or lifting yourself off the seat periodically as you bicycle doesn't help, it would be a good idea to cut down on bicycling during the conception-attempting period. Numb genitals don't perform as desired. If the numbness (and/or tingling) doesn't go away, see your doctor.

Relax. This is important for both you and your partner. Stress doesn't just affect your libido and performance, it also affects your testosterone levels and your sperm production. The less you worry about it, the more easily you'll conceive. So relax and enjoy trying!

Now That You've Read the Ending . . .

It's time to start at the beginning. Once your preconception period is behind you, and conception's taken care of, flip back to Chapter 1 to get started on your pregnancy reading. Have fun!

◆ ◆ ◆

Appendix

COMMON TESTS DURING PREGNANCY

Your practitioner may omit some of these tests or add others, depending on your medical history and his or her professional opinion. For more information on the individual topics, see the index.

TEST AND WHEN PERFORMED	PROCEDURE	REASON
Blood type. First visit.	Examination of blood drawn from your arm.	To determine blood type, Rh type, and Kell factor.
Hematocrit or hemoglobin. First visit and again at 20 weeks.	Examination of blood drawn from your arm.	If test shows iron deficiency or anemia, iron supplementation is necessary.
Rubella titer. First visit.	Examination of blood drawn from your arm.	To check for immunity to rubella (German measles).
Syphilis test (VDRL). First visit.	Examination of blood drawn from your arm.	If syphilis infection is present, prompt treatment will prevent harm to fetus.
HIV test. First visit.	Examination of blood drawn from your arm.	Diagnosis and treatment can help the mother and reduce the risk of transmitting HIV to the fetus.
Hepatitis B screen. First visit.	Examination of blood drawn from your arm.	If hepatitis B infection is present, the mother can be treated prenatally, and the infant can be treated immediately after birth.
Pap smear. First visit.	Cervical secretions are collected on a swab and examined under a microscope for abnormal cells.	To check for cervical cancer, or other cell abnormalities.

TEST AND WHEN PERFORMED	PROCEDURE	REASON
Gonorrhea culture and genital herpes. First visit.	Vaginal secretions are collected on a swab and cultured in the lab.	If infection is present, it can be treated.
Chlamydia test. First visit.	Area around cervix, urethra, or rectum is swabbed to check for possible infectious organisms.	If infection is present, it can be treated.
Bacteria in urine. First visit.	Urine specimen is examined.	Bacteria in urine can indicate an infection, which would then be treated.
Drug screen. First visit.	Urine specimen is examined.	Any abuse of illicit drugs during pregnancy is hazardous and should be treated promptly.
Blood pressure. Each visit.	Blood pressure is measured with cuff and stethoscope, or with electronic device.	To screen for pregnancy-induced hypertension, or preeclampsia.
Sugar (glucose) in the urine. Each visit.	A specially treated "dipstick" is dipped in a specimen of urine.	Persistent high levels of sugar in the urine could be an indication of gestational diabetes and require further testing.
Albumin (protein) in the urine. Each visit.	A specially treated "dipstick" is dipped in a specimen of urine.	High protein levels in the urine could indicate a bladder infection or might be related to preeclampsia.
Triple Screen (MSAFP). Between weeks 15 and 18.	Examination of blood drawn from your arm.	Prenatal diagnosis screening test to check for the *possibility* of fetal defect and the need for more testing.
Glucose tolerance test. At 28 weeks (usually earlier and more often in diabetics).	Examination of blood drawn from your arm after drinking a special glucose drink.	To test for gestational diabetes.
Group B step (GBS) test. Around 37 weeks.	A swab of the area around the vagina and rectum is examined. Urine is also examined.	To screen for GBS, which can be treated during labor to protect the newborn.

NON-DRUG TREATMENTS DURING PREGNANCY

SYMPTOMS	TREATMENT	PROCEDURE
Aching back	Warmth	Take a long warm (not hot-as-you-can-stand-it) bath, morning and evening. Apply a heating pad wrapped in a towel for up to 15 minutes, 3 or 4 times a day.
	Preventive measures	Exercise, proper body mechanics, good posture; see page 209.
Bruises due to injury	Ice pack	Use a commercial ice pack you store in the freezer; a sealed zip-lock plastic bag filled with ice cubes and a few paper towels to absorb the melting ice; or an un-opened can of frozen juice or package of vegetables. Apply for 30 minutes; repeat 30 minutes later if swelling or pain persists, and as needed.
	Cold compresses	Dip a soft cloth in a basin of ice cubes and cold water, wring it out, and place over affected site. Rechill when cold dissipates.
Bruises on hands, wrists, feet	Cold soaks	Place a tray or two of ice cubes in a basin (a Styro-foam bucket or cooler is best) of cold water and immerse the injured part for 30 minutes; repeat 30 minutes later if necessary.
Burns	Cold compresses	See Bruises. Do not apply ice directly to a burn.

SYMPTOMS	TREATMENT	PROCEDURE
Colds	Saline nose drops	Use a commercial preparation or a solution of ¼ teaspoon salt in 8 ounces water (measure carefully). Put a few drops in each nostril, wait 5 to 10 minutes, and blow your nose.
	Vicks VapoRub	Follow package directions.
	Additional fluids	Drink 8 ounces liquid every hour, including water, juices, soups. Hot fluids, particularly chicken soup, are best. Limit milk intake only if recommended by your doctor.
	Inhalation	Use a steam vaporizer, humidifier, or steaming kettle; prepare a tent by draping a sheet over an open umbrella which is resting on a chair back; place humidifier on chair. Spend 15 minutes 3 or 4 times a day under tent; extend the time to 30 minutes if you aren't Ùoo uncomfortable. (Don't stay under the tent if you become uncomfortably warm.) Keep the humidifier near your bedside when you are sleeping or resting.
	Nasal strips	Follow package directions.
Coughing, due to colds or flu	Inhalation	See Colds.
	Additional fluids	See Colds.
Diarrhea	Additional fluids	Drink 8 ounces liquid every hour, including water, diluted fruit juice (but not prune juice), clear soups.

SYMPTOMS	TREATMENT	PROCEDURE
Fever (Call your practitioner the same day if you have a fever over 100°F in the absence of cold or flu symptoms; call right away for a fever over 102°F. In addition to these non-drug treatments, begin bringing down any fever over 100°F promptly by taking acetaminophen.)	Cooling bath	Use a tub of tepid water and gradually cool it by adding ice cubes. Stop immediately if shivering begins.
	Sponge bath	Soak towels in bowl containing 2 quarts water, 1 pint rubbing alcohol, and 1 quart ice cubes; apply cold towels to the skin. Use a plastic sheet to catch drips. Stop if shivering begins.
Hemorrhoids	Sitz bath	Sit in just enough hot water (hotter than your usual bath) to cover the affected area for 20 to 30 minutes, 2 or 3 times daily.
Itchy abdomen or skin elsewhere	Preventive measures	Avoid long hot showers and baths, and soaps that are drying. Try oatmeal baths. Use a good moisturizer, spread on while you are still damp from the shower. For moisturizing indoor air, see page 457.
Itchy eye discharge	Warm soaks	Use a cloth dipped in warm, not hot, water (test it for comfort on your inner forearm), and apply to your eye for 5 or 10 minutes every 3 hours.
Muscle soreness, injury	Ice pack, cold compresses, or cold soaks for first 24 to 48 hours	See Bruises.

SYMPTOMS	TREATMENT	PROCEDURE
Muscle soreness, injury *(continued)*	After 48 hours, hot soaks, warm baths, or heating pad	Wet a towel thoroughly in warm water, then wring it out and place it over the affected site, covering all completely with a plastic bag. Place a heating pad over the plastic at a medium setting, being careful that it does not touch the wet towel. Apply for 1 hour twice daily.
Nasal congestion		See Colds.
Sinusitis	Alternating hot and cold compresses	Dip a cloth in hot water, wring it out, and apply to the painful area until the heat dissipates, about 30 seconds; then apply a cold compress until the cold dissipates. Continue alternating heat and cold for 10 minutes, 4 times daily.
Sore or scratchy throat	Gargle	Dissolve ¼ teaspoon salt in 8 ounces hot water (the temperature of tea) and gargle for 5 minutes; repeat as needed, or every 2 hours.

PREGNANCY CALORIE AND FAT REQUIREMENTS

Calorie and fat requirements vary according to an individual's weight and level of activity; factors such as metabolism also come into play. Though the following are merely rough guidelines, they can help you plan your daily fat intake during pregnancy. These servings take into account the fact that you will get at least one fat serving a day in dribs and drabs from "low-fat" foods.

Your Ideal Weight (pounds)	Your Activity Level*	Daily Calorie Needs**	Maximum Fat Intake (grams)	Maximum Full Fat Servings
100	1	1,500	50	2½
100	2	1,800	60	3½
100	3	2,500	83	5
125	1	1,800	60	3½
125	2	2,175	72	4
125	3	3,050	101	6
150	1	2,100	70	4
150	2	2,550	85	5
150	3	3,600	120	7½

*Score your activity level this way: 1 sedentary, 2 moderately active, 3 extremely active (very few pregnant women will fall into the extremely active category).
**See page 87.

SOURCES AND RESOURCES

"At Home" Childbirth Education. For those who can't attend classes, from The Childbirth Institute: (877) 31-BIRTH (312-4784). www. childbirthinstitute.com.

ALACE. For childbirth education information: PO Box 382724, Cambridge, MA 02238; (617) 441-2500; www. ALACE.com.

Alcoholics Anonymous. Provides information and materials: 468 Park Avenue South, New York, NY 10016; for referral to nearby AA meetings, check Alcoholics Anonymous listing in your local directory.

Alexander Technique. For information on this type of exercise: www. alexander technique.com.

American Board of Hypnotherapy. For information on hypnosis: (800) 872-9996; www.hypnosis.com/abh/abh.html.

American College of Nurse-Midwives. For information on nurse-midwifery: 818 Connecticut Avenue NW, Suite 900, Washington, DC 20006; (202) 728-9860.

American Massage Therapy Association. For information on safe pregnancy massage: (847) 864-0123; www. amtamassage.org.

American Oriental Bodywork Therapy Association. (856) 782-1616; www. healthy.net/aobta.

Association for Applied Psychophysiology and Biofeedback. For information on complementary medicine techniques: (303) 422-8436; www. aapb.org.

Association of Christian Childbirth Professionals. For childbirth education information: www. christianbirth.org.

Bradley: American Academy of Husband-Coached Childbirth. For childbirth education information: PO Box 5224, Sherman Oaks, CA 91413-5224; (800) 4-A-BIRTH (422-4784); www. bradley birth.com.

Center for Disease Control and Prevention's Traveler's Hotline. For information on health risks in different locales: (877) FYI-TRIP (394-8747); www. cdc. gov/travel.

City- or state-sponsored pregnancy, women's health, health, or environmental hotlines. For all kinds of pregnancy information: Provides information and referrals: check your local telephone directory (avoid hotlines that are sponsored by private clinics unless referred by your practitioner).

Doulas of North America. For information on doulas: (206) 324-5440; www. dona.com.

Food and Drug Administration (FDA). For all kinds of health information and referrals: Parklawn Building, 5600 Fishers Lane, Rockville, MD 20857. For food and drug safety information: (888) SAFE-FOOD (723-3366). For general health information, (888) INFO-FDA (463-6332); www.fda.gov.

Healthy Mother, Healthy Babies Coalition. Provides information on pregnancy safety: 409 12th Street SW, Washington, DC; (800) 424-8576.

International Association for Medical Assistance to Travelers (IAMAT). For tips for pregnant travelers: 417 Center Street, Lewiston, NY 14092; (716) 754-4883.

International Childbirth Education Association. For childbirth education information: PO Box 20048, Minneapolis, MN 55420; (612) 854-8660; www. icea.org.

La Leche League. For breastfeeding help: PO Box 1209, Franklin Park, IL 60131; (800) LA-LECHE (525-3243).

Lamaze International. For childbirth education information: 2025 M Street, Suite 800, Washington DC 20036-3309; (800) 368-4404; www. lamaze-child birth.com.

March of Dimes Resource Center. For information on prepregnancy and pregnancy; birth defects; genetics; drug use and environmental hazards during pregnancy: (888) MODIMES (663-4637); www. modimes.org.

Midwives Alliance of North America. For information about midwives: (888) 923-6262; www. mana.org.

National Acupuncture and Oriental Medicine Alliance. For information on complementary and alternative medicine: (253) 851-6896; www. acuall.org.

National Cocaine Hotline. For information and referrals for cocaine users and their families: (800) COCAINE (262-2463).

National Council on Alcoholism. Provides information and materials: 733 Third Avenue, New York, NY 10017; (800) NCA-CALL (622-2255) or your local or state affiliate.

National Institute for Occupational Safety and Health (NIOSH), Clearinghouse for Occupational Safety and Health Information. For information on safety on the job: 4676 Columbia Parkway, Cincinnati, OH 45226; (800) 35-NIOSH (356-4674); www. cdc.gov/niosh/homepage.html.

National Institute on Drug Abuse. For information and referrals for drug abusers and their families: (800) 662-HELP (662-4357).

National Library of Medicine. Provides a list of 300 health hotlines: 8600 Rockville Pike, Bethesda, MD 20894, ATTN: Health Hotlines; (301) 496-6308.

National Sanitation Foundation. For information on water safety: (800) NSF-MARK (673-6275).

Occupational Safety and Health Administration (OSHA). For information on job safety: 200 Constitution Avenue NW, Washington, DC 20210; (202) 693-1999; www.osha.gov.

Pesticide Hotline. Provides information on pesticides and their safe use, for the public and professionals: (800) 858-7378.

Sidelines National Support Network. For women with complicated pregnancies: PO Box 1808, Laguna Beach, CA 92652, (949) 497-2265; www. sidelines.org.

The American Academy of Pediatrics. For health information about babies and children:141 Northwest Point Blvd., PO Box 927, Elk Grove Village, IL 60009; (800) 433-9016.

The American College of Obstetricians and Gynecologists (ACOG) Resource Center. For information on pregnancy and women's health: 409 12th Street, SW, Washington DC 20024. Enclose a stamped, self-addressed, business-size envelope along with the subject of your request.

The American Seafood Institute. An industry source that can offer information on fish safety: (800) EAT-FISH (328-3474).

WIC. Provides low-income women with food: 3101 Park Center Drive, Alexandria, VA 22302; (703) 305-2746; www. fns.usda.gov/wic.

Women's Bureau of the U.S. Department of Labor. For information about work and family issues and pregnant women's rights: Washington, DC 20210; (800) 827-5335.

Pregnancy Notes

Our first baby? We are both <u>so</u> excited — we have waited a <u>very</u> long time?

It will be loved more than they will ever know and we will do our best to be great parents!!

Prenatal Test Results

Mom- not a carrier ot CF
        blood is good (A+)
        no diseases...
        healthy as can be

Gestational diabetes.
        Negative -

Weekly Weight Gain

Week 1: 149

Week 2: 151

Week 3:

Week 4:

Week 5: 153

Week 6:

Week 7:

Week 8:

Week 9: 154

Week 10:

Week 11:

Week 12: 156

Week 13: 158

Week 14:

Week 15:

Week 16:

Week 17: 160.8 (According to dr/81 kg total)

Week 18: 163.0

Week 19: 164

Week 20:

Week 21:

Week 22:

Week 23:

Week 24:

Week 25: 174

Week 26: 176

Week 27:

Week 28:

Week 29:

Week 30: 183

Week 31:

Week 32:

Week 33: 188

Week 34: 190

Week 35: 192

Week 36: 195

Week 37:

Week 38:

Week 39:

Week 40:

Week 41:

Week 42:

First Month

We tried twice during the middle
of the first week through the second
week of March... I was painting on
March 14th (in the master bath) and
something kept telling me to take a
pregnancy test... so I did... and it
was positive... and I didn't believe it,
so I ran to Jewel to get a different
one (test)... came home, took it and
it was positive... so I called Justin
@ work around 2:00pm to tell him the
exciting news... we hung up and I
ran to walgreens for one more test...
Sure enough... it was positive!!

My first doctor's appointment is
on March 26th @ 10:45am.

Symptoms as of week 2-3:
have a terrible cold... frequent headaches... achy breasts & body...

First Month

March 17th — we told our parents about the baby!! they were all very excited.. plus it happened so fast.

I get really bad headaches from the lack of caffine.. and feel ~~nausus~~ nauseas, but not all of the time, It comes in spurts.

My nipples are very tender...

March 20th — 5½ weeks
     Dr. Appt... it was exciting!
Blood Pressure is high 148/90
tested.. for STD's, HIV, blood count...ect
which is standard and I opted for
the cystic fibrosis test.. Due Date is
Friday, November 23, 2007
Next appt is April 24th.

Second Month

I am 8½ weeks now... and I feel great! I figured out that the prenatal vitamins I was taking were making me sick. So I stopped taking those.
I crave sweets! It is bad!! And I seem to eat much more.
I have gained about 4-5 pounds, my back hurts after sleep, and the sides of my thighs hurt after sitting. strange.
We just bought a baby name book. It is hard to choose!

So, we have picked names:
Girl = Teagan Melissa
Boy = Chase Anthony

April 24th, doctor's appt.
It went well... everything was great! My blood pressure is back

Second Month

to normal and all blood work
was good. Our next appointment
we get to hear our baby's heart
beat.

Third Month

I am now in my 13th week...
no changes really other than my
belly starting to grow. I seem
to still be a bit tired.

I get a little bit of cramping every
now and again, but the doc
says thats normal - just my
uterus growing.

↑ 3:45pm
May 22nd — my 13-5day checkup

Today was a big day!! We got
to hear our baby's heartbeat
for the first time. It was incredible,
it made this pregnancy feel so much
more real. It is truly amazing that
God gives the ability to a woman
to carry a life inside of her body!
This baby is a blessing and a joy!
I am loving him/her more each
moment!!

Third Month

Fourth Month

Today is Tuesday June 19, 2007
I had my monthly checkup today
@ 11:00am. It went well. The
doctor listened for the heartbeat. measured me.
He said "It Sounds like
a boy's heartbeat"... I could
not beleeve it!! this whole
time, I thought this baby
was/is a boy.

Everything is going well,
just a little tired every now
and again.

Almost ½ way there.

I am 17 weeks 5 days.
My ultrasound is on
July 5th @ 3:30.
Then July 17th @ 10:15 am

P.S. today we found Justin's baby
blanket

Fourth Month

Monday June 25, 2007, I had
to rush into the doctor's office - Sunday
I started cramping really bad...
but everything is OK :)

Wed. June 27, I felt the baby
move for the first time! It was
amazing!

19 weeks thursday 28th!!

July 1st - Baby is moving like
crazy when I sit to relax...
today you could feel the baby
from the outside of my belly!!

Fifth Month

July 5th - 1st ultrasound - we got to see our baby for the 1st time today, and it was amazing! Justin thinks he saw a pee-pee, which makes us feel more like it's a boy.

The baby has been going wild in my belly. especially in the morning and before bed. I still feel well...

My next appointment is July 17th... I think we will get the results of the ultrasound to see if everything was/is OK. - I think/pray so !!

July 23rd - Today we purchased the crib and over the weekend we had a beautiful mural painted by Betty-Boree's Tyne Paci's Aunt. It is amazing! But any who - the baby is moving like CRAZY!! I am looking more pregnant now as apposed to looking fat.

Fifth Month

_____

_____

_____

_____

_____

_____

_____

_____

_____

_____

_____

_____

_____

_____

_____

_____

_____

_____

_____

_____

_____

_____

_____

_____

Sixth Month

Next Appt: Tuesday ~~July,~~ August 14, 2007. We have had a few scares up til then. I had some really bad cramping on my right side down my leg.. it ended up being a urinary tract infection.

Doc Appt: Well, according to the doctor's the ultrasound results, the baby is BIG - in the 75th percentile so, doctor Khafu wants to do another ultrasound when I am 34 weeks to see the size.. & we may go early. All is good though! I feel great.. getting sleepy again. The baby has days where it moves a ton and others where he/she's sleepy & not much movement.

Next Doc Appt. Sept 11.

First baby shower given by Joan is 8/24/07 @ Maurus table..

Sixth Month

The shower came 3 went, it was small but fun! We got lots of good prizes for the baby!

Next shower Sept. 1st... thrown by Grammy, Missi, 3 Meg. @ Merichkas. It was just family (Freund side) but great. I ended up in the (28 wks) hospital around 6:00 or so... I was having some REALLY bad burning in my belly 3 swelling on my hands 3 feet.

Next shower is in Sept (15th)

Seventh Month

Sept. 11- 9:45pm - Doctors Appt...
It went well, I had the
Gestational diabetes test done--
twice.. and it came back
negative. The doctor said I
am where I should be. I have
gained 33 lbs !!
      the baby gets the
hiccups almost everynite! I
love it.
      The next doc. appt is
Oct. 14th. it is my last 4 week
from then they will be more
frequent. At that appt. I will
have another ultrasound to see
the size of the baby, along
with the group B strep test.

I am getting Nervous. In
10 weeks or less. We are going
to be parents !!

Seventh Month

Eighth Month

Oct. 11th Check up & Ultrosound
4:00 pm... 34 weeks-

So, we just got back and
the doctors are estimating the
baby's size to be 6 lbs. 02 oz.
he says that if the baby gets
to be 9 lbs. C-SECTION. My
next appt. is Oct. 30th. I
have "Group B Strep" & another
Ultrasound then..

The baby moves ALL of the
time! Sitting in my ribs on
the right side. I still feel the
baby is a boy - we will see
soon enough!!

Eighth Month

Ninth Month

Oct. 28th... this baby is crazy! loves to move and kick my ribs. baby sits on my right side... it HURTS! Sleep is getting less & less. I feel like I am squishing the baby. Everyone says I look great - all belly!

Lots of swelling - it's bad! 45 lbs today I have gained. Jus & I are getting realey excited!

Ninth Month

Labor and Delivery

Postpartum

INDEX